Volume 2

Atlas of Ultrasonography
Second Edition

Volume 2

Atlas of Ultrasonography
Second Edition

Edited by

Kenneth J.W. Taylor, M.D., Ph.D.

Professor of Diagnostic Radiology
Yale University School of Medicine
New Haven, Connecticut

Drawings by

Caroline R. Taylor, M.D.

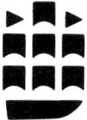

CHURCHILL LIVINGSTONE
New York, Edinburgh, London, and Melbourne   1985

Acquisitions editor: William R. Schmitt
Copy editor: Donna C. Balopole
Production editor: Karen Goldsmith Montanez
Production supervisor: Sharon Tuder
Compositor: Waldman Graphics, Inc.
Printer/Binder: The Murray Printing Co.

Second Edition © Churchill Livingstone Inc. 1985
First Edition © Longman Inc. 1978

All rights reserved. No part of this publication may be reproduced, stored in a retrieval system, or transmitted in any form or by any means, electronic, mechanical, photocopying, recording or otherwise, without prior permission of the publishers (Churchill Livingstone Inc., 1560 Broadway, New York, N.Y. 10036).

Distributed in the United Kingdom by Churchill Livingstone, Robert Stevenson House, 1-3 Baxter's Place, Leith Walk, Edinburgh EH1 3AF and by associated companies, branches and representatives throughout the world.

Printed in USA

ISBN 0-443-08424-6

9 8 7 6 5 4 3 2 1

Library of Congress Cataloging in Publication Data
Main entry under title:

Atlas of ultrasonography.

   Previous ed. published as: Atlas of gray scale ultrasonography. 1978.
   Bibliography: p.
   Includes index.
   1. Diagnosis, Ultrasonic—Atlases. I. Taylor, Kenneth J. W. [DNLM: 1. Ultrasonics—diagnostic use—atlases. WB 17 A8825]
RC78.7.U4A79   1985   616.07'543   84-17619
ISBN 0-443-08424-6

Manufactured in the United States of America

To Caroline

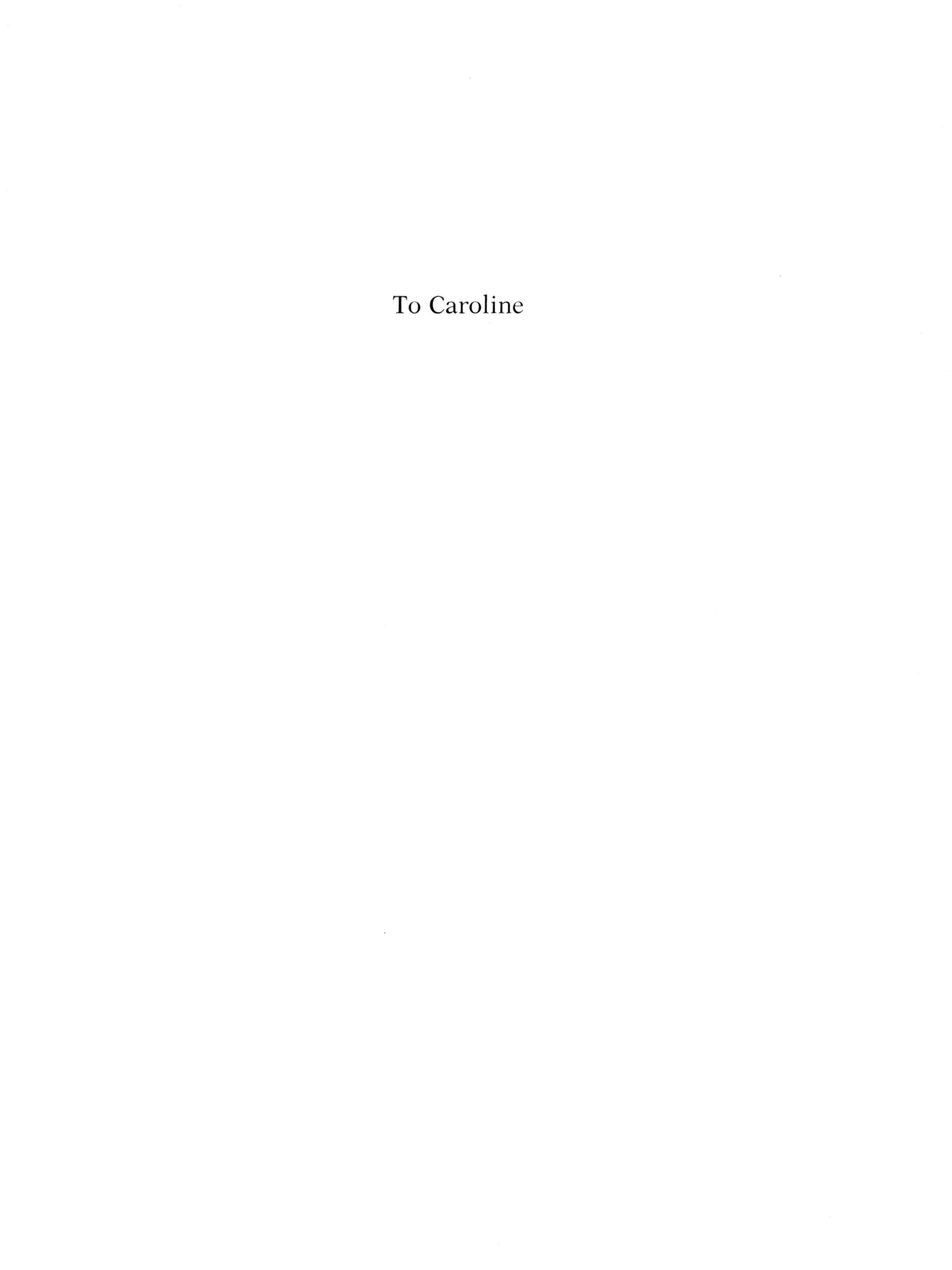

Contributors

K.T. Evans, F.R.C.P., F.R.C.R.
Professor of Radiology, University Hospital of Wales, Heath Park, Cardiff, Great Britain

Peter A. Grannum, M.D.
Assistant Professor of Obstetrics and Gynecology, Yale University School of Medicine, New Haven, Connecticut

G.J. Griffiths, M.B., B.Ch., D.Ch., F.R.C.R.
Consultant Radiologist, Royal Gwent Hospital, Department of Radiology, Newport, Gwent, Great Britain

Paula Jacobson, RT, RDMS
Chief Technologist, Ultrasound Section, Yale New Haven Hospital, New Haven, Connecticut

Frederick W. Kremkau, Ph.D.
Associate Professor of Diagnostic Radiology, Yale University School of Medicine, New Haven, Connecticut

Eric Mannes, M.D.
Assistant Clinical Professor of Diagnostic Radiology, Middlesex Memorial Hospital, Middletown, Connecticut

Kara Mayden, RT, RDMS
Sonographer, Department of Obstetrics and Gynecology, Yale University School of Medicine, New Haven, Connecticut

Peter R. Mueller, M.D.
Department of Radiology, Massachusetts General Hospital, Associate Professor, Harvard Medical School, Boston, Massachusetts

Dorothea Peck, M.D.
Associate Clinical Professor of Diagnostic Radiology, Yale University School of Medicine, New Haven, Connecticut

W.B. Peeling, M.B., F.R.C.S.
Consultant Urologist, Department of Urology, St. Woolos Hospital, Newport, Gwent, Great Britain

Tina Richman, M.D.
Assistant Clinical Professor of Diagnostic Radiology, Yale University School of Medicine, New Haven, Connecticut

E.E. Roberts, D.C.R.
Instructor in Diagnostic Techniques, Department of Radiology, University Hospital of Wales, Heath Park, Cardiff, Great Britain

Arthur T. Rosenfield, M.D.
Professor of Diagnostic Radiology, Yale University School of Medicine, New Haven, Connecticut

Joseph F. Simeone, M.D.
Department of Radiology, Massachusetts General Hospital, Associate Professor, Harvard Medical School, Boston, Massachusetts

Bruce D. Simonds, M.D.
Assistant Clinical Professor of Diagnostic Radiology, Yale University School of Medicine, New Haven, Connecticut

James Sivo, RT, RDMS
Assistant Chief Technologist, Ultrasound Section, Yale New Haven Hospital, New Haven, Connecticut

Caroline R. Taylor, M.D.
Assistant Professor, Yale University School of Medicine, New Haven, Connecticut; Director of Radiology, Veterans Administration Hospital, West Haven, Connecticut

Kenneth J.W. Taylor, M.D., Ph.D.
Professor of Diagnostic Radiology, Yale University School of Medicine, New Haven, Connecticut

Marge Tortora, RDMS
Sonographer, Department of Obstetrics and Gynecology, Yale University School of Medicine, New Haven, Connecticut

C. Whitley Vick, M.D.
Assistant Professor, Department of Radiology, Medical College of Virginia, Richmond, Virginia

Preface

The major problem with writing any modern book is the need for a frequent update. Enormous strides in knowledge and improvements in technology in ultrasound during the past seven years made a major revision inevitable.

Not all the scans are real-time despite the fact that such equipment is predominently used. The books on so-called "real-time" ultrasound merely show static frames, like those from a static scanner but of more limited geometry. Further, where pathologic entities have been accumulated over a period of twelve years, the scan quality is that available at the time.

Since the first edition of this atlas, there has been a great increase in familiarity with ultrasound scans, especially in obstetrics, and thus we have used direct labeling for some figures instead of line drawings. It is notable that there has been a great increase in the size of this book, but even now, it is far from comprehensive.

I owe an enormous debt of gratitude to my co-authors, many of whom are faculty or former fellows at Yale. I am particularly grateful to Dr. Griffiths and his colleagues for their chapter on per rectal scanning of the prostate, a technique which they have pioneered.

I would like to thank Professor Rhys Davies and Dr. P.N.T. Wells for providing me with the facilities in Bristol University during my sabbatical, which provided me with the peace and respite from clinical duties that I needed to complete this work. My special thanks go to Karen Zarkades who edited and typed this manuscript, often translating my transatlantic tapes into reasonable chapters. I also thank Cheryl Wilcox, my administrative assistant, for editing and checking so many references.

I hope this book will be a source of education to physicians, especially residents preparing for their boards, and for sonographers preparing for their registry. I thank our own sonographers, especially their supervisor Paula Jacobson, for providing me with so many of these scans.

I thank my wife Caroline not only for the line drawings but especially for encouraging me to continue and complete this work when I was daunted by the sheer magnitude of it. Finally, I would like to thank Donna Balopole and her co-workers at Churchill Livingstone for their collaboration in the production of this book.

Kenneth J.W. Taylor

Contents

Volume 1

1. Basic Principles of Diagnostic Ultrasound 1
   Kenneth J.W. Taylor and Frederick W. Kremkau

2. Physical Basis of Artifacts 23
   Kenneth J.W. Taylor and Frederick W. Kremkau

3. Gynecology 37
   Kenneth J.W. Taylor

4. Obstetrics 183
   Peter A. Grannum, Marge Tortora, Kara Mayden, and Kenneth J.W. Taylor

5. The Breast 329
   Kenneth J.W. Taylor and Dorothea Peck

6. The Neonatal Head 373
   Eric Mannes, James Sivo, and Kenneth J.W. Taylor

7. The Liver 429
   Kenneth J.W. Taylor

   Index

Volume 2

8. The Gallbladder and Biliary Tree 541
   Kenneth J.W. Taylor

9. The Pancreas 623
    Kenneth J.W. Taylor and Bruce D. Simonds

10. The Spleen 693
    Kenneth J.W. Taylor

11. The Urinary Tract 733
    Arthur T. Rosenfield and Tina Richman

12. Renal Masses, Cystic Disease, Trauma, and Disorders
    of the Bladder and Prostate 839
    Arthur T. Rosenfield and Tina Richman

13. The Adrenal Gland 931
    Tina Richman and Arthur T. Rosenfield

14. The Prostate 947
    G.J. Griffiths, W.B. Peeling, K.T. Evans, and E.E. Roberts

15. The Testes 965
    C. Whitley Vick

16. The Retroperitoneum 989
    Kenneth J.W. Taylor

17. The Bowel 1023
    Kenneth J.W. Taylor

18. The Thyroid and Parathyroid Glands 1053
    Joseph F. Simeone and Peter R. Mueller

19. The Vascular System 1081
    Kenneth J.W. Taylor and Paula Jacobson

20. The Thorax 1125
    Kenneth J.W. Taylor

    Index

8 The Gallbladder and Biliary Tree

KENNETH J.W. TAYLOR

Normal Anatomy (8.1 and 8.2)

8.1 Landmarks and Examination Technique

Ultrasonic examination of the gallbladder and biliary tree is one of the most widely accepted applications of the modality. Ultrasound has largely replaced oral cholecystography (OCG) as a screening examination for gallbladder disease, while ultrasound of the bile ducts should be the initial imaging procedure in the jaundiced patient.

Nevertheless, pitfalls abound in the sonographic diagnosis of gallbladder disease and the examination technique must be meticulous. The limitations of the modality must be recognized and other modalities used when necessary to overcome these limitations.

The gallbladder is pear-shaped, and the gallbladder fossa lies in the main lobar fissure. Thus, the neck of the gallbladder is connected to the porta hepatis by the fissure, which can be used as a landmark (Fig. A).

The patient must be examined in the fasting state, using a subcostal or intercostal approach. Dilatation in response to fasting is an important physiological characteristic of the normal gallbladder. Failure to distend on fasting is highly suggestive of disease. The thickness of the gallbladder wall can only be assessed in the fasting state. Furthermore, bile contained within the gallbladder lumen acts as an essential contrast medium to delineate the walls of the gallbladder and any contained gallstones.

Longitudinal scans through the right upper quadrant are performed to identify the long axis of the gallbladder lumen (Fig. A). Hundreds of sections through the gallbladder are made in this plane, searching for abnormality. The length of the normal gallbladder is virtually always less than 13 cm, although this measurement is too variable to be of much diagnostic use. Certainly, a hydropic gallbladder can be smaller. Whether a manual scanner or a real-time device is used, the sonographer must view hundreds of sections even though few may be retained as hard copy.

It is also essential to examine the gallbladder in different planes, especially to avoid artifacts due to side lobes. The gallbladder is next scanned in the transverse plane (Fig. B). Again, numerous sections are viewed although only a few are retained on hard copy. The transverse diameter of the gallbladder should be less than 4 cm. Finally, the position of the patient is changed to left posterior oblique (LPO) or decubitus (Fig. C). This movement encourages contained stones to roll toward the fundus of the gallbladder, where they can be imaged more easily. This change in position also demonstrates free movement of any gallstones, which is an important criterion for their reliable diagnosis.

In our laboratory, an examination is never limited to the gallbladder alone. Coexistence of disease in the bile ducts and pancreas justifies careful examination of the liver, biliary tree, and pancreas in any patient with gallbladder symptoms. In addition, symptoms may be due to disease in adjacent organs. A major advantage of ultrasound over OCG and other one-organ examinations is the ease with which the entire area and many different organs can be surveyed.

In the symptomatic patient, concomitant physical examination is essential to elicit the "ultrasonic Murphy's sign." The point of maximum tenderness must be located and correlated with the position of the gallbladder.

There are wide variations in the shape, size, and position of the normal gallbladder. The gallbladder may be deeply buried in the liver or may be freely mobile on a mesentery suspended from the undersurface of the liver. In the latter case, the gallbladder may be found on the left side of the abdomen and may vary with the patient's position to form a "wandering gallbladder."

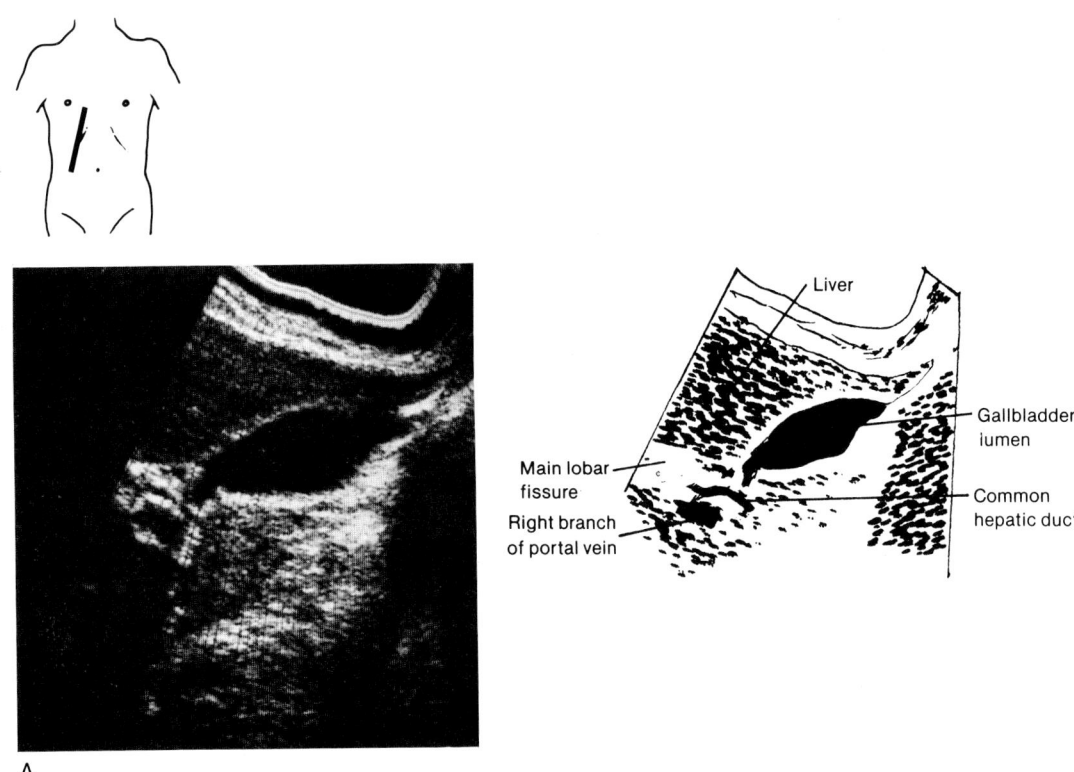

A

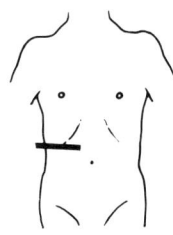

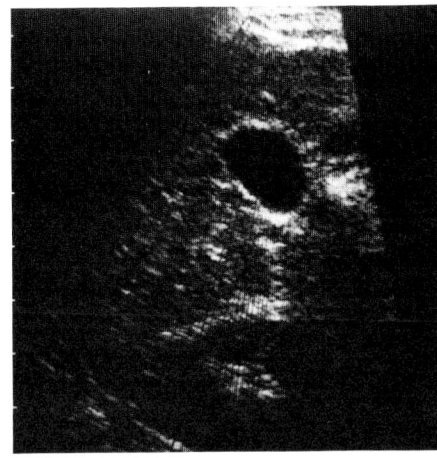 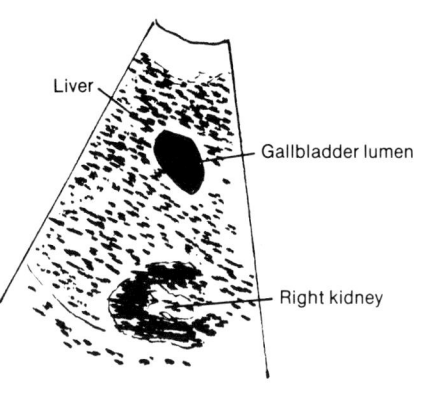

B

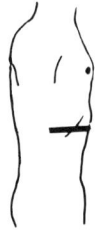

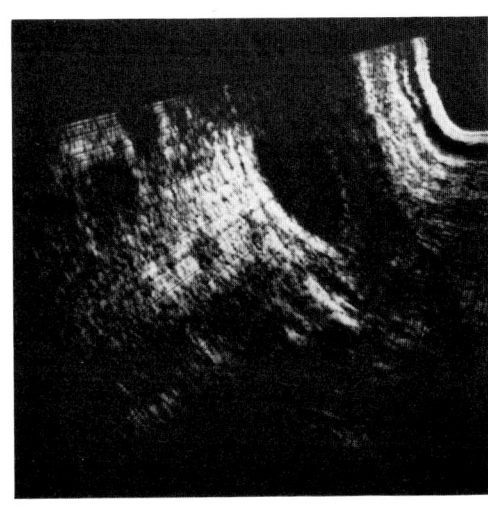 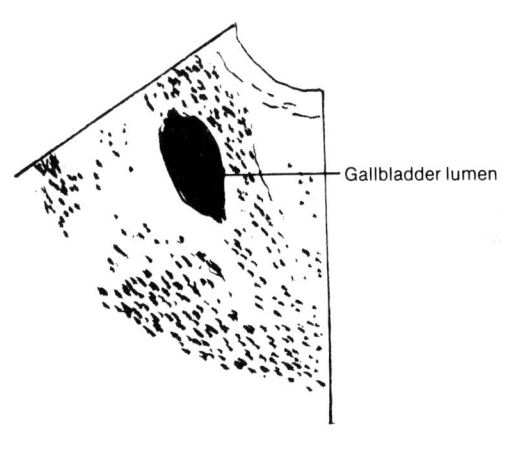

C

8.2 Gallbladder Neck and Cystic Duct

The normal appearance of the gallbladder neck should be noted (Fig. A). A shadow emanates from the neck of the gallbladder due to beam splitting by reflection and refraction. This should not be confused with a stone impacted in the neck of the gallbladder.

An oblique ultrasonogram along the costal margin shows the lumen of the gallbladder converging into the cystic duct (Fig. B). The spiral valve arrangement can be seen and there is a slight shadow from this area.

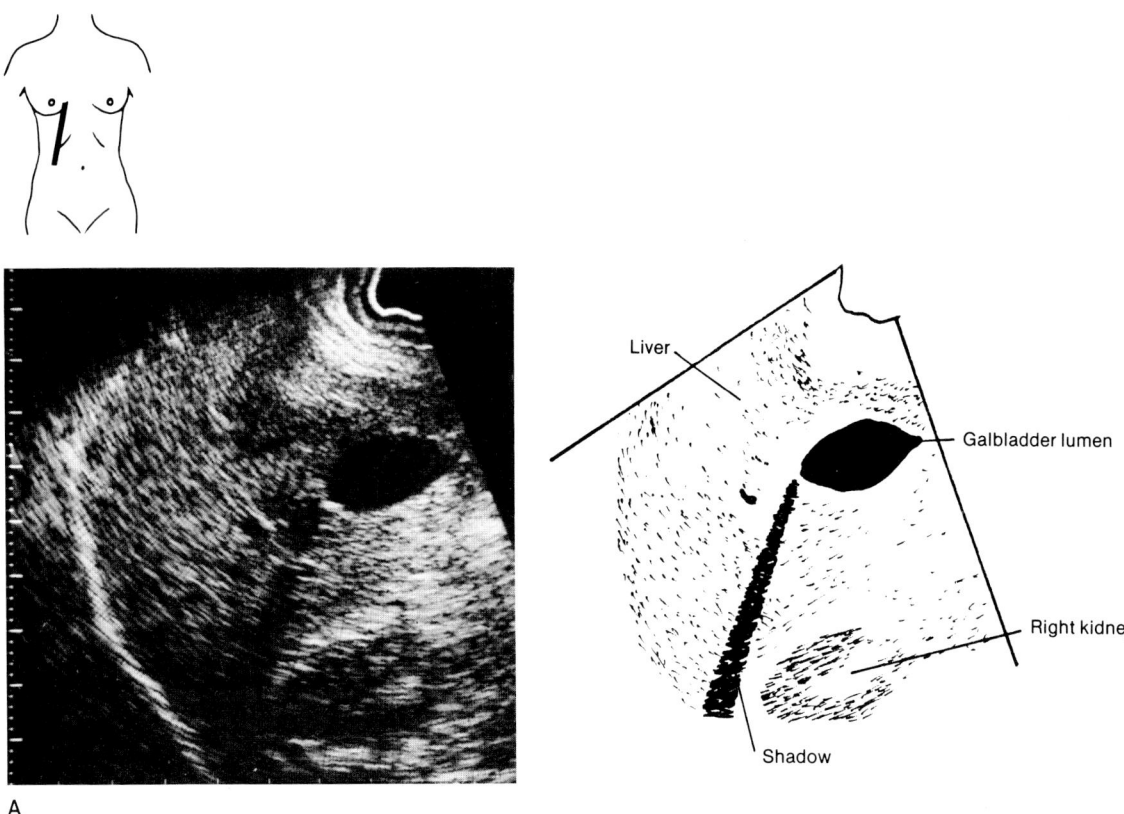

A

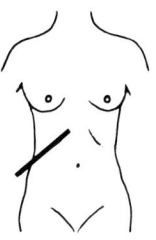
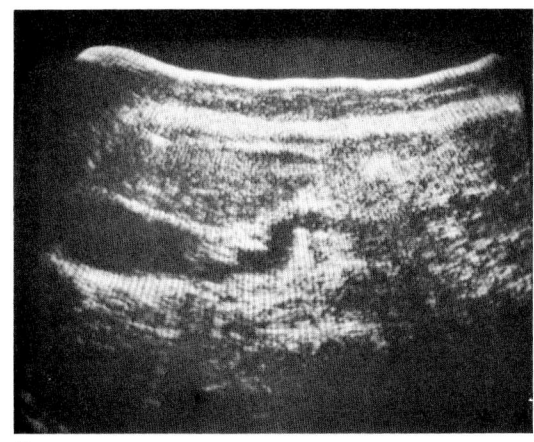

B

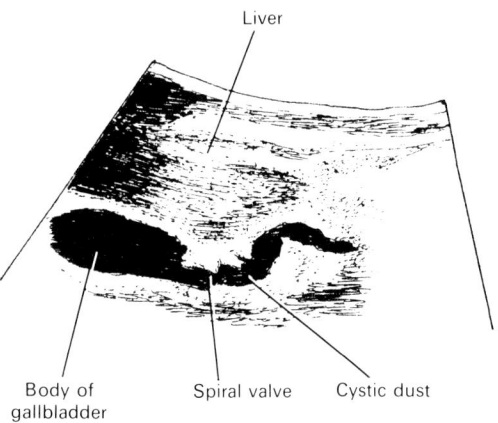

Liver

Body of gallbladder | Spiral valve | Cystic dust

8.3 Junctional Fold Simulating Gallstone

A 27-year-old man was referred for ultrasonography to exclude gallstones. The longitudinal (Fig. A) and the transverse scan (Fig. B) demonstrated a small projection on the wall of the gallbladder, with shadowing on either side of it. Movement of the patient demonstrated no evidence of free movement of the mass. Furthermore, careful inspection demonstrated that the shadows were on either side of the mass and not immediately distal to it, allowing differentiation from an adherent gallstone. A further longitudinal section demonstrated an apparent septation of the gallbladder (Fig. C).

Sukov et al.[1] reported the presence of a fold at the junction of the body and infundibulum of the gallbladder and termed this the junctional fold. They noted that this could simulate the appearance of an intraluminal polyp or calculus. In their series, this structure ranged from 3 to 5 mm and produced an acoustic shadow in some patients. Careful observation and real-time examination should prevent misinterpretation of this fold as either a polyp or a gallstone.

Folds in the gallbladder also produce apparent anatomic variations. When the fundus of the gallbladder is folded over, it is called a "phrygian cap" while a proximal fold produces "Hartmann's pouch." Folds may produce apparent septation, as in this patient. These variations are best appreciated by dynamic scanning which allows the continuity of the gallbladder lumen to be followed.

REFERENCE

1. Sukov RJ, Sample WF, Sarti DA, et al: Cholecystosonography—the junctional fold. Radiology 133:435–436, 1979

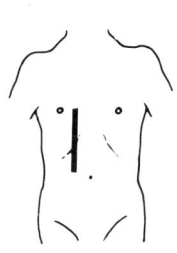
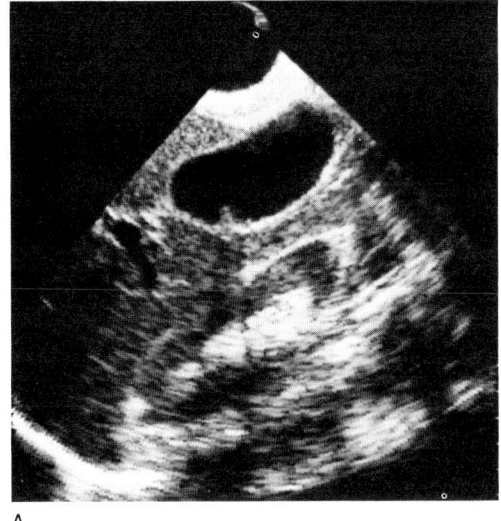
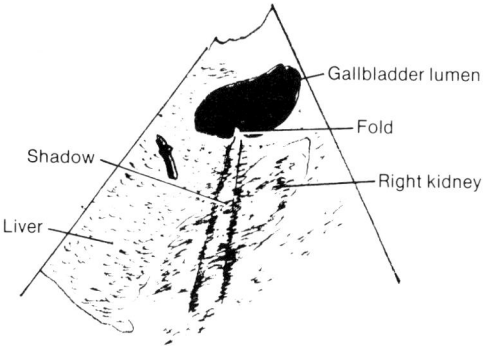

A

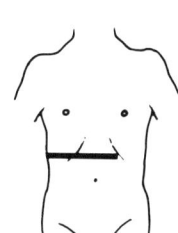
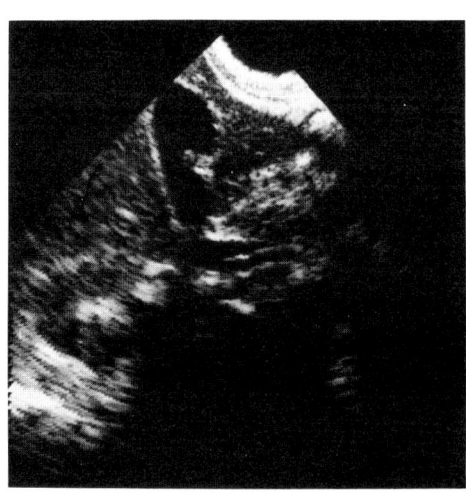
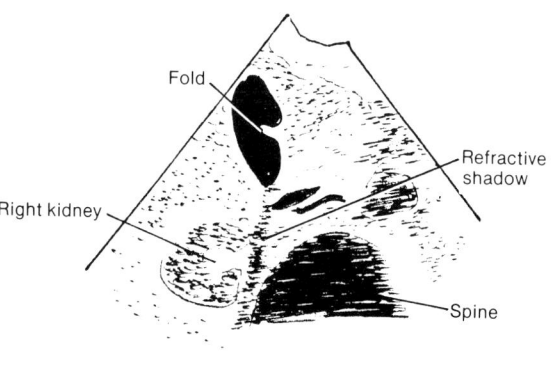

B

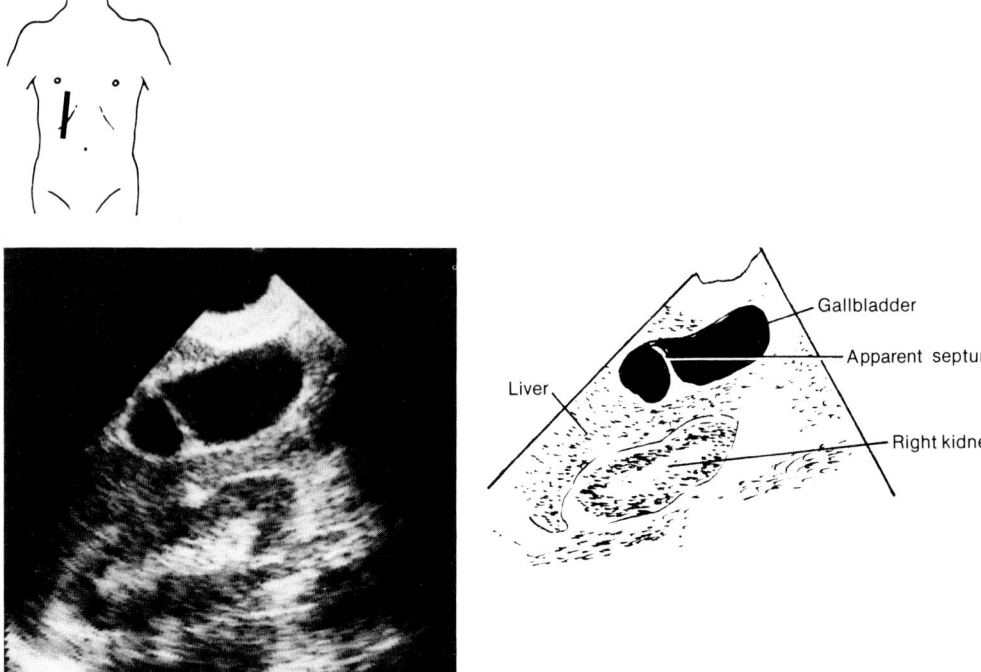

C

548

8.4 Acute Cholecystitis

A 37-year-old woman presented with a 2-day history of right upper quadrant pain, nausea, and vomiting. Extreme tenderness was elicited on subcostal palpation. An ultrasound scan of the gallbladder in the sagittal plane demonstrated thickening (arrow) of the gallbladder wall with a sonolucent rim.

As illustrated by other case histories, gallbladder wall thickening is a nonspecific finding, occurring commonly in alcoholics, in patients with hepatitis, and in those with acute cholecystitis.[1] ^{99m}Tc-HIDA or other biliary imaging agents appear to provide much more specific studies for the diagnosis of acute cholecystitis.[2] However, in some series it has been reported that only 30 percent of patients with right upper quadrant pain prove to have acute cholecystitis.[3] Thus, a nonspecific method such as ultrasound, which allows one to survey the adjacent organs, is very helpful in the differential diagnosis of acute cholecystitis. Physical examination, in addition to the sonographic appearances, adds considerably to the specificity. With the typical clinical history, tenderness located over the gallbladder and a thickened gallbladder wall, with or without gallstones, are persuasive evidence of acute cholecystitis.

Ralls et al.[4] evaluated the "ultrasonic Murphy's sign" prospectively in 427 consecutive patients. Sensitivity of the sign for the diagnosis of acute cholecystitis was 63 percent with a specificity of 93.6 percent. The positive predictive value was 72.5 percent and the negative predictive value was 90.5 percent. They concluded that Murphy's sign was a useful, although imperfect, indicator of acute cholecystitis.

REFERENCES

1. Schlaer WJ, Leopold GR, Scheible FW: Sonography of the thickened gallbladder wall: a non-specific finding. AJR 136:337–339, 1981
2. Weissman HS, Frank MS, Bernstein LH, Freeman LM: Rapid and accurate diagnosis of acute cholecystitis with ^{99m}Tc-HIDA cholescintigraphy. AJR 132:523–528, 1979
3. Laing FC, Federle MP, Jeffrey RB, Brown TW: Ultrasonic evaluation of patients with acute right upper quadrant pain. Radiology 140:449–455, 1981
4. Ralls PW, Halls J, Lapin SA, et al: Prospective evaluation of the sonographic Murphy sign in suspected acute cholecystitis. J Clin Ultrasound 10:113–115, 1982

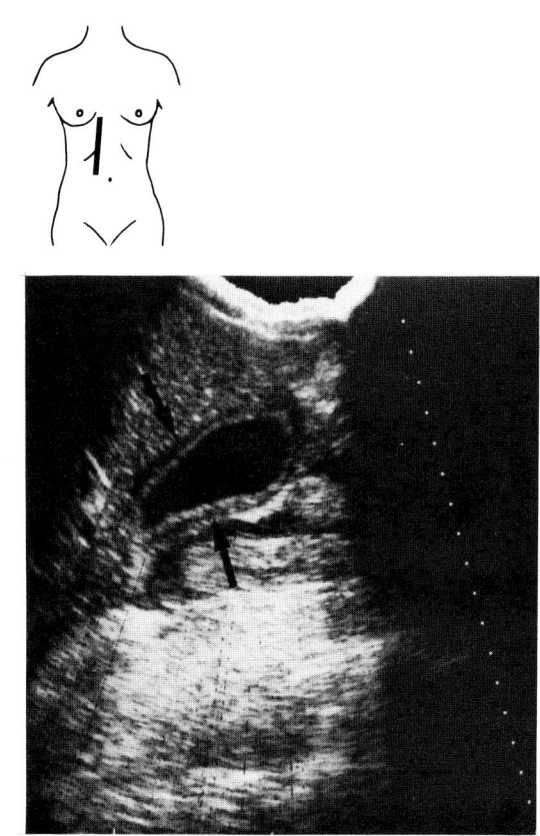

Gallstones (8.5 to 8.8)

8.5 Classic Gallstones

The diagnosis of gallstones by ultrasound can be highly accurate, but different appearances demand different degrees of confidence. Highly specific appearances are considered here. A longitudinal ultrasound scan showed multiple opacities within the lumen of the gallbladder (Fig. A). These opacities exhibited distal shadowing due to their high attenuation. Repositioning the patient in the decubitus position resulted in free movement of these stones to the dependent position (Fig. B). With the patient again supine, the stones returned to their dependent position (Fig. C).

Reliable criteria for the ultrasonographic diagnosis of gallstones include the presence of opacities within the lumen of the gallbladder, distal shadowing, and free movement. When all these criteria are satisfied, the specificity approaches 100 percent.[1] A nonshadowing opacity may be due to technical factors considered previously. Attempts to elicit shadowing should be made by choosing a transducer which focuses in the plane of the gallbladder, using a higher frequency, and/or decreasing the gain settings.[2] If less than 2 mm in diameter, stones may be too small to shadow because of diffraction of the beam around them. However, several small stones may aggregate to form a shadow. Also, the significance of such small particles is questionable since particles less than 2 mm in diameter can pass down the extrahepatic ducts.

Free movement of gallstones differentiates them from fixed anomalies of the gallbladder wall, such as polyps or adenomyomas. Stones may not move because of impaction, especially in the neck of the gallbladder. If this is suspected, the patient can be turned prone and hit lightly over the right lumbar region to dislodge the stone. If the stone cannot be dislodged, an equivocal report is given since the appearances of the spiral valve and the refractive shadow are similar to those of a gallstone impacted in the gallbladder neck. Under these circumstances, other modalities such as ^{99m}Tc-HIDA can be used to diagnose cystic duct obstruction. If chronic cholecystitis is suspected, OCG is valuable.

REFERENCES

1. Crade M, Taylor KJW, Rosenfield AT, et al: Surgical and pathologic correlation of cholecystosonography and cholecystography. AJR 131:227–229, 1978
2. Taylor KJW, Jacobson P, Jaffe CC: Lack of an acoustic shadow on scans of gallstones: a possible artifact. Radiology 131:463–465, 1979

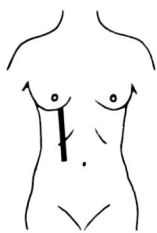

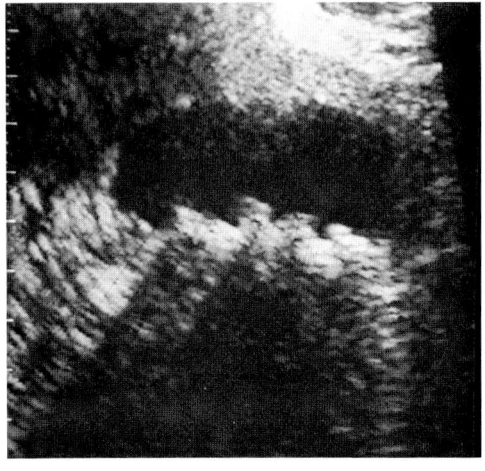

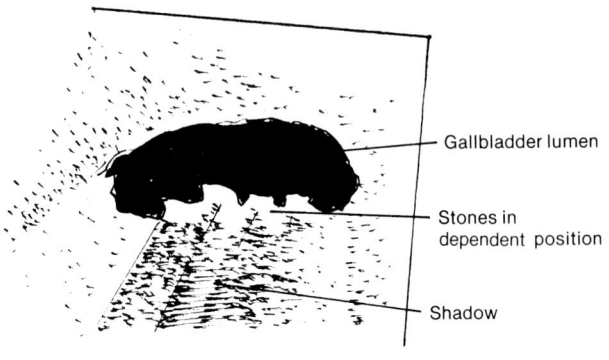

A

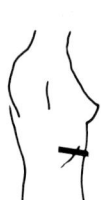

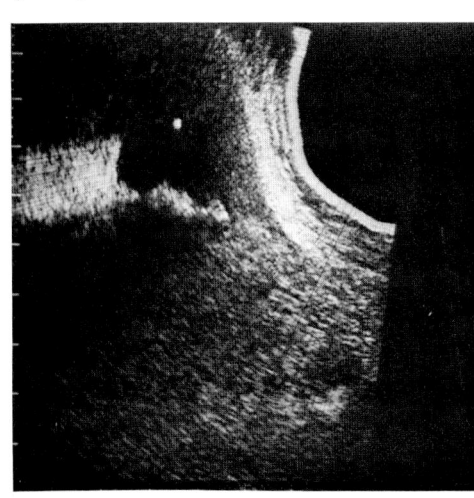

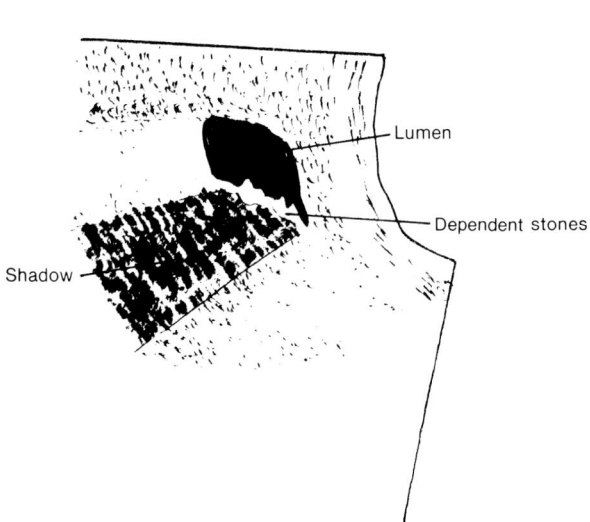

B

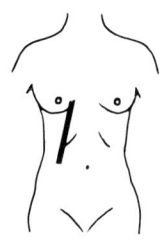

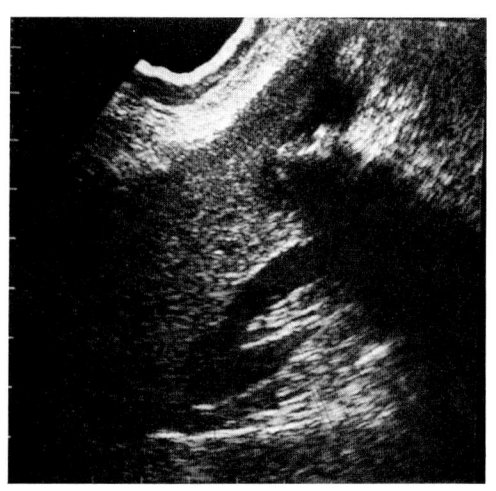

C

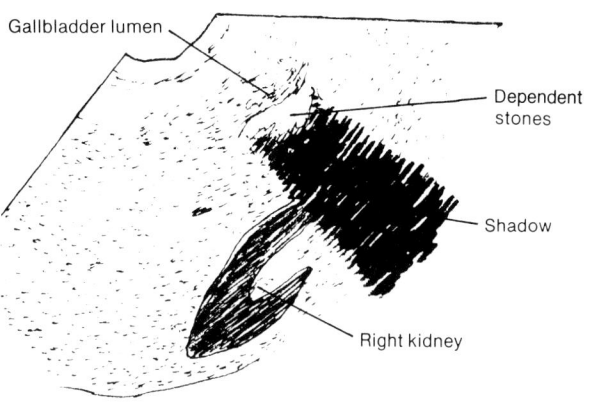

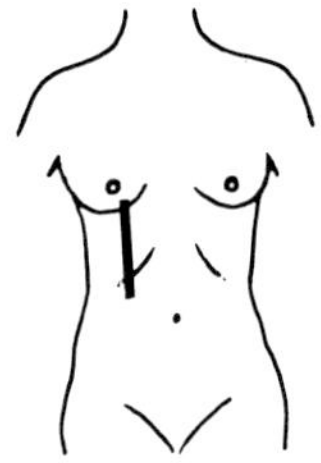

8.6 Gallstones in Septate Gallbladder

A septate gallbladder containing gallstones was an incidental finding in a 65-year-old woman referred for exclusion of metastatic disease to the liver. A definite line was seen passing through the lumen of the gallbladder, as shown in the figure. Two opacities were clearly seen in the gallbladder. These produced distal shadowing due to high attenuation (absorption and scatter) within them. These also moved with gravity, exhibiting all of the classic appearances of gallstones.

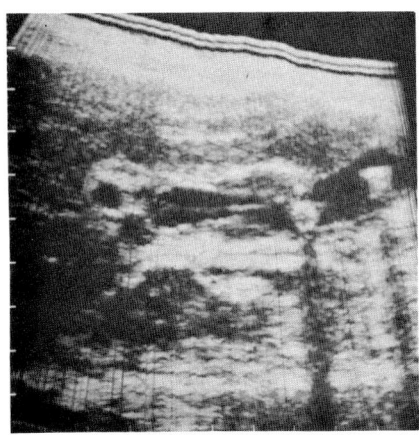
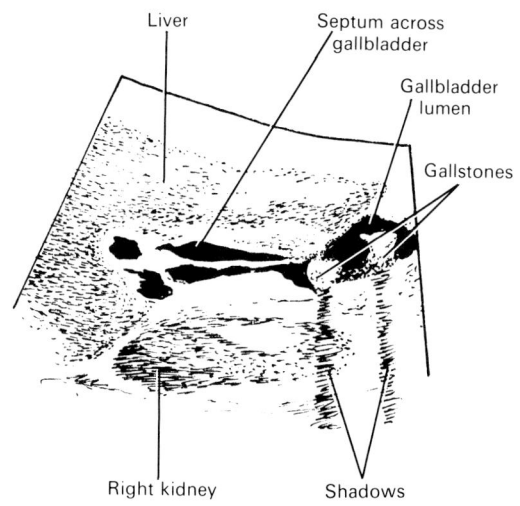

8.7 Floating Gallstones

Floating gallstones are occasionally seen. This 60-year-old patient with acute cholecystitis was referred for gallbladder examination. A scan of the gallbladder in the decubitus position demonstrated a stone (arrowed, Fig. A) with marked distal shadowing from the superior aspect of the gallbladder. There was free movement of this floating stone. At surgery, flocculent calcareous material was found in the gallbladder. Pathologic examination showed this to be a gallstone. Another example is shown in Figure B.

Scheske et al. reported 400 patients in whom only three demonstrated floating gallstones.[1] In all patients, the ultrasound examination had been performed soon after an oral cholecystogram. They suggested that gallstones only float in the presence of contrast medium. The specific gravity of bile varies from 1.010 to 1.040 but increases to 1.030–1.085 when contrast is present. The specific gravity of the lightest cholesterol stone[1] is around 1.040 to 1.085. However, other authors including ourselves have noted floating gallstones in the absence of contrast,[2] as in these patients. It is probable that this phenomenon is related to air which may be contained within gallstones.

REFERENCES

1. Scheske GA, Cooperberg PL, Cohen MM, et al: Floating gallstones: the role of contrast media. J Clin Ultrasound 8:227–231, 1980
2. Carroll B, Sommer FG: Letter to the editor. J Clin Ultrasound 9:A–30, 1981

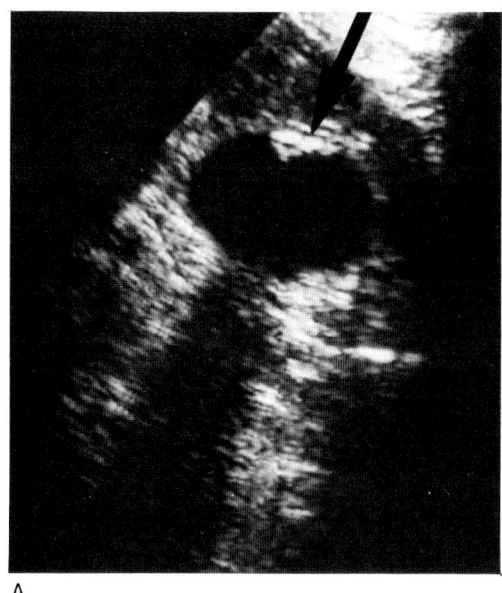

A

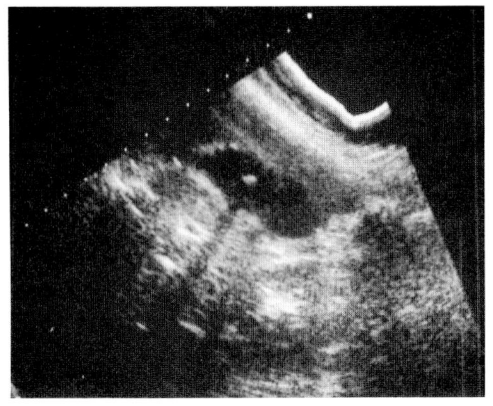
B

8.8 Gallstones Due to Hemolytic Anemia

A 4-year-old child was admitted for splenectomy. When patients with hemolytic anemias are admitted for splenectomy, the protocol at this institution is to perform ultrasound of the upper abdomen including the spleen and the gallbladder in order to exclude stones.

A decubitus sonogram of the gallbladder demonstrated physiological dilatation of the gallbladder and a definite stone opacity (arrowed in the figure). This opacity moved with gravity and demonstrated distal shadowing. These appearances are diagnostic of a gallstone. A cholecystectomy was performed at the same time as the splenectomy.

The prevalence of cholelithiasis in sickle cell disease is 10–70 percent. Sarnaik et al. reported on 226 patients, aged 2–18 years, with sickle cell anemia.[1] Gallstones were demonstrated in 27 percent and the mean age of patients with gallstones was 11.5 years. The presence of gallstones increased with age and patients with gallstones had higher bilirubin levels.

REFERENCE

1. Sarnaik S, Slovis TL, Corbett DP, et al: Incidence of cholelithiasis in sickle cell anemia using the ultrasonic gray-scale technique. J Pediatr 96: 1005–1008, 1980

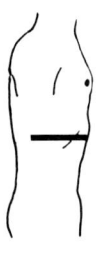
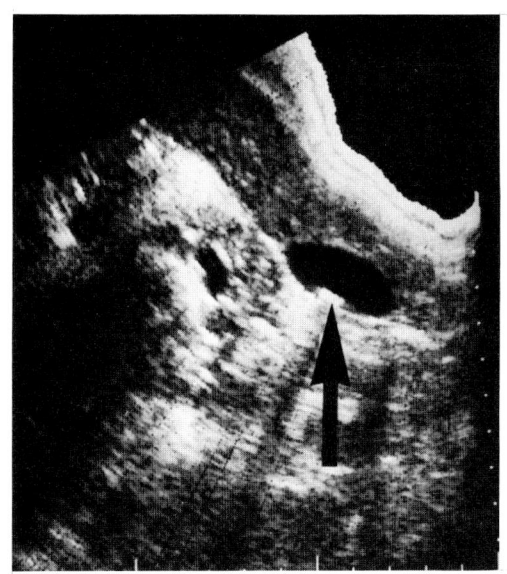

Chronic Cholecystitis (8.9 and 8.10)

8.9 Chronic Cholecystitis and Cholelithiasis

Ultrasonic nonvisualization of the gallbladder lumen has been shown to indicate pathology.[1] In the fasting patient, physiological dilatation of the gallbladder should be observed, and, if the gallbladder lumen is not demonstrated, three possibilities exist:

1. The gallbladder is congenitally absent. This condition has an incidence of only 0.03 percent.
2. The patient is not fasting and has eaten a fatty meal. This possibility can be checked by rescanning the patient after confirmed fasting.
3. The gallbladder is small and contracted with a thickened wall due to cholecystitis and is incapable of physiological distention.

In clinical practice, by far the most common cause of ultrasonic nonvisualization of the gallbladder lumen is contraction of the gallbladder due to chronic cholecystitis. Such gallbladders almost invariably contain stones and, instead of the lumen being demonstrated, a highly reflective opacity is seen within the gallbladder fossa with distal shadowing.

A 40-year-old woman presented with symptoms suggesting biliary tract disease. The gallbladder was not visualized on oral cholecystography.

A paramedian ultrasound section 6 cm to the right of the midline showed a reflective opacity within the liver substance, with shadowing across the upper pole of the right kidney (Fig. A). Surgery disclosed chronic cholecystitis and cholelithiasis.

A transverse sonogram showed a reflective, shadowing opacity anterior to the right kidney, just lateral to the head of the pancreas (Fig. B). The normal gallbladder lumen was not visualized. The pancreas and great vessels were well-demonstrated.

In such patients, it is important to differentiate air in the duodenum causing a shadow from pathology of the gallbladder producing a shadow. Again, the absence of the normal gallbladder lumen indicates definite pathology.

A further example of ultrasonic nonvisualization of the gallbladder lumen was seen on a transverse scan (Fig. C). An opacity was seen in the gallbladder fossa which shadowed distally. The surgical specimen of a small contracted gallbladder and gallstones is shown in Figure D.

It should be noted that the gallbladder often lies in a fossa on the undersurface of the liver. This helps to differentiate the pathologic gallbladder from colon since this fossa is occupied only by the gallbladder.

REFERENCE

1. Crade M, Taylor KJW, Rosenfield AT, et al: Surgical and pathologic correlation of cholecystosonography and cholecystography. 131:227–229, 1978

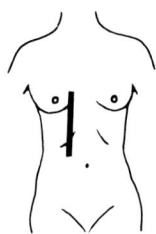
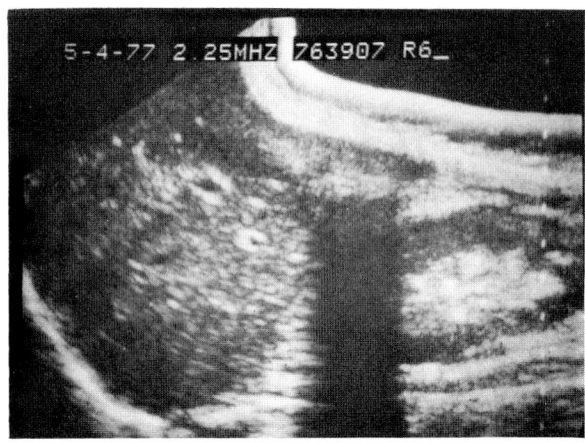
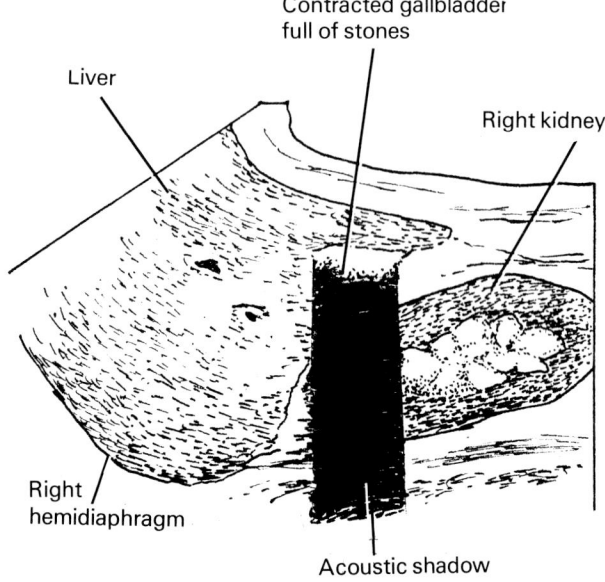

A

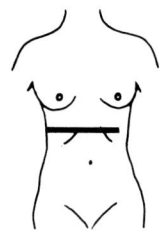
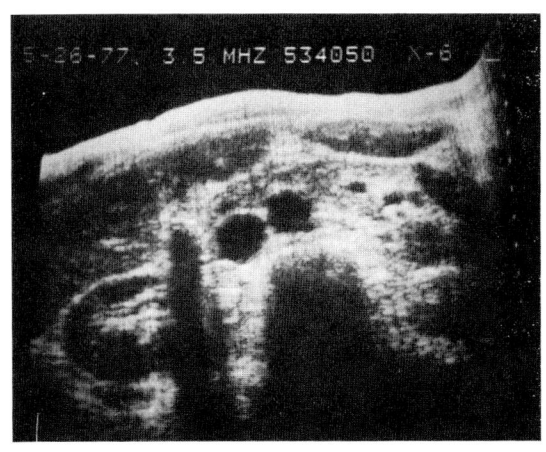
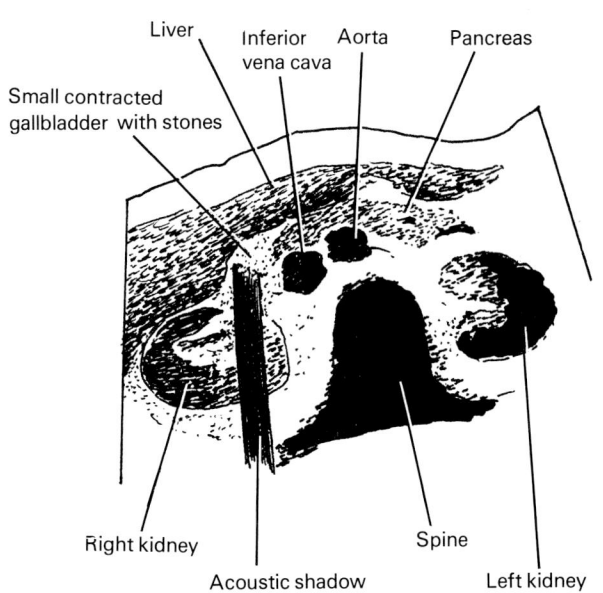

B

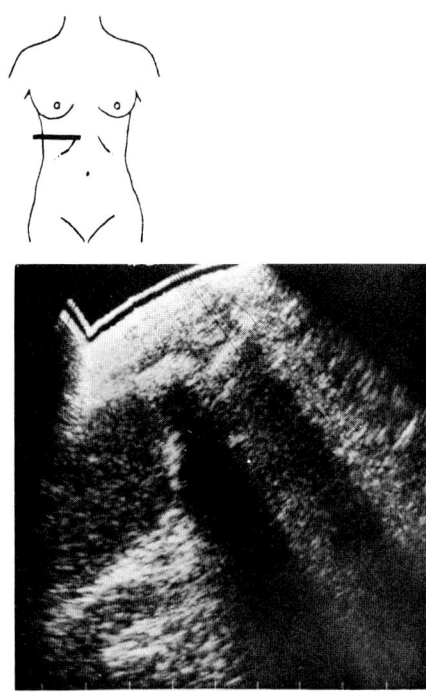

C

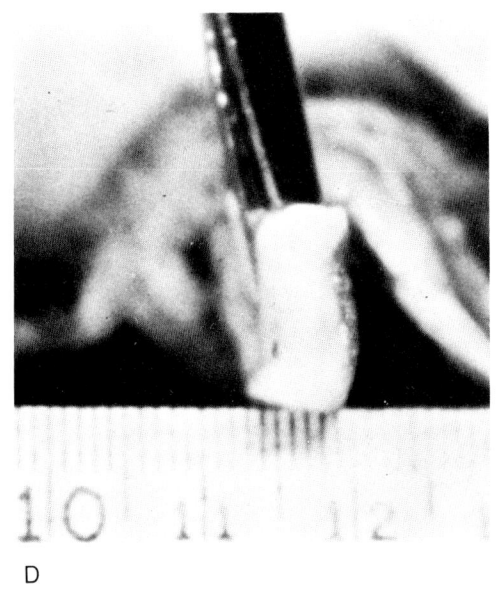

D

8.10 Ultrasound and ERCP

A 46-year-old woman presented with transient jaundice and epigastric pain. A longitudinal ultrasound scan (Fig. A) demonstrated a highly echogenic, shadowing mass within the gallbladder fossa, without evidence of any normal lumen. The transverse scan (Fig. B) again demonstrated an echogenic mass producing shadowing from the gallbladder fossa. These appearances were consistent with chronic cholecystitis producing a small, contracted gallbladder.

Subsequently, endoscopic retrograde cholangiopancreatography (ERCP) demonstrated a small but distensible gallbladder (Fig. C) on an oblique view. The bile ducts were of normal caliber and common duct stones were demonstrated.

This demonstrates the difference between physiological and iatrogenic distention of the gallbladder lumen. Absence of physiological distention of the gallbladder in response to fasting is virtually diagnostic on ultrasound scans of chronic cholecystitis. However, this does not imply that the gallbladder is incapable of distention in response to iatrogenic infusion of contrast material. In the same way, the size of the biliary vessels seen on ERCP may bear little relation to their size in the physiological state without distention by contrast material.

Surgery revealed a small, contracted gallbladder containing multiple gallstones. This case demonstrates that ERCP is not a good method for demonstrating gallstones within the gallbladder but is highly effective for demonstrating stones in the bile ducts. In contrast, small stones in the bile ducts are seldom successfully imaged by ultrasound.

(ERCP figure courtesy of Morton I. Burrell, M.D., Yale University School of Medicine.)

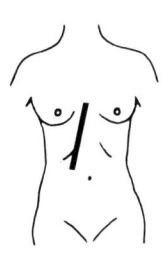

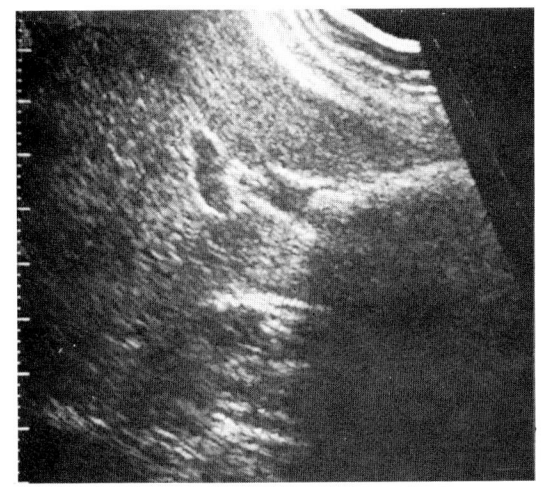

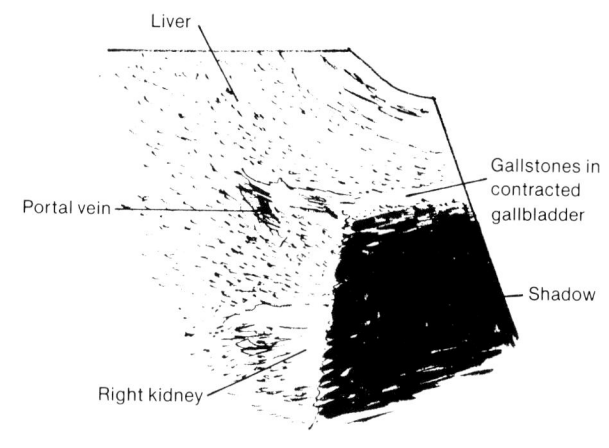

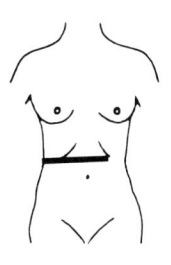

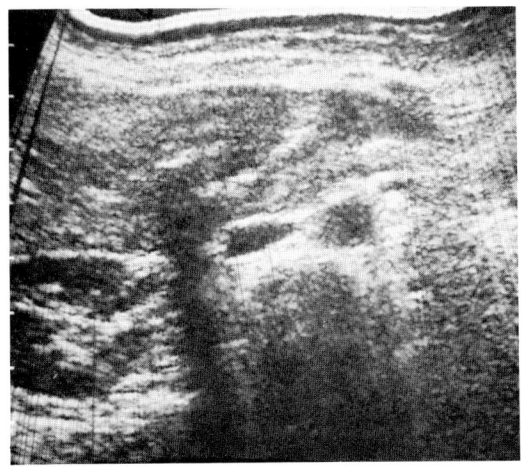

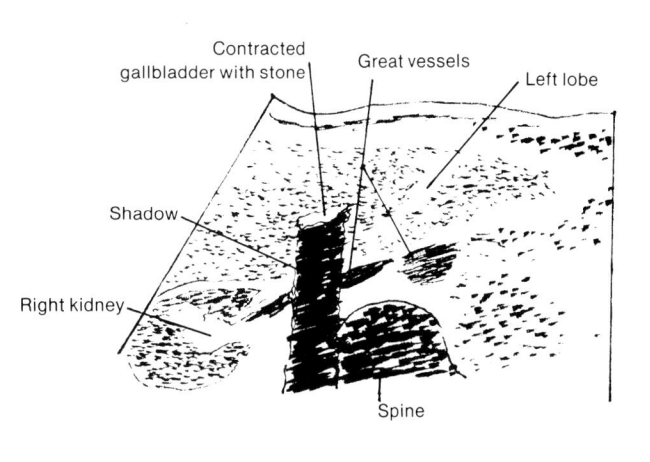

A

B

563

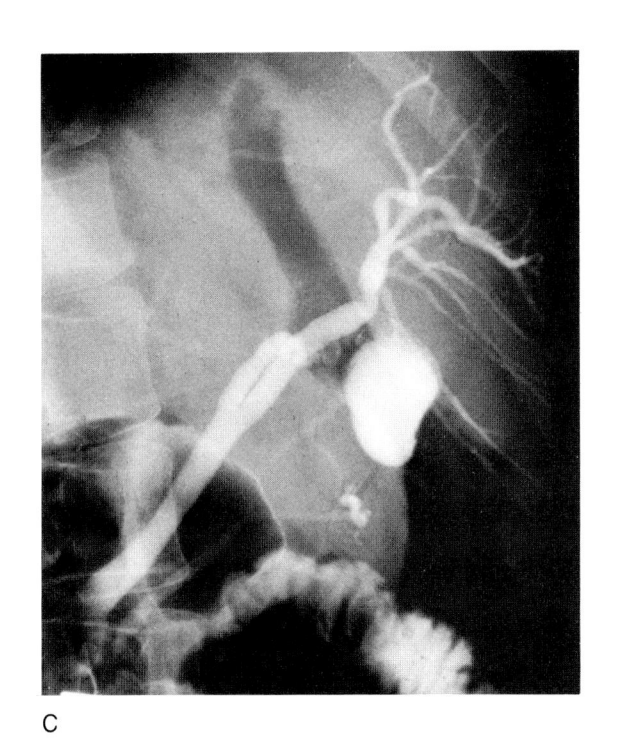

C

8.11 Porcelain Gallbladder

A calcified gallbladder was an incidental radiographic finding in a 44-year-old woman. A longitudinal ultrasound scan showed a densely reflective gallbladder wall (arrowed in the figure) with distal shadowing. The differential diagnosis included chronic cholecystitis and cholelithiasis, porcelain gallbladder, and emphysematous cholecystitis. In all of these instances, gross pathology of the gallbladder is present.

A porcelain gallbladder is a rare occurrence in which there is calcification in the wall of a gallbladder affected by chronic inflammatory disease. An increased incidence of carcinoma of the gallbladder has been recognized. Etala found 26 patients with porcelain gallbladders among 78 patients with carcinoma of the gallbladder in a series of 1,786 cholecystectomies.[1] In this study, 61 percent of patients with porcelain gallbladders had carcinoma. It appears that a porcelain gallbladder is only rarely found in carcinoma of the gallbladder, but patients with porcelain gallbladders have a high incidence of carcinoma.[2]

REFERENCES

1. Etala E: Cancer de la vesicula biliar. Prensa Med Argent 49:2283–2299, 1962
2. Berk RN, Armbuster TG, Saltzstein SL: Carcinoma in the porcelain gallbladder. Radiology 106:29–31, 1973

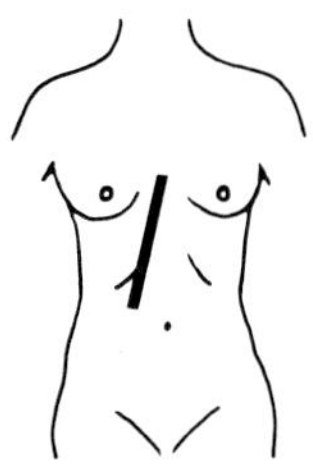

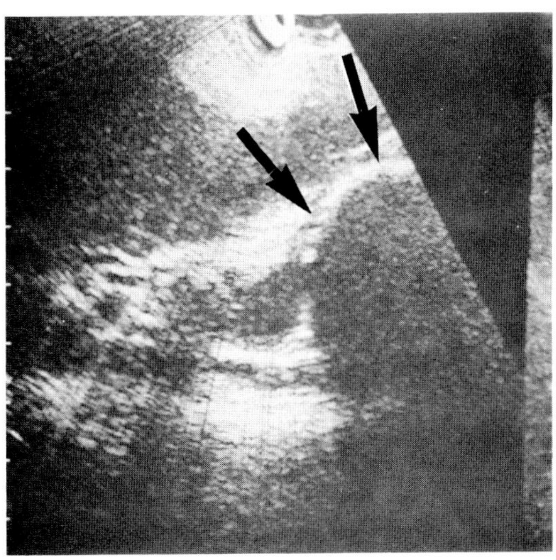

8.12 Empyema with Pericholecystitic Abscess

A 44-year-old woman presented with an unknown septic focus. Transverse ultrasound examination through the gallbladder fossa (Fig. A) using an intercostal sector scan showed the gallbladder lumen to be half-filled wih fine debris. Such appearances may be due to an empyema of the gallbladder, but any other fine, granular contents of the gallbladder may produce these appearances.

A further transverse section through the gallbladder (Fig. B) showed the gallbladder as well as another fluid-filled cavity within the liver substance. This raised the possibility of an abscess cavity surrounding the gallbladder, suggesting that this was an empyema of the gallbladder with spread to surrounding tissues.

At surgery, an empyema of the gallbladder was found with perforation of the wall and a pericholecystitic abscess.

Kane described five cases of gangrenous cholecystitis in which the sonogram demonstrated thickening of the gallbladder wall with intraluminal echoes.[1] Localized peritoneal fluid collections were also found. Bergman et al. also described pericholecystitic abscesses due to perforation of an empyema with bile leakage.[2] This is a life-threatening condition that is most important to recognize.

REFERENCES

1. Kane RA: Ultrasonographic diagnosis of gangrenous cholecystitis and empyema of the gallbladder. Radiology 134:191–194, 1980
2. Bergman AB, Neiman HL, Kraut B: Ultrasonographic evaluation of pericholecystitic abscesses. AJR 132:201–203, 1979

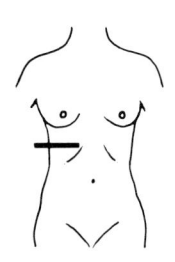

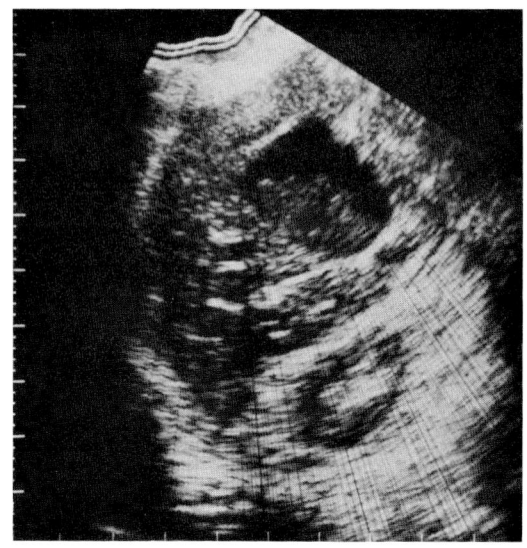

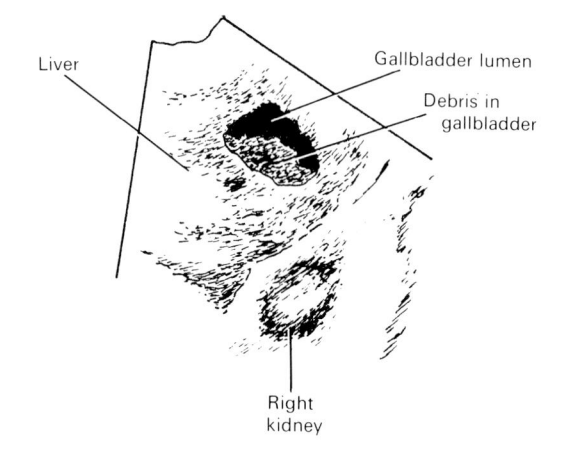

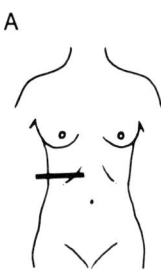

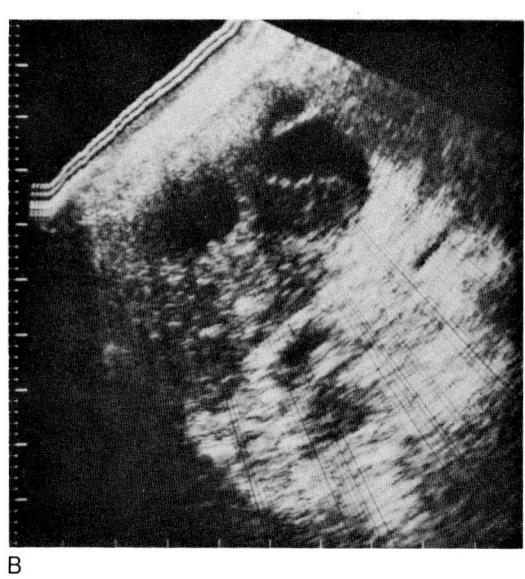

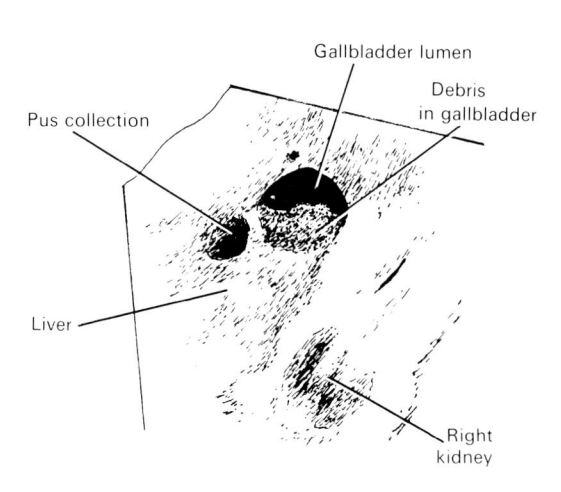

A

B

Gallbladder Wall Thickening (8.13 and 8.14)

8.13 Nonspecific Thickening

A 28-year-old patient was terminally ill with Hodgkin's disease. The liver was grossly enlarged and although no focal disease was seen on ultrasound, diffuse malignancy was certain. An ultrasound scan was requested to exclude renal obstruction in this patient with probable hepatorenal syndrome.

A parasagittal sonogram (Fig. A) demonstrated gross thickening of the gallbladder wall, with a definite sonolucent rim and a right pleural effusion. A magnified view of the gallbladder wall is shown in Figure B. There was no evidence of gallstones or tenderness on clinical examination. A ^{99m}Tc-HIDA examination demonstrated very poor liver function at 40 minutes, and absence of gallbladder activity with renal excretion (Fig. C). In the absence of adequate hepatic excretion, nonvisualization of the gallbladder has no diagnostic meaning.

The patient died from hepatorenal failure the following day. Postmortem examination revealed a grossly thickened and edematous gallbladder wall. There was extensive ascites and edema of the abdomen and thorax, with nodal compression of the inferior vena cava.

The literature on the value of thickening of the gallbladder wall for the diagnosis of acute cholecystitis illustrates the pitfalls that exist. Thickening of the gallbladder wall, especially with a sonolucent rim, has been considered a reliable sign of acute cholecystitis.[1] However, in a large study of normal patients it was reported that thickened gallbladder walls (between 3 and 5 mm), may be found in 3.5 percent of fasting normal patients.[2] Subsequently, numerous other causes of thickening of the gallbladder wall have been demonstrated. In this patient, extensive liver disease was present, resulting in hypoalbuminemia. This patient also had widespread edema and ascites of the rest of the body; gallbladder edema in this case was merely one manifestation of that generalized condition. Thus, it should be recalled that thickening of the gallbladder wall may be due to edema, but edema is not always due to acute cholecystitis.

(This case and Scans A & B and Fig. C taken from Crade M, Taylor KJW, Viscomi GN: Need for care in assessing gallbladder wall thickening. AJR 135:423–424, 1980. © 1980 Am Roentgen Ray Soc.)

REFERENCES

1. Handler SJ: Ultrasound of gallbladder wall thickening and its relation to cholecystitis. AJR 132:581–585, 1979
2. Finberg HJ, Birnholz JC: Ultrasound evaluation of the gallbladder wall. Radiology 133:693–698, 1979
3. Shlaer WJ, Leopold GR, Scheible FW: Sonography of the thickened gallbladder wall: a non-specific finding. AJR 136:337–339, 1981

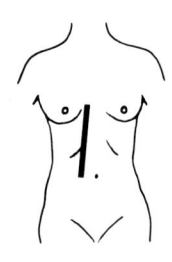

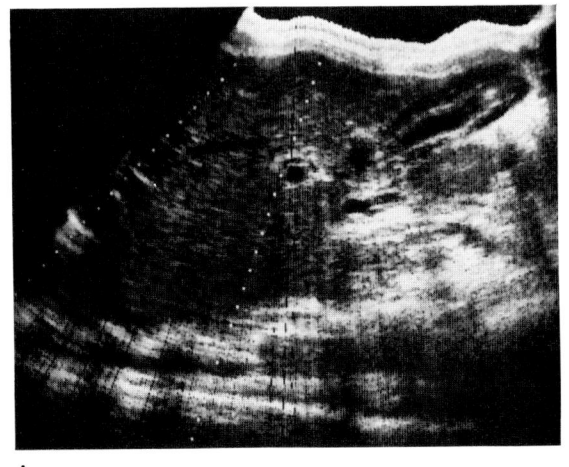

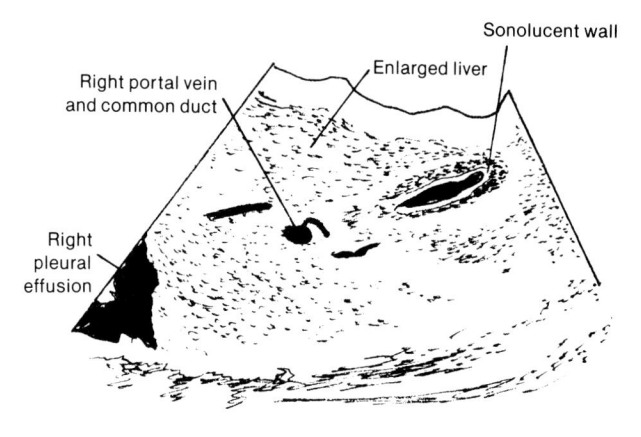

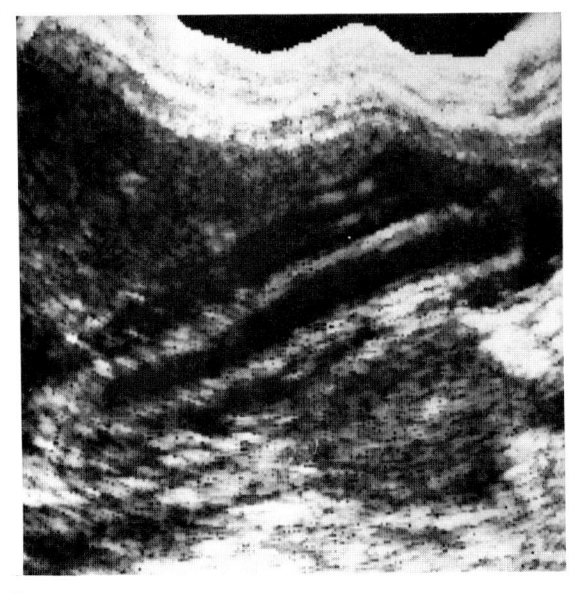

A

B

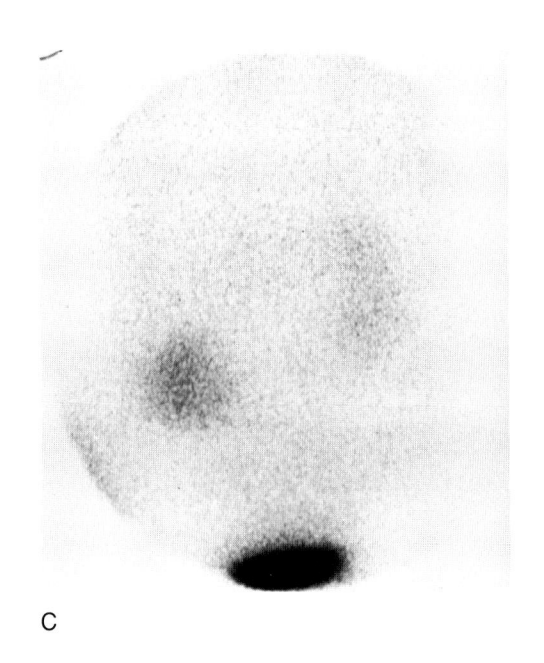

C

8.14 Rapid Change

A 33-year-old patient presented with transient jaundice postpartum. There had been substantial blood loss during the delivery, necessitating transfusion of 3 pints of blood. On clinical examination, there was no evidence of any tenderness. She was referred for ultrasound examination to determine the cause of her jaundice. A transverse sonogram in the decubitus position (Fig. A) demonstrated gross thickening of the gallbladder wall with a sonolucent rim. Repeat examination 4 days later (Fig. B) demonstrated a normal gallbladder wall without evidence of thickening.

This patient again demonstrated the nonspecific causes for gallbladder wall thickening.[1] Her transient jaundice was almost certainly due to the blood transfusion and, despite the highly abnormal ultrasound appearances, she had no symptoms or signs suggestive of acute cholecystitis. The marked edema of the gallbladder wall could have been due to a transient overload associated with her transfusion which also resulted in some ascites. Whatever the cause, rapid resolution occurred.

(This case and scans taken from Crade M, Taylor KJW, Viscomi GN. Need for care in assessing gallbladder wall thickening. AJR 135:423–424, 1980. © 1980 Am Roentgen Ray Soc.)

REFERENCE

1. Shlaer WJ, Leopold GR, Scheible FW: Sonography of the thickened gallbladder wall: a non-specific finding. AJR 136:337–339, 1981

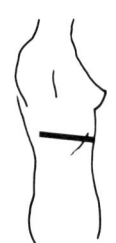

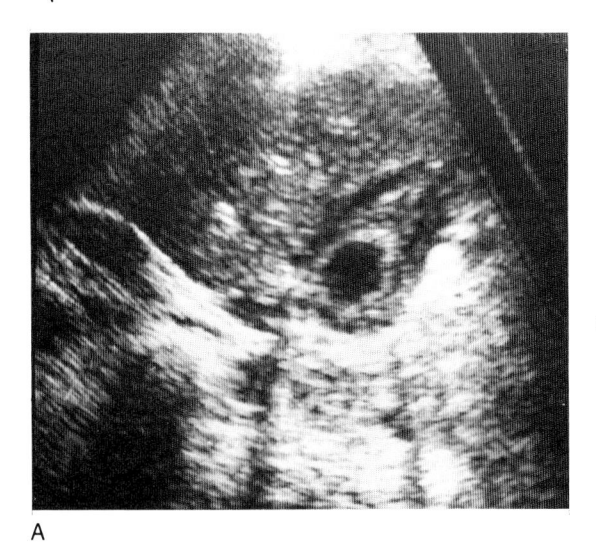

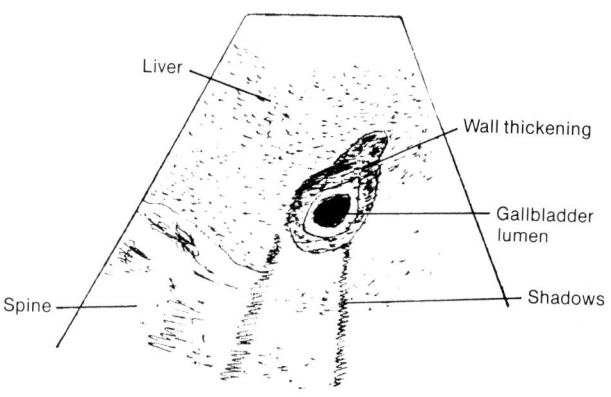

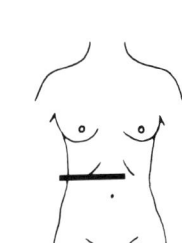

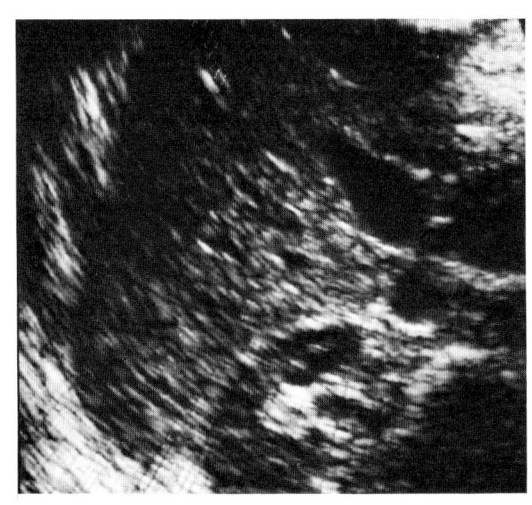

A

Liver	Wall thickening
	Gallbladder lumen
Spine	Shadows

B

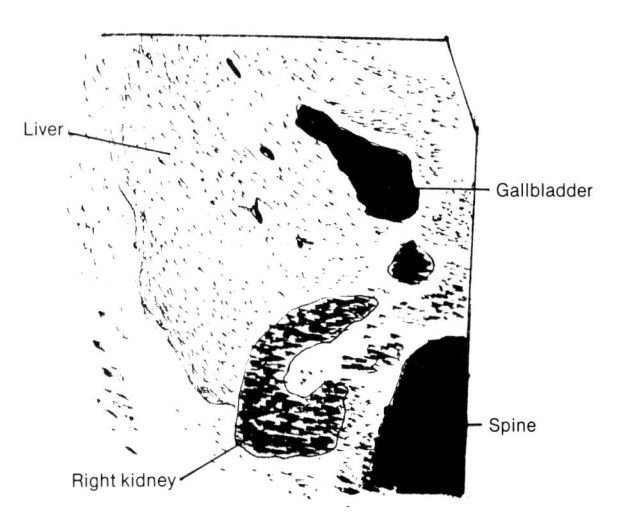

Liver	Gallbladder
Right kidney	Spine

8.15 Biliary Gravel and Sludge

A 40-year-old woman presented with symptoms of biliary tract disease. The ultrasound examination was carried out with the patient fasting.

A transverse sonogram showed the gallbladder lumen which was physiologically dilated (Fig. A). The gallbladder was half full of fine particulate debris which showed no evidence of distal shadowing. Note that the pancreas and prevertebral vessels were well seen.

A paramedian sonogram through the right upper quadrant showed the physiologically dilated gallbladder, which was also half full of particulate material (Fig. B). Note that in both scans the particulate matter layered with gravity. Such patients should be examined in both the erect and left decubitus positions to determine whether the material contained within the gallbladder moves rapidly with gravity after changes in the patient's position.

A sonogram in the decubitus position is shown in Figure C. The particulate matter within the gallbladder layered immediately, in contrast to viscous, slow-moving sludge.

The significance of gravel in the gallbladder is still being evaluated. Sludge may certainly occur in a normal gallbladder subjected to biliary stasis, but the presence of gravel suggests biliary tract disease and gallstones may be obscured by gravel. In a follow-up of 145 patients at this center, gallstones were found in only 60 percent of patients coming to surgery with nonshadowing material in the gallbladder. However, in the remaining 40 percent there was evidence of acute or chronic cholecystitis, either at surgery or on pathologic examination. These appearances should suggest the possibility of empyema of the gallbladder, in which the particulate matter is due to pus within the gallbladder lumen. This must be excluded on clinical grounds.

However, most patients with particulate matter within the gallbladder do not come to surgery because of the absence of clinical symptoms and signs. This particulate matter may pass spontaneously without symptoms. For this reason, the full significance of this particulate matter has yet to be determined.

Filly et al. investigated the origin of gallbladder sludge in vitro. They found that filtering sludge removed its echogenicity and examination of the filtrate showed it to be predominantly microcrystals of calcium bilirubinate and cholesterol.

Positional change of sludge is slow. This suggests high-viscosity bile which is seen in biliary obstruction, acute and chronic cholecystitis, fistulae, hyperalimentation, or other conditions usually associated with biliary stasis. However, biliary stasis occurs in pregnancy without formation of sludge.

REFERENCE

1. Filly RA, Allen B, Minton MJ, et al: In vitro investigation of the origin of echoes within biliary sludge. J Clin Ultrasound 8:193–200, 1980

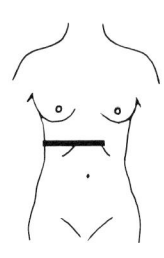

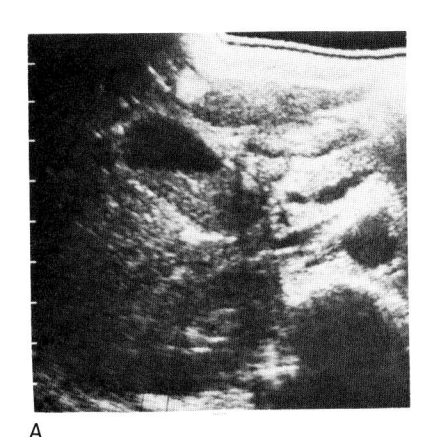

A

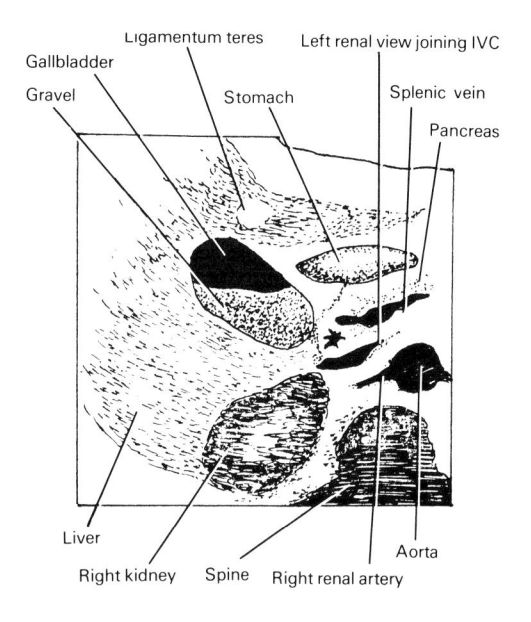

B

Gravel — Gallbladder — Ligamentum teres — Stomach — Left renal view joining IVC — Splenic vein — Pancreas

Liver — Right kidney — Spine — Right renal artery — Aorta

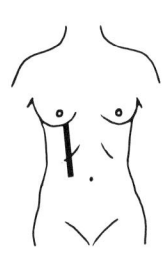

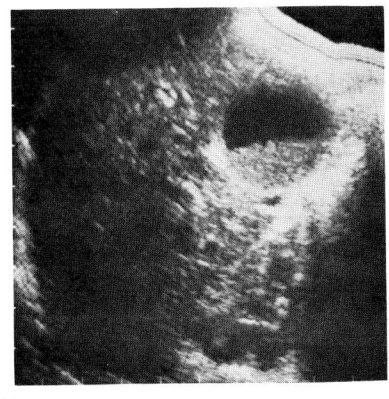

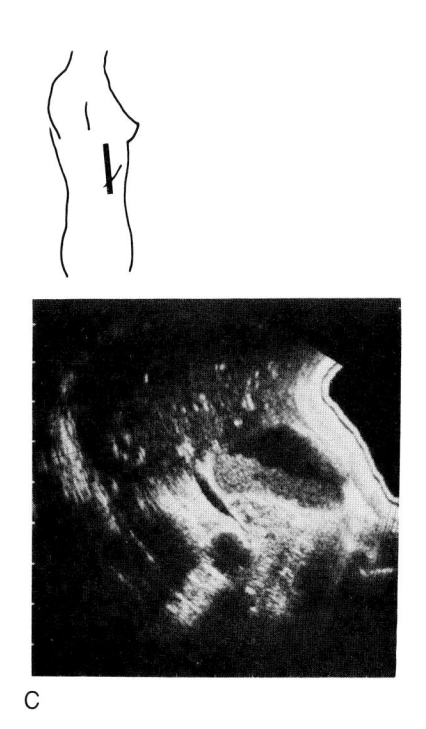

C

Hydrops of Gallbladder (8.16 and 8.17)

8.16 Adult

A 43-year-old man who was known to have Hodgkin's disease presented with a mobile, palpable mass in the right hypochondrium. The sonogram, taken in the paramedian plane 6 cm to the right of the midline, showed the palpable mass to be pyriform in shape and cystic (Fig. A). There was a definite shadow from the neck of the gallbladder, which is found in all gallbladders and is not due to a gallstone impacted in the neck. From its shape and state of distention, the gallbladder appeared to be obstructed. The appearances were consistent with a mucocele of the gallbladder.

In another patient, a paramedian sonogram showed marked dilatation of the gallbladder; the longitudinal axis measured 16 cm (Fig. B). In the author's experience to date, 13 cm is the upper limit of normal. However, many hydropic gallbladders are smaller than this.

A transverse sonogram of the patient shown in Figure B demonstrated a markedly distended gallbladder lying anterior to the right kidney (Fig. C). Note the very constant relationship between the gallbladder lumen, the duodenum which contains an air bubble, and the head of the pancreas passing from the lateral to the medial aspect.

At surgery, hydrops of the gallbladder due to a stone impacted in the cystic duct was confirmed. Such stones may be missed on ultrasound examination.

Physiological distention of the gallbladder may look very similar to a hydrops. If the gallbladder is easily palpable and may be balloted, this confirms the presence of a hydrops. An obstructed gallbladder tends to be more spherical than one which is physiologically distended. This can also be differentiated by a repeat scan after a fatty meal, or by ^{99m}Tc-HIDA examination, which is highly sensitive for the diagnosis of cystic duct obstruction.

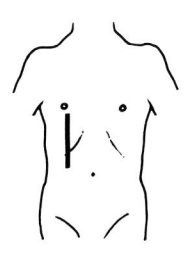

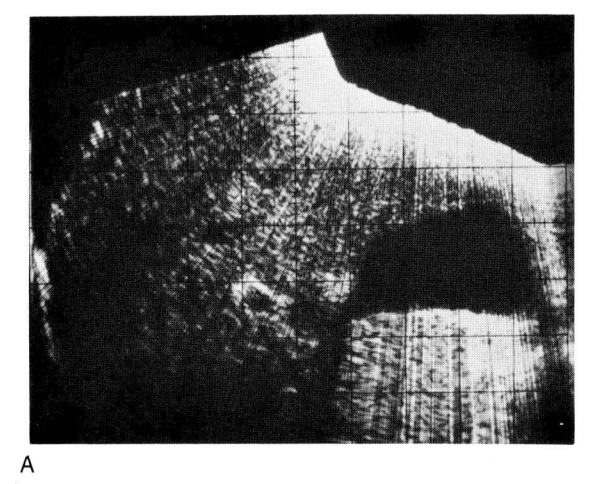

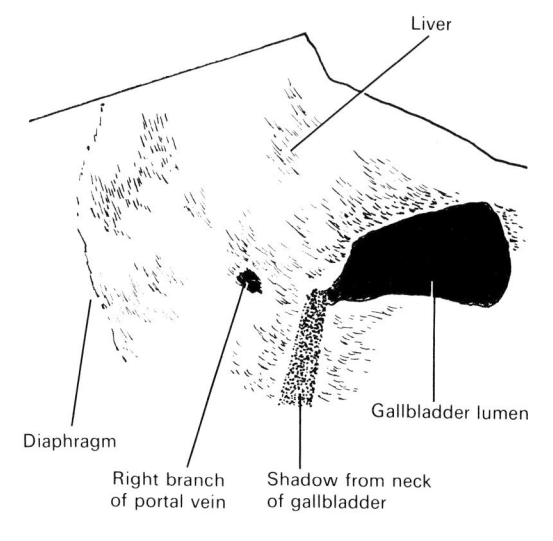

A

Liver

Diaphragm
Right branch of portal vein
Shadow from neck of gallbladder
Gallbladder lumen

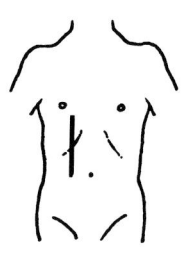

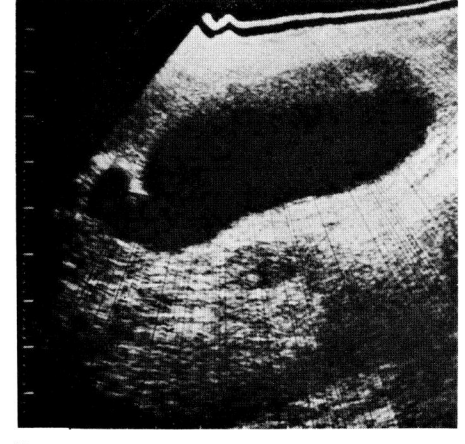

B

578

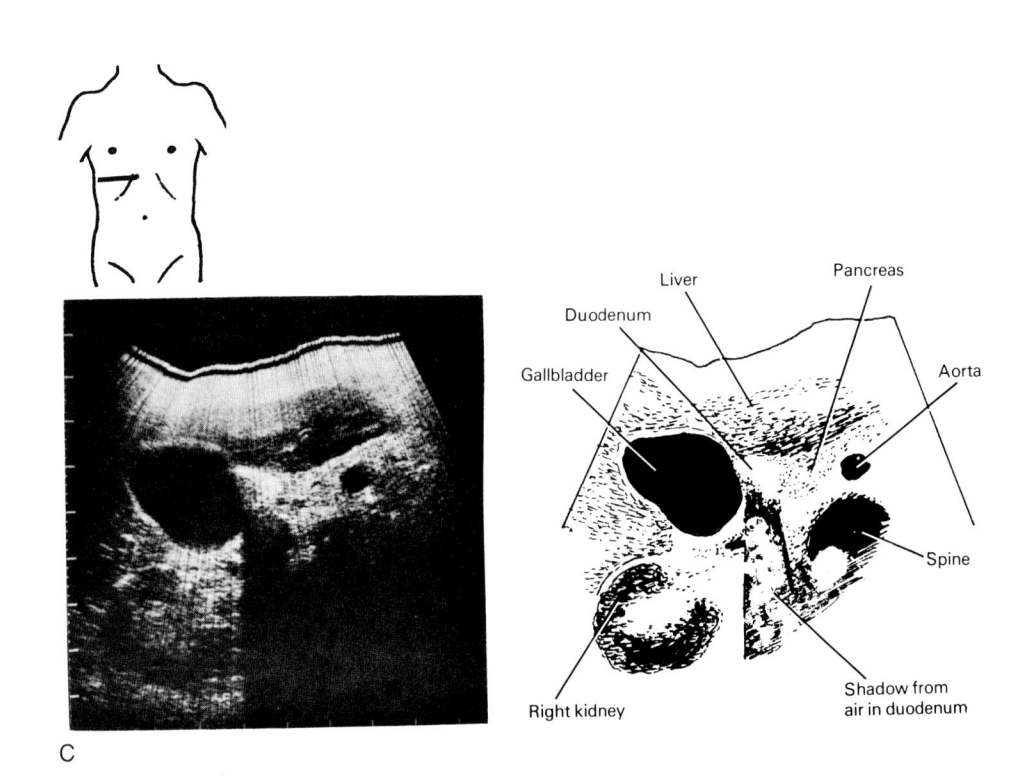

C

8.17 Pediatric

A 4-year-old child was admitted with a fever of 40°C (104°F) of 7 days' duration and was treated successfully with oral and intramuscular penicillin. On admission, cervical lymphadenopathy and an erythematous throat were noted, but there was no abnormality in the abdomen. During the next 3 days, a palpable mass became apparent in the right hypochondrium which appeared to be a tense, distended gallbladder. The sonogram showed a distended gallbladder on longitudinal (Fig. A) and transverse section (Fig. B). At surgery, the ultrasound finding of hydrops of the gallbladder was confirmed and the patient treated by cholecystostomy and cholecystectomy. The rarity of gallstones in children makes a hydrops unusual. However, in this child no gallstones were present and obstruction of the cystic duct was due to inspissation of bile associated with prolonged pyrexia and dehydration.

Physiological distention must be differentiated from hydrops. A tense gallbladder which can be ballotted on palpation is evidence of pathologic tension. If doubt exists, the patient should be re-examined after a fatty meal.

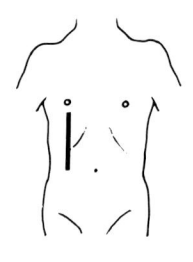

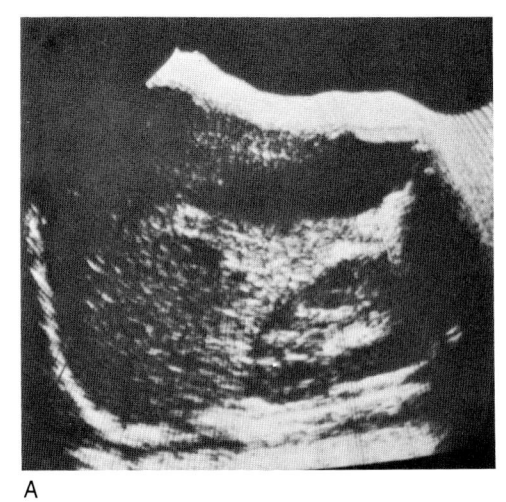

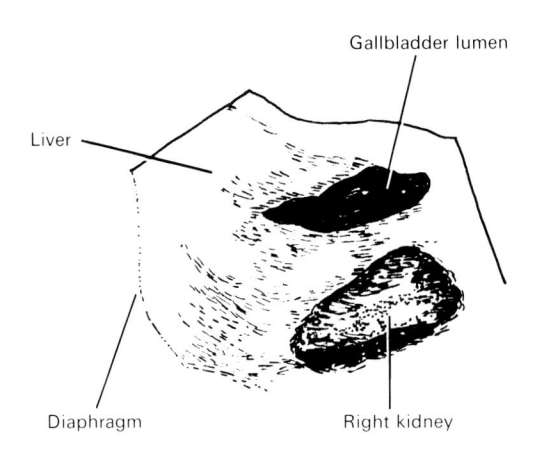

A

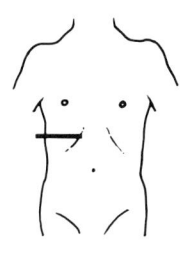

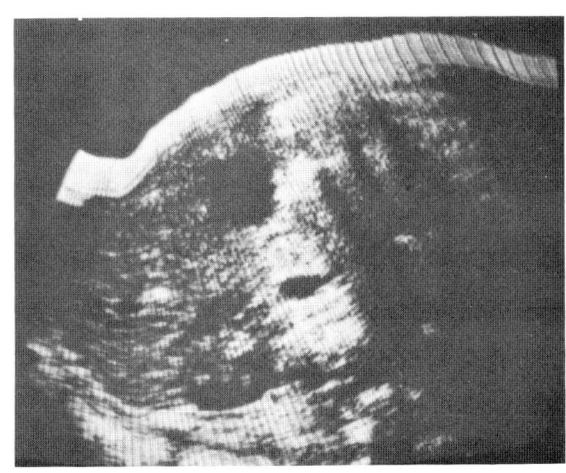

B

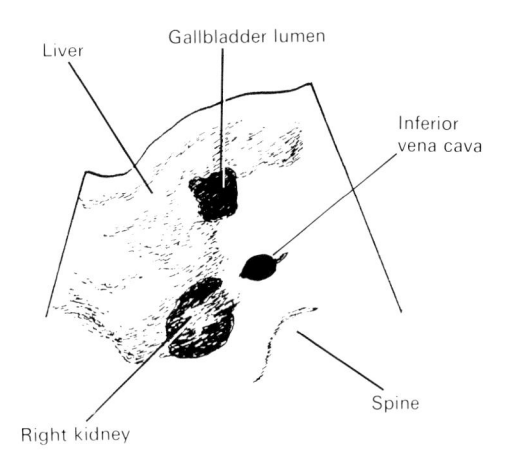

Liver
Gallbladder lumen
Inferior vena cava
Right kidney
Spine

581

Carcinoma (8.18 and 8.19)

8.18 Occult Carcinoma

A 76-year-old woman presented with right upper quadrant pain and was admitted for routine cholecystectomy. Ultrasound examination demonstrated typical shadowing opacities (arrow) within the lumen of the gallbladder, which also had a thickened wall. This appeared to be merely acute on chronic cholecystitis. At surgery, the ultrasound findings were confirmed and a cholecystectomy was performed. After the patient had been discharged, the pathologist's report revealed adenocarcinoma of the gallbladder, which had not been apparent at surgery.

Accurate distinction by sonography between inflammatory and neoplastic changes of the gallbladder appears to be impossible.[1] Pathologically, carcinoma of the gallbladder may be either infiltrating or fungating. The infiltrating type is more common and produces a diffuse thickening and induration of the gallbladder. These appearances may closely simulate those of a purely inflammatory lesion.

A fungating tumor fills the lumen of the gallbladder and invades the walls. At diagnosis, most of these tumors have invaded the liver and extended to obstruct the cystic duct, bile duct, and regional lymph nodes, producing obstructive jaundice. Many of these patients present with nonspecific symptoms mimicking chronic cholecystitis.

The mean survival of patients with carcinoma of the gallbladder is less than 5 months from diagnosis, with a 4 percent 5-year survival rate. Even when the tumor is found fortuitously at surgery, only 3 percent of patients have a long survival.[2]

REFERENCES

1. Yeh H-C: Ultrasonography and computed tomography of carcinoma of the gallbladder. Radiology 133:167–173, 1979
2. Piehler JM, Crichlow RW: Primary carcinoma of the gallbladder. Surg Gynecol Obstet 147:929–942, 1978

583

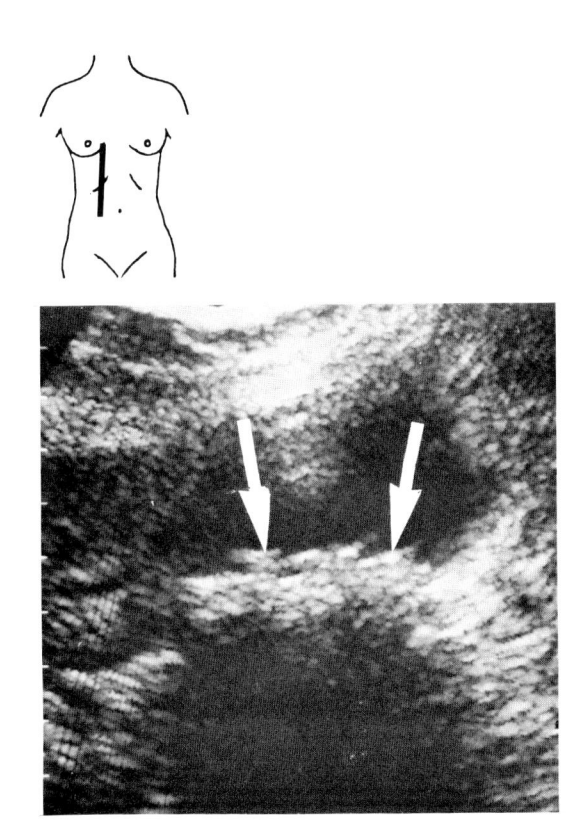

8.19 Advanced Carcinoma

A 80-year-old white woman presented with weight loss and a large, palpable mass in the right upper quadrant. A liver/spleen scan demonstrated a large cold area in the right upper quadrant coinciding with the palpable mass. The longitudinal sonogram through the right upper quadrant, shown in the figure, demonstrated an irregular solid mass in the lower border of the liver, anterior to the right kidney. The gallbladder was not visualized separately from this mass, but it was impossible to tell whether the gallbladder was merely compressed by the mass or whether the mass represented a carcinoma of the gallbladder. The presence of a shadowing opacity within the mass supported the diagnosis of a carcinoma of the gallbladder. This possibility deterred suggestions of a cutting needle biopsy of the mass. A fine-needle biopsy specimen of the mass disclosed a mixture of adenocarcinoma and squamous carcinoma cells consistent with carcinoma of the gallbladder. In view of evidence of spread into the liver and the patient's refusal of further treatment, she was discharged home and died 6 weeks later.

Carcinoma of the gallbladder constitutes up to 3 percent of all cancers and is the most common malignancy of the biliary system. The prevalence increases with age and is most common in 60–70-year-old women. Gallstones are present in up to 90 percent of patients with carcinoma of the gallbladder.[1]

In 1924, Blalock[2] suggested that surgery should be avoided if this diagnosis could be made preoperatively. More than half a century later, the 5-year survival rate is still only 4 percent.

Gallbladder carcinomas spread widely throughout the liver substance and metastasize early to the periportal nodes. Although the differentiation of liver tumor from carcinoma of the gallbladder is not possible based on ultrasound appearances alone, the finding of gallstones within a mass should raise strong suspicion of a gallbladder carcinoma.

The sonographic features reported include a diffusely echogenic gallbladder associated with complete replacement by tumor, localized or diffuse thickening of the gallbladder wall, or a polypoid mass within the gallbladder lumen.[3–5] In view of the appalling prognosis, a conservative approach to this tumor is still desirable, especially when there is evidence of local spread to the liver or distant spread producing obstructive jaundice. A fine-needle biopsy now allows a definitive preoperative diagnosis and in this patient precluded the need for exploratory surgery. Thus, her terminal weeks were spent at home rather than in the hospital recovering from major, futile surgery.

REFERENCES

1. Fraumeni JF Jr: Cancer of the pancreas and biliary tract: epidemiological considerations. Cancer Res 35:3437–3446, 1975
2. Blalock AA: A statistical study of 888 cases of biliary tract disease. Johns Hopkins Hosp Bull 35:391, 1924
3. Yeh H-C: Ultrasonography and computed tomography of carcinoma of the gallbladder. Radiology 133:167–173, 1979
4. Palma LD, Rizzatto G, Pozzi-Mucelli RS, et al: Grey-scale ultrasonography in the evaluation of carcinoma of the gallbladder. Br J Radiol 53:662–667, 1980
5. Raghavendra BN: Ultrasonographic features of primary carcinoma of the gallbladder: report of five cases. Gastrointest Radiol 5:239–244, 1980

585

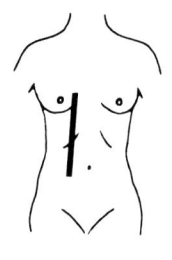

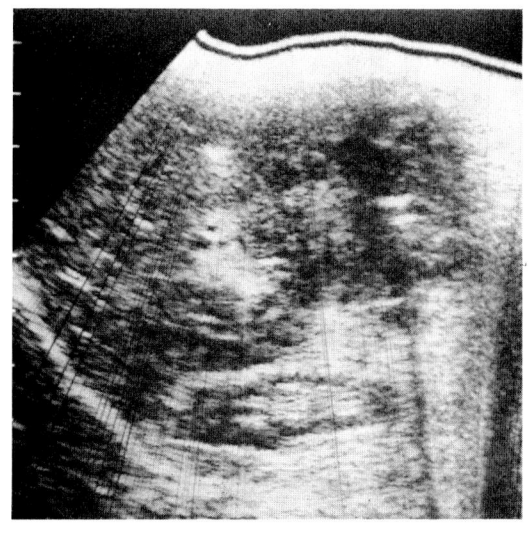

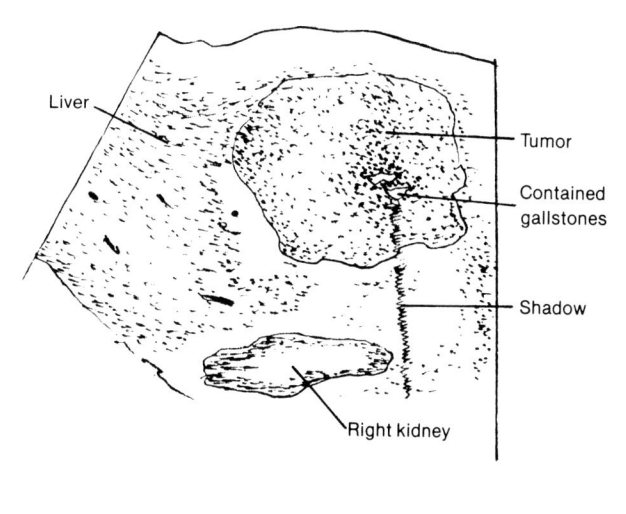

8.20 Gallbladder Wall Tumor: Neoplastic or Inflammatory?

A 60-year-old man presented with symptoms suggesting a pulmonary embolus and was found to have a right pleural effusion. He was referred for ultrasound examination to exclude a subphrenic abscess.

A sagittal ultrasound scan demonstrated no evidence of subphrenic abscess, but did demonstrate gallstones. Of note was a solid mass 4 × 2 cm in the inferior wall of the gallbladder, shown in the figure. Tenderness was elicited over the site of the gallbladder as localized by ultrasound. The differential diagnosis included papilloma, adenoma, carcinoma, or inflammatory mass of the gallbladder.

Subsequent cholecystectomy disclosed acute and chronic cholecystitis. The gallbladder contained a single, large stone and there was a perforation of the inferior and posterior wall. This appeared to be due to perforation of the gallbladder which had subsequently healed.

The nonspecific appearances of gallbladder masses have been reported.[1] It appears to be impossible to differentiate between inflammatory and neoplastic masses by ultrasound alone.

REFERENCE

1. Crade M, Taylor KJW, Rosenfield AT, et al: The varied ultrasonic character of gallbladder tumor. JAMA 241:2195–2196, 1979

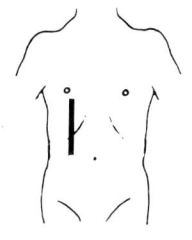

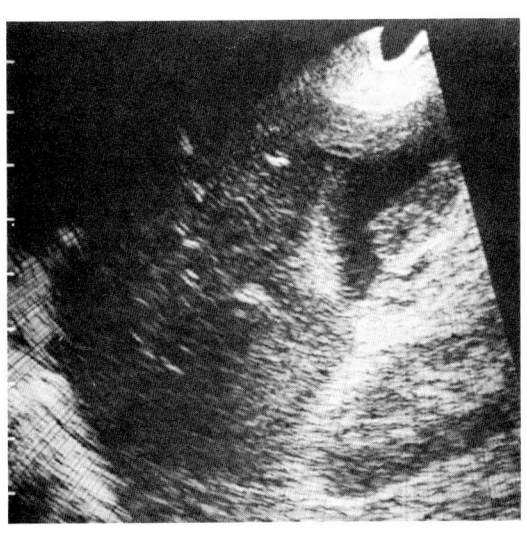

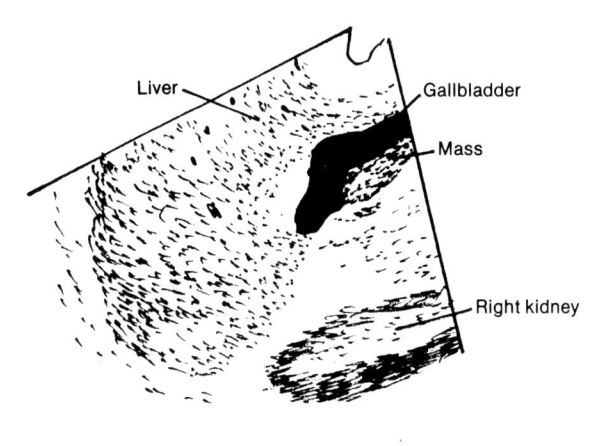

Liver
Gallbladder
Mass
Right kidney

8.21 Distended Cystic Duct and Gallbladder

An elderly man was referred for ultrasound examination of the biliary tree following episodes of fever and right upper quadrant pain which simulated acute cholecystitis. An oblique subcostal scan (Fig. A) in the plane of the costal margin showed the gallbladder fundus and body along its longitudinal axis, converging into the neck of the gallbladder and passing into a dilated cystic duct. This duct was 1.5 cm in diameter and the mucosal folds which form part of the spiral valve were seen in the wall of the duct. This spiral valve was optimally seen in a slightly lower section through the gallbladder lumen (Fig. B).

Surgery revealed an obstructed cystic duct due to cholangiocarcinoma.

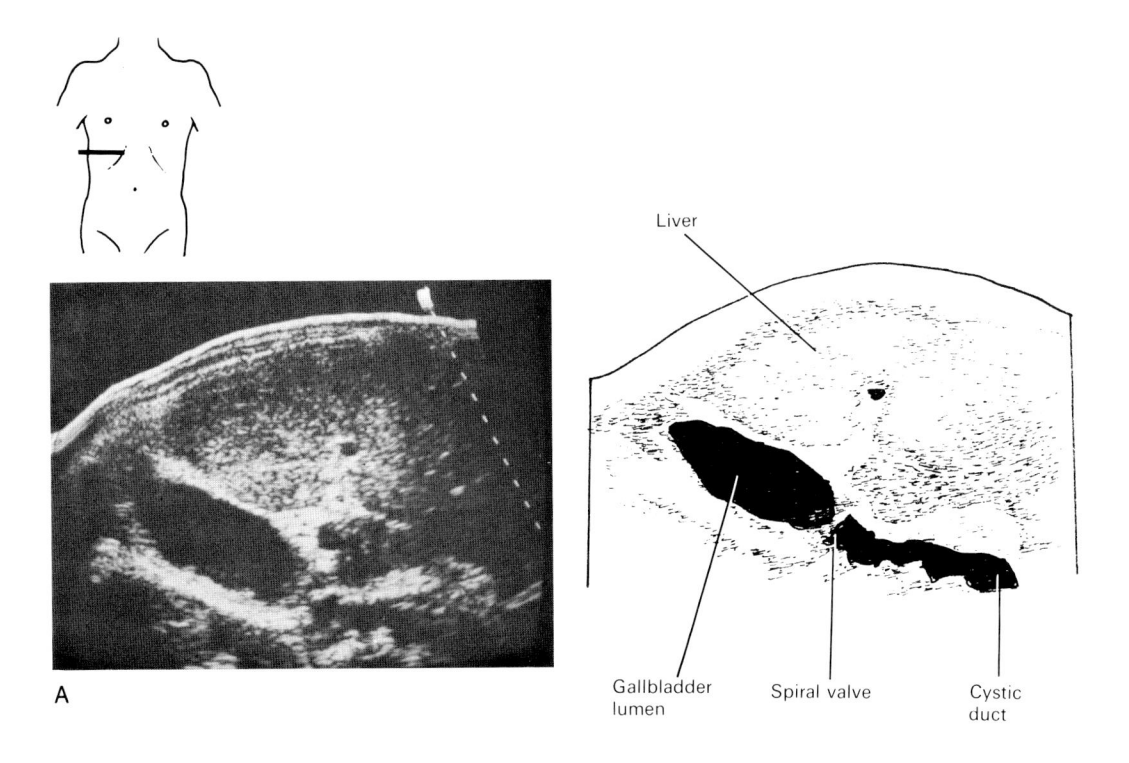

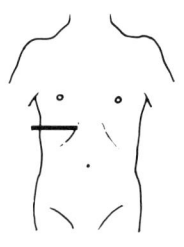

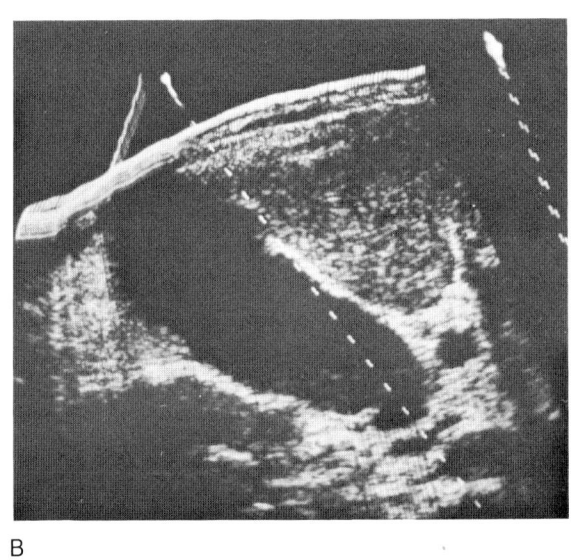

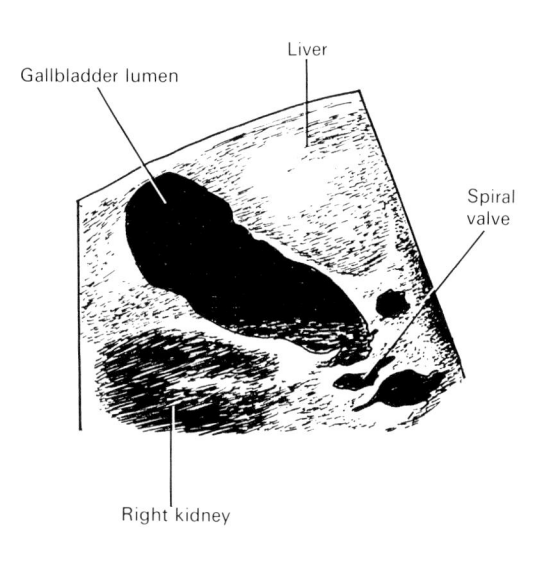

B

Gallbladder lumen
Liver
Spiral valve
Right kidney

589

8.22 Extrahepatic Ducts

ANATOMY

Ultrasound examination of the extrahepatic ducts commences with the patient in the supine position, although a left-side-down oblique or decubitus view may often be helpful.[1,2] Because the junction of the cystic and common hepatic ducts is seldom apparent on ultrasound, the term "common duct" (CD) is used to describe either the common hepatic or the common bile duct. The plane of the common duct is established by identifying the portal vein and the common duct anterior to it (Fig. A). This plane usually approximates a line perpendicular to the costal margin. The common hepatic duct is seen anterior to the right branch of the portal vein in virtually every patient. The right hepatic artery (arrowed, Fig. B) may be seen between the common duct and the portal vein. As the common duct is traced inferiorly, it passes posterior to the first part of the duodenum to reach the deep aspect of the head of the pancreas anterior to the IVC. The distal duct may be well-seen embedded in the pancreatic head (Fig. C), especially when water distention of the stomach has been used to display the pancreas. However, the frequent occurrence of air in the duodenum often obscures the mid portion of the duct.

NORMAL CALIBER

The upper limit of the normal caliber for the extrahepatic bile ducts has steadily decreased over recent years. Differences among reports by various authors are partly related to the different levels at which the duct was measured. Cooperberg[3] examined 100 normal subjects and found the largest internal diameter of the common duct anterior to the right portal vein to be 4 mm. Sample et al.[4] followed up 129 patients with jaundice. Using 6 mm as the upper limit for the diameter of the normal common duct, there were 4 false-positives (3.1 percent) and 10 false-negatives (7.7 percent). If the upper limit of normal was increased to 10 mm, the false-positive rate dropped to zero, but the false-negative rate increased to 16 percent. Thus, he concluded that 6 mm should be regarded as the upper limit of normal for the common bile duct. It must be noted that measurements were made in different positions (common hepatic duct vs. common bile duct) in these two series.

In a further study, Cooperberg et al.[5] used 4 mm as the upper limit for the common duct anterior to the right portal vein. Of 170 patients studied, 14 had common hepatic ducts larger than 4 mm without evidence of current obstruction on radiologic examination. However, 13 of these 14 had a history of recent calculus (7/13), or had had a previous cholecystectomy (6/13).

There is evidence that the common duct increases in size with age. In an autopsy study, Mahour et al.[6] found that the outer diameter of the common bile duct increased from 6.2 mm at age 35 to 8.5 mm at the age of 75.

In the most recent study to be published, Niederau et al. reported a survey on the size of the common duct in 830 healthy blood donors.[7] The mean diameter was 2.5 ± 1.1 mm at the porta hepatis and 2.8 ± 1.2 mm at the widest point in the lower part of the duct. None had a duct greater than 7 mm and the duct was less than 4 mm in 95 percent of this population. There was a slight, but significant, increase in size with age and weight. In contrast, in 73 patients with gallstones, the upper duct measured 3.8 ± 2.0 mm and the lower duct was 4.8 ± 2.2 mm.

POSTCHOLECYSTECTOMY

Conventional surgical wisdom has long indicated that the common duct is larger after cholecystectomy, since the duct acts as a reservoir. Graham et al. followed up 57 asymptomatic patients for 16 months after cholecystectomy for gallstones.[8] Eighty-four percent had a common duct 4 mm or smaller. Similar results by Mueller et al.[9] showed that 93 percent of asymptomatic patients had normal-sized ducts before and 6 months after cholecystectomy. Graham et al.[10] defined 36 symptomatic patients with a common duct larger than 4 mm. In 23 patients (64 percent) an obstructing cause was found at surgery. In 20 patients with common ducts of less than 4 mm, only 3 (15 percent) had choledocholithiasis.

In contrast, Niederau et al.[7] measured the ducts in 55 patients after cholecystectomy. The upper portion of the duct was 5.2 ± 2.3 mm and the lower part, 6.2 ± 2.5 mm. Thus, 58 percent of patients had ducts larger than the normal of 4 mm, compared with 18 percent of those with gallstones. These authors concluded that dilatation was not due to past or present obstruction, but due to the common duct acting as a reservoir.

Thus, although there are conflicting reports in the literature, we believe that a dilated duct cannot merely be ascribed to the postcholecystectomy state but suggests past or present obstruction and warrants further investigation if the patient is symptomatic.

OTHER TECHNIQUES FOR IMAGING THE BILIARY VESSELS

Many other techniques are available for imaging the biliary system, although in the jaundiced patient, ultrasound has the best potential cost/benefit ratio. Where both the level and cause of the obstruction are demonstrated by ultrasound alone, no other imaging procedure may be necessary before surgery. However, in many patients, transhepatic cholangiography is required to demonstrate the level and cause of the obstruction in those in whom an initial ultrasound examination demonstrates only that the biliary vessels are dilated. It is important to precede a transhepatic cholangiogram with an ultrasound examination, since technical success is virtually guaranteed if the ducts are dilated. ERCP requires greater expertise and is invasive, but also shows exquisite anatomy and is usually reserved for patients with problems not resolved by the initial ultrasound, such as suspected gallstones within the ducts. Intraoperative cholangiography is particularly useful to investigate the possibility of ductal stones at the time of surgery.

We long ago abandoned intravenous cholangiography (IVC) as an acceptable technique in terms of risk vs. benefit. A recent review[11] found only 55 percent of examinations to be adequate, and the accuracy was only 60 percent. CT is not as widely available as ultrasound, but is as effective in diagnosing dilatation of the biliary tree. In addition, CT allows display of pancreatic tumors concealed from the ultrasound beam by gas. Because CT is more expensive, it should be used only if ultrasound examination is unsuccessful or in the very obese patient. Finally, the newer biliary imaging agents are especially useful for demonstrating patency of the ducts. These agents can be used in the jaundiced patient despite very high levels of serum bilirubin.

DISCREPANCY BETWEEN CONTRAST CHOLANGIOGRAPHY AND ULTRASOUND MEASUREMENTS

When the caliber of bile ducts is measured, first by contrast cholangiogram and then by ultrasound using no contrast media, a definite discrepancy is found. For example, intrahepatic ducts of 3 mm are within normal limits, but would be abnormal on a sonogram. Similarly, a common duct of 8 mm is definitely abnormal on an ultrasound scan, although it would be normal on a cholangiogram. Sauerbrei et al.[12] reported five factors that contribute to this discrepancy.

1. Measurement at different locations (common duct vs. CBD)
2. Choleretic effect of IV contrast in intravenous cholangiography
3. Pressure effect of injected contrast material in transhepatic cholangiography
4. X-ray magnification factor
5. Reverberation artifact minifying the ductal lumen on ultrasound

In conclusion, ultrasound is a highly valuable method for the initial investigation of the jaundiced patient; it has been accepted for nearly 10 years.[13] Less successful is the precise localization of the level of the biliary obstruction and the determination of its cause. Nevertheless, these are apparent in more than 50 percent of patients.

REFERENCES

1. Behan M, Kazam E: Sonography of the common bile duct: value of the right anterior oblique view. Am J Roentgenol 130: 701–709, 1978
2. Parulekar SG: Ultrasound evaluation of the common bile duct size. Radiology 133:703–707, 1979
3. Cooperberg PL: High-resolution real-time ultrasound in the evaluation of the normal and obstructed biliary tract. Radiology 129:477–480, 1978
4. Sample WF, Sarti DA, Goldstein LI, et al: Gray scale ultrasonography of the jaundiced patient. Radiology 128:719–725, 1978
5. Cooperberg PL, Li D, Wong P, et al: Accuracy of common hepatic duct size in the evaluation of extrahepatic biliary obstruction. Radiology 135:141–144, 1980
6. Mahour GH, Wakim KG, Ferris DO: The common bile duct in man: its diameter and circumference. Ann Surg 165:415–419, 1967
7. Niederau C, Muller J, Sonnenberg A, et al: Extrahepatic bile ducts in healthy subjects, in patients with cholelithiasis and in postcholecystectomy patients: a prospective ultrasonic study. J Clin Ultrasound 11:23–27, 1983
8. Graham MF, Cooperberg PL, Cohen MM, Burhenne HJ: The size of the normal common hepatic duct following cholecystectomy: an ultrasonographic study. Radiology 135:137–139, 1980
9. Mueller PR, Ferrucci JT Jr, Simeone JF et al: Postcholecystectomy bile duct dilatation: myth or reality? AJR 136:355–358, 1981
10. Graham MF, Cooperberg PL, Cohen MM, Burhenne HJ: Ultrasonographic screening of the common hepatic duct in symptomatic patients after cholecystectomy. Radiology 138:137–139, 1981
11. Goodman MW, Ansel HJ, Vennes JA, et al: Is intravenous cholangiography still useful? Gastroenterology 79:642–645, 1980
12. Sauerbrei EE, Cooperberg PL, Cohen MM, Bur-

henne HJ: Dynamic changes in the calibre of the major bile ducts, related to obstruction. Radiology 135:215–216, 1980

13. Taylor KJW, Carpenter DA: Grey scale ultrasonography in the investigation of obstructive jaundice. Lancet 1:586–587, 1974

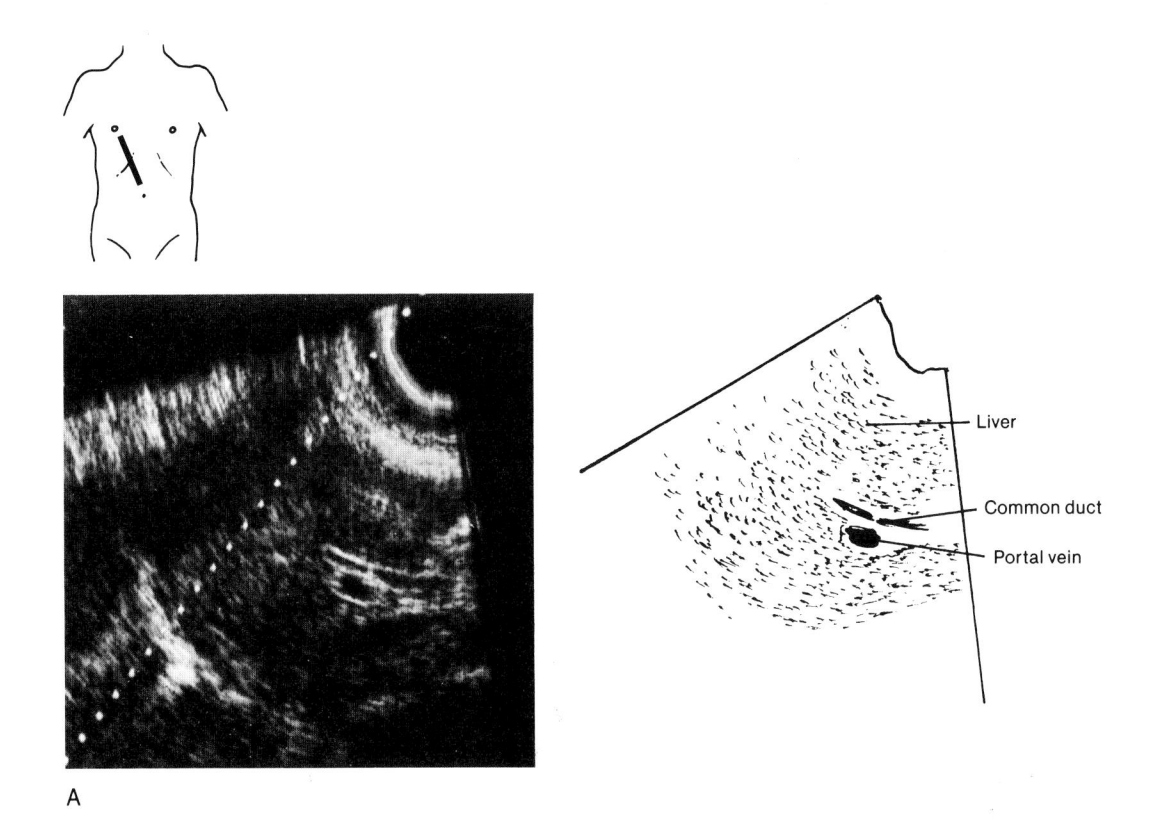

A

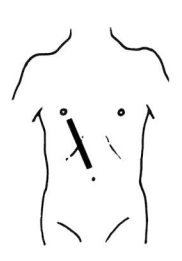

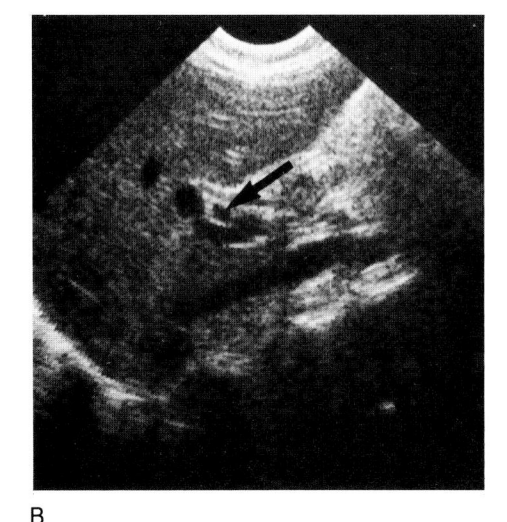

B

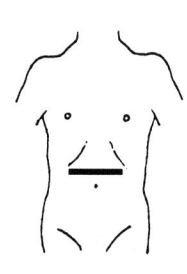

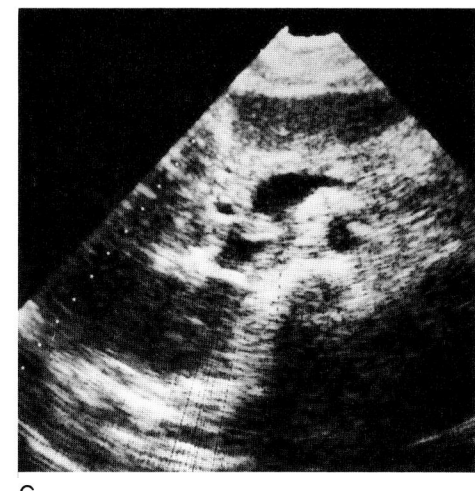

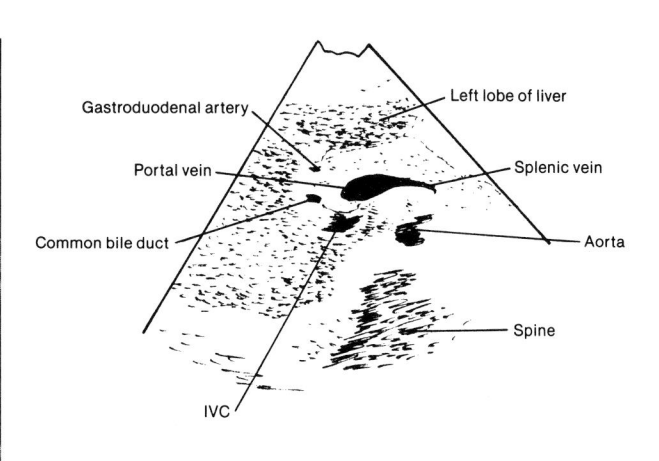

Gastroduodenal artery
Portal vein
Common bile duct
Left lobe of liver
Splenic vein
Aorta
Spine
IVC

C

594

Biliary Dilatation (8.23 to 8.25)

The low capacity of the biliary vessels and the high volume of bile production imply that biliary dilatation must occur soon after obstruction. However, the presence of the gallbladder will delay biliary dilatation since it acts as a reservoir for bile and also actively absorbs fluid. The gallbladder, therefore, decompresses the distended biliary vessels. Thus, after cholecystectomy or in a patient with a nonfunctioning gallbladder, an earlier onset of biliary dilatation may be expected. Zeman et al.[1] investigated the time course of the onset of dilatation after acute common duct obstruction in cholecystectomized dogs. The intrahepatic ducts were dilated within 3 hours of obstruction, before elevation of the serum bilirubin level. The presence of a gallbladder could delay this time sequence. Experiments by Shawker et al.[2] on monkeys with intact gallbladders supported this concept. In their study, dilatation of the common duct was apparent 24 hours after obstruction and reached a maximum at 48 hours with subsequent dilatation of the intrahepatic ducts.

The early onset of dilatation helps to explain the extraordinary sensitivity of biliary dilatation as a criterion of obstruction, since biliary dilatation can occur even before the onset of jaundice.

REFERENCES

1. Zeman RK, Taylor KJW, Rosenfield AT, et al: Acute experimental biliary obstruction in the dog: sonographic findings and clinical implications. AJR 136:965–767, 1981
2. Shawker TH, Jones BL, Girton ME: Distal common bile duct obstruction: an experimental study in monkeys. J Clin Ultrasound 9:77–82, 1981

8.23 Effect of Fatty Meal

A 75-year-old patient presented with abdominal pain 3 years after cholecystectomy. A longitudinal ultrasound scan perpendicular to the costal cartilage demonstrated the common bile duct, which was dilated to a maximum diameter of 8 mm (Fig. A). A transverse section (Fig. B) showed the dilated common hepatic duct anterior to the right portal vein. To investigate further the possibility of common duct obstruction, the patient was given a fatty meal and rescanned. An oblique longitudinal scan (Fig. C) showed that the duct had reduced to 4 mm. This reduction in size was also seen on a transverse sonogram (Fig. D).

Simeone et al.[1] investigated the effect of a fatty meal on patients with normal and enlarged common ducts. In both volunteers and patients with a duct of normal caliber, there was no change or decrease in size in response to a fatty meal. In 12 patients with a mildly dilated common hepatic duct after cholecystectomy (6–10 mm), 8 reduced to 5 mm or less after a fatty meal and 4 increased or remained enlarged. In each of these four patients, obstructive biliary pathology was present. Thus, if the duct increases in size after a fatty meal, the presence of obstruction is suggested. When the duct decreases to a normal size in response to a fatty meal as in this patient, this suggests that the duct is not obstructed.

Rapid changes in the caliber of ducts in response to the passage of stones have been reported both by intravenous cholangiography[2] and ultrasound.[3] Gooding[4] reported acute biliary dilatation associated with the passage of a stone with resolution in 43 hours. Thus, it appears that both physiological and pathologic processes can contribute to dynamic changes in the caliber of the extrahepatic ducts.

REFERENCES

1. Simeone JF, Mueller PR, Ferrucci JT, et al: Sonography of the bile ducts after a fatty meal: An aid in detection of obstruction. Radiology 143:211–215, 1982
2. Sullivan FJ, Eaton Jr SB, Ferrucci JT Jr, et al: Cholangiographic manifestations of acute biliary colic. N Engl J Med 288: 33–35, 1973
3. Scheske GA, Cooperberg PL, Cohen MM, Burhenne HJ: Dynamic changes in the calibre of the major bile ducts, related to obstruction. Radiology 135:215–216, 1980
4. Gooding GAW: Acute bile duct dilation with resolution in 43 hours: an ultrasonic demonstration. J Clin Ultrasound 9:201–202, 1981

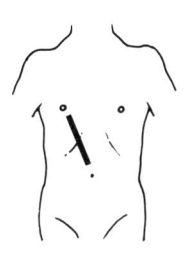

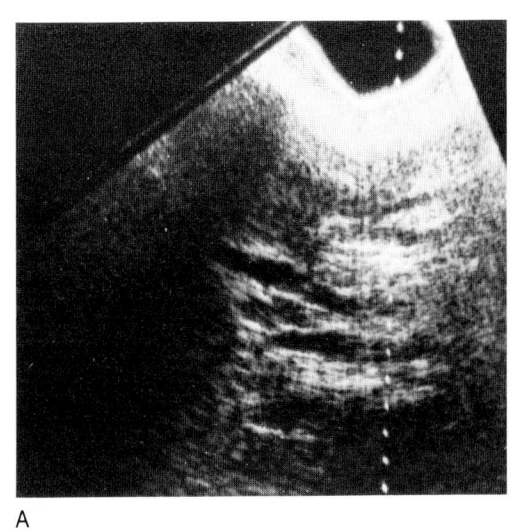

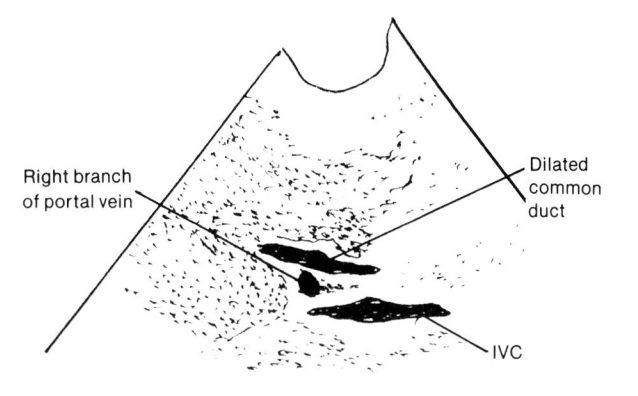

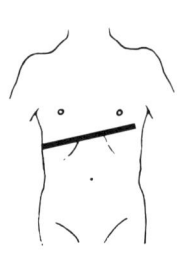

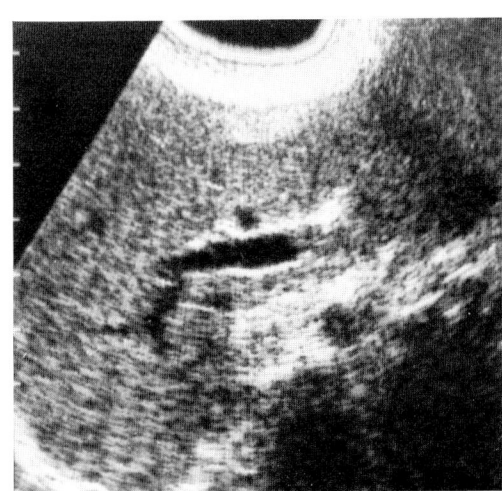

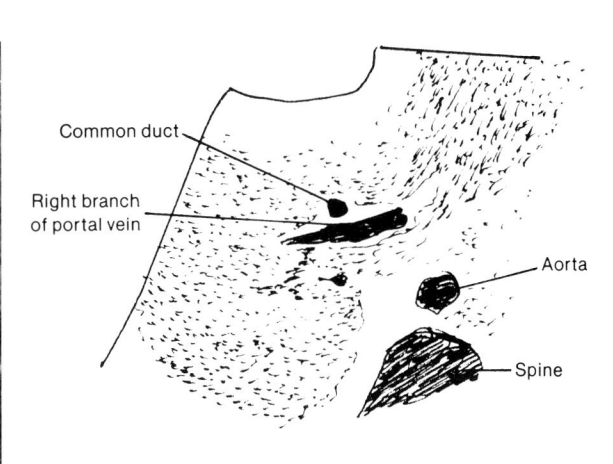

A

B

597

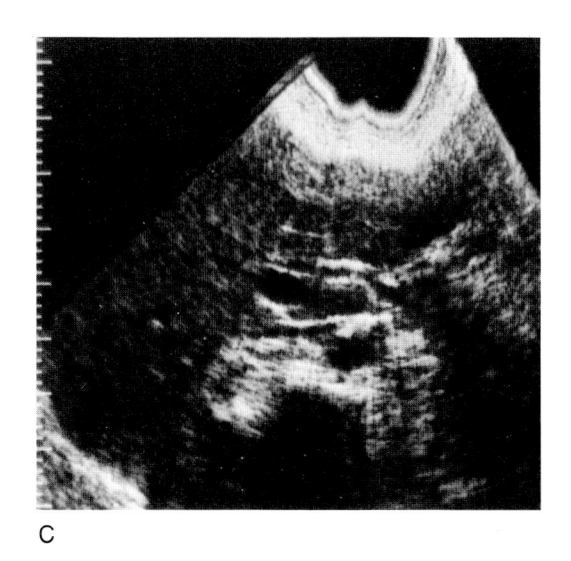

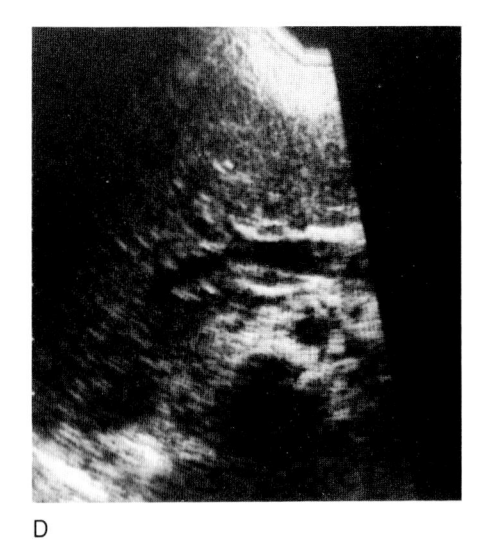

C

D

8.24 Dilated Ducts Due to Carcinoma of the Pancreas

A 60-year-old man presented with painless jaundice of 3 weeks' duration. Transverse (Fig. A) and longitudinal (Fig. B) sections through the liver revealed marked distention of the intrahepatic biliary ducts, indicating an extrahepatic site of biliary obstruction.

A longitudinal sonogram 2 cm to the right of the midline (Fig. B) showed a dilated common bile duct containing small stones. This duct could be traced inferiorly for 7 cm before ending in an ill-defined mass partially obscured by intestinal gas. The common bile duct and entire biliary tree were therefore obstructed in the region of the pancreas.

A transhepatic cholangiogram was unsuccessful, but laparotomy revealed a small carcinoma of the head of the pancreas causing biliary obstruction.

Ultrasound is a highly sensitive technique for the detection of dilatation of the extrahepatic bile ducts. It is less satisfactory for determining the level and cause of the obstruction, which may require transhepatic cholangiography. In our series of jaundiced patients followed up from 1973 to 1976, biliary dilatation occurred in all 44 patients with pancreatic cancer.[1] The obstructing mass was only seen in 33 (75 percent).[2] Nevertheless, display of dilated ducts alone is valuable, since it defines the population in whom transhepatic cholangiography will be technically successful and diagnostic.

REFERENCES

1. Taylor KJW, Rosenfield AT, Spiro HM: Diagnostic accuracy of gray scale ultrasonography for the jaundiced patient: a report of 275 cases. Arch Intern Med 139:60–63, 1979
2. Sullivan FJ, Eaton Jr SB, Ferrucci JT Jr, et al: Cholangiographic manifestations of acute biliary colic. N Engl J Med 288:33–35, 1973

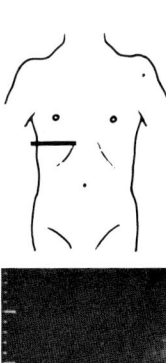

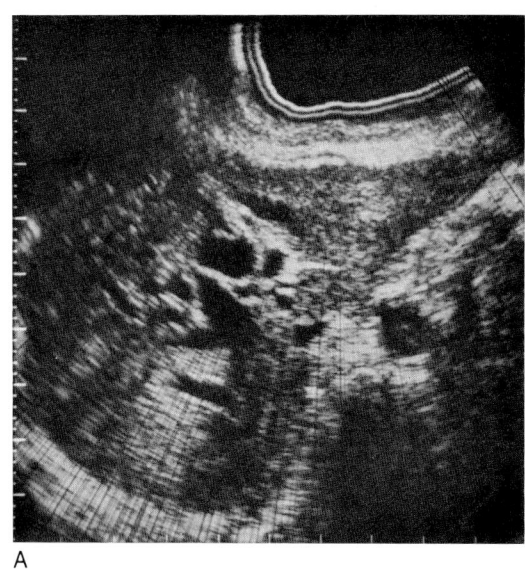

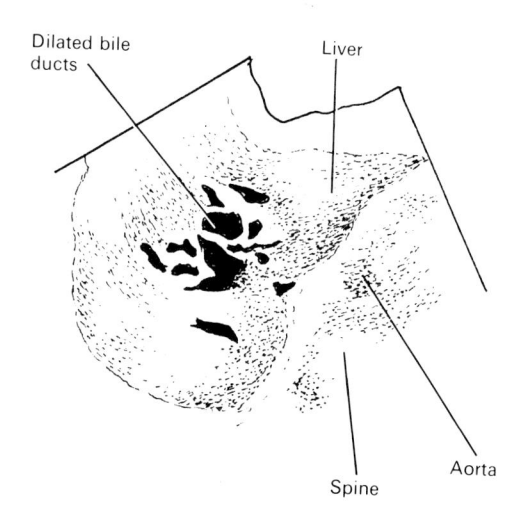

A

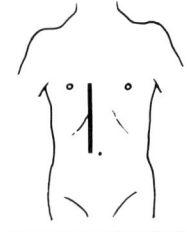

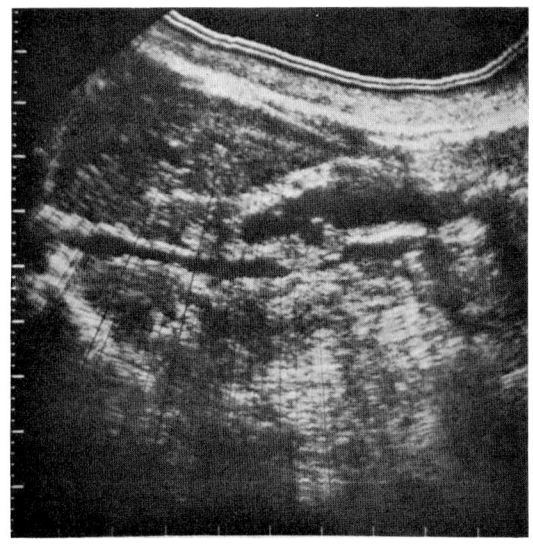

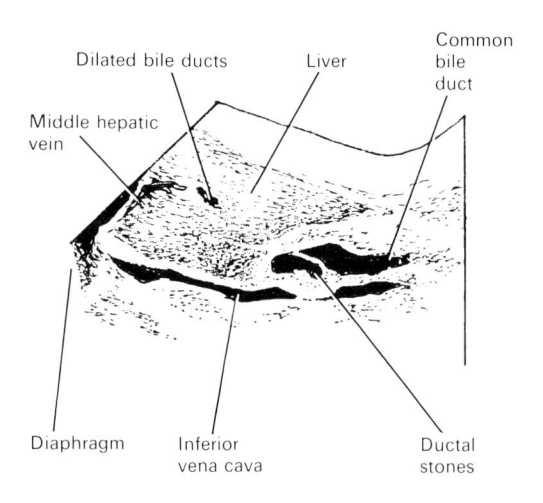

B

8.25 Disparate Biliary Dilatation

A 56-year-old white woman presented with jaundice. Her serum bilirubin level was 7 mg/dl and the clinical problem was whether her jaundice was due to hepatitis or was obstructive in nature. The SGOT level was 420 U and the alkaline phosphatase was 490 IU/dl.

A longitudinal sonogram showed gross dilatation of the common bile duct to 20 mm (Fig. A). The gallbladder was spherical, but not enlarged. Sections through the liver showed minimal dilatation of the intrahepatic ducts (Fig. B).

At surgery, a hard mass was felt in the pancreas, and biopsy specimens showed this to be a carcinoma. The CBD measured 25 mm. The pancreatic mass was bypassed.

This case illustrates several important points about imaging the jaundiced patient. Ultrasound is extraordinarily sensitive for detecting dilatation of the intrahepatic as well as the extrahepatic ducts. In our original series of 275 jaundiced patients, we achieved a sensitivity of 94 percent, a specificity of 100 percent, and an overall accuracy of 96.5 percent.[1] The false-negative results were mainly due to gallstones which we suggested were acting as intermittent ball valves. These results were obtained mainly on observation of the intrahepatic ducts, since the sonographic anatomy of the normal common duct was unknown during much of that time.

These results have been recently illuminated by manometric pressure and perfusion studies during percutaneous transhepatic cholangiography (PTC) by van Sonnenberg et al.[2] These authors reported 104 successful PTC manometric pressure recordings. Normal pressures within the biliary tree varied from 5 to 18 cm saline. Perfusion in these patients showed neither elevated pressure nor ductal distention. In addition, pain was not produced.

In dilated systems, there was an approximate linear relation between duct size and pressure, but with some notable exceptions. Higher pressures appeared to have some predictive value for subsequent bile leakage.

Eight of 104 patients had elevated pressure due to obstruction without dilatation. Four of these patients had stones in the distal common duct. This finding concurs with the false-negative results in our series. In van Sonnenberg's series, two patients had infiltrating intrahepatic metastases which limited the capacity of the biliary tree to dilate, one had sclerosing cholangitis, and another had recently undergone surgery for a periampullary tumor.

Four of 104 patients had a dilated nonobstructed duct with normal pressure and 2 of these had had a prior cholecystectomy. It was suggested that chronic dilatation occurred due to prior stone passage, periampullary fibrosis, and/or infection leading to loss of elasticity of the duct walls. These patients had normal pressure, although one had abnormal results of a perfusion study.

In this patient, the intrahepatic ducts were only minimally dilated, despite the gross dilatation of the extrahepatic ducts. This has been termed disparate biliary dilatation and is an important entity.[3] In this author's experience, the combination of dilated extrahepatic ducts with completely normal intrahepatic ducts is rare. However, where there is difficulty in recognizing the presence of minimal intrahepatic duct dilatation, it appears that this is a relatively common condition. In this patient, the intrahepatic ducts were definitely abnormal and the diagnosis of biliary obstruction could be made based on their appearance alone.

The same phenomenon has been described in

the CT literature. Shanser et al.[4] described six patients with obstructive jaundice in whom dilated extrahepatic ducts were seen with normal intrahepatic ducts. However, the ultrasonic diagnosis of biliary obstruction is made by observing intrahepatic ducts with any recognizable lumen. Structures of this size would not have been imaged by the CT scanners employed by the authors.

Dilatation of the common bile duct before the intrahepatic ducts can be partly explained in terms of Laplace's Law. At constant pressure, the force exerted on the wall is directly proportional to the diameter of the cylinder.[5] However, this does not account for the vast differences seen in various patients with long-standing obstruction.

The intrahepatic ducts may be constrained by decreased compliance of the liver in patients with cirrhosis. However, disparate biliary dilatation may also be seen in patients with normal livers.

REFERENCES

1. Taylor KJW, Rosenfield AT, Spiro HM: Diagnostic accuracy of gray scale ultrasonography for the jaundiced patient. A report of 275 cases. Arch Intern Med 139:60–63, 1979
2. van Sonnenberg E, Ferrucci JT, Neff CC, et al: Biliary pressure: manometric and perfusion studies at percutaneous transhepatic cholangiography and percutaneous biliary drainage. Radiology 148:41–50, 1983
3. Zeman RK, Dorfman GS, Burrell MI, et al: Disparate dilatation of the intrahepatic and extrahepatic bile ducts in surgical jaundice. Radiology 138:129–136, 1981
4. Shanswer JD, Korobkin M, Goldberg HI, et al: Computed tomographic diagnosis of obstructive jaundice in the absence of intrahepatic ductal dilatation. AJR 131:389–392, 1978
5. Compton RA: Bursting forces within the human body. Radiology 107:77–80, 1973

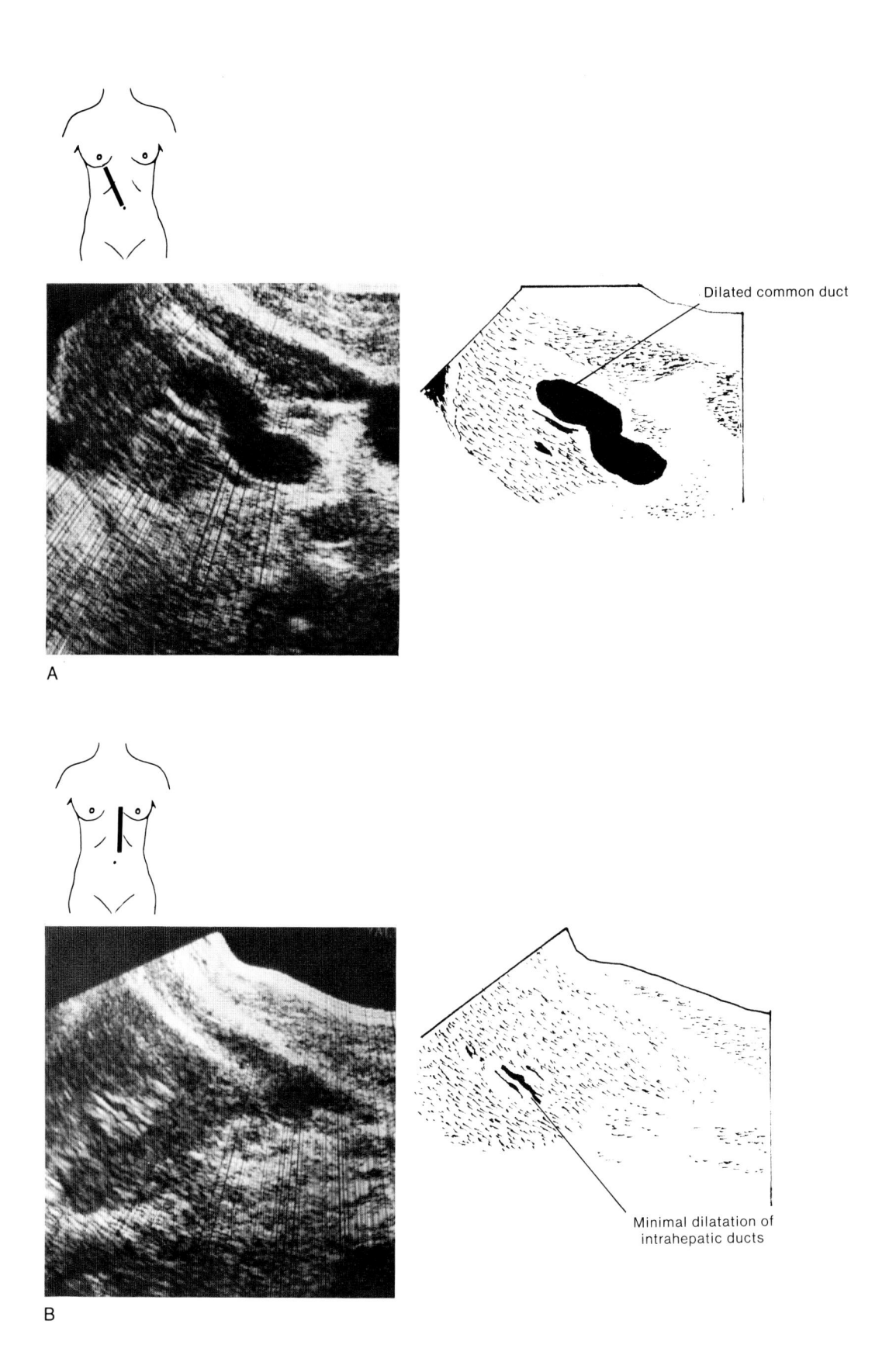

A

B

604

8.26 Choledocholithiasis

A 54-year-old woman presented with right upper quadrant pain and sudden onset of jaundice, obstructive in nature. The paramedian ultrasound section 2 cm to the right of the midline (Fig. A) showed a dilated tube, the common bile duct lying anterior and parallel to the inferior vena cava. A definite opacity was seen within the duct, which cast a shadow distal to the opacity. These appearances indicated the presence of a ductal stone. Dilatation of the whole of the common bile duct implied a further obstruction at the ampulla. The liver substance showed distention of the intrahepatic biliary canaliculi.

A transverse section (Fig. B) showed the lumen of the gallbladder immediately lateral to the dilated common bile duct. Both contained stones. At surgery, gallstones were found in the gallbladder and common bile duct, and impacted in the ampulla.

Choledocholithiasis occurs in 10 percent of patients with cholecystitis and in 2–4 percent of patients following cholecystectomy.[1,2] Patients are frequently referred for ultrasound examination to exclude the presence of common duct stones, especially after cholecystectomy. Since it is a tomographic technique, ultrasound is poorly suited to this purpose.

In our series of jaundiced patients,[3] ductal stones were only detected in 25 percent of patients. With modern, real-time instrumentation, the ducts can be examined more effectively if they are dilated. Common duct stones cannot be excluded with any acceptable degree of clinical confidence, especially in nondilated ducts. In contrast, if duct stones are visualized, they are then found at surgery. That is, ultrasound has a very low sensitivity but a high specificity for the diagnosis of ductal stones. It is important to appreciate that gallstones and duct stones occur commonly in association with other, more sinister conditions. The demonstration of a ductal stone does not necessarily indicate that the obstruction is due to a more distal stone. It is also important to appreciate that when stones are demonstrated in dilated ducts, the obstructing cause is usually more distal.

Recently, Mueller et al.[4] have reiterated the limitations of ultrasound in the diagnosis of choledocholithiasis. In 87 patients with choledocholithiasis, their preoperative sensitivity was only 13 percent. In this series, only 64 percent of patients with ductal stones had dilated extrahepatic ducts, and no stones were seen in nondilated ducts.

The choice of modality for visualizing ductal stones depends on the expertise available in a particular institution. ERCP is effective but requires considerable experience. Transhepatic cholangiography is technically easier. The newer hepatobiliary imaging agents can be used to document the patency of the ducts.

REFERENCES

1. Greenwald RA, Pereiras R, Morris SJ, Schiff ER: Jaundice, choledocholithiasis and a nondilated common duct. JAMA 240:1983–1984, 1978
2. Glenn F: Postcholecystectomy choledocholithiasis. Surg Gynecol Obstet 134:249–252, 1972
3. Taylor KJW, Rosenfield AT, Spiro HM: Diagnostic accuracy of gray scale ultrasonography for the jaundiced patient: a report of 275 cases. Arch Intern Med 139:60–63, 1979
4. Cronan JJ, Mueller PR, Simeone JF, et al: Prospective diagnosis of choledocholithiasis. Radiology 146:467–469, 1983

606

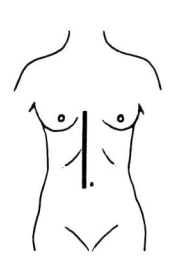

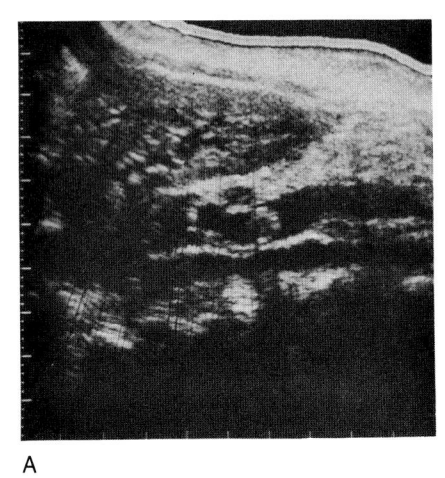

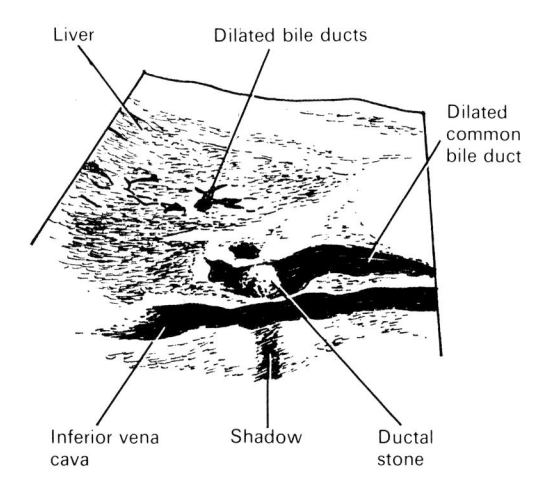

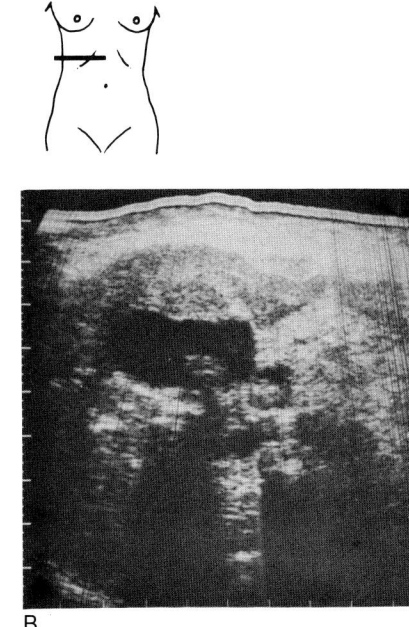

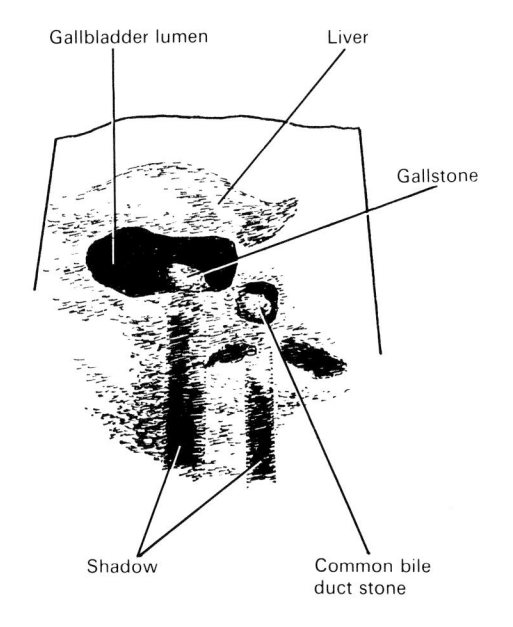

8.27 Ascaris Worms

A 62-year-old woman presented with right upper quadrant pain and jaundice. Five years prior to admission she had undergone a cholecystectomy and was admitted with a presumptive diagnosis of a common duct stone. Longitudinal ultrasound scans (Figs. A and B) demonstrated nonshadowing linear structures within a dilated common duct (arrowed). This was further investigated by an intravenous cholangiogram (Fig. C). Tomography disclosed a long linear foreign body (arrowed) within a dilated and tortuous common duct. Appearances were consistent with ascaris worms.

Medical treatment was contraindicated in this patient since dead worms are extremely hard to extricate from the common duct, whereas live worms are easily extracted. Surgery confirmed the presence of the worms and they were removed.

Ascariasis is a parasitic infection caused by the giant round worm *Ascaris lumbricoides*. The adult worm may be up to 30 cm long and up to 5 mm in diameter. Food contaminated by feces harboring the parasite eggs allows the larvae to develop in the small gut. Penetrating the mucosa, they are arrested in the lungs and migrate up the respiratory tree to be swallowed into the gastrointestinal tract. The larvae can do considerable damage to the lung, resulting in a disease resembling viral pneumonitis. Bronchial asthma and peribronchitis may occur. In the intestine, the worms cause a slight inflammatory reaction and may penetrate the intestinal wall to give rise to peritonitis. As in this patient, they may become impacted in the biliary tract or the pancreatic duct.

(Case and figures courtesy of Ramon Gonzales, M.D., Yale University School of Medicine.)

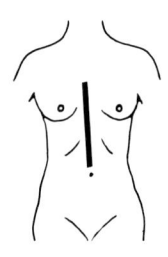

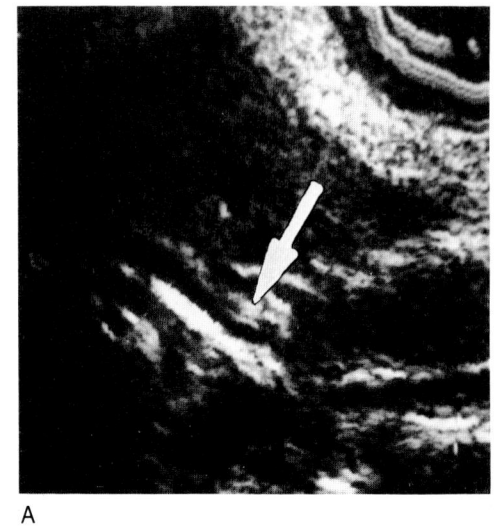

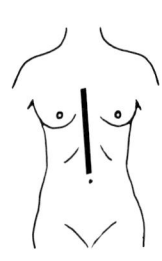

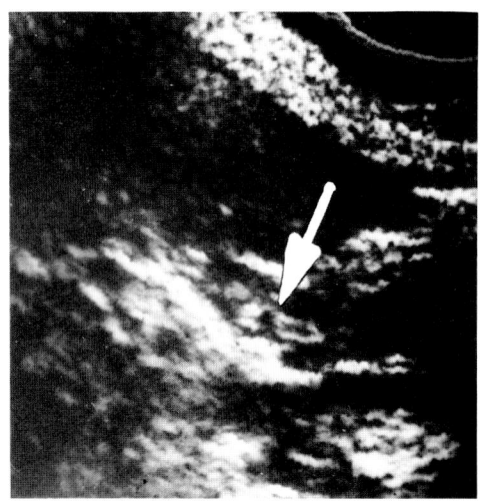

A

B

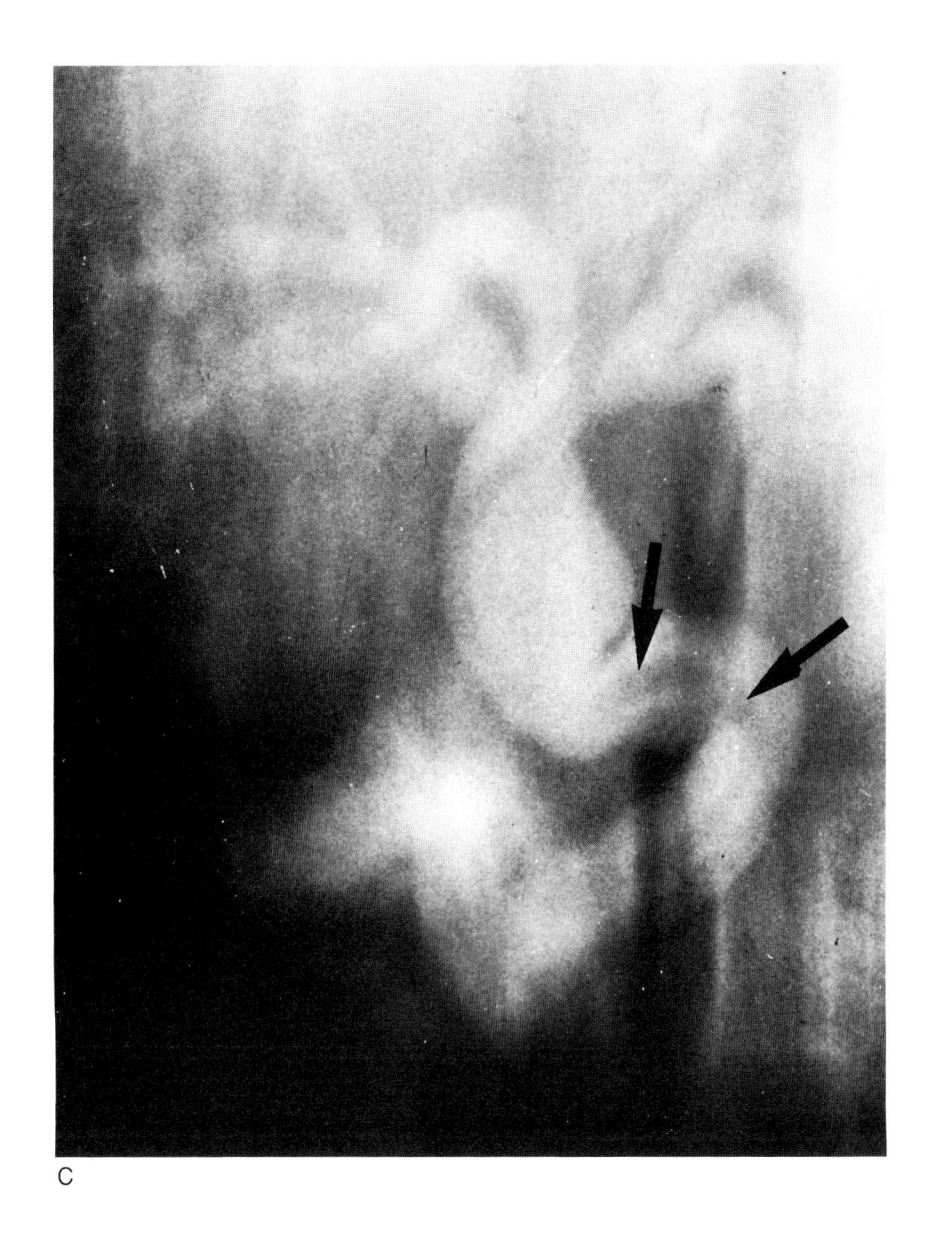

C

8.28 Obstruction by Common Duct Tumor

A 79-year-old patient presented with painless jaundice. Ultrasound examination demonstrated dilated intrahepatic and extrahepatic bile ducts. The common bile duct was dilated to a diameter of 11 mm. Two focal cystic areas were seen in the liver, which appeared to be incidental cysts. At surgery, a cholecystojejunostomy was performed with temporary relief of the patient's jaundice. However, he returned 3 months later with a 3-day history of malaise, nausea, vomiting, acholuric stools, and fever. Blood analysis disclosed a white cell count of 14,000 mm^3 and a total bilirubin level of 1.8 mg/dl.

Repeat ultrasound examination at this time revealed gross dilatation of both the intrahepatic and extrahepatic bile ducts. A longitudinal sonogram showed the common duct dilated to a maximum diameter of 20 mm (Fig. A). Nonshadowing material was seen in the lower end of the common duct, suggesting tumor or blood clot. A transverse sonogram confirmed the presence of this mass within the lower end of the common duct and dilatation of the pancreatic duct (Fig. B). There was, therefore, recurrent obstruction of the common bile duct by periampullary tumor and failure of the cholecystojejunostomy bypass.

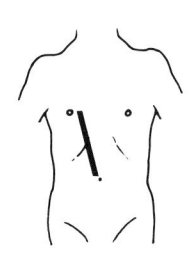

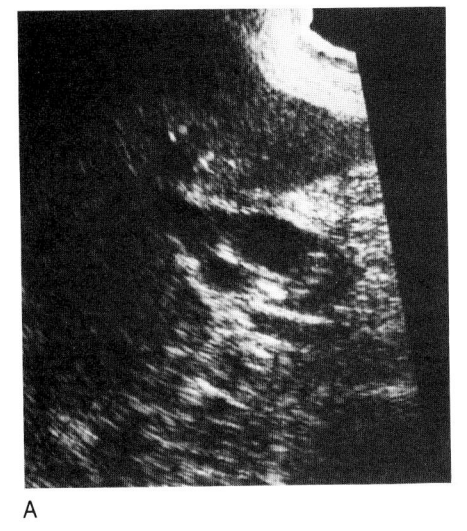

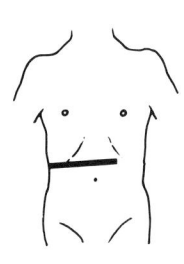

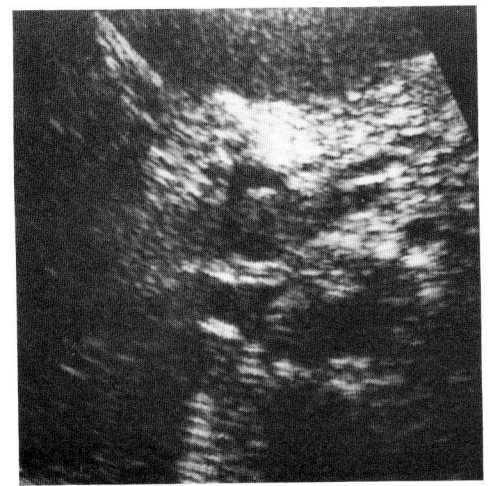

A

B

8.29 Anicteric Biliary Dilatation—Unilateral Obstruction

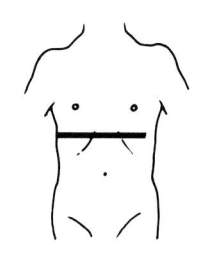

A 67-year-old man presented with a history of a 30-lb weight loss. His alkaline phosphatase level was slightly elevated at 105 IU/dl, but the serum bilirubin level was within normal limits. He was referred for ultrasound examination to exclude a carcinoma of the pancreas. The pancreas was normal but a transverse sonogram of the liver demonstrated dilatation of the left hepatic ducts (Fig. A). In the region of the portal vein, an echogenic mass was seen which was considered most likely to be a cholangiocarcinoma (Fig. B). However, examination of a biopsy specimen showed this to be an adenocarcinoma, metastatic to the porta hepatis.

Anicteric intrahepatic biliary dilatation has been reported by several authors[1,2] and may occur under several different conditions:

1. As a preicteric phase in which there is subtotal obstruction of the biliary tree with dilatation.
2. When there is unilateral biliary obstruction, as in this patient.
3. When biliary dilatation has been prolonged and has been surgically relieved. There may be persistent biliary dilatation following surgery, which on occasion we have followed for several years.

(This case and scans taken from Zeman R, Taylor KJW, Burrell MI, et al: Ultrasound demonstration of anicteric dilatation of the biliary tree. Radiology 134:689–692, 1980.)

REFERENCES

1. Zeman R, Taylor KJW, Burrell MI, et al: Ultrasound demonstration of anicteric dilatation of the biliary tree. Radiology 134:689–692, 1980
2. Weinstein DP, Weinstein BJ, Brodmerkel GJ: Ultrasonography of biliary tract dilatation without jaundice. AJR 132:729–734, 1979

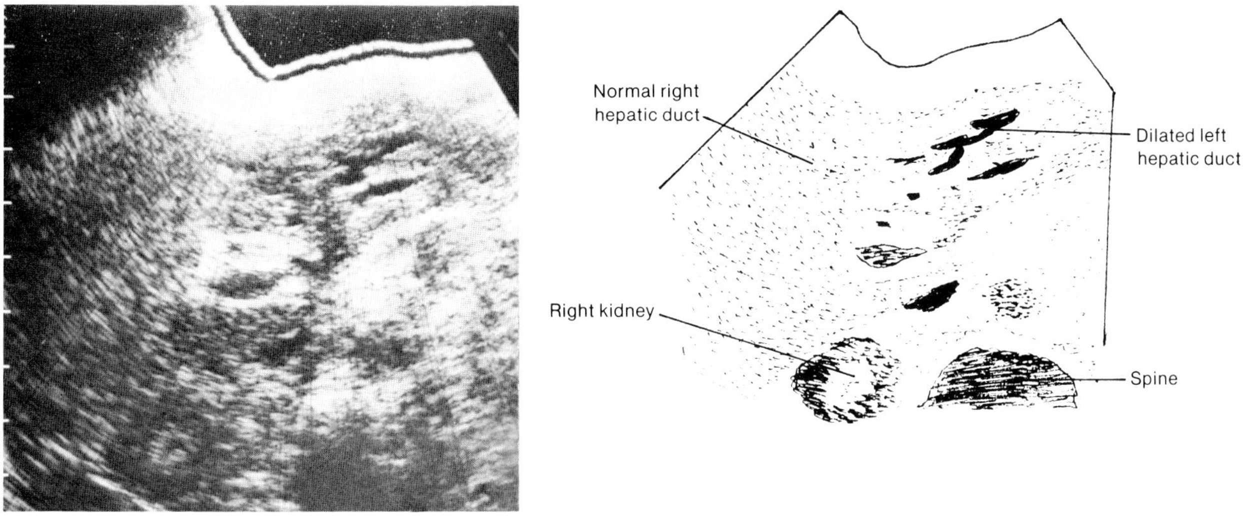
Normal right hepatic duct
Dilated left hepatic duct
Right kidney
Spine

A

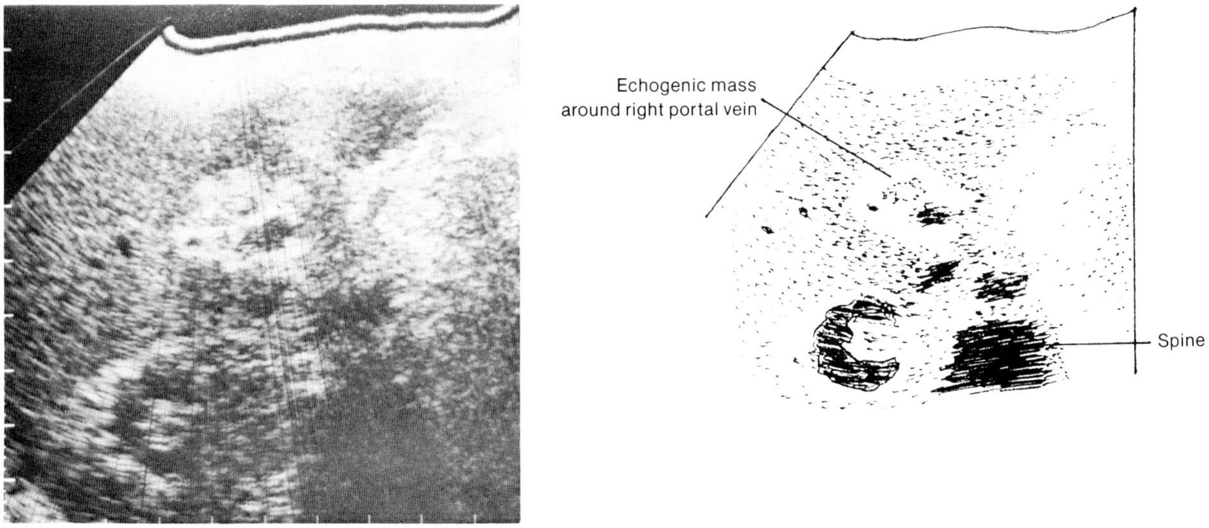
Echogenic mass around right portal vein
Spine

B

8.30 Pneumobilia

A 50-year-old man had undergone a choledochojejunostomy to bypass a tumor of the pancreatic head. After such procedures, air in the intrahepatic bile ducts is common. A transverse scan (Fig. A) shows very high level echoes throughout the left lobe of the liver, with some evidence of distal shadowing. A longitudinal scan (Fig. B) demonstrates highly echogenic biliary radicals, again with some evidence of shadowing.

Air in the biliary tree is usual after biliary enteric bypass procedures and it acts as a contrast agent, which delineates the biliary vessels that are not normally apparent. It is difficult to evaluate the liver parenchyma in the presence of extensive shadowing. Minimal quantities of air in the ducts produce enhanced echogenicity without shadowing.

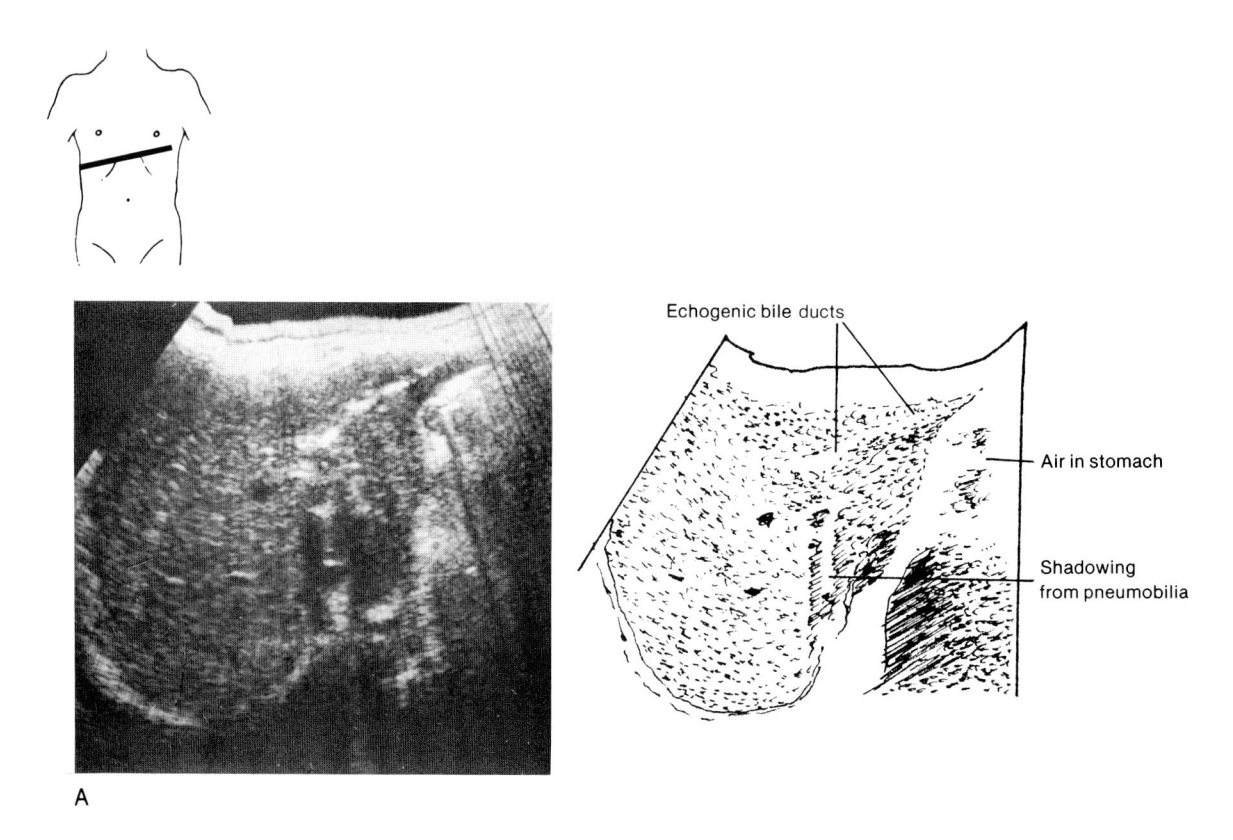

A

Air in bile ducts

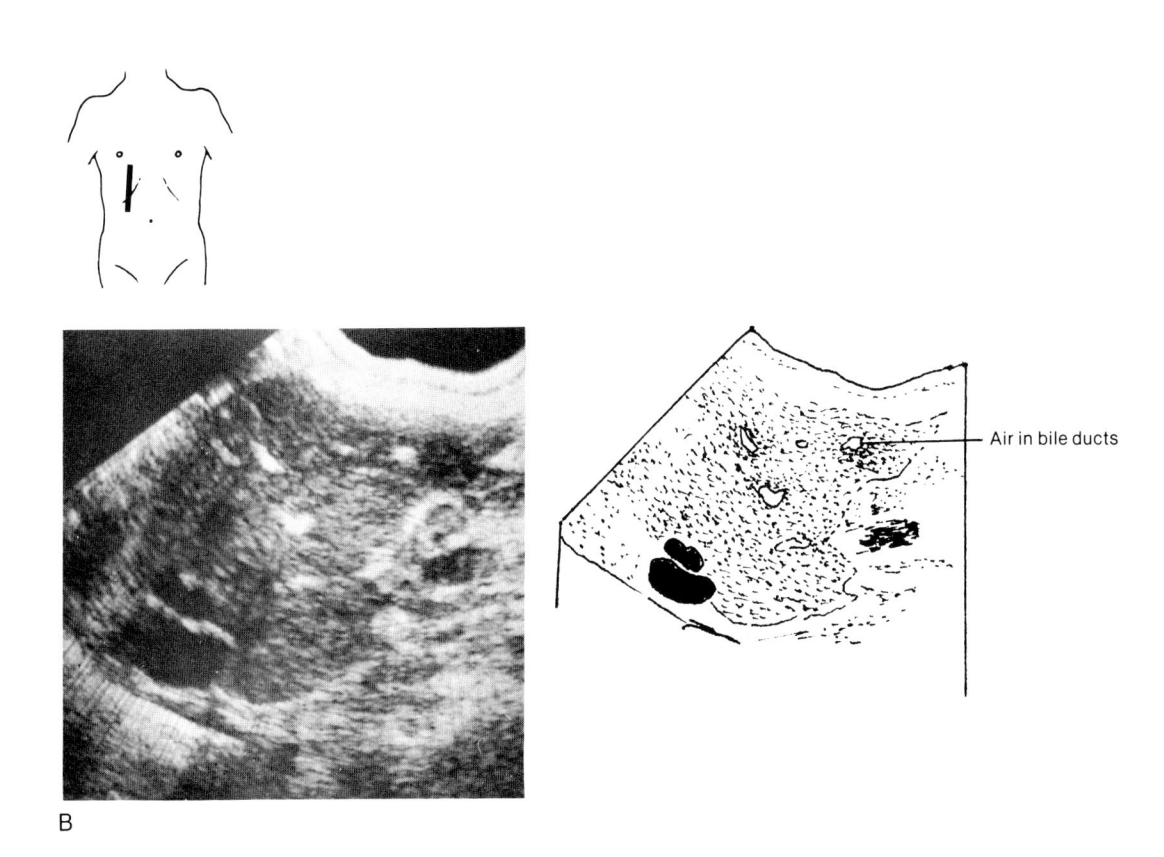

B

Congenital Biliary Dilatation (8.31 and 8.32)

8.31 Caroli's Disease

A 2-year-old boy was admitted with a history of diarrhea, steatorrhea, jaundice, hepatomegaly, and intermittent fever. His SGOT level was mildly elevated to 146 U/dl. The transverse sonogram (Fig. A) demonstrated saccular dilatation of the intrahepatic ducts (arrowed). In addition, the liver appeared abnormally echogenic, suggesting fibrosis or an inflammatory process. This was believed to be consistent with Caroli's syndrome. At this time, 99^mTc-HIDA was not available and the patient was referred for a transhepatic cholangiogram (Fig. B). This confirmed intrahepatic saccular dilatation of the biliary radicals (arrowed), a characteristic of Caroli's disease.

Caroli's disease is a segmental, saccular cystic dilatation of the intrahepatic biliary vessels. There is usually free communication between these ectatic ducts and the common bile duct, in contrast with the cysts seen in polycystic liver disease which do not communicate with the biliary tree.

Although most cases of Caroli's disease are not associated with cirrhosis or portal hypertension, some are associated with congenital hepatic fibrosis. The presenting symptoms and signs of pain, jaundice, and fever are due to cholelithiasis, bile stasis in the ectatic ducts, and cholangitis.[1]

(ERCP courtesy of Morton I. Burrell, M.D., Yale University School of Medicine; Figs. A and B from DiPietro MA, Taylor KJW: Imaging of idiopathic biliary duct dilatation. J Clin Gastroenterol 2:299–304, 1980.)

REFERENCE

1. Bass EM, Funston MR, Shaff MI: Caroli's disease: an ultrasonic diagnosis. Br J Radiol 50:366–369, 1977

617

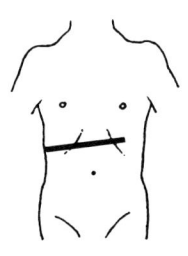

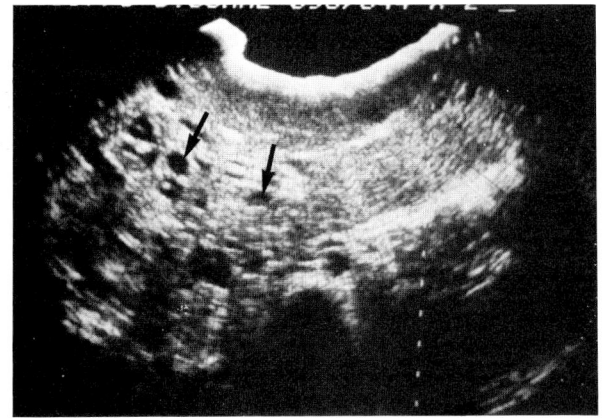

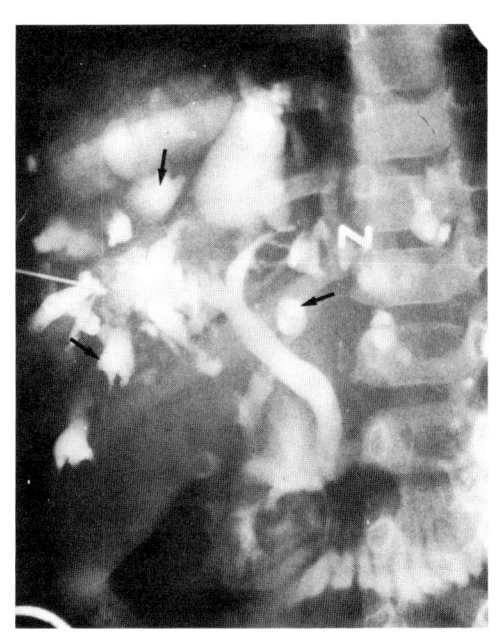

8.32 Choledochal Cyst

A 2-year-old girl presented with an 8-month history of pruritus. Her total serum bilirubin was 3.3 mg/dl (direct was 1.8 mg/dl) with a serum SGOT level of 111 U/dl. The liver was enlarged and tender. A longitudinal sonogram (Fig. A) in the region of the porta hepatis demonstrated a large cystic mass without evidence of intrahepatic duct dilatation. Multiple small vessels could be seen emptying into the cyst.

A subsequent ^{99m}Tc-HIDA examination showed an area of decreased activity in the right upper quadrant which subsequently filled with activity, confirming that the cyst communicated with the biliary tree. An intraoperative cholangiogram (Fig. B) demonstrated a markedly dilated common bile duct without drainage into the duodenum. Liver biopsy specimens disclosed acute and chronic pericholangitis and biliary stasis. The excised cyst showed fibrous tissue in the wall with no epithelium and little muscle, indicative of a choledochal cyst.

The liver in this patient appeared to be normal in texture. Eight percent of choledochal cysts are associated with Caroli's syndrome (8.31), which can be excluded by the normal liver texture seen on the sonogram.

Choledochal cysts have been classified according to the site of dilatation[1] (Fig. C). The most common sort is Type I which is dilatation of the common bile duct. The cystic duct and gallbladder are usually normal. Type II is a diverticulum from the common bile duct and Type III is an invagination of the distal duct into the duodenum.

The classic presentation of choledochal cysts includes the presence of a right upper quadrant mass with pain and intermittent jaundice. However, this presentation occurs in only 5–25 percent of patients.[1-3] In one series, 70 percent of patients presented with at least one of these symptoms, with jaundice present in 42 percent.[4]

(This case and Scan A and Fig. B taken from DiPietro MA, Taylor KJW. Imaging of idiopathic biliary duct dilatation. J Clin Gastroenterol 2:299–304, 1980.)

REFERENCES

1. Rosewarne MD: Cystic dilatation of the intrahepatic bile ducts. Br J Radiol 45:825–827, 1972
2. McNulty JG: Congenital and hereditary disorders of the liver. pp. 174–176. In Potchea EJ, ed: Radiology of the Liver. W.B. Saunders, Philadelphia, 1977.
3. Mowat AP: Liver Disorders in Childhood. Butterworths, Boston, 1979
4. Klotz D, Cohn BD, Kottmeier PK: Choledochal cysts: diagnostic and therapeutic problems. J Pediatr Surg 8:271–283, 1973

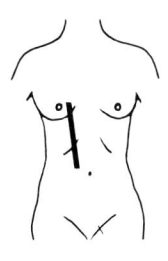

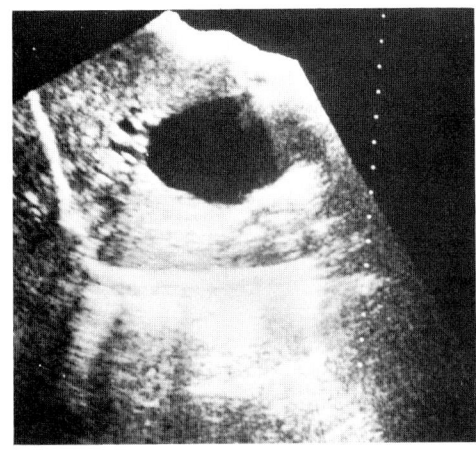

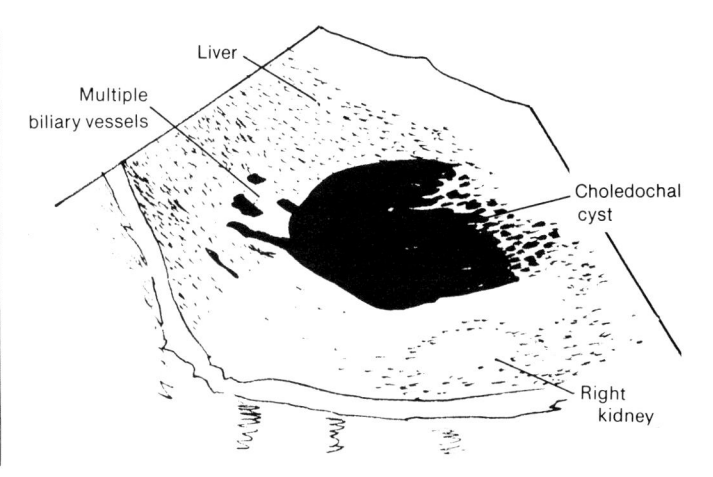

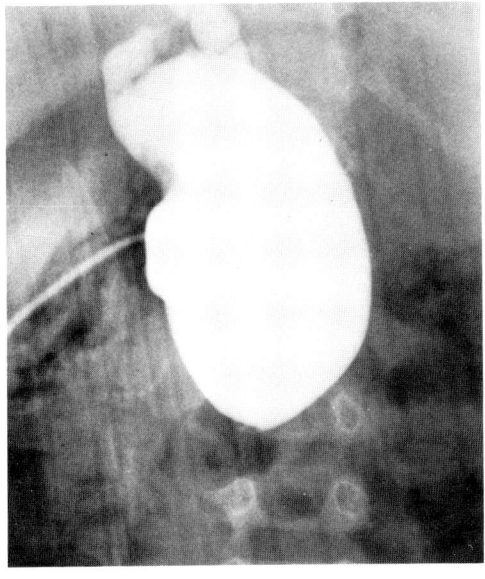

A

B

Type I   Type II   Type III

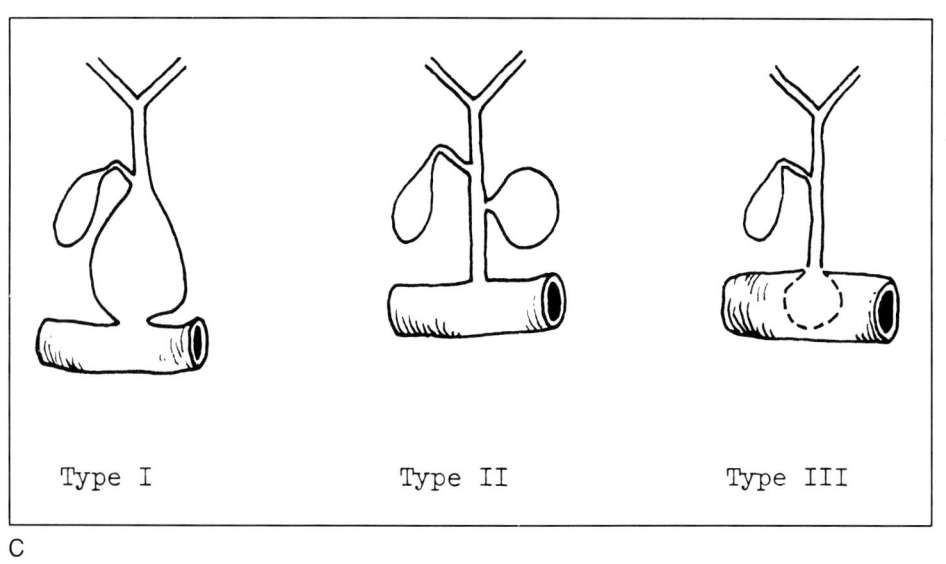

C

8.33 Congenital Biliary Atresia

A term infant was noted to be jaundiced at birth, and investigation revealed alpha-trypsin deficiency. Her jaundice persisted and at 1 month there was a total serum bilirubin level of 16 mg/dl and a direct bilirubin level of 10 mg/dl. She was referred for ultrasound scanning to determine the cause of her cholestasis.

A parasagittal sonogram demonstrated no evidence of dilatation of the intrahepatic ducts. The portal vein was identified and a tubular structure was seen anterior to it (Fig. A). Careful examination of this structure during real time sequence demonstrated pulsation, indicating that it was the hepatic artery. Further detailed scanning, despite vigorous patient movement, failed to identify the common hepatic duct. Several examinations were performed to search for the gallbladder, with the infant in the fasting state. At no time was a gallbladder identified.

The patient was referred for a ^{99m}technetium HIDA scan. This demonstrated good concentration in the hepatic parenchyma, but no evidence of extrahepatic excretion. Excretion into the bladder was noted (Fig. B).

Specimens from a closed liver biopsy demonstrated changes associated with cholangitis with fibrosis of the biliary radicals. The findings were consistent with those of biliary atresia.

At surgery, a distended gallbladder was found, suggesting that the infant had not fasted before our study, as requested. However, biliary atresia was confirmed.

Infants with biliary atresia are frequently not jaundiced at birth because of maternal clearance of bilirubin. However, they become jaundiced on the 2nd or 3rd day of life. Persistent obstruction progresses to biliary cirrhosis, beginning by 1 month of age and becoming irreversible at 3–4 months. Portal hypertension, ascites, and hemorrhage from esophageal varices are frequent complications. Death by the age of 2 years used to be the rule; new surgical treatment is improving the prognosis in a small percentage of these patients.

Biliary atresia is unknown in embryos, stillborns, or premature infants. Modern theory suggests that biliary atresia is due to an inflammatory process, possibly due to a viral infection, in which there is obliterative change in both the intra- and extrahepatic ducts, presumably in the prenatal period. A wide spectrum of different pathology results, and histologic appearances may be indistinguishable from what was called neonatal hepatitis.

The incidence of biliary atresia is 1:16,000 live births, with equal male and female prevalence. In view of the early onset of irreversible changes, it is important that clinical evaluation commence early, with a view to early treatment. The combination of ultrasound and the newer hepatobiliary agents allow the presumptive diagnosis to be made. Special care should be taken to avoid the pitfall of mistaking the hepatic artery for the common duct. The absence of a gallbladder is a useful additional indicator of possible biliary atresia, although the gallbladder may be present in this condition.

SUGGESTED READING

Bergsma D: Birth Defects Compendium, second edition. Alan R. Liss, New York, 1979.

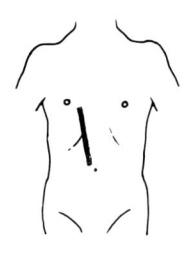

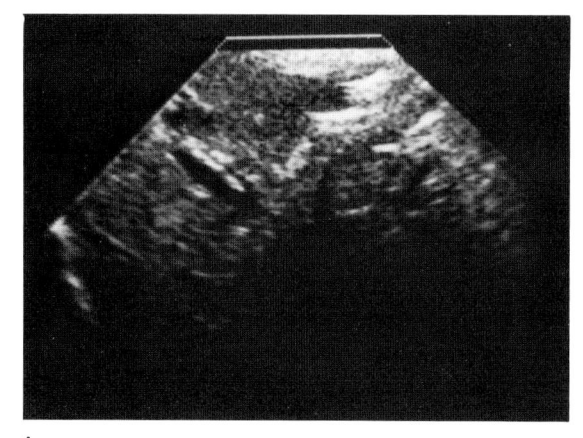

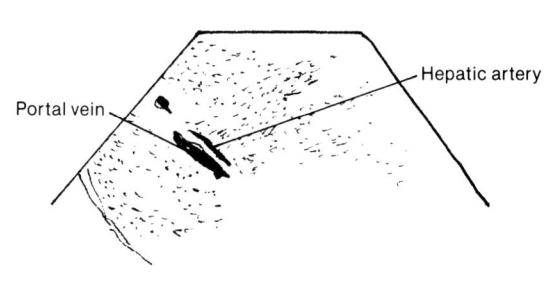

A

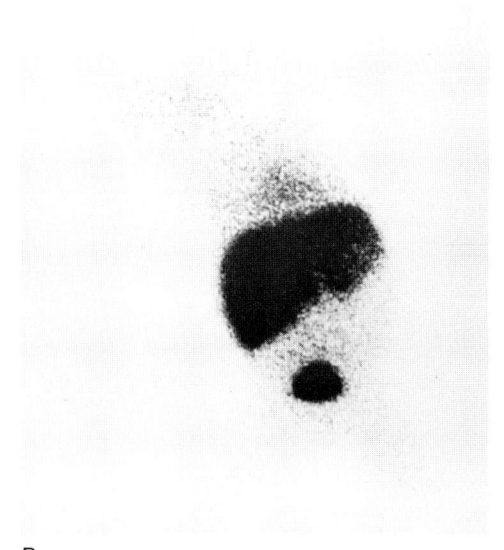

Portal vein
Hepatic artery

B

622

9 The Pancreas

KENNETH J.W. TAYLOR and BRUCE D. SIMONDS

The pancreas is a retroperitoneal organ shaped like a tadpole, with a bulbous head, thin neck, elongated body and tail. The head is situated deeply in the right paravertebral gutter and is a peninsula surrounded on three sides by the C loop of the duodenum. From this deep position of the head of the pancreas, the gland is draped over the vertebral column so that part of the body of the pancreas in the midline may, in thin patients, be extremely superficial. As the pancreas extends towards the left, it again passes deeply posteriorly into the left paravertebral gutter, crossing the retroperitoneum across the upper pole of the left kidney to reach the hilum or upper pole of the left kidney.

Earlier scintigraphic techniques demonstrated that the pancreas has a very variable shape and orientation. Classically, the head of the pancreas lies to the right of the body of the second lumbar vertebra and the body and tail pass upwards and to the left to the hilum of the spleen. The pancreas may, however, lie virtually transversely or may be U-shaped. Real-time ultrasound demonstrates that the pancreas is quite mobile, moving both up and down and anteroposteriorly with physiological movements. Enlargement of the liver may rotate the pancreas so that it is virtually vertical. Due to all these variations in the position of the pancreas, it is essential to use reliable and stable vascular landmarks to identify the organ.

9.1 Examination Technique

ANATOMY AND SCANNING

Patients are scanned as early as possible in the morning after an overnight fast, thus minimizing the problems of intestinal gas and stomach contents while simultaneously allowing effective examination of the gallbladder and biliary tract. Water distention of the stomach is particularly helpful, especially when there is suspicion of a pancreatic mass which could be due to stomach contents or duodenum. The pancreas is usually examined in deep suspended inspiration so that the descent of the liver helps provide an acoustic window.

It is important to use mainly a linear or sector rather than compound scanner, both to avoid artifacts and to prevent loss of resolution due to biologic movement. Compound scans can produce pseudotumors, particularly in the head of the pancreas (arrowed, Fig. A). A linear or sector scan of the pancreas eliminates such artifacts.

The vascular anatomy, important in the identification of the pancreas on a transverse scan, is shown in Figure B. The splenic vein constitutes the essential landmark as it crosses the midline structures anterior to the superior mesenteric artery (SMA) and joins the superior mesenteric vein (SMV) to form the portal vein. This confluence occurs posterior to the neck of the pancreas; the head of the pancreas lies toward the right. A small mass of tissue passes deep to the portal vein as a prolongation from the head of the pancreas. This is the uncinate process, which is best seen in a longitudinal plane. It is important to ensure that the splenic vein has been identified rather than the left renal vein, which is posterior to the SMA but concentric with the splenic vein.

The examination continues with a longitudinal parasagittal section (Fig. C) commencing in the plane of the inferior vena cava (IVC) which locates the head of the pancreas. The head of the pancreas lies on the anterior surface of the IVC, just caudal to the crossing of the IVC by the portal vein. In this position the lower end of the common bile duct passes deep to the head of the pancreas while the gastroduodenal artery lies on its superficial surface (Fig. D). Thus, the best vascular demarcation of the head of the pancreas is the interval between the gastroduodenal artery and the common bile duct.

The scanning arm or real-time transducer is then moved toward the left and the SMV is identified running in the root of the mesentery (arrowed, Fig. E). This vein has a longitudinal course and ends in a bulbous termination due to its fusion with the splenic vein to form the portal vein behind the neck of the pancreas. At this point, the tissue lying superficial to the termination of the SMV is the neck of the pancreas, while the tissue lying deep to the SMV is the uncinate process of the pancreas. It should be recalled that the vascular interval between the IVC and the SMV also contains the third part of the duodenum, the left renal vein, and numerous lymph nodes. Masses derived from these structures are therefore included in the differential diagnosis of tumors of the uncinate process.

A longitudinal section in the plane of the aorta demonstrates the body of the pancreas (Fig. F).

The tail of the pancreas is the most difficult area of the organ to display because of the frequent occurrence of gas in the stomach which obscures this region. A number of techniques can be used to permit visualization of this area in the large majority of patients.

Transverse scans often demonstrate the tail of the pancreas extremely well, particularly after the use of water to distend the stomach (arrowed, Fig. G). A further valuable technique is an oblique longitudinal scan (see Fig. 9.2B). For this technique, a longitudinal scan is performed with the transducer tilted to the left. The degree of this tilt can be determined on transverse scan by noting the approximate angle the tip of the tail makes with the body of the pancreas. Again, this scan is optimally performed after fluid distention of the stomach. As the transducer is rotated toward the left, the aorta and SMA are visualized and further rotation reveals the tail of the pancreas, with the left kidney posterior and the stomach anterior.[1] A popular technique described in the literature involves placing the patient prone. In this position, the tail of the pancreas lies anterior to the hilum of the left kidney and is well-visualized (arrowed, Fig. H), particularly after water distention of the stomach.[2] It has been our experience, however, that the prone position is the least successful of the methods described. The relationship of the tail of the pancreas to the kidney is extremely variable and numerous other masses may confuse the operator: stomach contents, an extension of the spleen, colon, or accessory spleen. Thus, we believe that it is better to use a technique in which the continuity of the tail of the pancreas with the rest of the organ can be demonstrated to permit positive identification.

WATER DISTENTION OF THE STOMACH

Water distention of the stomach is invaluable, both for demonstrating the anatomy of the pancreas and for clarifying any abnormal appearances.[3] Despite this, it is not universally used. The technique does take time and patience to perform, but the results are worth the effort.

The pancreas is frequently obscured by gas and, as seen from the schema in Figure B, this gas lies not in the small bowel but usually in the stomach. It can therefore be replaced by the judicious administration of water. In practice, the patient drinks approximately 12 ounces of water. We usually turn the patient into a left-side-down decubitus position. The water is then drunk through a straw, thereby diminishing the number of air bubbles imbibed. If the patient is scanned immediately, numerous bubbles are seen within the stomach; time must be allowed for their dissolution. The scanning plane can be adjusted to utilize gas-free intervals. By manipulating the transducer, these acoustic windows can be used to optimal effect. As is usual in ultrasound scanning, an intelligent, appropriate scanning technique must be adopted and used in a flexible way. The rigid technique which has been advocated in the literature (scanning at fixed 1-cm intervals) must be abandoned.

The use of the water technique allows dramatic improvement in the visualization of the pancreas, often from being completely obscured to being optimally demonstrated (Figs. I and J). Tilting the patient toward the right encourages the flow of water through the duodenum and outlines the head of the pancreas (Fig. K). Masses due to the duodenum or stomach contents are also clarified after distention with water.

The final technique that can be used to visualize the pancreas is the erect position.[4] The patient is asked to stand and transverse and longitudinal scans are performed. The advantage of this position is that air in the stomach tends to rise above the level of the pancreas into the fundus of the stomach while the liver falls inferiorly, producing an acoustic window to the pancreas. Air-containing gut tends to fall away from the pancreatic bed and there may be a dramatic improvement in visualization of the pancreas. In our laboratory this technique is designated LCE (last chance erect). In practice, the use of all these techniques allows adequate visualization of the pancreas in more than 90 percent of patients.[5] Modern instrumentation allows visualization of the pancreatic duct in more than 80 percent of the normal population.[6] The duct is often slightly dilated, so that a lumen of 2 mm is normal (Fig. L). Pathologic dilation may occur in both inflammatory and neoplastic conditions. However, ultrasound is generally inadequate to demonstrate fine ductal anatomy and does not compete with the value of ERCP (endoscopic retrograde cholangiopancreatography).

ROLE OF OTHER IMAGING MODALITIES

CT is probably the technique most frequently used to visualize the pancreas. It is technically easier than ultrasound, but is also more time-consuming and certainly less economical. In the majority of patients, ultrasound in experienced hands is capable of producing images at least as good as those produced by CT. Patients with pancreatic cancer usually have marked weight loss and tend to be thin, and the ultrasound images may be significantly superior to those produced by CT. We strongly believe, therefore, that there is a role for ultrasound imaging, particularly to exclude a carcinoma of the pancreas. In a prospective study of patients referred with the clinical suspicion of pancreatic cancer, we were able to exclude the diagnosis with a specificity of 98 percent.[6] In addition, until the fourth-generation CT scanners, it was not possible to delineate a small tumor of the pancreas which produced no abnormality of size or contour. Thus, small tumors of the pancreas visualized by ultrasound may not show on a CT scan. Conversely, a bulbous pancreatic tail, which is a normal variant, may be misinterpreted as a tumor on an older CT scanner, yet the normal texture seen on an ultrasound scan excludes the presence of a tumor.

REFERENCES

1. Taylor KJW, Jacobson P, Talmont CA, et al: Manual of Ultrasonography. Churchill Livingstone, New York, 1980.
2. Goldstein HM, Katragadda CS: Prone view ultrasonography for pancreatic tail neoplasms. Am J Roentgenol 131:231, 1978
3. Crade M, Taylor KJW, Rosenfield AT: Water distention of the gut in the evaluation of the pancreas by ultrasound. Am J Roentgenol 131:348–349, 1978
4. Crade M, Jacobson P, Taylor KJW: The upright position while giving water for evaluation of pancreas. J Clin Ultrasound 6:353–354, 1978
5. Taylor KJW, Buchin PJ, Viscomi G, Rosenfield AT: Ultrasonographic scanning of the pancreas. Radiology 138:211–213, 1981
6. Parulekar SG: Ultrasonic evaluation of pancreatic duct. J Clin Ultrasound 8:457–463, 1980

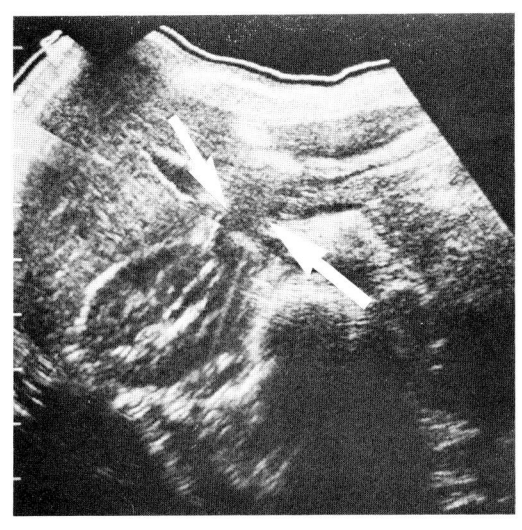

A

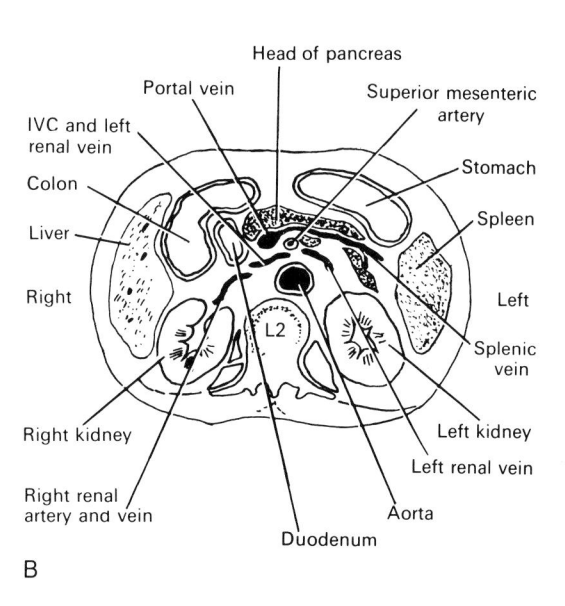

Head of pancreas
Portal vein
Superior mesenteric artery
IVC and left renal vein
Stomach
Colon
Spleen
Liver
Right
Left
Splenic vein
Right kidney
Left kidney
Left renal vein
Right renal artery and vein
Aorta
Duodenum

B

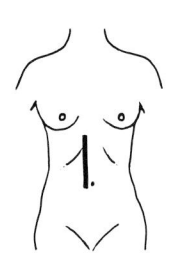

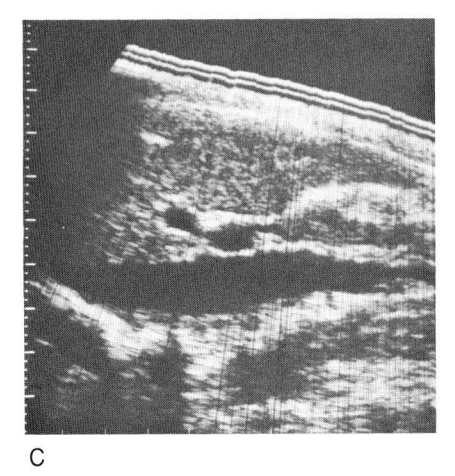

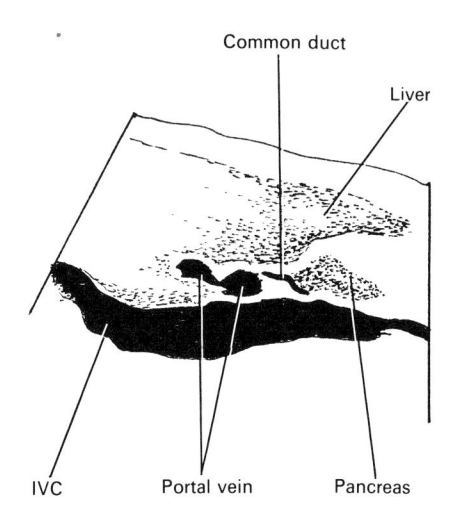

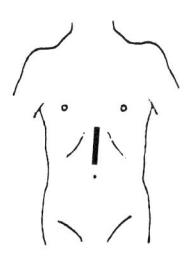

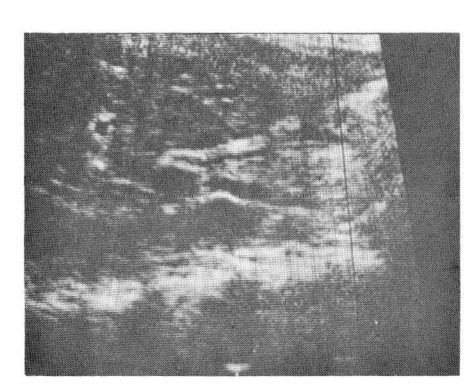

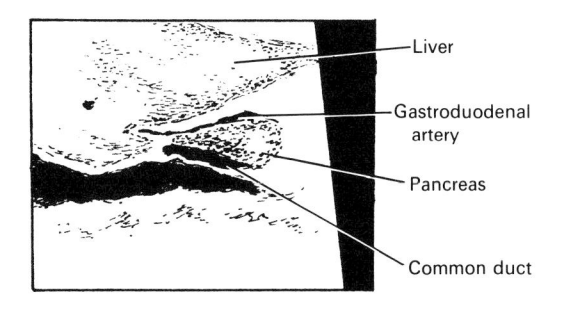

C

D

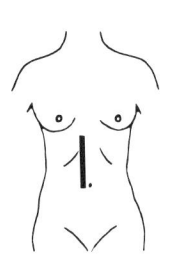

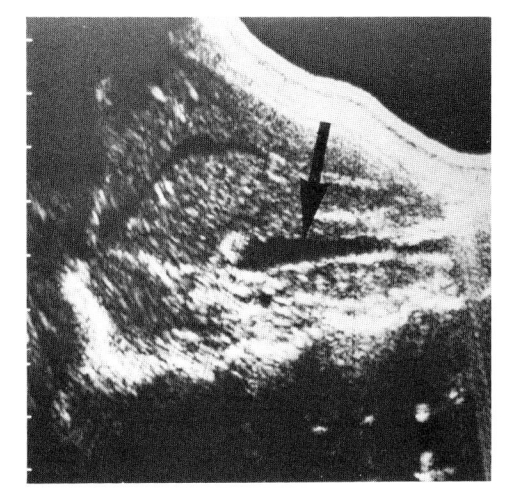

E

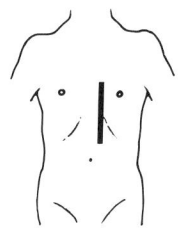

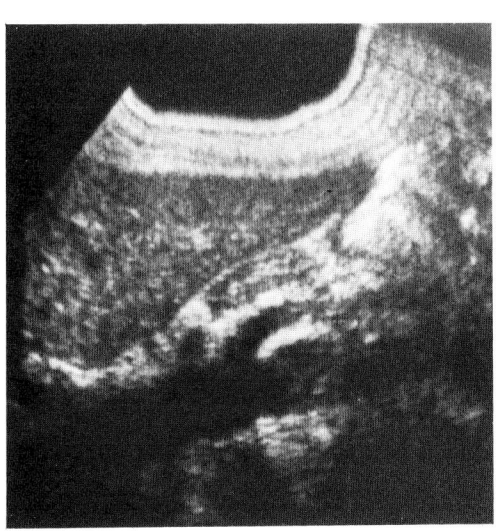

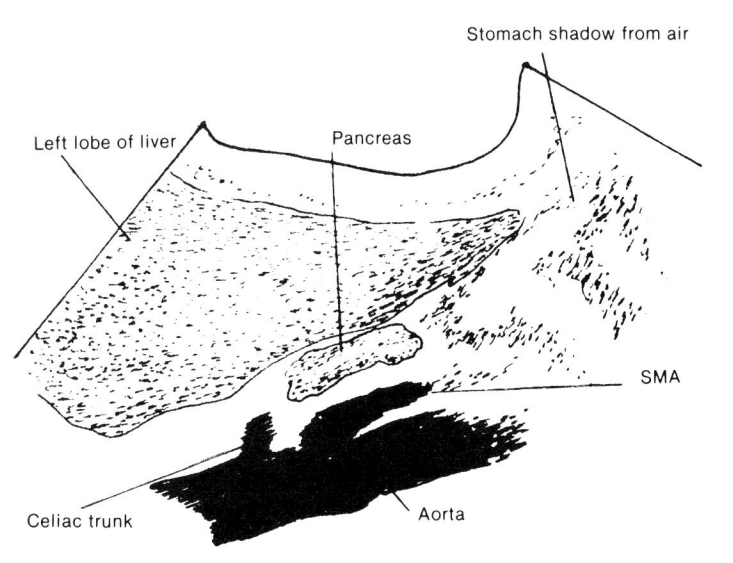

F

Stomach shadow from air
Left lobe of liver
Pancreas
SMA
Celiac trunk
Aorta

629

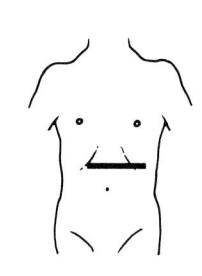

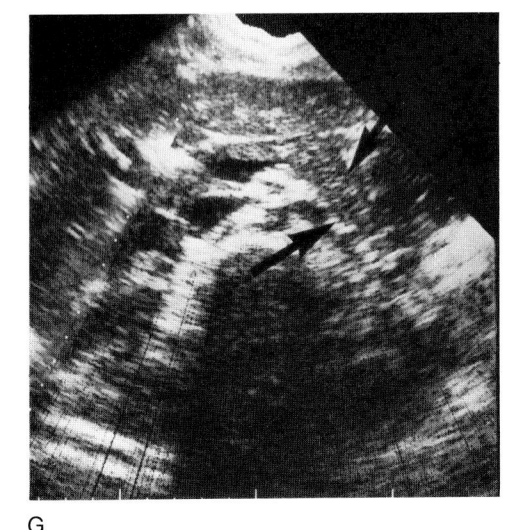

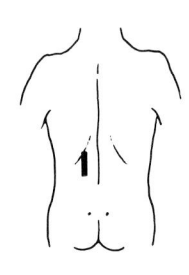

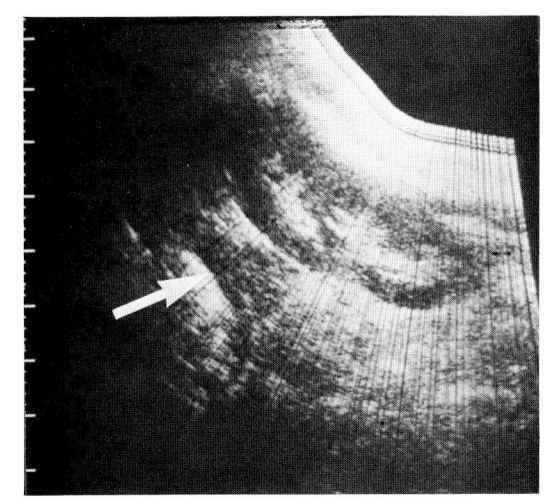

G

H

I

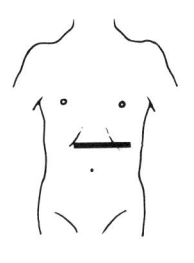

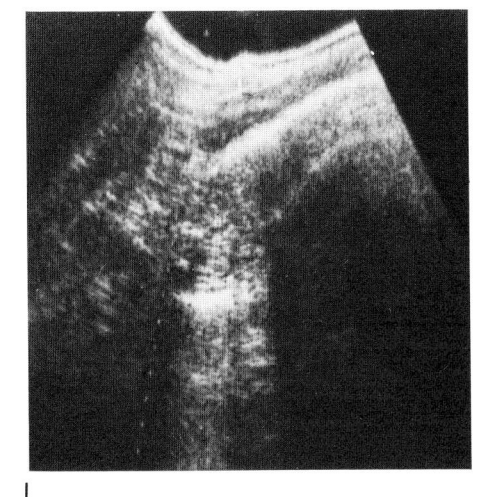

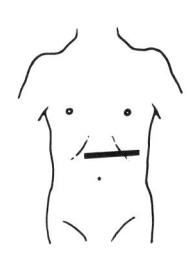

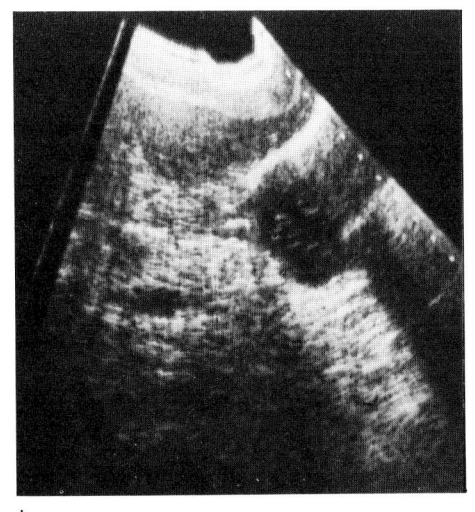

J

631

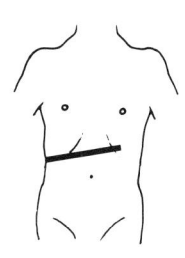

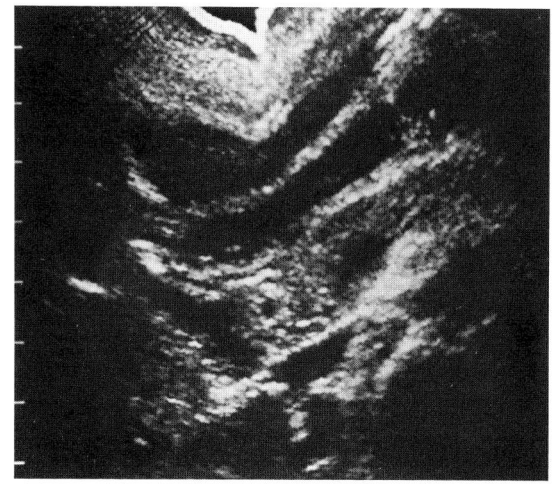

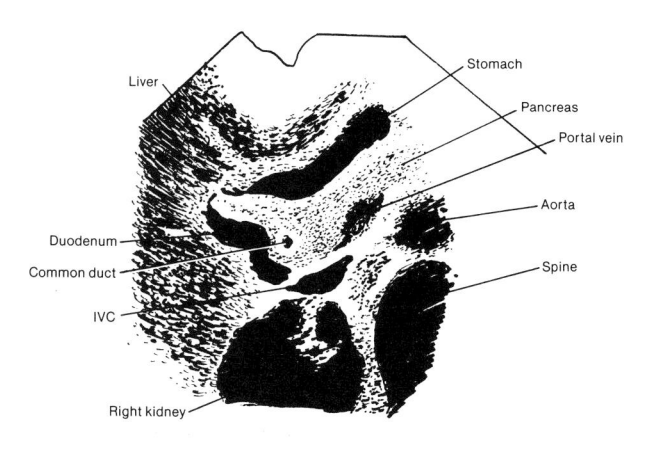

K

Liver	Stomach
	Pancreas
	Portal vein
Duodenum	Aorta
Common duct	Spine
IVC	
Right kidney	

L

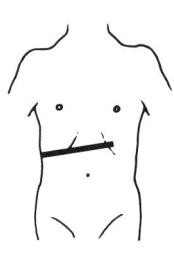

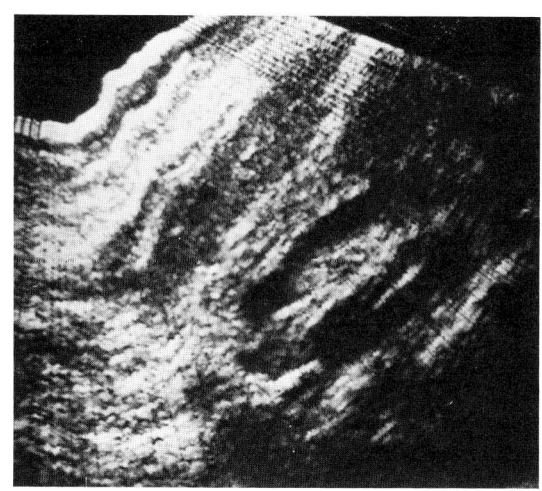

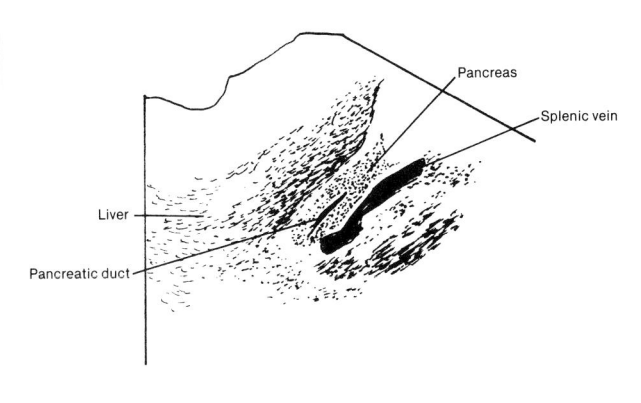

	Pancreas
	Splenic vein
Liver	
Pancreatic duct	

Normal Variants (9.2 to 9.4)

9.2 Bulbous Tail Simulating Tumor

The shape and contour of the pancreas are extremely variable. An important variant is a bulbous tail which may simulate a tumor, particularly when demonstrated on one of the older CT scanners.

A 60-year-old patient was referred for scanning to exclude a pancreatic cancer. The transverse sonogram (Fig. A) and the oblique parasagittal scan (Fig. B) demonstrated a markedly bulbous tail, although the texture was completely normal. A second-generation CT scan may merely demonstrate an enlarged pancreatic tail indistinguishable from tumor. Initially, we subjected these patients to ERCP and even angiography to exclude the presence of a tumor but invariably this proved to be a normal variant.[1] We therefore developed considerable confidence in excluding a pancreatic tumor based on the echogenicity of the mass. In our experience to date, all exocrine pancreatic tumors have been less echogenic than normal pancreatic texture.

This is an important variant of which sonographers should be aware. We know anecdotally of patients who, based on results of CT scan, have undergone a partial pancreatectomy for a presumed tumor of the pancreas. In a number of other patients, this variation has led to unnecessary pancreatic biopsy. The fourth generation CT scanners demonstrate the normal glandular components in optimal patients and thereby allow a more reliable exclusion of a pancreatic tumor. However, since many hospitals still have second-generation CT scanners, it is important that this normal variant be appreciated.

REFERENCE

1. Gorelick FS, Spiro HM: The gastrointestinal view of the indications and efficacy of ultrasound examination. p. 1. In Taylor KJW (ed): Gastrointestinal Disease, Clinics in Diagnostic Ultrasound, volume 1. Churchill Livingstone, New York, 1979

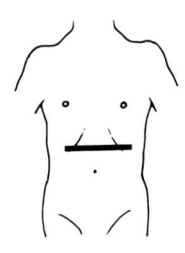

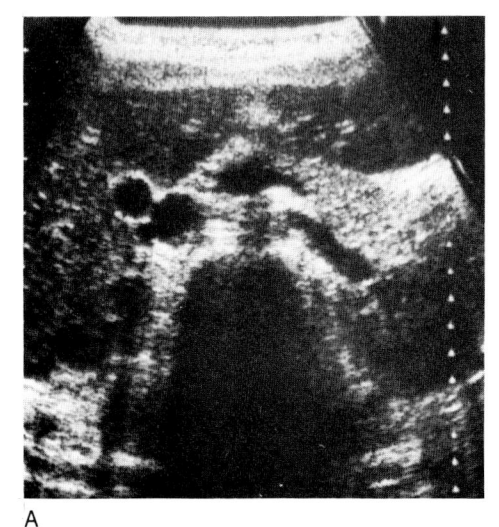

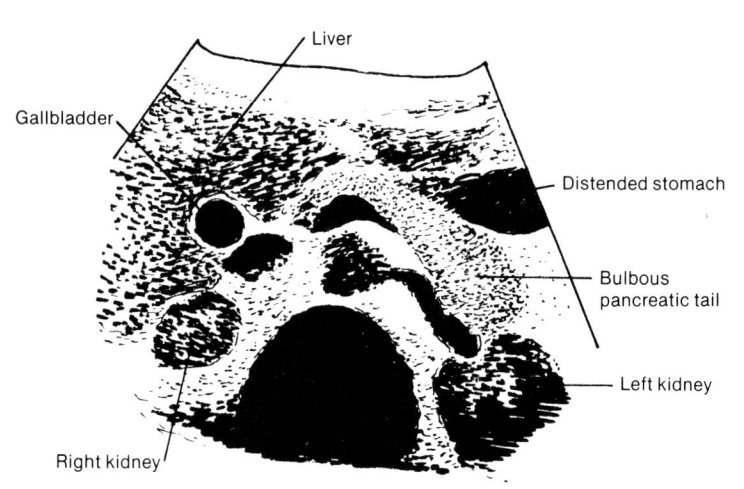

A

	Liver
Gallbladder	
	Distended stomach
	Bulbous pancreatic tail
Right kidney	Left kidney

B

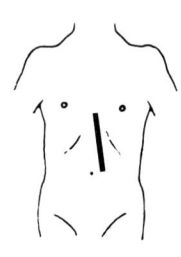

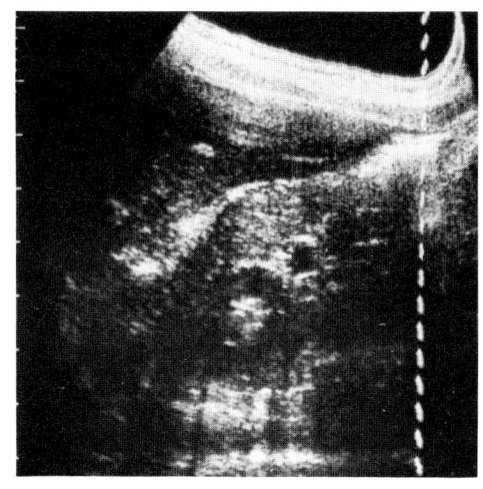

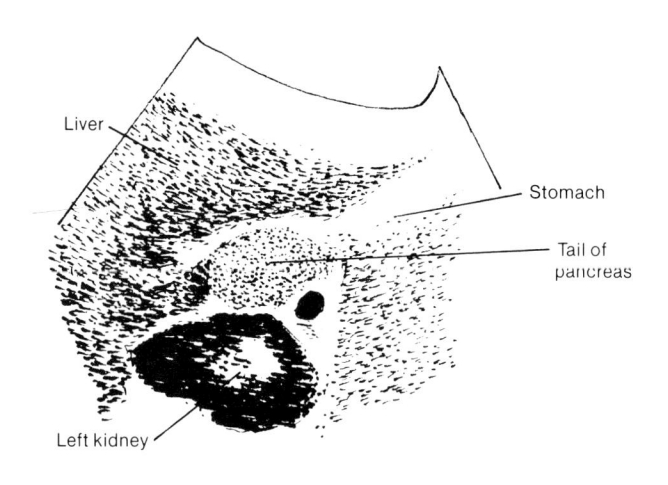

	Liver
	Stomach
	Tail of pancreas
Left kidney	

9.3 Displacement by Hepatomegaly

A 46-year-old woman presented with known primary biliary cirrhosis. Ultrasound demonstrated marked hepatomegaly. The transverse sonogram demonstrated displacement of the pancreas toward the left, as seen in the figure. Note that the portal vein is formed anterior to the aorta rather than the inferior vena cava.

There is considerable variation in the position of the pancreas and the only reliable means for its identification are the vascular landmarks. Enlargement of the liver displaces the pancreas to the left and rotates it so that it may lie almost in an anterior–posterior axis.

Anatomic dissection and CT scans tend to leave the student with the impression that the pancreas is a static, rigidly fixed retroperitoneal organ. Real-time ultrasound scanning demonstrates vividly the ease with which the pancreas moves with biologic movement. The pancreas moves (an average of 4 mm) anteroposteriorly with each aortic pulsation. It also moves craniocaudally with respiration. Hepatomegaly produces a permanent displacement of the pancreas and again indicates the need for flexible scanning technique to display the anatomy based on the recognition of the vascular landmarks, in whatever position they may lie.

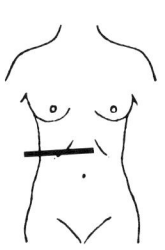

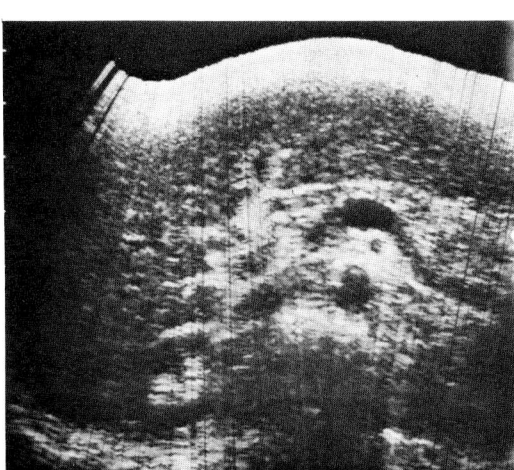

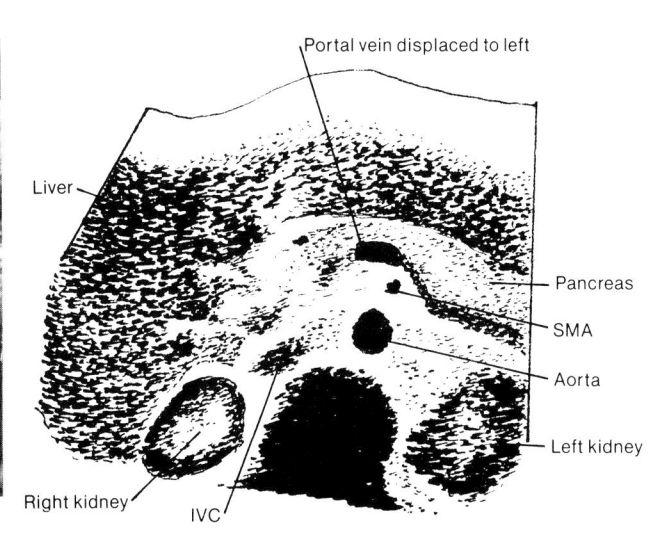

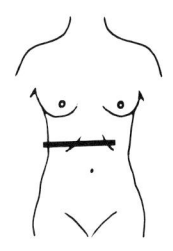

9.4 Superficial Location

The pancreas is usually considered to be a deeply retroperitoneal organ. However, as is apparent on the transverse scan, the body of the pancreas normally may be comparatively superficial since it is draped over the vertebral bodies and great vessels. In thin patients, the pancreas may be extremely superficial.

A 68-year-old woman was referred for ultrasound examination of the pancreas because of back pain and weight loss—symptoms suggestive of a pancreatic cancer. A transverse ultrasound scan showed that the pancreas was entirely normal, but was very superficially located so that the body of the pancreas was within a centimeter of the anterior abdominal wall (Fig. A).

This normal variant should be compared with a pathologic displacement of the pancreas superficially by a retropancreatic mass almost invariably due to malignant involvement. Figure B shows a mass around the aorta and the pancreas dislocated anteriorly. A fine-needle biopsy specimen of the mass yielded adenocarcinoma cells and a primary tumor was located in the stomach. Peripancreatic nodes occur commonly in lymphoma or as metastases from gut or lung primaries.[1] These nodes may present as a pulsating, epigastric mass simulating an aortic aneurysm. These patients usually undergo ultrasound as an initial diagnostic procedure. Recognition of the nature of the mass and expeditious percutaneous biopsy permit a histologic diagnosis within 24 hours of presentation.

REFERENCE

1. Schnur MJ, Hoffman JC, Koenigsberg M: Gray-scale ultrasonic demonstration of peripancreatic adenopathy. J Ultrasound Med 1:139–143, 1982

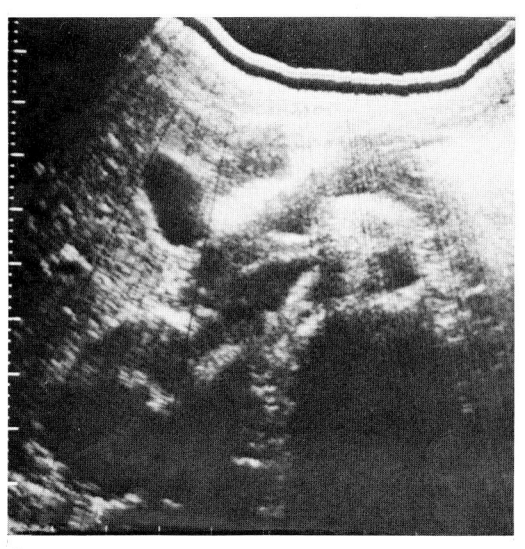

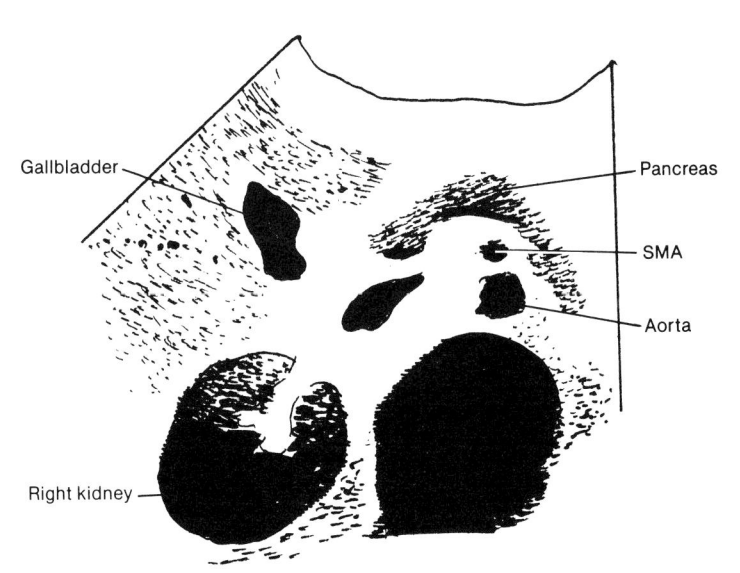

A

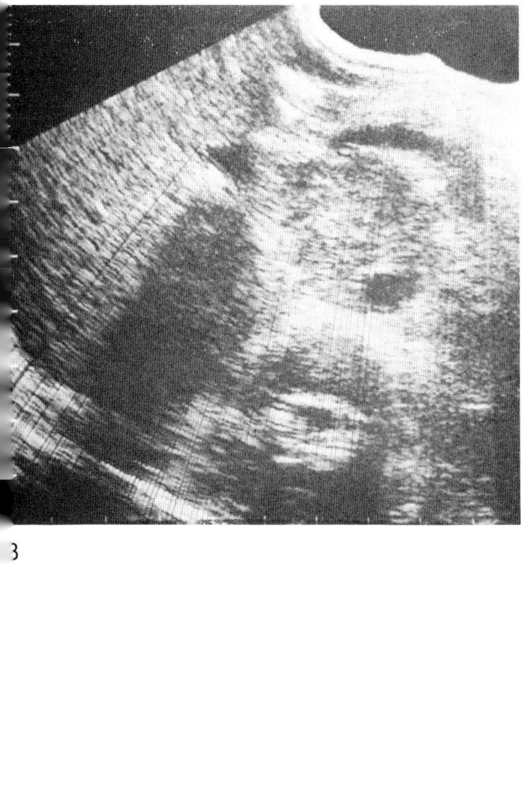

3

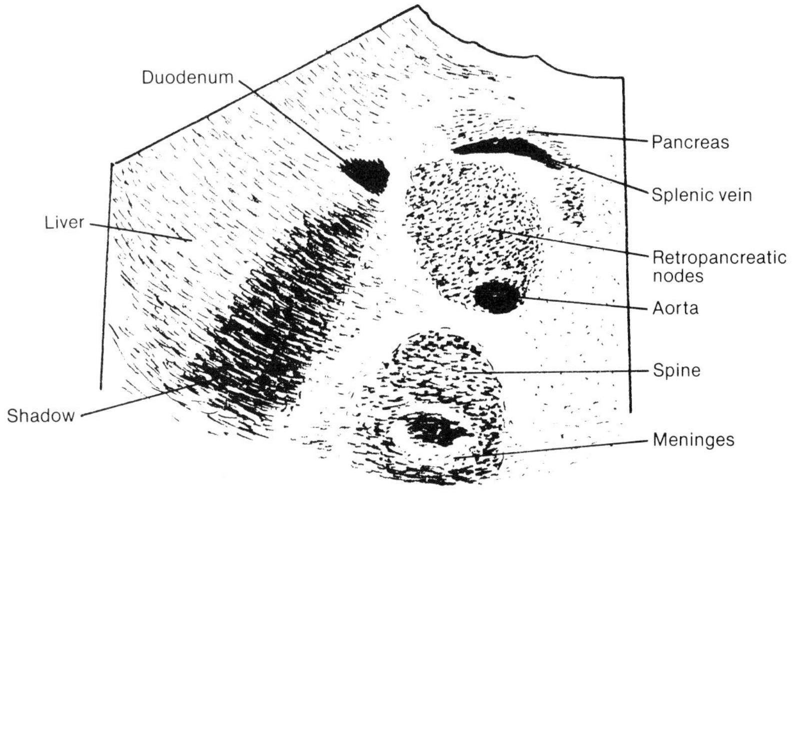
Duodenum
Pancreas
Splenic vein
Liver
Retropancreatic nodes
Aorta
Spine
Shadow
Meninges

9.5 Fatty Infiltration of the Pancreas

A 54-year-old business executive had an incidental finding of a fatty pancreas on CT (Fig. A) and ultrasound (Fig. B).

Frequently in elderly patients a large echogenic pancreas is seen, and yet at postmortem examination little or no glandular tissue is present. In such patients the pancreas is partially replaced by fat. By ultrasound alone, both the glandular tissue and the fat appear echogenic so that the amount of residual glandular tissue cannot be estimated. CT allows the glandular tissue to be adequately differentiated from the infiltrating fat.

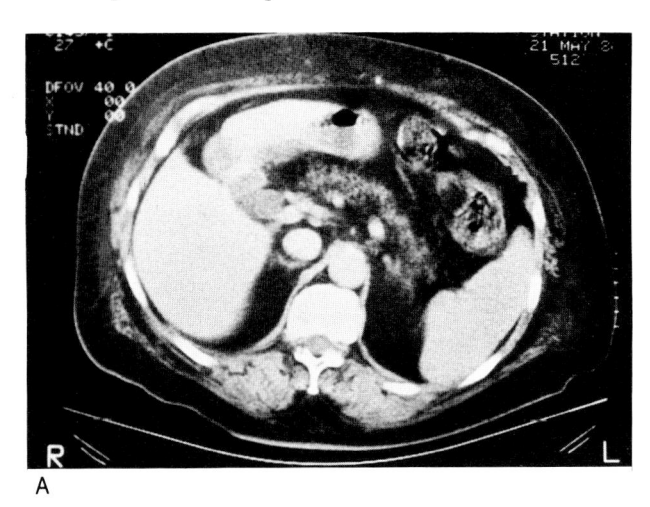

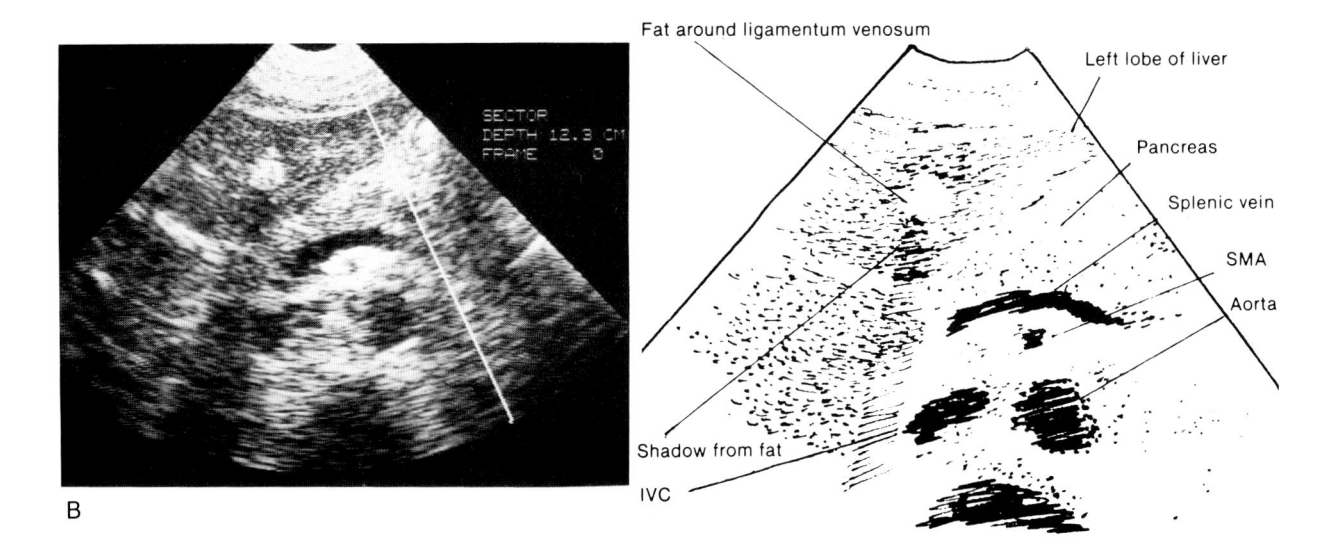

9.6 Cystic Fibrosis

A 13-year-old patient presented with known cystic fibrosis and a long history of chronic respiratory infections due to the pulmonary manifestations of her disease. There was some evidence of pancreatic dysfunction and she was maintained on Pancrease.

A longitudinal sonogram (Fig. A) showed a highly echogenic mass which was the neck of the pancreas lying superficial to the SMV and limited above by the celiac axis. The transverse scan (Fig. B) again demonstrated a highly echogenic pancreas, suggesting abnormality.

Phillips et al. noted increased echogenicity of the pancreas in 20 patients with cystic fibrosis.[1] Shawker et al. used quantitative echo amplitude analysis to compare the echo amplitude from pancreatic tissue in patients with cystic fibrosis with that of the normal population.[2] Their studies confirmed that the pancreas was significantly more echogenic in patients with cystic fibrosis.

REFERENCES

1. Phillips HE, Cox KL, Reid MH, et al: Pancreatic sonography in cystic fibrosis. AJR 137:69–72, 1981
2. Shawker TA, Parks SI, Linzer M, et al: Amplitude analysis of pancreatic B-scans: a clinical evaluation of cystic fibrosis. Ultrasonic Imaging 2:55–66, 1980

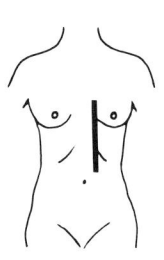

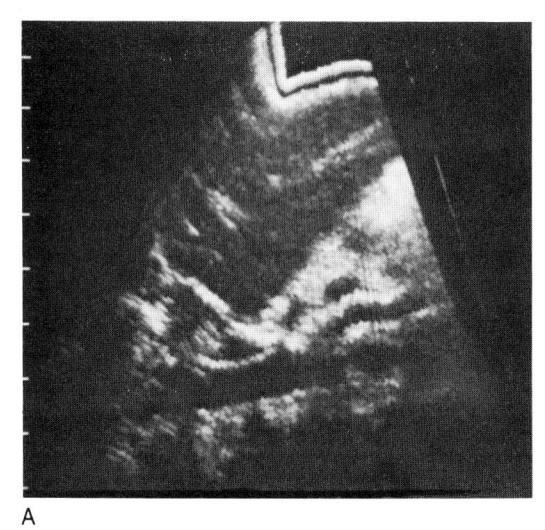

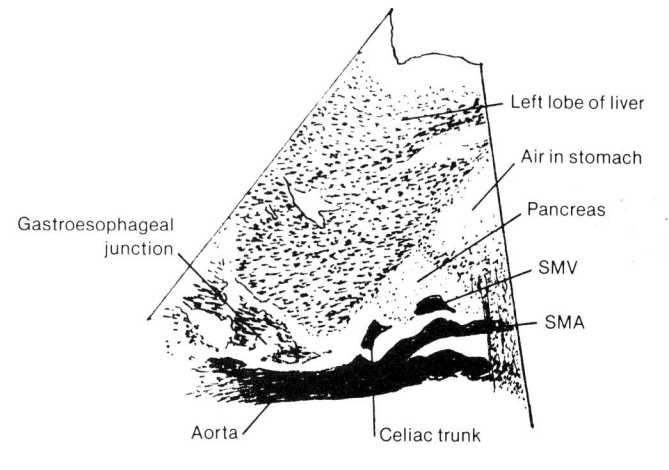

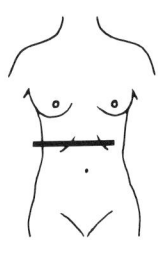

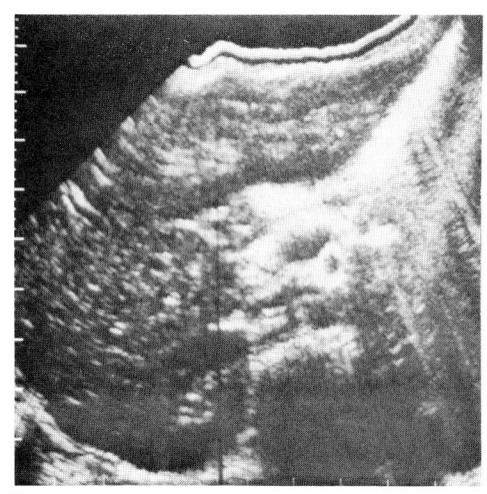

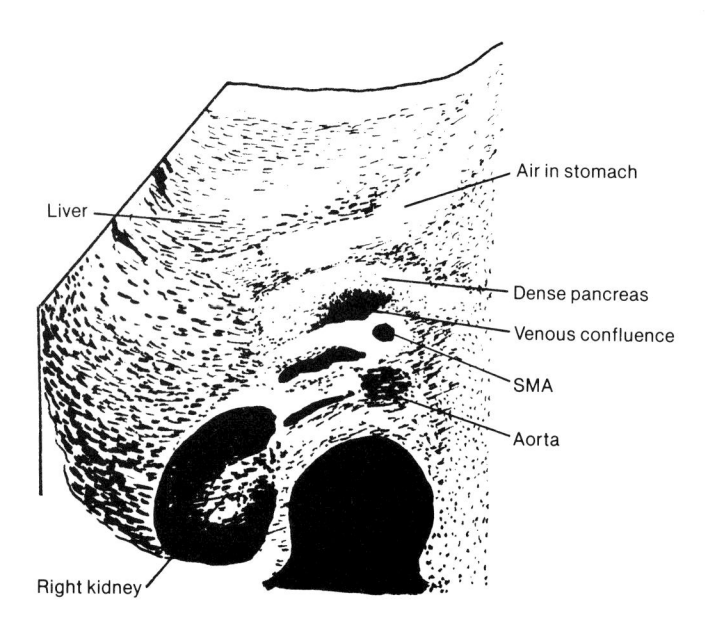

A

Left lobe of liver
Air in stomach
Pancreas
SMV
SMA
Gastroesophageal junction
Aorta
Celiac trunk

B

Liver
Air in stomach
Dense pancreas
Venous confluence
SMA
Aorta
Right kidney

Pancreatitis (9.7 to 9.9)

9.7 Acute Pancreatitis

A middle-aged alcoholic with acute pancreatitis demonstrated diffuse enlargement of the head, neck, body, and tail of the pancreas on sonogram. Note that in addition to the enlargement of the organ, it returned lower level internal echoes than the liver, indicating edema of the pancreas. The diagnosis of pancreatitis was made based on both a diffuse enlargement of the gland and a decrease in echogenicity. When there is only a localized enlargement of the gland, the differentiation between localized pancreatitis and carcinoma may be difficult. Observing the more prominent attenuation of carcinoma may allow this differentiation.

In Figure A, a parasagittal section over the inferior vena cava shows marked compression of its anterior surface by an enlarged head of the pancreas, which measured about 4 cm. Figure B is a sagittal section over the aorta which demonstrates the body of the pancreas lying between the left lobe of the liver and the superior mesenteric vein.

A transverse scan (Fig. C) demonstrates the diffuse enlargement of the gland. The left renal vein is seen passing between the superior mesenteric artery and the aorta. The vena cava is seen as a slitlike structure due to compression from the enlarged pancreas.

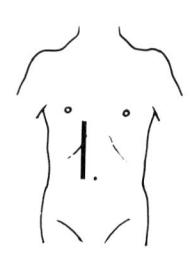

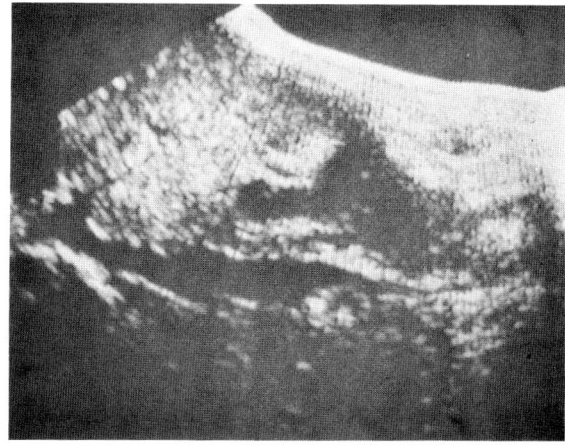

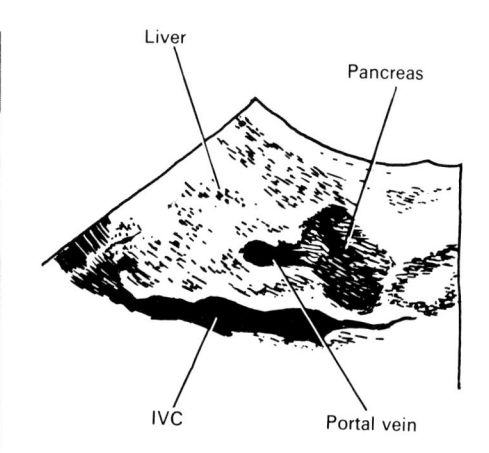

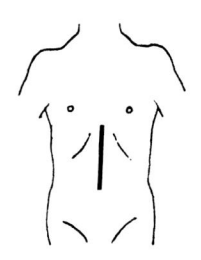

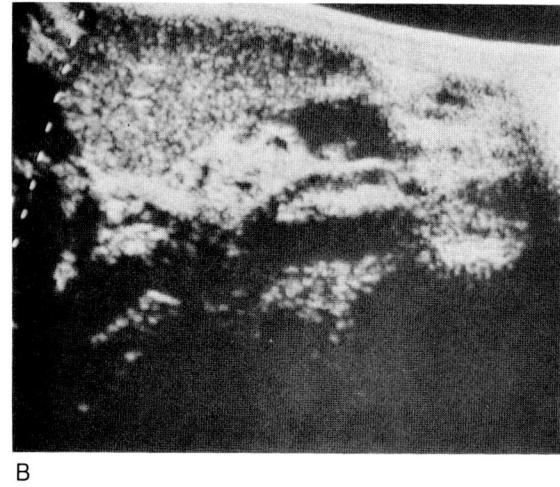

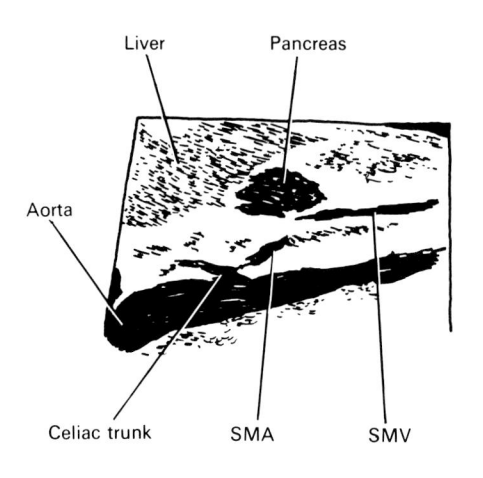

B

Liver	Pancreas
Aorta	
Celiac trunk	SMA	SMV

C

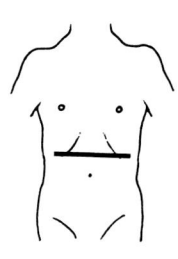

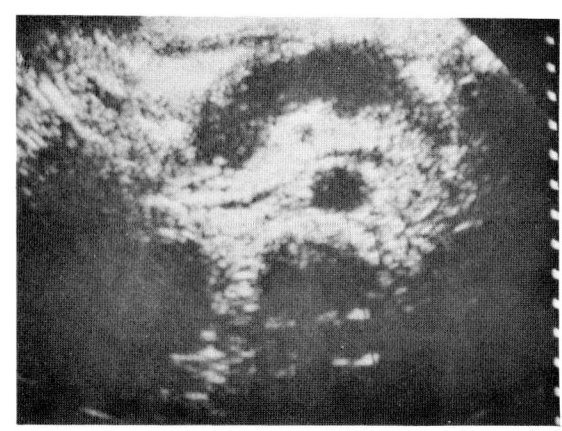

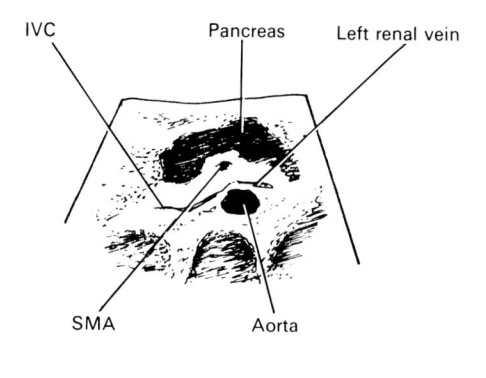

| IVC | Pancreas | Left renal vein |
| SMA | Aorta |

9.8 Acute Superimposed on Chronic Pancreatitis

A transverse ultrasonogram shows diffuse enlargement of the head and body of the pancreas which also had an abnormal consistency. Most of the gland returned lower level echoes than the liver substance and this was consistent with edema in acute pancreatitis. In addition, there are areas of high-level echoes appearing as white flecks, especially in the head. This suggested fibrosis in the gland and these appearances are characteristic of acute pancreatitis superimposed on chronic inflammatory disease.

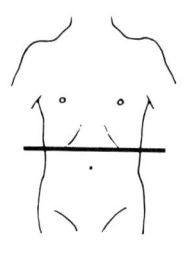

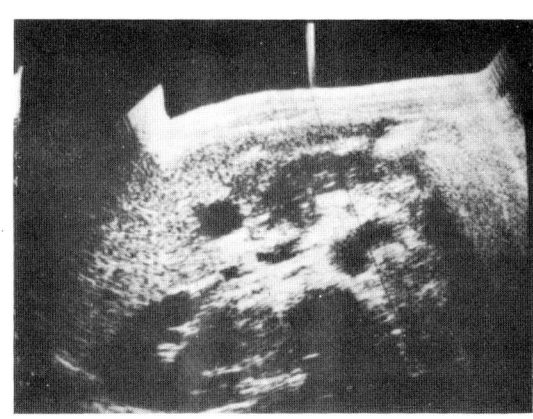

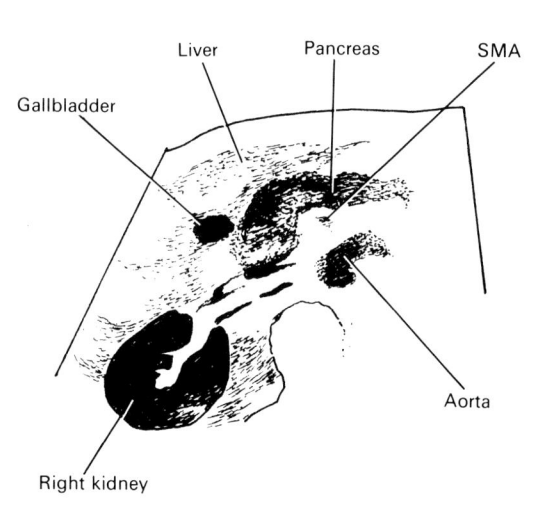

9.9 Chronic Pancreatitis

A 40-year-old chronic alcoholic with a long history of recurrent pancreatitis entered the hospital with a mild acute exacerbation. A transverse echogram (Fig. A) demonstrated a diffusely enlarged gland but with relatively stronger internal echoes than normal, indicative of chronic inflammatory change, probably secondary to fibrosis in the gland. Again note the superior mesenteric artery and vein which are landmarks for the pancreas. A sagittal section (Fig. B) of the aorta demonstrated the vertically oriented celiac trunk and the origin of the superior mesenteric artery just caudad. The pancreas lay between the superior mesenteric artery and the left lobe of the liver and immediately anterior to the splenic vein, which was seen in cross-section. Note that the celiac trunk marks the cephalad limit of the pancreas. The irregular margin of the pancreas was seen on both scans and is another indication of chronic change.

Ultrasound is insensitive for the demonstration of chronic pancreatitis. CT is far superior for imaging the calcifications characteristic of chronic pancreatitis.

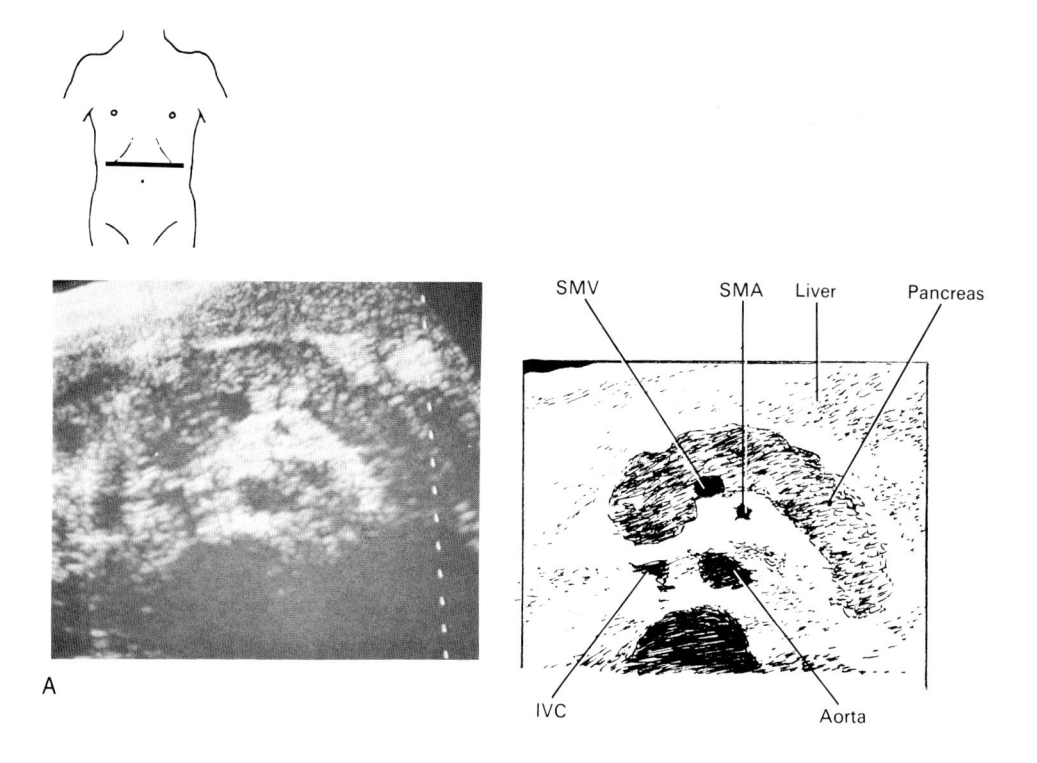

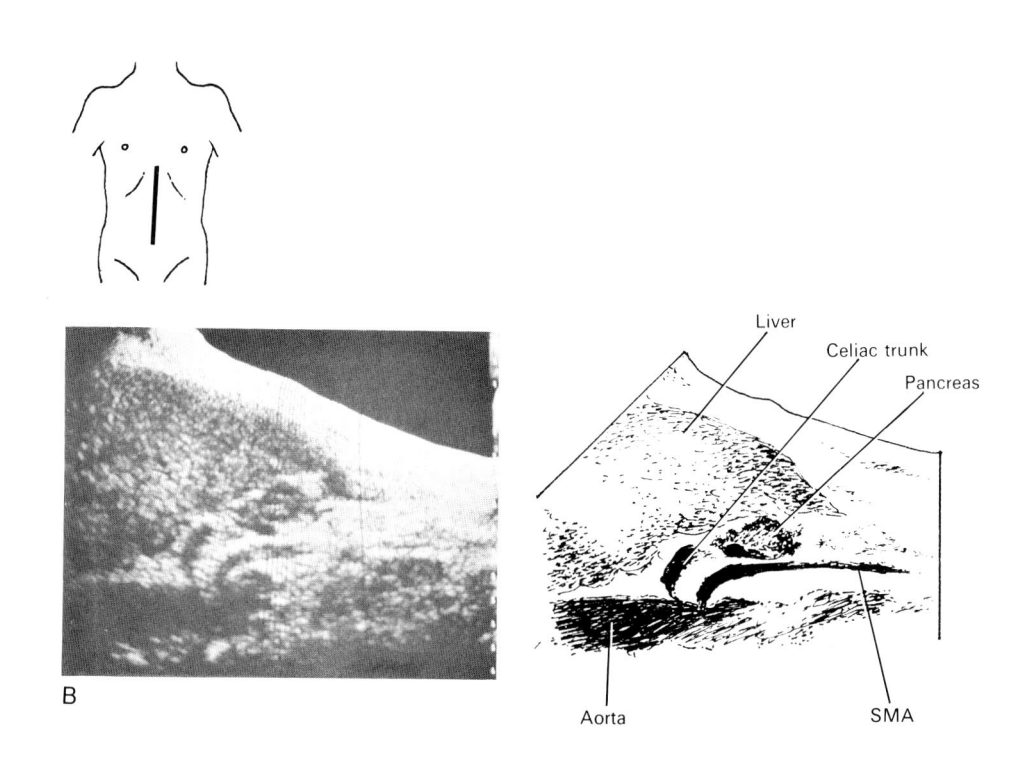

B

Liver
Celiac trunk
Pancreas
Aorta
SMA

9.10 Pancreatic Lithiasis

A 44-year-old man with a long history of recurrent pancreatitis secondary to alcoholism was admitted for investigation of chronic abdominal pain. A transverse sonogram (Fig. A) demonstrated a markedly dilated pancreatic duct (arrowheads), which was irregular in contour and contained at least one stone (arrowed). Gross dilatation of the pancreatic duct was also seen on a parasagittal section (arrowed, Fig. B).

A normal pancreatic duct can be visualized in approximately 82 percent of the population.[1] Parulekar found that the mean diameter of the duct was 1.3 mm and that the upper limit of normal was 2 mm. Dilatation of the duct may occur in both acute and chronic pancreatitis and also when the duct is obstructed by carcinoma of the pancreas.

Gosink and Leopold described four cases of stones occurring in a dilated pancreatic duct.[2] Pancreatic duct stones are the result of chronic pancreatitis and are part of the process of pancreatic calcification. Isikoff and Hill described two patients with pseudocysts distal to pancreatic duct stones.[3]

REFERENCES

1. Parulekar SG: Ultrasonic evaluation of the pancreatic duct. J Clin Ultrasound 8:457–463, 1980
2. Gosink BB, Leopold GR: The dilated pancreatic duct: ultrasonic evaluation. Radiology 126:475, 1978
3. Isikoff MB, Hill MC: Ultrasonic demonstration of intraductal pancreatic calculi: a report of 2 cases. J Clin Ultrasound 8:449–452, 1980

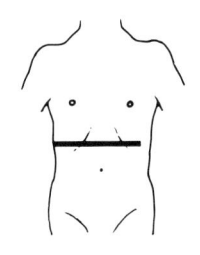

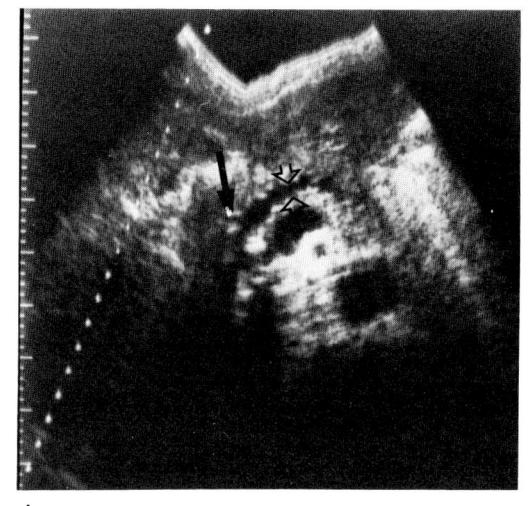

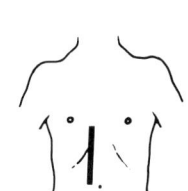

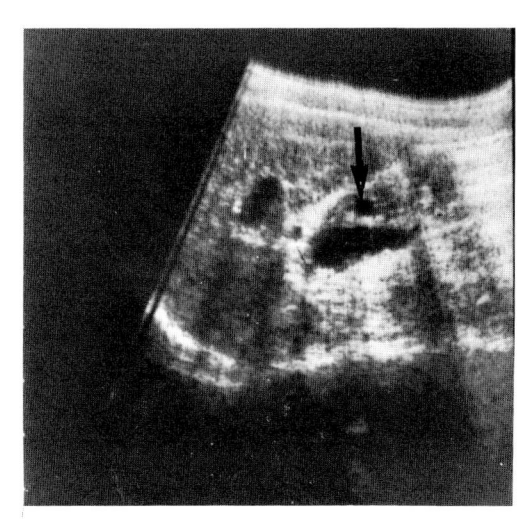

A

B

647

9.11 Puestow Procedure

A 46-year-old woman was referred for evaluation of recurrent pancreatitis. She had experienced periodic epigastric discomfort for 10 years associated with nausea and vomiting. This resulted in a cholecystectomy, at which time gallstones were found. Six months after the surgery, her abdominal discomfort recurred and laparotomy disclosed hemorrhagic pancreatitis. In the previous 5 years, the patient had been hospitalized approximately six times per year for recurrent pancreatitis. She had no history of jaundice, fever, chills, or weight change. There was a history of heavy alcohol use (more than 1 pint of liquor per day) for 4 years prior to her first attack of pancreatitis.

In 1977, ERCP showed chronic pancreatitis with dilated ducts and the patient underwent a Puestow procedure. In this operation, the pancreas is filleted and anastomosed to a loop of small bowel. ERCP in 1980 (Fig. A) demonstrated ampullary stenosis with a 1-inch stricture from the proximal portion of the pancreatic duct (arrowed). More distally, the duct was dilated (arrowheads), followed by a dilated duct with probable stones and drainage of dye into the jejunum. The transverse sonogram (Fig. B) showed a slightly enlarged pancreas, but no other gross abnormality. Water distention of the stomach has produced excellent visualization of the pancreas.

Ultrasound is adequate for imaging the size, contour, and texture of the pancreas, but ERCP was required in this patient to demonstrate the changes in the ducts, on which the diagnosis depended.

(Fig. A courtesy of Dr. M. Burrell, Yale University.)

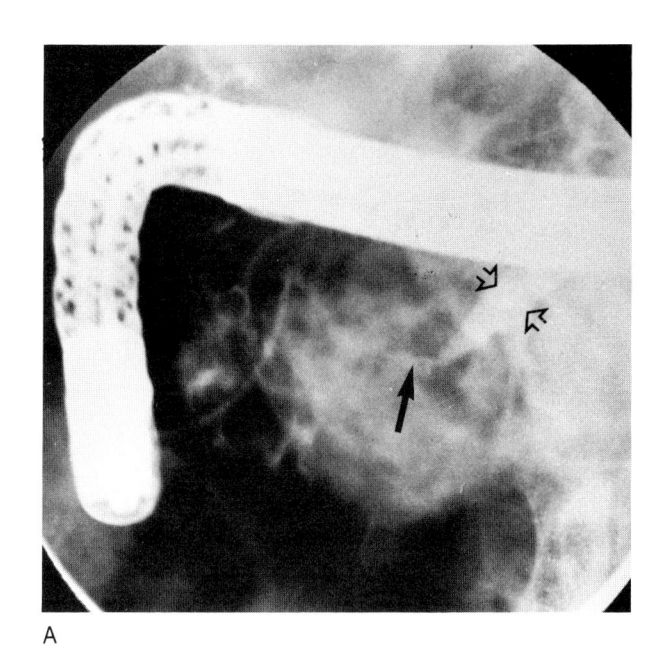

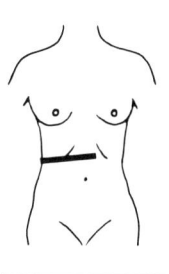

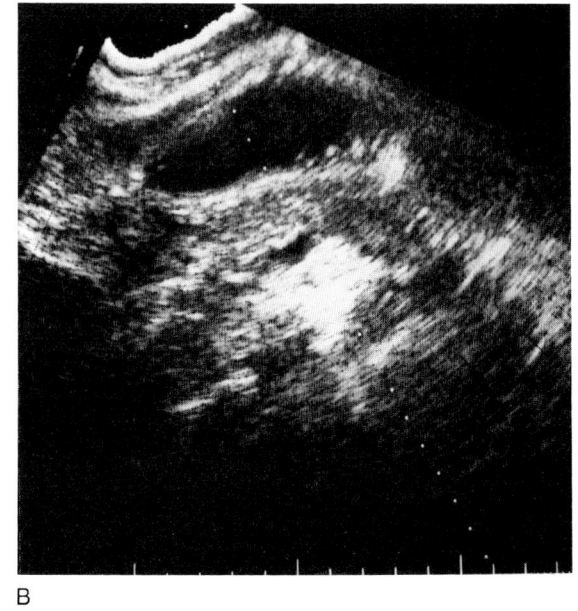

A

B

Pseudocyst (9.12 and 9.13)

9.12 Spontaneous Drainage

A middle-aged chronic alcoholic presented with a normal serum amylase level and an enlarging mass in the epigastrum. A sagittal section (Fig. A) over the inferior vena cava revealed a large cystic mass just caudad to the portal vein. A transverse section (Fig. B) showed a large pseudocyst in the head of the pancreas medial to the gallbladder. It is important in diagnosing pseudocysts of the head of the pancreas to locate the gallbladder to avoid a mistaken identity. Transverse and sagittal sonograms (Figs. C and D) from a follow-up examination 2 months later demonstrated a decrease in the size of the pseudocyst.

The term pseudocyst describes both the chronic, thick-walled variety and the more transient peripancreatic inflammatory effusion.[1] Pseudocysts can form rapidly and resolve spontaneously.[2] Indications for conservative treatment include a pseudocyst less than 5 cm in diameter, or an observation time of less than 6 weeks from the attack of pancreatitis.[1] A pseudocyst may dissect away from the pancreas and present in a distant location.[3]

REFERENCES

1. Bradley EL III, Clements JL Jr, Gonzalez AC: The natural history of pancreatic pseudocysts: a unified concept of management. Am J Surg 137:135–141, 1979
2. Sarti DA: Rapid development and spontaneous regression of pancreatic pseudocysts documented by ultrasound. Radiology 125:789–793, 1977
3. Conrad MR, Landay MJ, Khoury M. Pancreatic pseudocysts: unusual ultrasound features. AJR 130:265–268, 1978

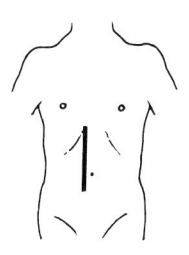

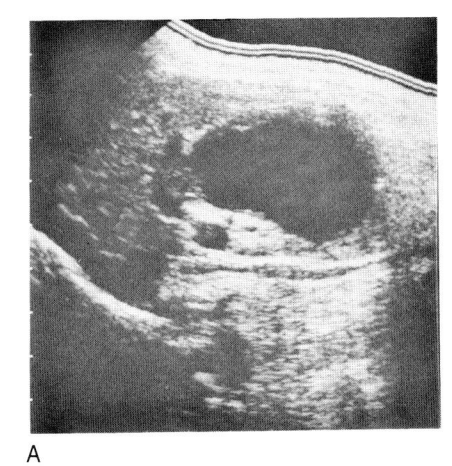

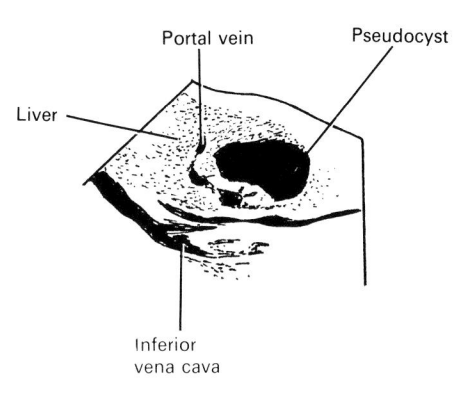

A

Portal vein — Pseudocyst
Liver
Inferior vena cava

B

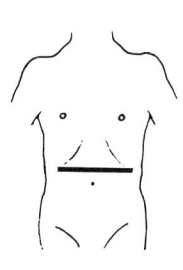

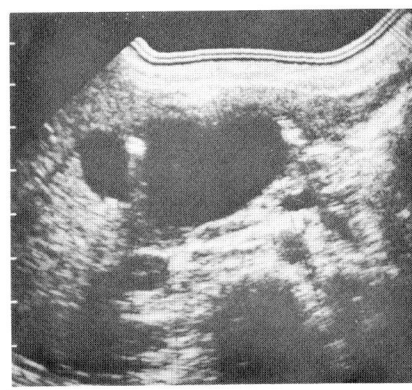

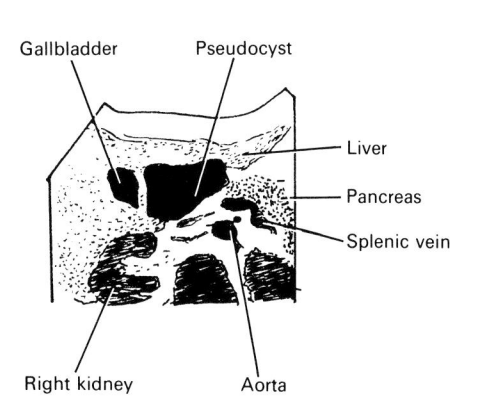

Gallbladder — Pseudocyst
Liver
Pancreas
Splenic vein
Right kidney — Aorta

651

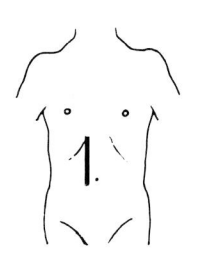

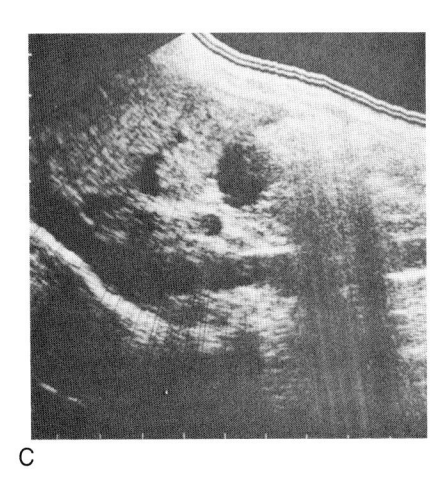

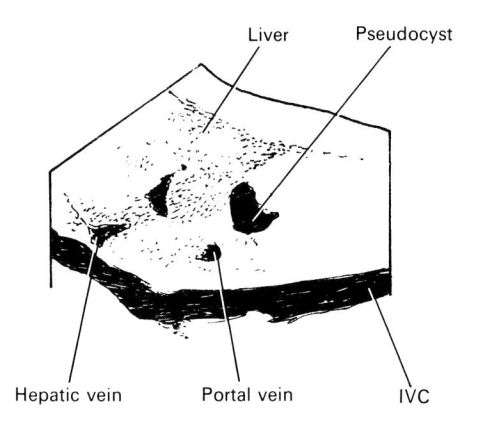

C

	Liver	Pseudocyst
Hepatic vein	Portal vein	IVC

D

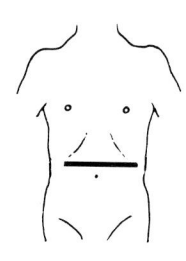

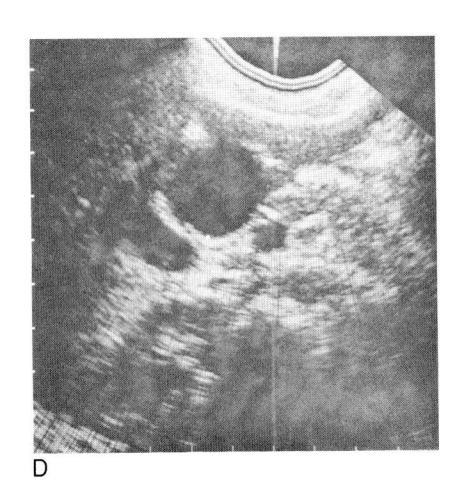

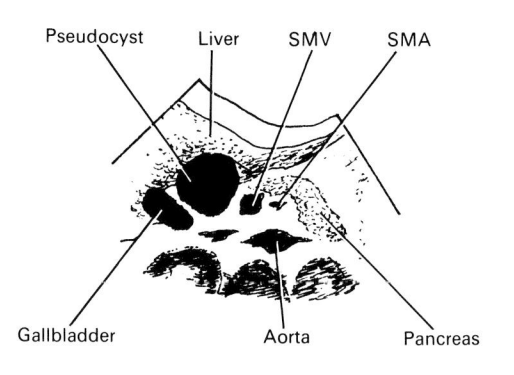

Pseudocyst	Liver	SMV	SMA
Gallbladder		Aorta	Pancreas

9.13 Traumatic Pseudocyst

A 24-year-old man took a case of beer and his speedboat out on Long Island Sound. Having drunk the beer, he drove his boat into a rock at high speed, impaling his epigastrium on the steering wheel.

On admission his serum amylase level was elevated to 190 u/dl and his serum lipase level was 2.6 u/ml. The serum alcohol level was 150 mg/dl. The abdomen was nontender but demonstrated voluntary guarding. Under observation, his abdomen became silent and more diffusely tender. His serum amylase level increased to 850 u/dl and serum lipase level decreased to 1.2 u/ml.

A transverse sonogram 2 days after admission demonstrated a focal injury to the tail of the pancreas (Fig. A). A longitudinal scan demonstrated a complex mass below the left lobe of the liver (Fig. B). This complex mass became more cystic with time, although the patient's clinical course was still benign (Fig. C). A longitudinal sonogram 1 week later demonstrated that the mass had increased in size to 16 × 6 × 7 cm and showed some septation (Fig. D). His serum amylase level continued to increase to 2,300 U/dl. The patient underwent exploratory laparotomy and was found to have a fractured pancreas. A distal pancreatectomy and cystogastrostomy were performed and the patient made an uneventful recovery.

Pseudocysts are very well documented when evaluated by ultrasound, although acute pancreatitis may be accompanied by paralytic ileus, which interferes with ultrasound visualization. Subsequent scans show development of a pseudocyst. Few surgeons operate on acute pancreatitis, so that failure to visualize the early phlegmon is seldom clinically significant. Ultrasound is capable of predicting whether the contents of the pseudocyst are fluid or whether a solid phlegmon is present. Surgical drainage should not be undertaken until the contents are relatively echo free. However, the sonologist should avoid the temptation to predict the maturity of the pseudocyst wall. To perform a cystogastrostomy, surgeons need a well-organized fibrous wall which can hold sutures. Generally, a mature wall takes about 6 weeks to form after an attack of pancreatitis, but the maturity of the wall cannot be predicted from sonogram.

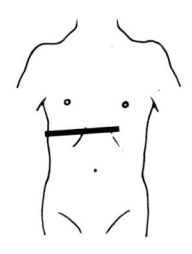

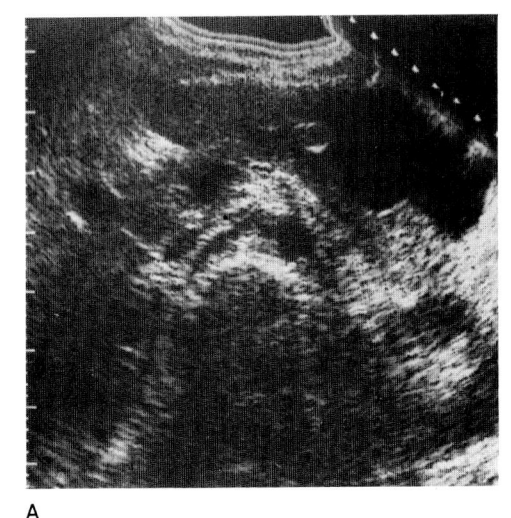

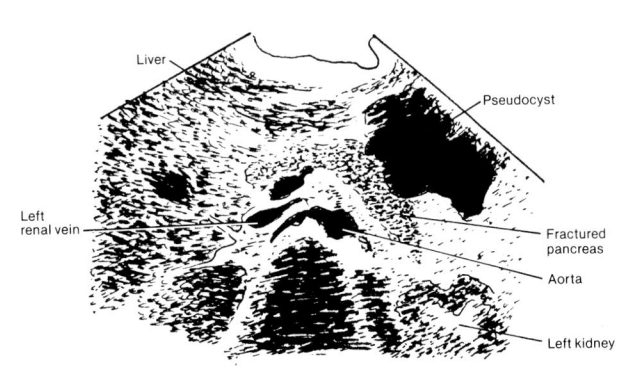

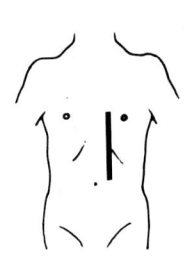

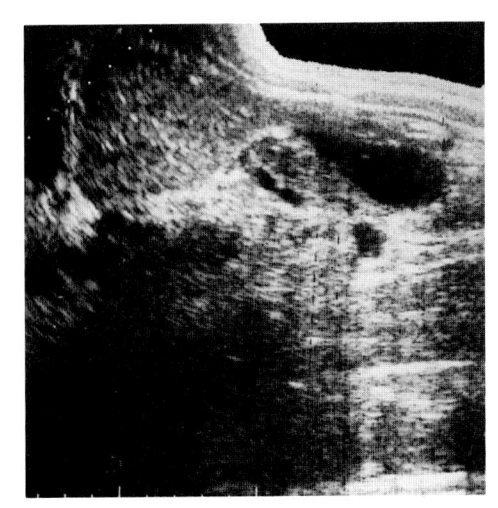

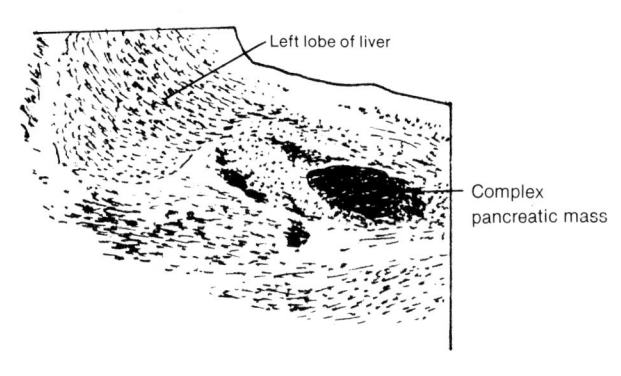

A

B

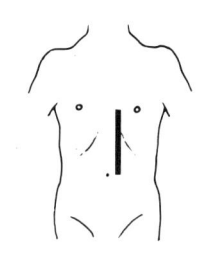

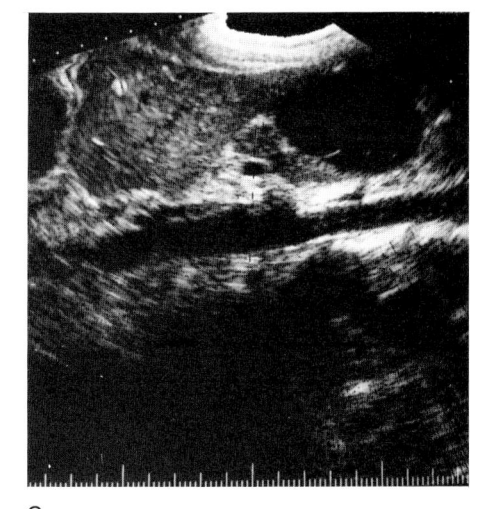

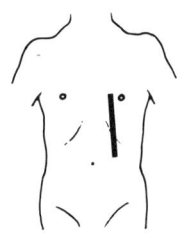

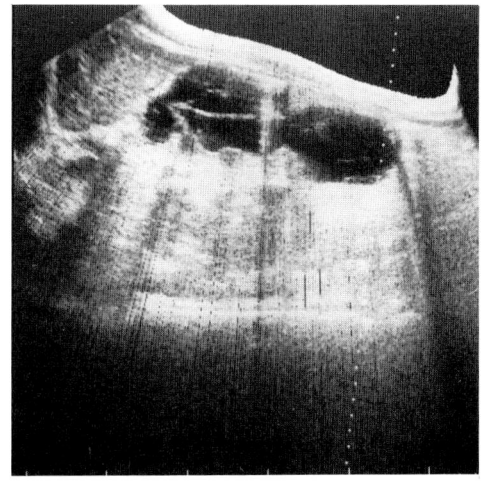

C

D

Hematoma (9.14 and 9.15)

9.14 Pediatric

A 6-year-old boy received a blow to the epigastrium and was admitted with severe abdominal pain. He developed signs of blood loss and was referred for ultrasound to rule out a retroperitoneal hematoma.

A transverse sonogram showed a septate cystic mass in the region of the tail of the pancreas anterior to the left kidney (Fig. A). This was presumed to be a hematoma, although a pancreatic effusion probably contributed to it. Since his condition was stable, he was treated conservatively. A repeat scan 5 days later showed a decrease in the size of the fluid collection (Fig. B). He was discharged and followed up as an outpatient. A third ultrasound scan 2 weeks later (Fig. C) demonstrated almost complete resorption of the mass.

This again demonstrates the nonspecific appearances of fluid collections, but a presumptive diagnosis can often be made from the clinical history. Aspiration of this mass might have infected it and was inappropriate unless the patient had developed fever.

Slovis et al. reported three cases of pancreatic pseudocysts and effusion in children.[1] They suggested the treatment of such fluid collections should be more conservative than is conventional in adults. Many children with pancreatic trauma are victims of child abuse. However, unlike most adults, the pancreas is intrinsically normal before trauma and spontaneous resolution of fluid collections can be expected in most patients.

REFERENCE

1. Slovis TL, VonBerg VJ, Mikelic V: Sonography in the diagnosis and management of pancreatic pseudocysts and effusions in childhood. Radiology 135:153–155, 1980

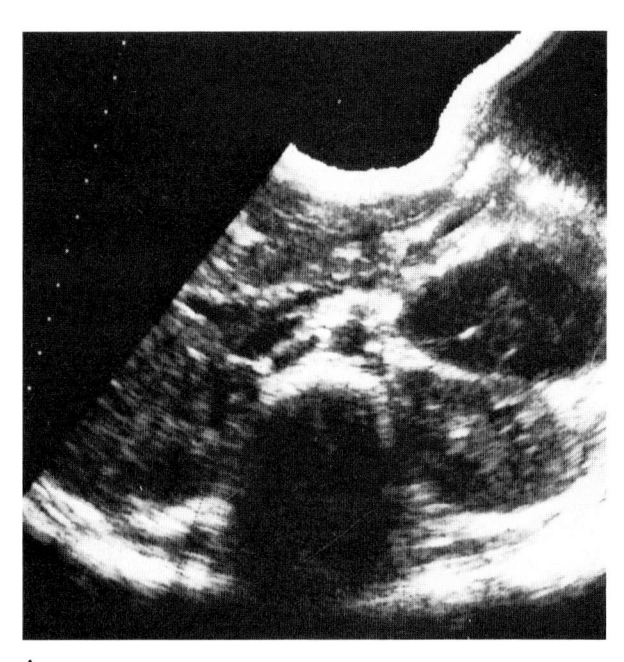

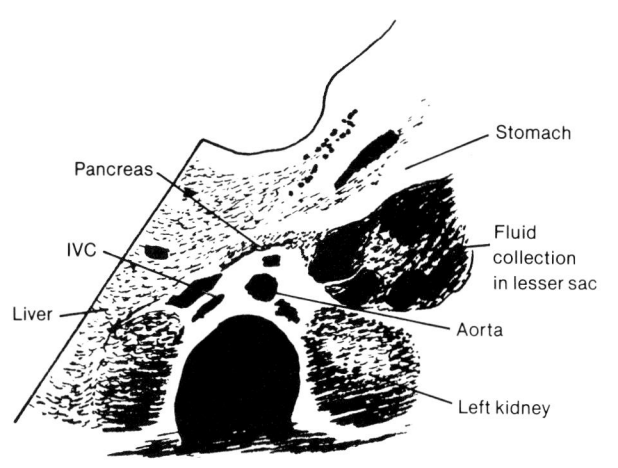

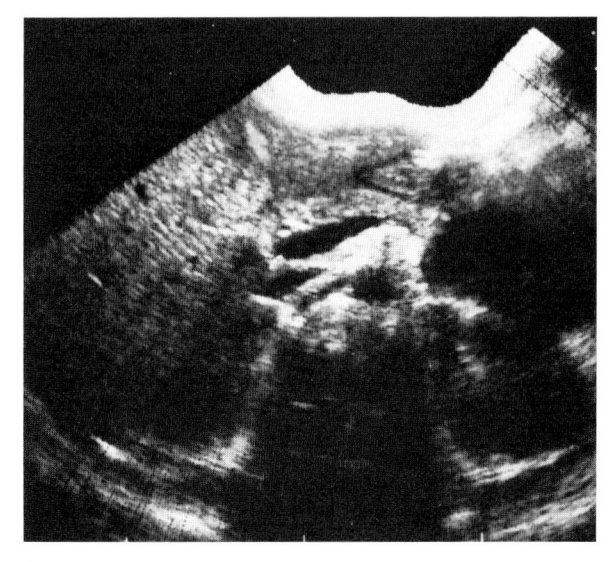

A

B

657

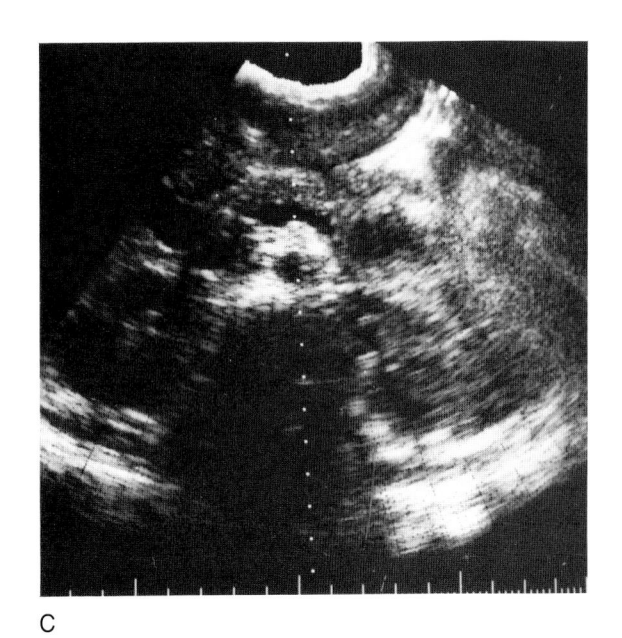

C

9.15 Infected Hematoma

A 61-year-old man presented with an inferior wall myocardial infarction, complicated by congestive heart failure and heart block requiring a balloon pump. He underwent mitral valve replacement; a perforated diverticulum of the sigmoid colon required sigmoid resection and colostomy. He was admitted for colostomy closure. Following surgery, he developed a chemical pancreatitis and was referred for ultrasound. The ultrasound scan shown in the figure revealed a large, complex mass in the hilum of the spleen, which was considered to be a pseudocyst. However, almost immediately after the examination he became hypotensive and was found to have a white cell count of 17,000/mm^3, presumably due to septic shock from a pancreatic abscess. Exploratory laparotomy disclosed an infected intra-abdominal hematoma which was drained successfully.

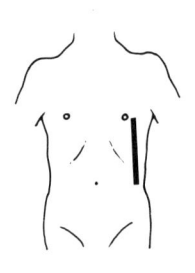

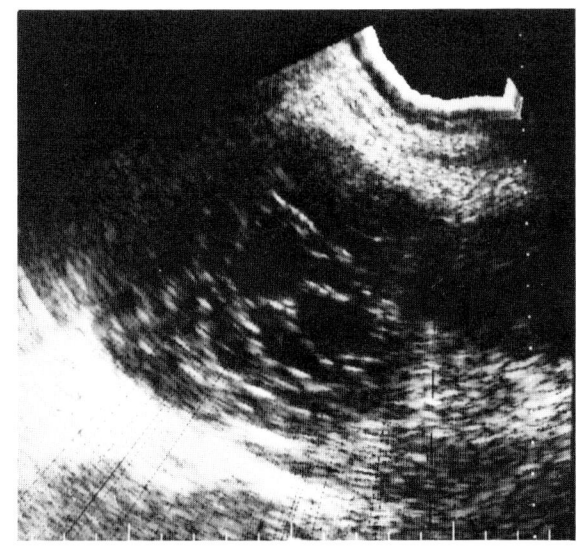

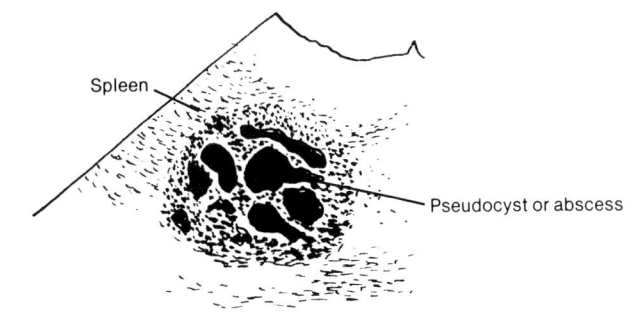

9.16 Peripancreatic Abscess

A 53-year-old white woman underwent subtotal pancreatectomy and splenectomy for chronic pancreatitis induced by alcohol abuse. She developed a fistula postoperatively, which necessitated laparotomy. At this time a peripancreatic abscess with seeding from the transverse colon was found. She did well for 2 months, when she again presented with fevers, shaking, chills, and abdominal pain.

Examination revealed an ill, thin patient with a temperature of 104°. The abdomen was soft and there was a drain in the left upper quadrant sinus tract which exuded a small amount of yellow pus. The longitudinal ultrasonogram, shown in the figure, demonstrated a complex mass anterior to the aorta consistent with a pseudocyst or a pancreatic abscess.

Repeated exploration demonstrated an abscess around the pancreas and an 80 percent pancreatectomy was performed. Her recovery was complicated again by the development of a sinus tract between the pancreatic bed and the left transverse colon.

This case demonstrates the nonspecific ultrasound appearances of fluid collections. A pseudocyst cannot be differentiated from a pancreatic abscess on scan appearances alone. Patients with pancreatic abscesses tend to be very sick and often moribund. Diagnostic aspiration is the best way to establish the nature of a fluid collection.

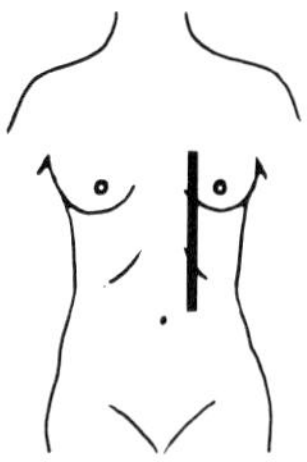

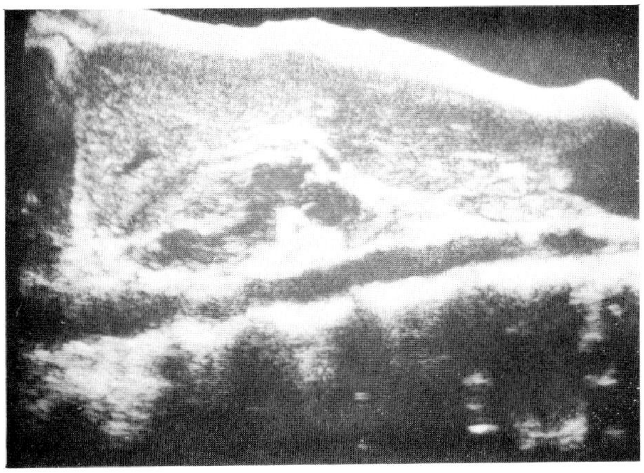

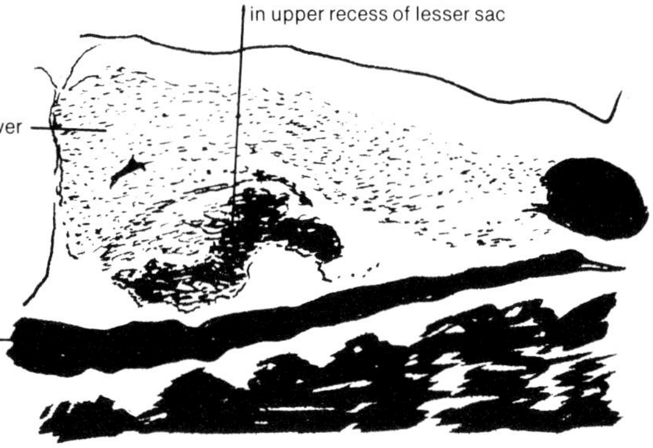
Abscess or pseudocyst
in upper recess of lesser sac
Liver
Aorta

Cystadenoma (9.17 and 9.18)

9.17 Microcystic Cystadenoma

An 82-year-old woman presented with anemia and was found to have an upper abdominal mass. The patient had lost 10 lbs, had no back pain, and a good appetite. Physical examination showed slight jaundice. The total bilirubin was 4.2 mg/dl (direct 0.76). A barium enema gave negative findings and results of a liver/spleen scan were normal. Upper GI studies demonstrated widening of the duodenum, suggesting a mass in the pancreas. The mass was separate from the kidneys and calcification was seen in the right paravertebral area (arrowed, Fig. A).

A longitudinal sonogram demonstrated a huge mass in the head and the uncinate process of the pancreas causing the superior mesenteric vein to be displaced anteriorly (Fig. B). Free ascites was seen. There was hydrops of the gallbladder and dilatation of the intrahepatic bile ducts (Fig. C).

At surgery a large pancreatic tumor was found involving the entire head and body of the pancreas, with the duodenal sweep draped over it. Small cysts were biopsied, but no definite malignancy was found. The patient then underwent a Roux-en-Y procedure. Microscopic examination revealed a microcystic cystadenoma of the pancreas.

Cystic neoplasms of the pancreas are differentiated into microcystic and macrocystic tumors. In the microcystic variety, the cysts are generally less than 2 cm in diameter and have no malignant potential. In contrast, a macrocystic tumor has cysts which are greater than 2 cm in diameter and are premalignant. Both tumors occur more frequently in women.

Microcystic adenomas often occur in the head of the pancreas, as in this patient and may produce obstructive jaundice. They are well-circumscribed and may be calcified. The CT and ultrasonic appearances have been described.[1]

REFERENCE

1. Wolfman NT, Ramquist NA, Karstaedt N, et al: Cystic neoplasms of the pancreas: CT and sonography. AJR 138:37–41, 1982

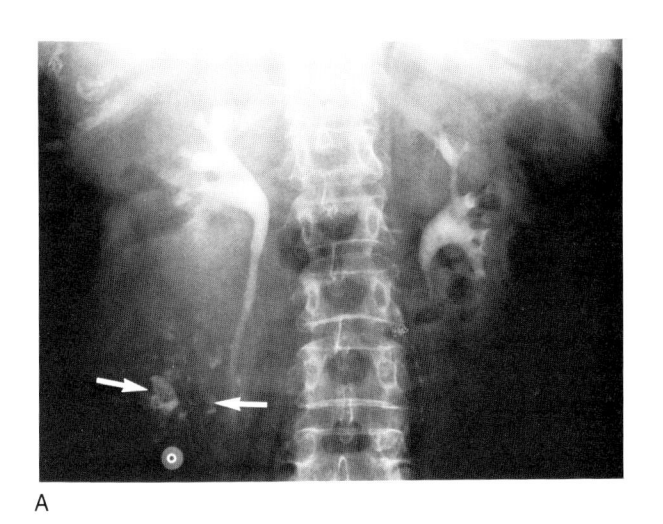

A

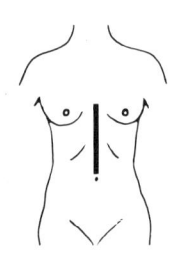

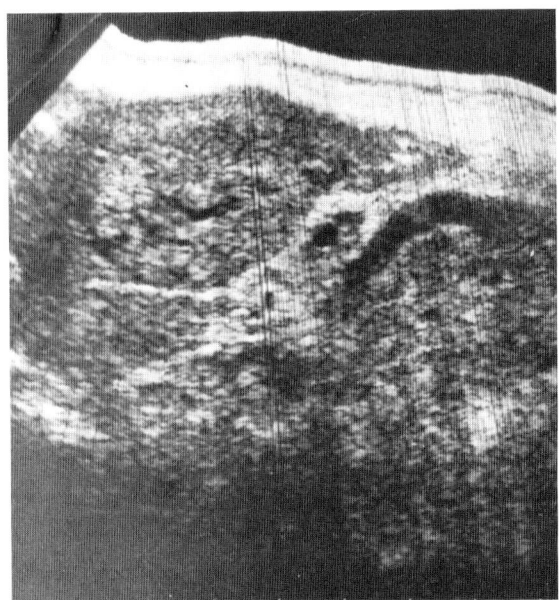

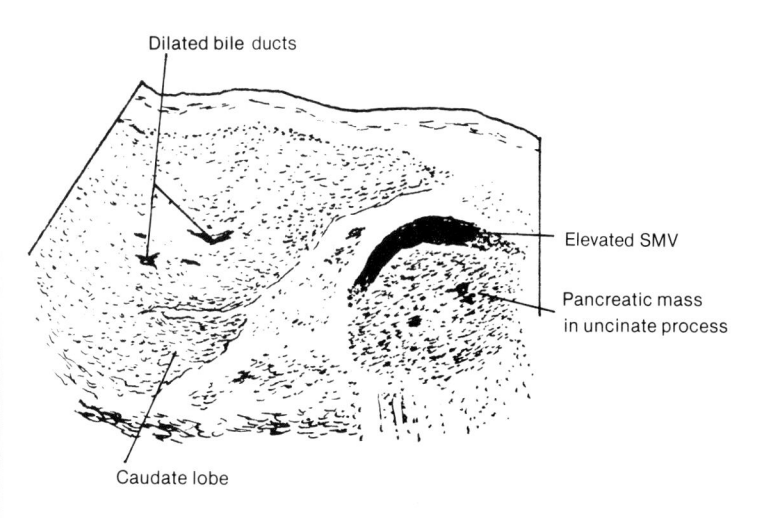

B

Dilated bile ducts

Elevated SMV

Pancreatic mass in uncinate process

Caudate lobe

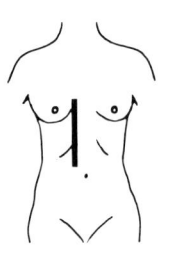

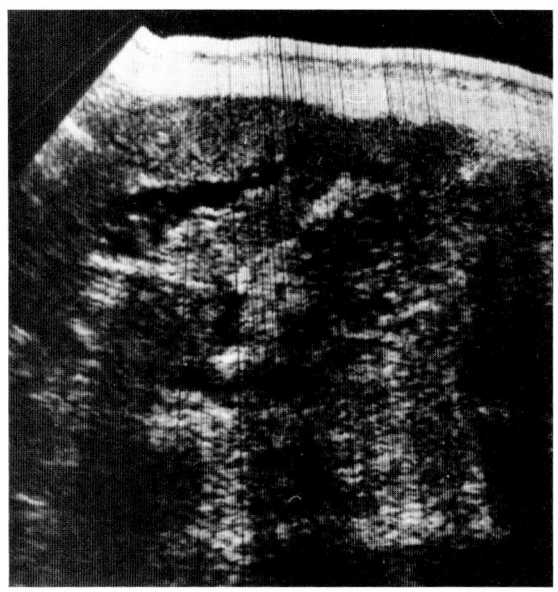

C

9.18 Cystadenocarcinoma

A 67-year-old woman presented with a pulsating, epigastric mass which appeared clinically to be an aortic aneurysm. A longitudinal sonogram to the left of the midline showed a complex epigastric mass lying superficial to the great vessels (Fig. A). With the patient prone, a large cystic component was seen anterior to the left kidney (Fig. B). These appearances were consistent with either an immature pseudocyst or a cystadenocarcinoma arising from the pancreas or, more commonly, the ovary.

A first-generation CT scan (Fig. C) confirmed the predominantly cystic nature of this mass and an angiogram further demonstrated its vascularity. Surgery revealed a cystadenocarcinoma arising from the body and tail of the pancreas.

A further example of a cystadenocarcinoma is seen in Figures D and E, a sonogram and a CT scan, respectively, showing the mixed cystic and solid components (arrowed).

Cystadenocarcinoma is the malignant counterpart of a macrocystic cystadenoma. It is a rare tumor which occurs more commonly in women than in men and usually affects a younger age group. It is less malignant than its adenocarcinoma counterpart, with 5-year survivals of approximately 40 percent.

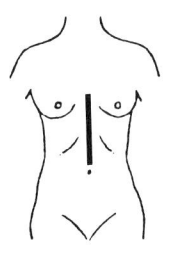

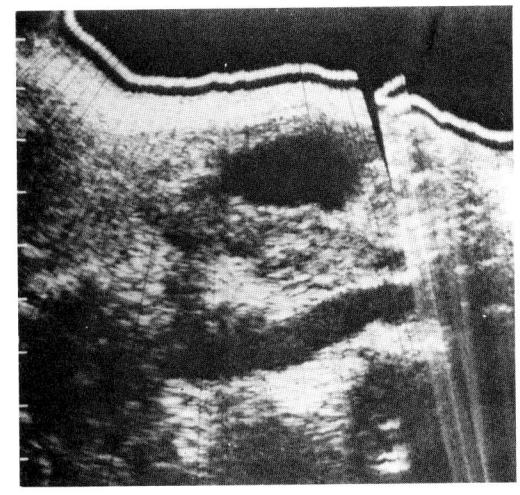

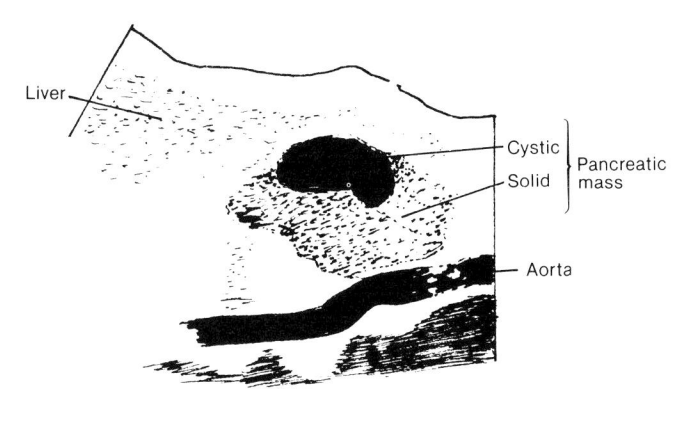

A

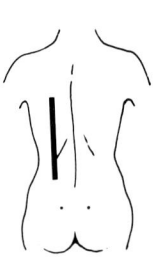

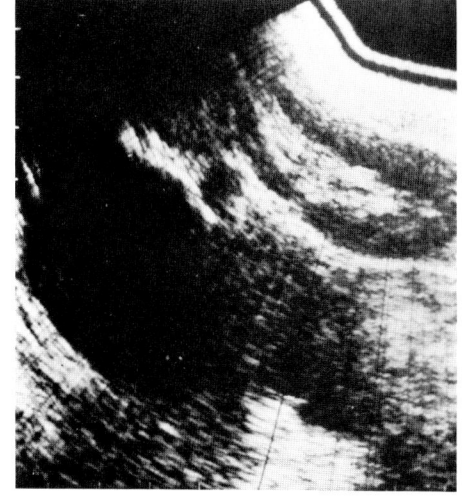

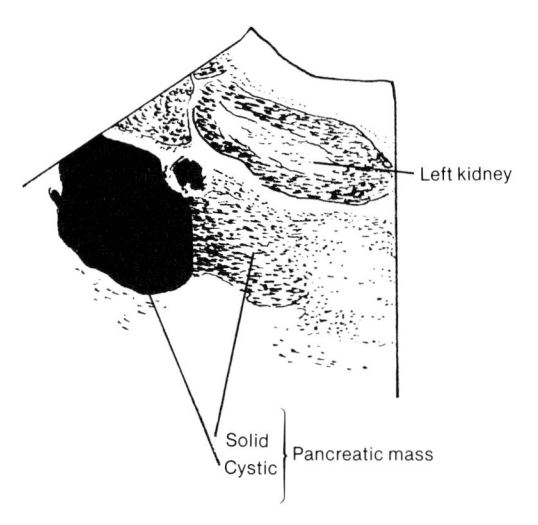

Left kidney

Solid
Cystic } Pancreatic mass

B

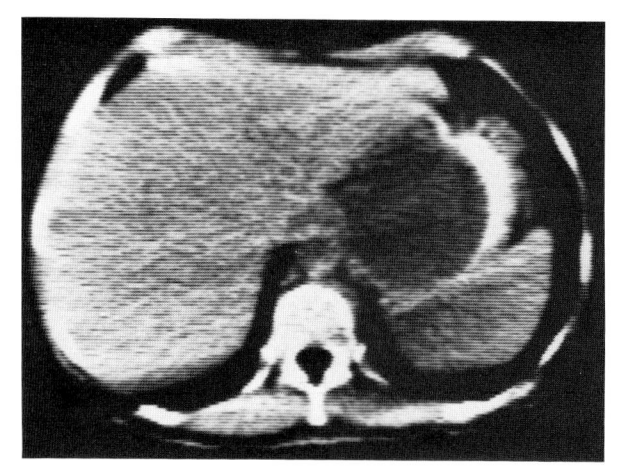

C

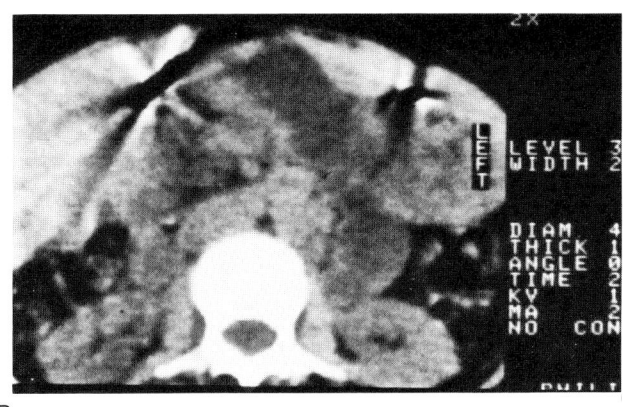

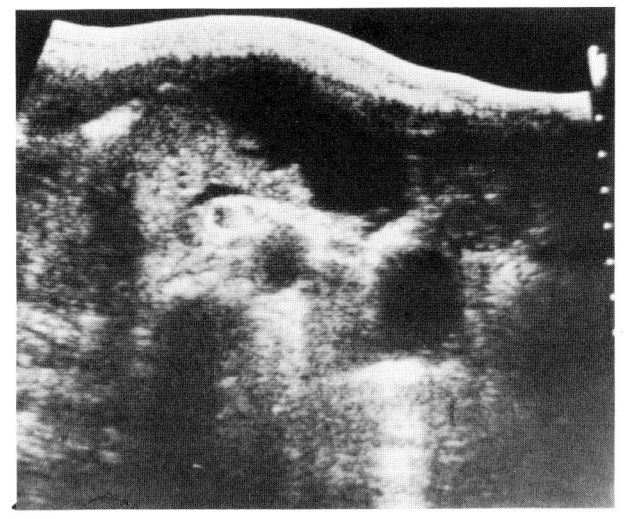

D

E

Carcinoma (9.19 to 9.23)

Carcinoma of the pancreas is one of the few malignant diseases that has shown a disturbing increase in prevalence. During the past 40 years, most countries throughout the world have reported a fourfold increase in the incidence of this disease.[1] There are few known etiologic factors, although an increased incidence has been reported in asbestos workers and in smokers. More recently, it has been suggested that coffee drinking may be a modest risk factor.[2]

Despite advances in radiotherapy and chemotherapy, the prognosis remains appalling, with 5-year survival rates of virtually zero and 12-month survival of 5 percent or less.[3] With the exception of patients with periampullary tumors, survival after radical surgery appears to be no greater than with chemotherapy and radiotherapy.

Approximately 70 percent of all carcinomas of the pancreas occur in the head, and less than 10 percent in the tail. Carcinomas of the tail almost invariably present so late that metastatic disease is already present. Thus, better delineation of the pancreatic tail by CT has little or no impact upon patient management, nor does it improve survival. Ultrasound adequately displays the head of the pancreas and tumors arising from it. Ultrasound is also an extremely sensitive way of detecting dilatation of the extra- and intrahepatic bile ducts and can image dilation of the pancreatic duct. These effects may, of course, occur as a result of benign as well as malignant obstruction. However, ultrasound is an effective screening technique for the diagnosis of pancreatic cancer, with a sensitivity of 94 percent and a specificity of 96–99 percent.[4–6]

The radiologic literature frequently refers to the patient with pancreatic cancer as having painless jaundice. In a review of 15,000 patients with this disease, Gudjonsson et al. demonstrated that the most common symptoms of pancreatic cancer were pain and weight loss, often accompanied by common gastrointestinal symptoms such as nausea, vomiting, and anorexia.[3] These symptoms are also common in the elderly so that, in practice, many patients are referred for ultrasonic evaluation and, in our experience, less than 10 percent have the disease. Thus, a negative predictive value of 99 percent is a most important aspect of the sonogram.

The lack of efficacy of surgery for the diagnosis and therapy of pancreatic cancer has encouraged the use of percutaneous biopsy for tissue diagnosis.[7] This is a particularly rewarding procedure, which may preclude the necessity for exploratory laparotomy with its attendant morbidity and mortality.

Percutaneous biopsy allows a tissue diagnosis in less than 24 hours, and the patient can often be discharged home for outpatient therapy.

CT or ultrasound can be used to localize the pancreatic mass and a fine needle, usually 22-gauge, is used to obtain small tissue fragments for cytologic or histologic study. Fine needles appear able to traverse gut or stomach with impunity and multiple passes can be made until a diagnosis has been reached. Even if the patient requires subsequent surgery for gastrointestinal bypass of the pancreatic tumor, a preoperative diagnosis is still valuable. It has been demonstrated that the immediate operative diagnosis of pancreatic cancer may be incorrect in up to 25 percent of patients.[3] A preoperative diagnosis of malignancy allows the surgeon to evaluate the patient's ability to withstand a Whipple procedure and saves the time required for intraoperative biopsy.

REFERENCES

1. Silverberg E: Cancer statistics, 1977. Cancer 27:6–21, 1979
2. MacMahon B, Yen S, Trichopoulos D, et al: Coffee and cancer of the pancreas. N Engl J Med 304:630–633, 1981

3. Gudjonsson B, Livstone EM, Spiro HM: Cancer of the pancreas: diagnostic accuracy and survival statistics. Cancer 42:2494–2506, 1978
4. DiMagno EP, Malagelada J-R, Taylor WF, et al: A prospective comparison of current diagnostic tests for pancreatic cancer. N Engl J Med 297:737–742, 1977
5. Taylor KJW, Buchin PJ, Viscomi GN, et al: Ultrasonographic scanning of the pancreas. Prospective study of clinical results. Radiology 138:211–213, 1981
6. Pollock D, Taylor KJW: Ultrasound scanning in patients with clinical suspicion of pancreatic cancer: a retrospective study. Cancer 47:1662–1665, 1981
7. Goldstein HM, Zornoza J, Wallace S, et al: Percutaneous fine needle aspiration biopsy of pancreatic and other abdominal masses. Radiology 123:319–322, 1977

9.19 Head of the Pancreas

Carcinoma of the pancreas appears on a sonogram as an area of decreased echogenicity compared with the normal parenchyma. This differentiation is important since it allows the diagnosis of a small cancer which has not yet produced an increase in the size of the pancreas or alteration of its contour. Figure A shows such a small cancer, which proved to be only 2 cm in diameter at subsequent surgery. In such patients, ultrasound may be more sensitive than the older CT machines which are still widely used for diagnosis of this condition, often in preference to ultrasound.

Pancreatitis tends to involve the entire gland, while cancer is more focal. However, the appearances are nonspecific and only examination of a biopsy specimen will allow the ultimate differentiation between localized pancreatitis and carcinoma.

Periampullary tumors cause early onset of biliary dilatation which is accurately detected by ultrasound. This may occur before there is any elevation in serum bilirubin. Figure B shows a longitudinal section down the common duct. The duct is pathologically dilated and an obstructing mass is seen in the lower end. The differential diagnosis of such masses includes any periampullary tumor, whether derived from the pancreas, duodenum, or bile duct. The mass is well-delineated on a transverse sonogram, which also shows surrounding lobulated masses, probably due to peripancreatic lymphadenopathy (Fig. C).

Scans of the liver may demonstrate important additional information. Figure D shows intrahepatic dilatation of the bile ducts secondary to an obstructing pancreatic cancer. Liver metastases are frequently seen. In our experience, these may be either hypoechoic (Fig. E, arrowed) or hyperechoic (Fig. F). The presence of liver metastases is a most important observation, since it is definitive proof of the inoperability of the pancreatic cancer. Under these circumstances, a diagnosis may be more easily obtained by percutaneous biopsy of the liver than of the primary lesion. Finally, a periampullary tumor may obstruct the pancreatic duct, leading to pathologic dilatation (arrow, Fig. G).

In conclusion, a wide spectrum of findings is observed in patients with carcinoma of the head of the pancreas. The primary mass, which has a nonspecific appearance, may be 2 cm or larger, although these tumors are rarely more than 4–5 cm before they present with biliary obstruction or metastatic disease. A thorough evaluation of the biliary tree and liver should be performed by ultrasound and/or CT, since the dilated ducts within the liver make liver scintigraphy equivocal. It may also be difficult to exclude metastatic disease to the liver by ultrasound. When gross biliary dilatation is present, the refractive effects of the sound beam traversing dilated ducts produce such an uneven liver parenchyma that it may be difficult to exclude metastatic disease.

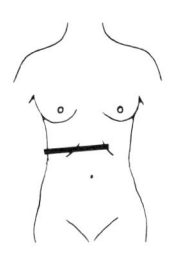

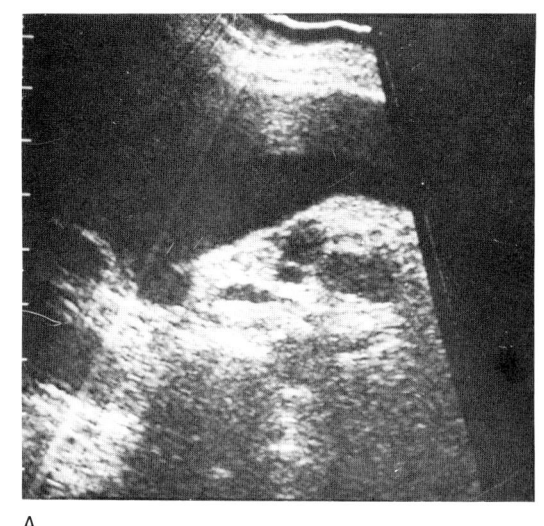

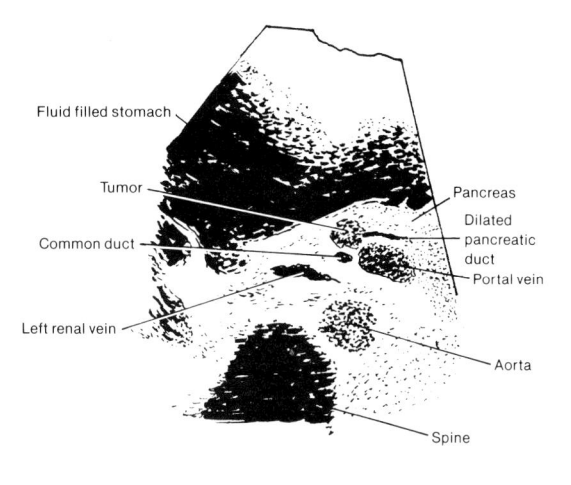

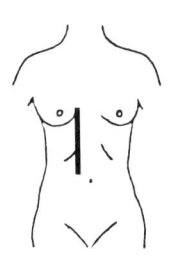

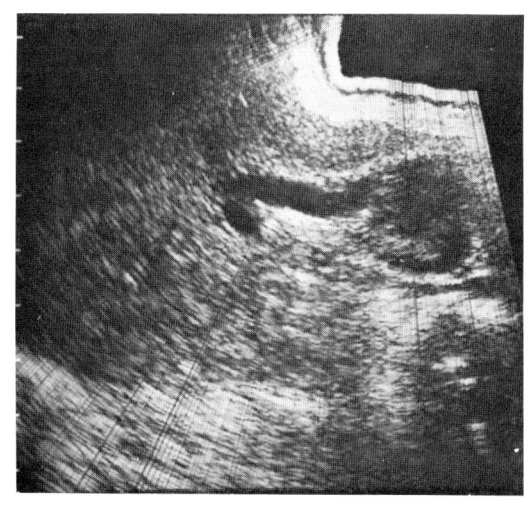

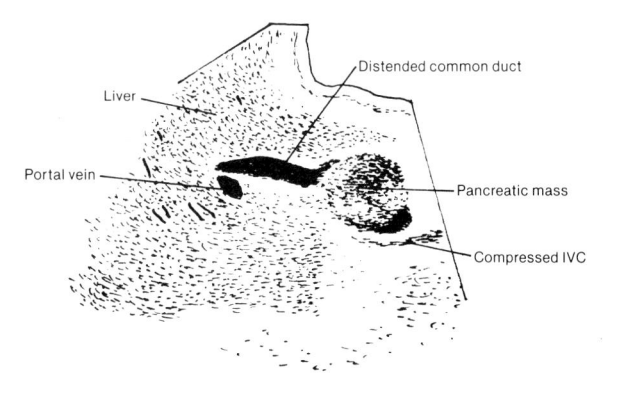

A

Fluid filled stomach
Tumor
Common duct
Left renal vein
Pancreas
Dilated pancreatic duct
Portal vein
Aorta
Spine

B

Liver
Portal vein
Distended common duct
Pancreatic mass
Compressed IVC

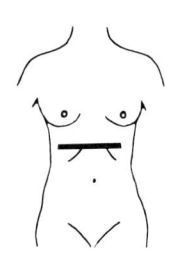

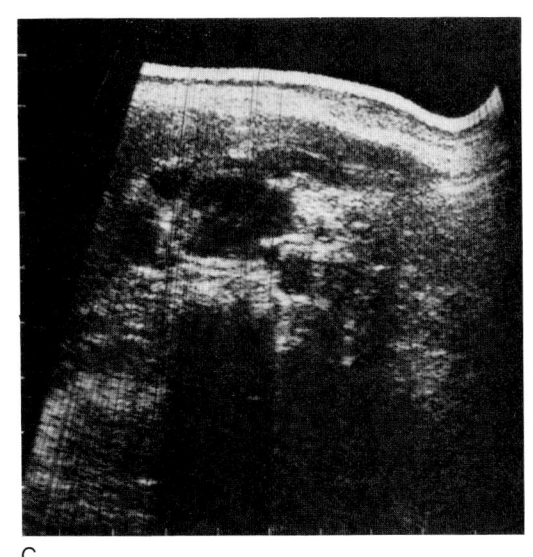

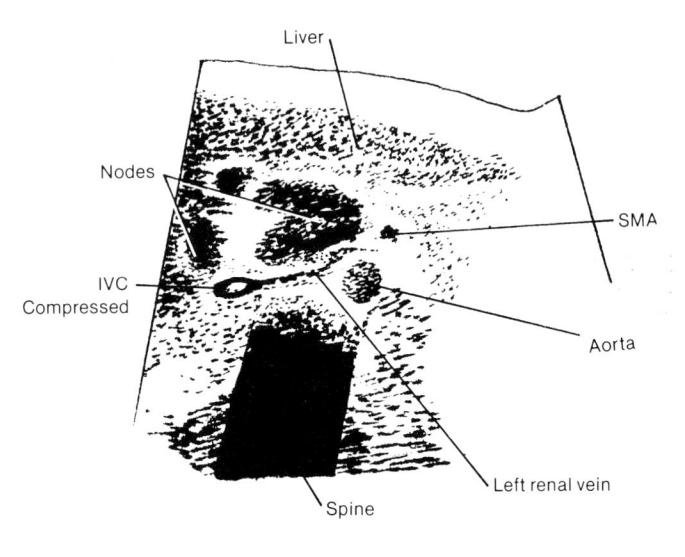

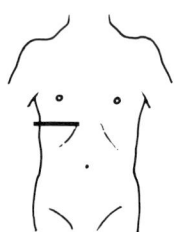

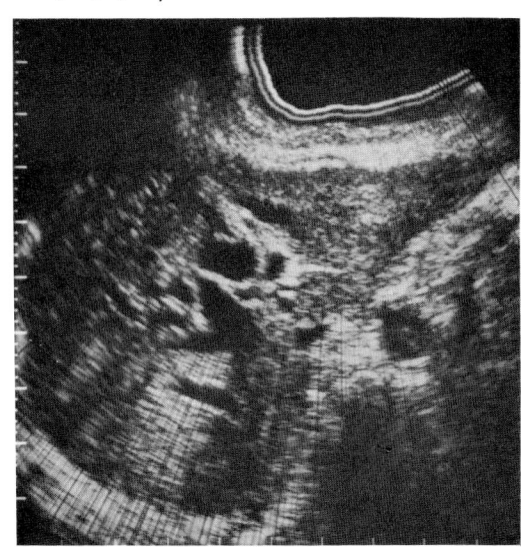

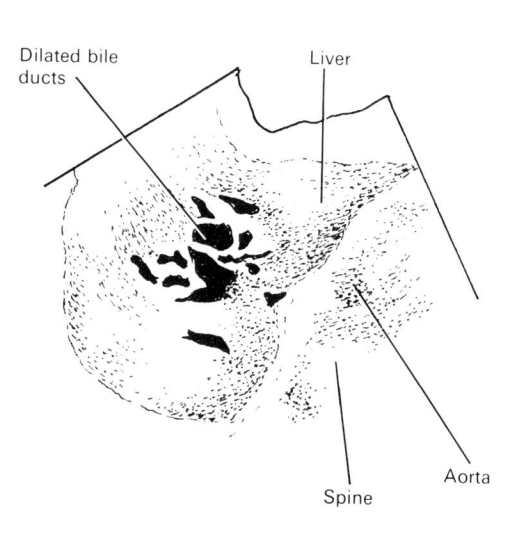

C

D

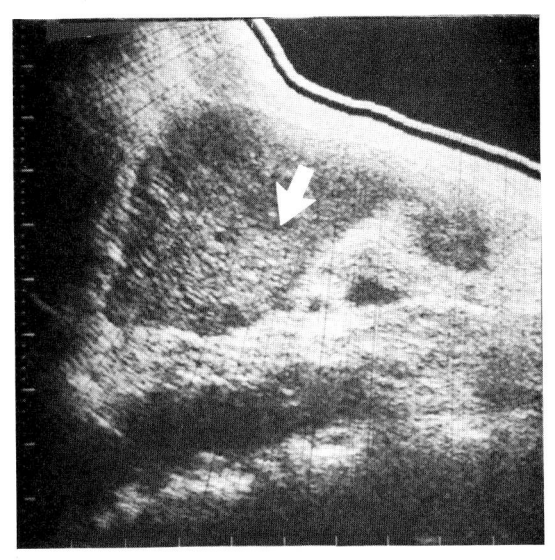

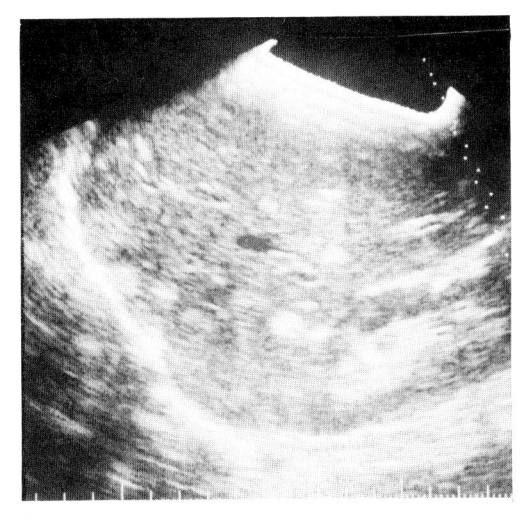

E

F

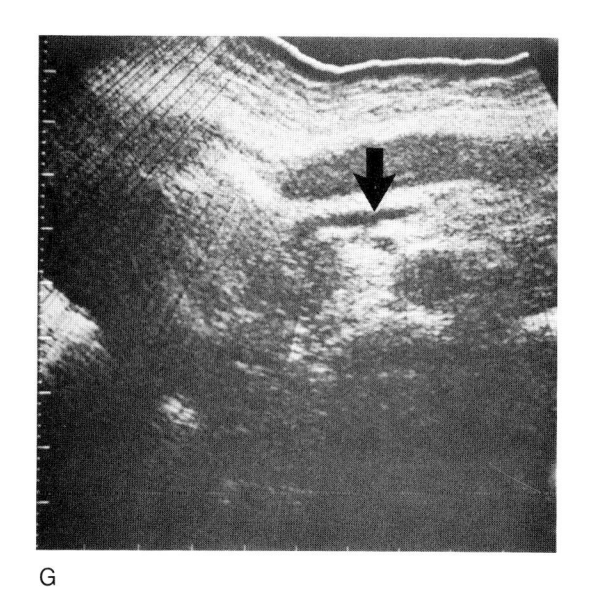

G

9.20 Tail of the Pancreas

A 60-year-old man with a history of weight loss and back pain was referred for ultrasound examination of the pancreas. The transverse sonogram in the figure showed the splenic vein coursing across the midline anterior to the superior mesenteric artery. The high-level echoes between the splenic vein and the liver represented the region of the neck of the pancreas. Just to the left of the splenic vein was an ill-defined, irregular solid mass which returned low-level echoes and represented a carcinoma arising at the junction of the body and tail of the pancreas.

Just to the left of the liver there was marked scattering and reverberation caused by the overlying air-containing bowel, making this region of the pancreas (the junction of the body and tail) the most difficult to visualize. However, additional techniques may be helpful. With the patient prone, scans through the acoustic window provided by the left kidney permitted visualization of the tail of the pancreas. In the decubitus position, the patient's liver and spleen may displace bowel gas and provide an acoustic window to the pancreas. Filling the stomach with fluid may also be very helpful. CT scanning may be valuable in this particular region. However, in this patient, who was thin, the pancreas was poorly outlined by CT. This problem is frequently encountered in patients with abdominal neoplasms who often have experienced marked weight loss.

Patients with carcinoma of the tail of the pancreas tend to present late and with nonspecific symptoms including back pain and weight loss. Metastases are almost invariably present. When metastases are documented by ultrasound, CT, or liver scintigraphy, or the primary tumor is clearly inoperable, fine-needle biopsy of the pancreas or of the liver is adequate to make the diagnosis and laparotomy is often unnecessary.[1] Mitty et al. reported the impact of fine-needle pancreatic biopsy in 53 patients. They attained a sensitivity of 86 percent, a specificity of 100 percent, and an overall accuracy of 89 percent.[2] Thirty laparotomies were avoided in 37 patients, resulting in estimated savings of $6,000 per patient.

REFERENCES

1. Ferrucci JT Jr, Wittenberg J, Mueller PR, et al: Diagnosis of abdominal malignancy by radiologic fine-needle aspiration biopsy. AJR 134:323–330, 1980
2. Mitty HA, Efremidis SC, Yeh HC: Impact of fine-needle biopsy on management of patients with carcinoma of the pancreas. AJR 137:1119–1121, 1981

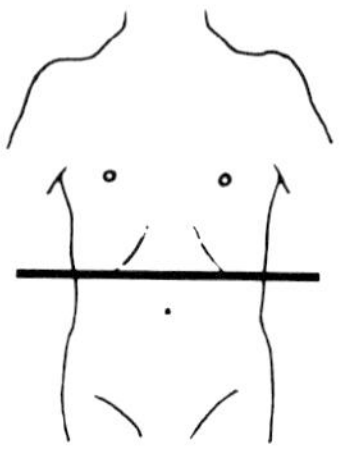

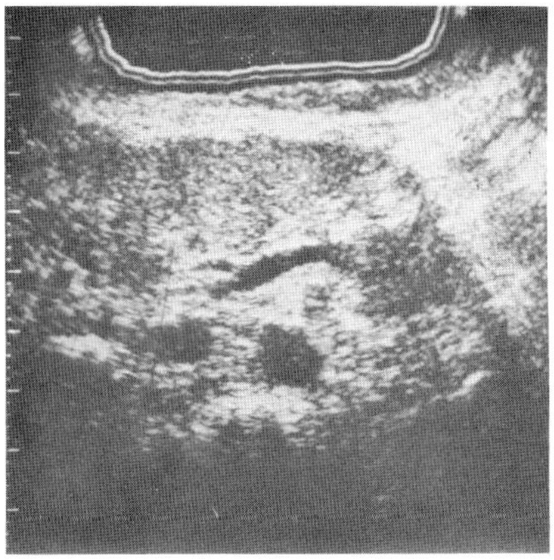

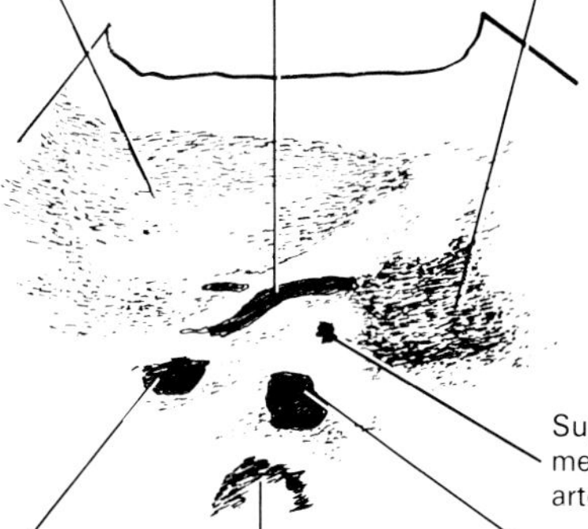
Liver
Splenic vein
Mass
Superior mesenteric artery
IVC
Spine
Aorta

9.21 Body and Tail of the Pancreas

A 60-year-old woman with a 20-lb weight loss developed left lateral chest pain and was investigated with an upper GI series which showed possible peptic ulcer disease. Treatment, however was unavailing, and she was admitted for further evaluation. Physical examination revealed an upper abdominal mass. A transverse sonogram showed an irregular 4-cm mass in the body and tail of the pancreas (Fig. A). This was confirmed on the longitudinal scan (Fig. B). Chest x-ray and liver/spleen scan showed normal findings and results of liver function tests were all within normal limits. ERCP demonstrated an obstruction of the main pancreatic duct, but a second-generation CT scan showed no definite tumor mass.

Laparotomy revealed tumor involvement of the body of the pancreas with extension to the celiac axis. Examination of a biopsy specimen demonstrated a poorly differentiated pancreatic adenosquamous carcinoma. Distal pancreatectomy and splenectomy were performed. After distal pancreatectomy, the patient was referred for simultaneous radiation and adriamycin therapy.

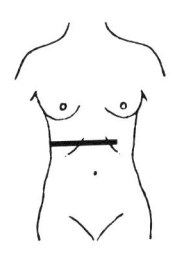

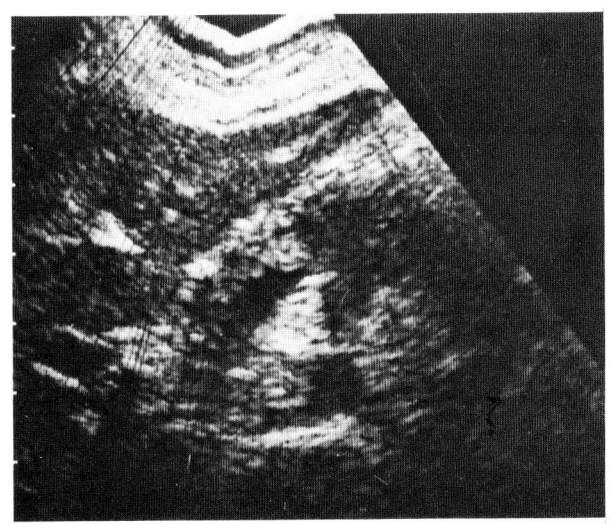

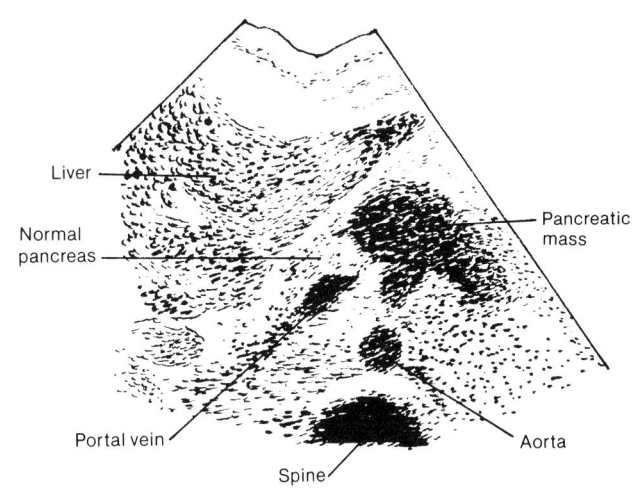

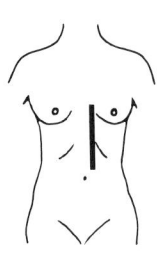

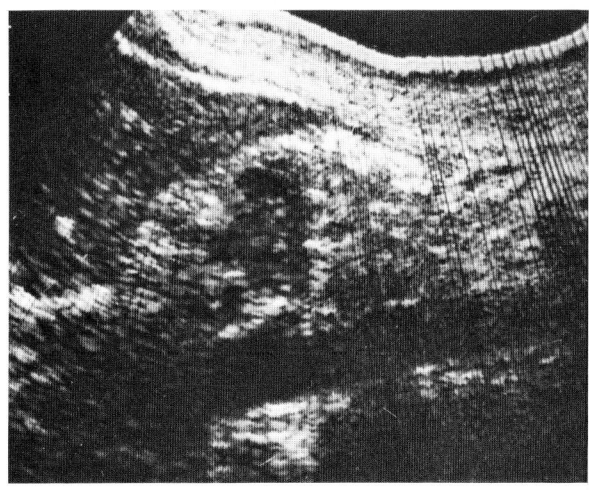

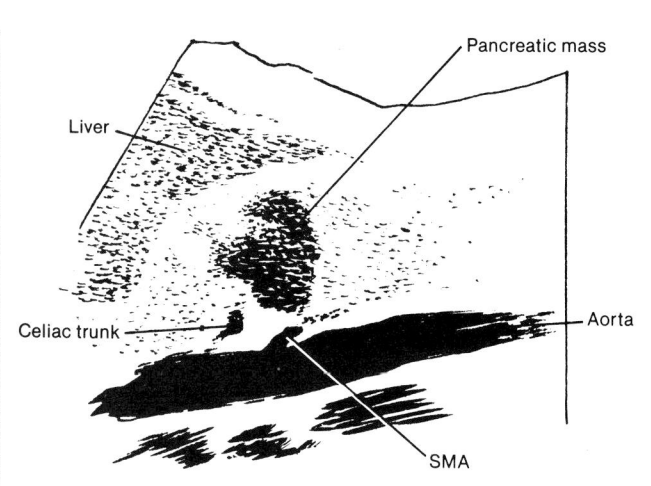

B

678

9.22 Nonfunctioning Islet Cell Carcinoma

A 69-year-old woman presented with massive GI bleeding and underwent exploratory laparotomy. Surgery disclosed a bleeding gastric ulcer. At that time a left upper quadrant mass was noted and was biopsied. It was considered to be either a microcystic adenoma or an islet cell adenoma of the pancreas. Subsequent arteriography showed that the spleen was enlarged and the splenic vein obstructed (Fig. A, curved arrow). Venous blood from the spleen drained by collateral vessels across the greater curvature of the stomach (arrowheads) and also the lesser curvature. A large mass was present in the tail of the pancreas and the pancreatic arteries were stretched and attenuated. A second exploratory laparotomy was undertaken, but radical removal of the mass was found impossible and a splenectomy was performed. The patient's history was remarkable for a "pancreatic cyst" which had been excised at another hospital 27 years before, but an adequate pathologist's report was lacking.

The left upper quadrant contained a rock-hard mass. A liver/spleen scan was unremarkable except for the absence of the spleen. Upper GI series demonstrated displacement of the stomach by a large abdominal mass. A transverse sonogram (Fig. B) showed an 18 × 18 cm mass in the left upper quadrant. A longitudinal scan (Fig. C) indicated its location anterior to the left kidney. This mass was fairly homogeneous and echogenic in texture. The patient's liver was displaced to the right and no liver metastases were seen.

Review of the microscopic sections did not allow differentiation between an islet cell adenoma and a carcinoma; it was believed that this distinction could only be made by evidence of distant spread of the tumor. The patient was treated with streptozotocin and 5-fluorouracil.

Her subsequent course has been downhill with the development of a malignant pleural effusion secondary to involvement of the left hemidiaphragm. In view of its behavior, this is a low-grade carcinoma.

Shawker et al. reported on 49 pancreatic islet cell tumors. Ultrasound was of little value for the diagnosis of beta-cell insulinomas, since the tumors tended to be small and the patients large.[1] Only 30 percent were detected by ultrasound, compared to 90 percent by angiography.[2] In Shawker's series, other functioning islet cell tumors were detected by ultrasound. Tumors associated with Zollinger-Ellison syndrome were detected by ultrasound in 42 percent of patients compared with 36 percent by CT[3] and 15 percent by angiography.[4]

Nonfunctioning islet cell tumors constitute 15 percent of all islet cell tumors, compared with insulinomas (60 percent) and gastrinomas (18 percent).[5] Nonfunctioning islet cell tumors are usually malignant. As in this patient, it is difficult to predict the malignant nature of these tumors except by the incidence of this invasive potential. They tend to be only slowly progressive, giving a 5-year survival rate of 44 percent.[5]

REFERENCES

1. Shawker TH, Doppman JL, Dunnick NR, et al: Ultrasonic investigation of pancreatic islet cell tumors. J Ultrasound Med 1:193–200, 1982
2. Fulton RE, Sheedy PF II, McIlrath DC, et al: Preoperative angiographic localization of insulin producing tumors of the pancreas. Am J Roentgenol 123:367–377, 1975

3. Dangaard-Petersen K, Stage JG: CT scanning in patients with Zollinger-Ellison syndrome and carcinoid syndrome. Scand J Gastroenterol 53:117, 1979
4. Mills SR, Doppman NR, Dunnick NR, et al: Evaluation of angiography in Zollinger-Ellison syndrome. Radiology 131:317–320, 1979
5. Kent RB III, van Heerden JA, Weiland LH: Nonfunctioning islet cell tumors. Ann Surg 193:185–190, 1981

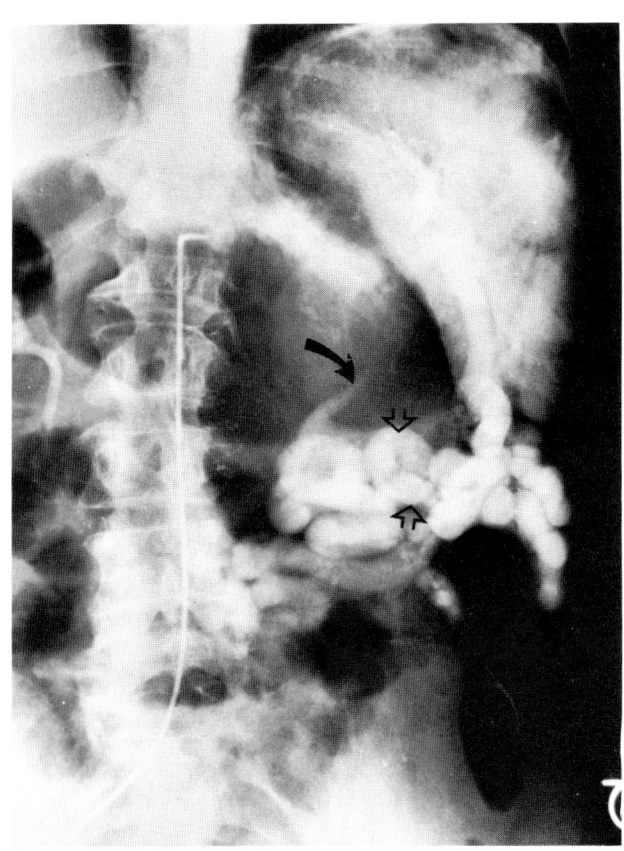

A

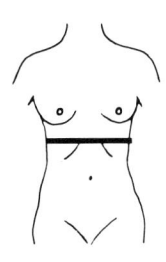

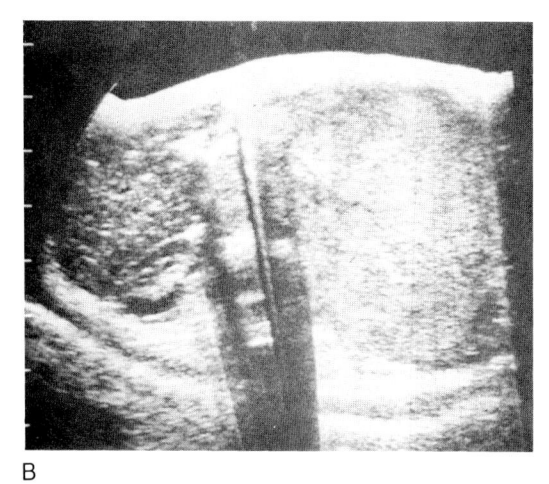

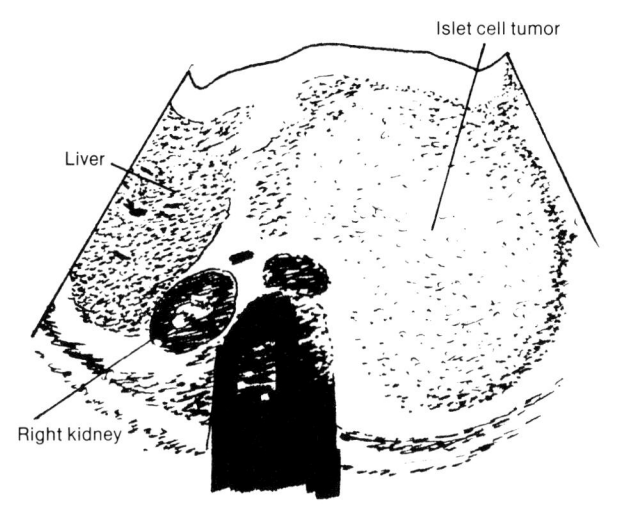

B

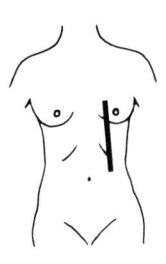

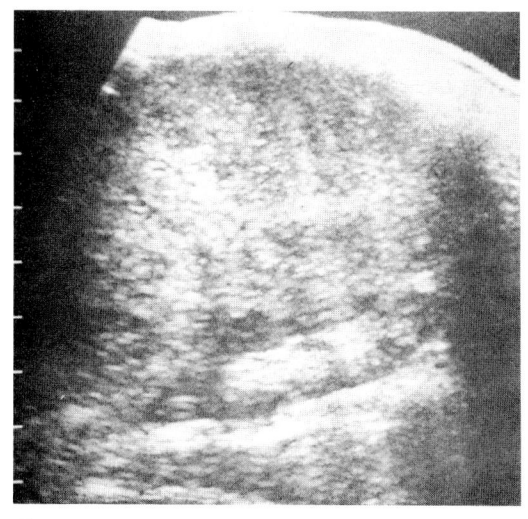

Liver
Islet cell tumor
Right kidney

C

Pancreatic Mass (9.23 and 9.24)

9.23 Pancreatitis or Tumor

A 55-year-old man presented with nausea, epigastric pain, weight loss, and jaundice. The serum bilirubin level was 15 mg/dl, the alkaline phosphatase 417 IU/dl, and serum glutamic oxaloacetic transaminase (SGOT) level was normal.

A transverse sonogram showed a mass in the body and tail of the pancreas (Fig. A). A longitudinal scan showed a grossly dilated common duct (Fig. B) and a further transverse scan showed a dilated pancreatic duct (Fig. C). The patient drank one to two alcoholic drinks per day. A transhepatic cholangiogram in the upright position demonstrated an obstruction in the region of the ampulla of Vater (arrowed, Fig. D). There is minimal irregularity in the cut-off of the duct.

At surgery, the entire pancreas was indurated, with swelling in the head of the pancreas. Transduodenal biopsy specimens showed only fibrosis. Multiple nodes were biopsied and failed to demonstrate tumor. The gallbladder was removed and a Roux-en-Y choledochojejunostomy was performed.

During the subsequent 10 months, the patient experienced progressive loss of weight and abdominal pain. Liver/spleen scan showed inhomogeneity of the left and right lobes of the liver. Ultrasound demonstrated liver metastases which were also confirmed by CT. Specimens from ultrasonically guided liver biopsy yielded adenocarcinoma cells consistent with a pancreatic primary.

This illustrates a frequent problem in the management of these patients. Differentiation between cancer and surrounding pancreatitis may be impossible for the radiologist as well as the surgeon, despite multiple biopsy attempts. At the time of surgery, as many as 25 percent of diagnoses by inspection and palpation alone may be in error.[1] This produces a major dilemma in deciding whether to perform radical as opposed to palliative surgery.

REFERENCE

1. Gudjonsson B, Livstone EM, Spiro HM: Cancer of the pancreas: diagnostic accuracy and survival statistics. Cancer 42:2494–2506, 1978

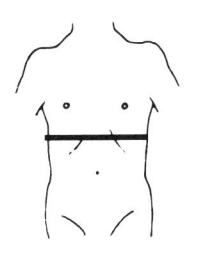

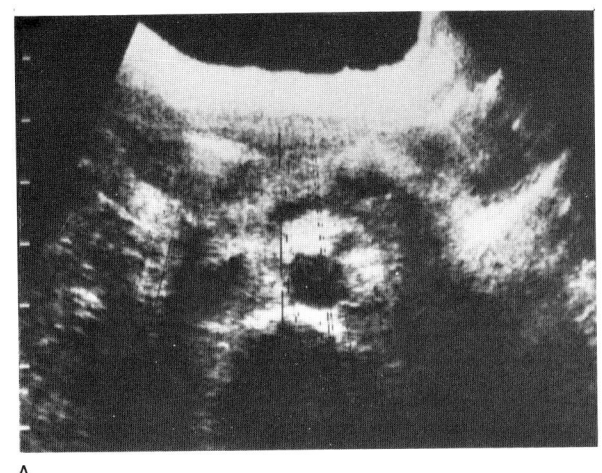

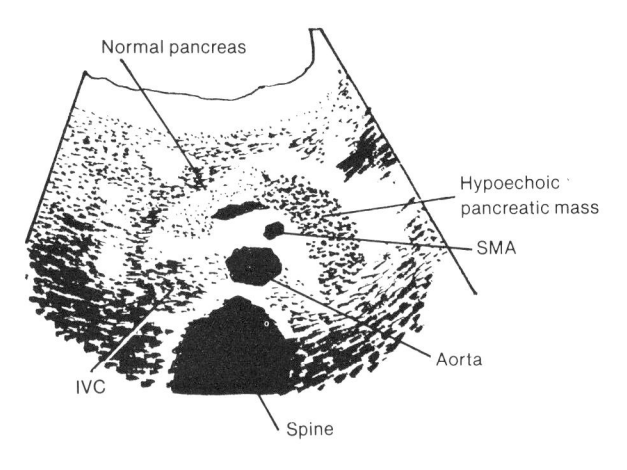

A

	Normal pancreas
	Hypoechoic pancreatic mass
	SMA
	Aorta
IVC	
	Spine

B

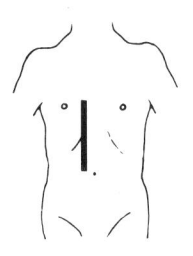

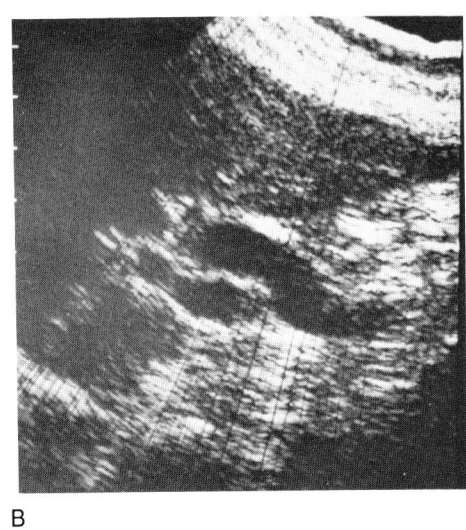

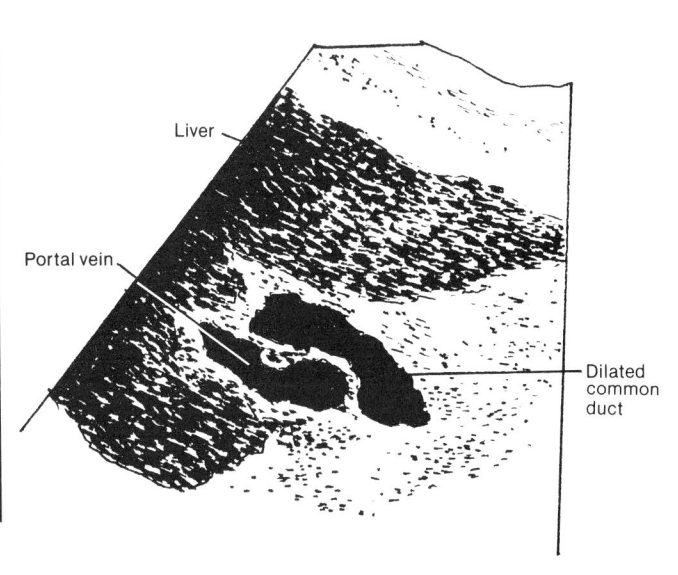

Liver	
Portal vein	
	Dilated common duct

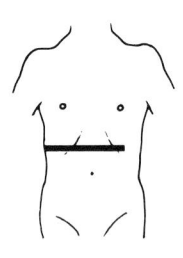

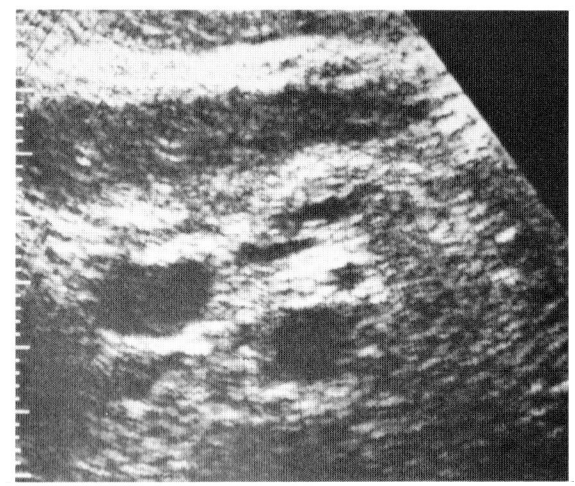

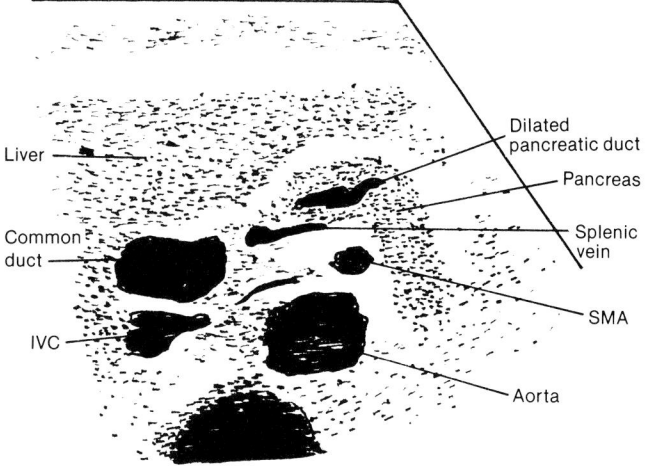

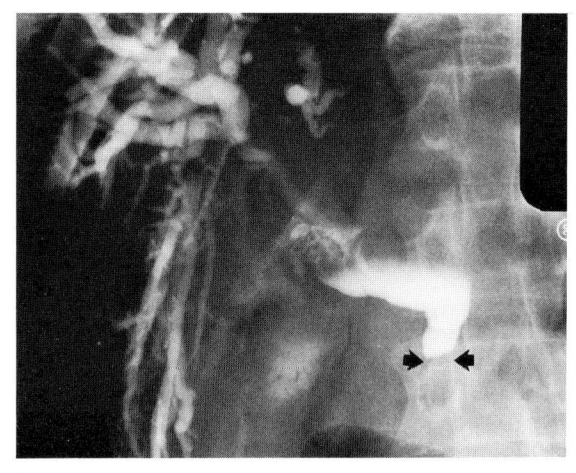

C

D

684

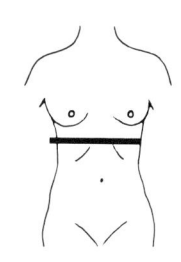

9.24 Pseudopancreatic Mass

A 50-year-old woman with a history of weight loss was referred for pancreatic scanning. The transverse sonogram (Fig. A) demonstrated a normal but rather thin pancreas, but a definite mass was seen at the junction of the body and tail. The possibility of a phlegmon or even a carcinoma was entertained. This morphology could also be related to stomach contents. The patient was then given 12 ounces of water to drink and the mass immediately disappeared, demonstrating that it had been produced by stomach contents (Fig. B).

This demonstrates the invaluable help that can be provided by the use of water ingestion.[1] Numerous difficult clinical problems would fail to be solved unless we used this technique. There is often dramatic improvement in the visualization of the pancreas; also, pseudomasses due to stomach and duodenum can be differentiated. The technique takes practice and often requires time and patience for dissolution of air bubbles. In a study on patients presenting with a clinical suspicion of cancer of the pancreas, we were able to visualize the pancreas adequately in 90 percent. This success in our laboratory can only be obtained through the liberal use of water ingestion.[2]

REFERENCES

1. Crade M, Taylor KJW, Rosenfield AT: Water distention of the gut in the evaluation of the pancreas by ultrasound. AJR 131:348–349, 1978
2. Taylor KJW, Buchin PJ, Viscomi GN, et al: Ultrasonographic scanning of the pancreas: prospective study of clinical results. Radiology 138:211–213, 1981

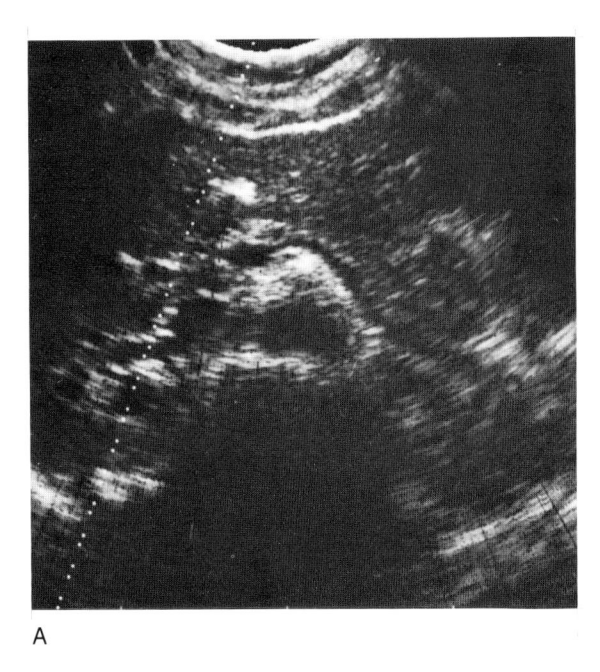

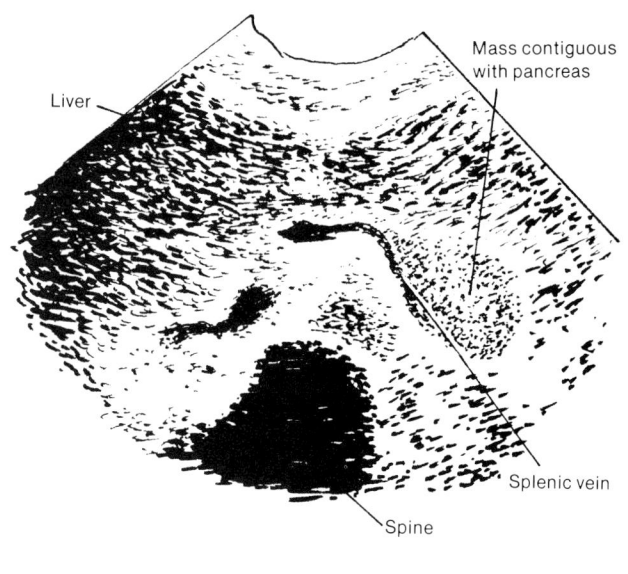

A

Mass contiguous
with pancreas

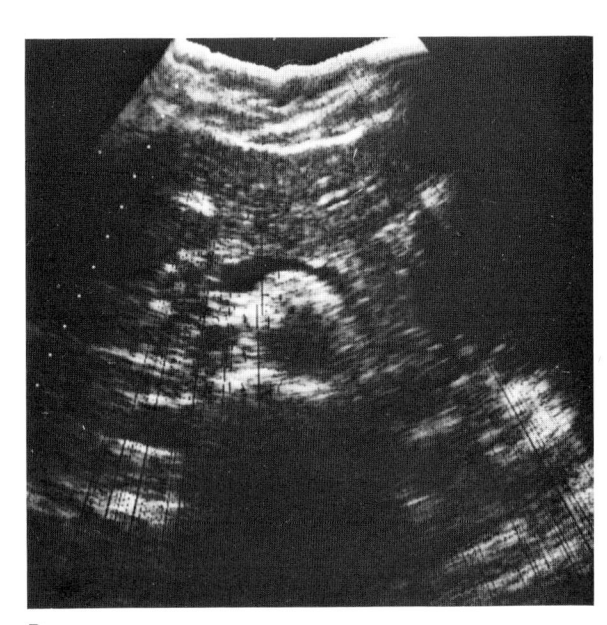

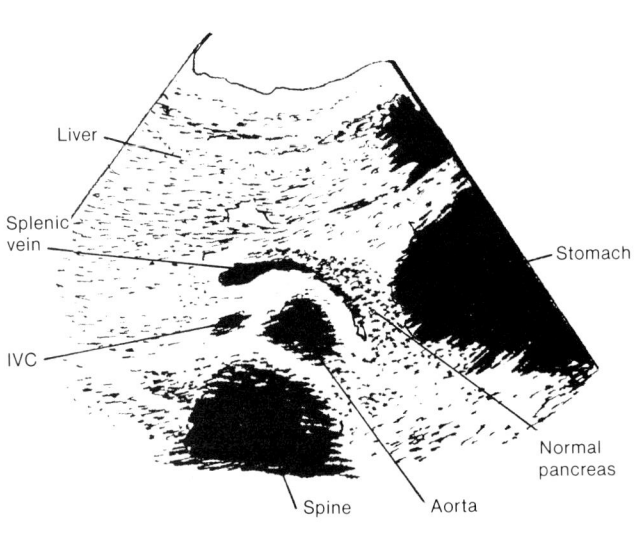

Liver

Splenic vein

Spine

B

Liver

Splenic
vein

Stomach

IVC

Normal
pancreas

Spine   Aorta

686

9.25 Pseudo Pseudocyst

Trauma to the pancreas is often sustained in motor vehicle accidents, especially by persons driving at high speeds without safety belts. On collision, the driver continues to travel forward onto the now stationary steering wheel. Pancreatic avulsion, aortic transection, and splenic rupture may occur.

This patient sustained such an injury, requiring exploratory laparotomy, repair of gut perforation, and splenectomy. Following surgery, chemical pancreatitis prompted referral for ultrasound scanning to rule out a pseudocyst.

The patient was swathed in bandages and limited scans were obtained between dressings. A transverse sonogram showed a well-demarcated cystic lesion lying anterior to the body of the pancreas (Fig. A). This was confirmed on the limited longitudinal scan (Fig. B) and was consistent with a pseudocyst.

A tube was then noted to be emerging from under the dressings and further investigation disclosed that the patient had a gastrostomy involving a Foley catheter. The "pseudocyst" proved to be the catheter balloon; deflating the balloon caused the pseudopseudocyst to disappear.

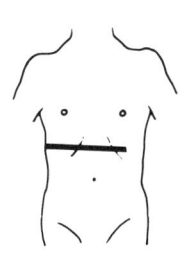

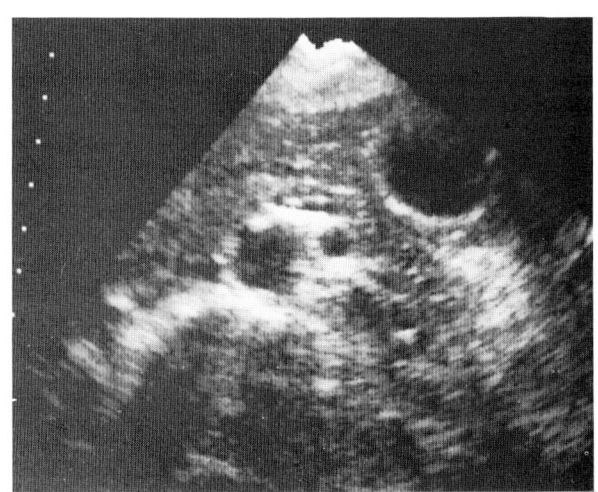

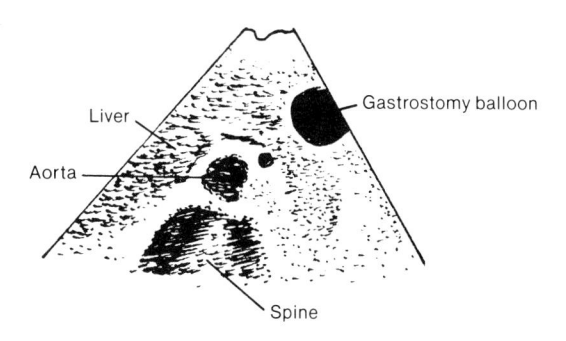

A

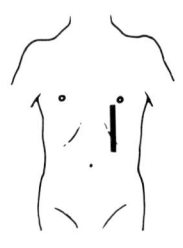

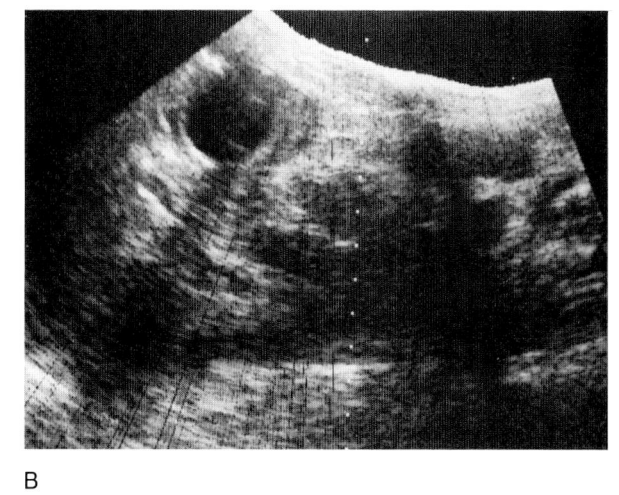

B

9.26 Liquefactive Necrosis (Pancreatic Sac)

A 42-year-old alcoholic man was admitted for recurrent nausea, vomiting, and abdominal pain. He had a long history of acute pancreatitis, and recurrent pseudocyst formation with spontaneous drainage. On admission, he reported a 90-lb weight loss over the preceding year. He had developed insulin-dependent diabetes. A longitudinal sonogram of the abdomen demonstrated an hypoechoic pancreatic mass (Fig. A). A transverse scan demonstrated a complex mass in the body of the pancreas (Fig. B).

ERCP showed a stricture of the intrahepatic part of the common bile duct. The proximal main pancreatic duct communicated freely with a large cystic structure which replaced the entire body and tail of the pancreas (Fig. C). A CT scan demonstrated the extent of the pancreatic sac with its contained contrast material (Fig. D).

At laparotomy, the pancreas was found to be completely destroyed and replaced by a sac containing debris the consistency of toothpaste. This mass did not displace the adjacent viscera. A Roux-en-Y gastrostomy was performed and the patient's recovery was uneventful.

Complications of pancreatitis include pancreatic phlegmon, pseudocyst, and abscess. Differentiation is important since the treatment varies. Ultrasound in this patient did not allow adequate differentiation between these entities and the pancreatic sac which was well-demonstrated by CT after contrast injection. Liquefactive pancreatic necrosis resulting in a pancreatic sac appears to be a distinct type of pseudocyst which totally replaces the pancreas and communicates with the ductal system.[1] This is in contrast to the common pseudocyst, which arises from the pancreas and displaces the duct.

(This case and Scans A and B and Figs. C and D taken from Burrell MI, Gold JA, Simeone J, et al: Liquefactive necrosis of the pancreas. The pancreatic sac. Radiology 135:157–160, 1980.)

REFERENCE

1. Burrell M, Gold JA, Simeone J, et al. Liquefactive necrosis of the pancreas. Radiology 135:157–160, 1980

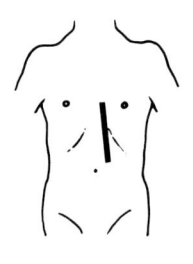

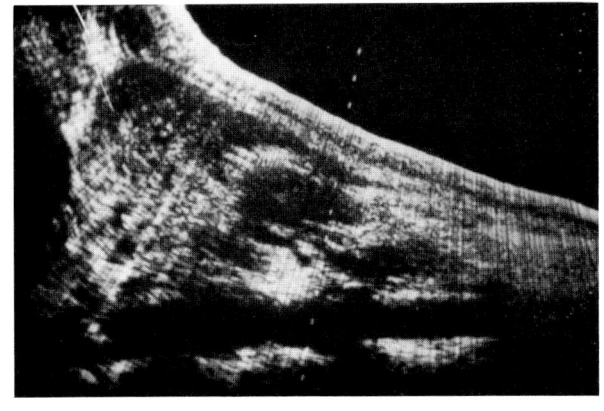

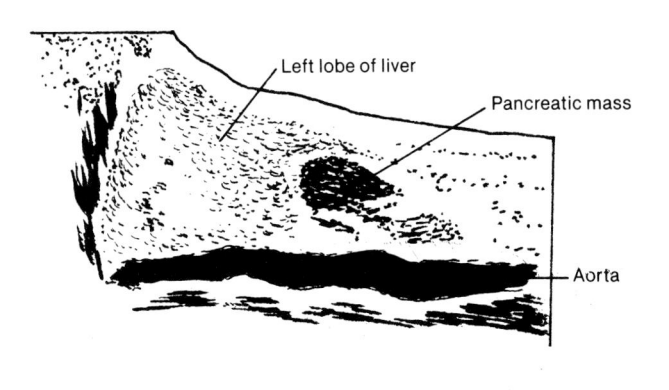

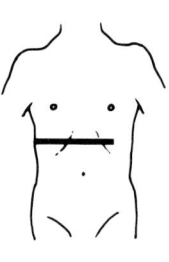

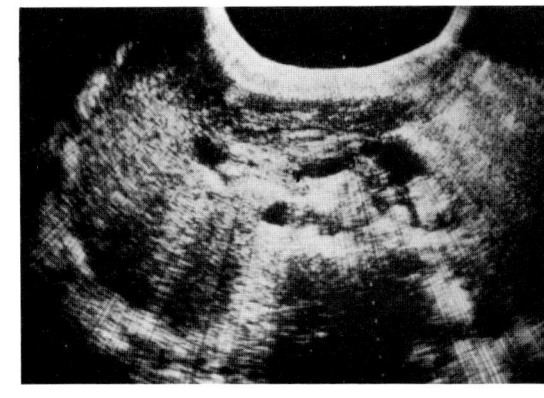

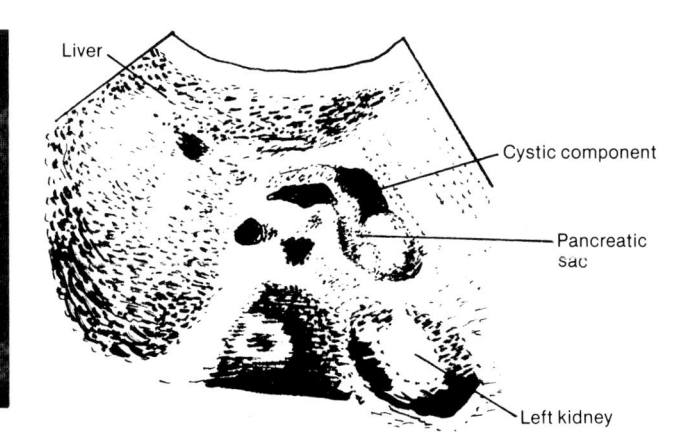

A

B

690

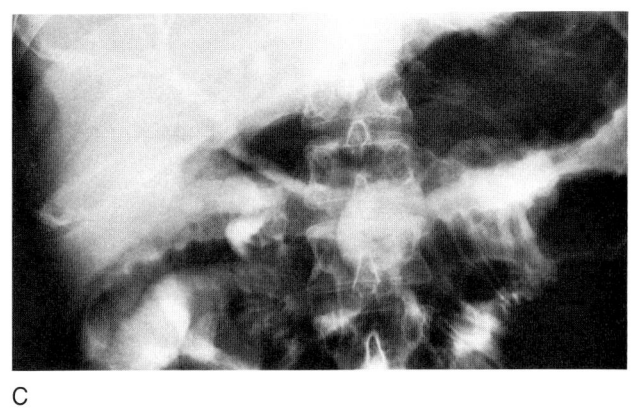

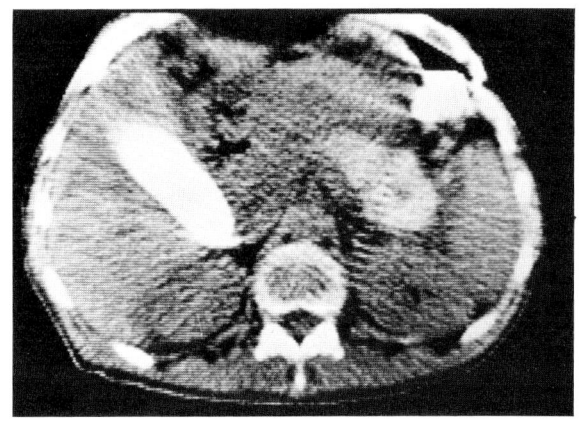

C

D

10 The Spleen

KENNETH J.W. TAYLOR

Scanning Techniques (10.1 to 10.3)

10.1 A-Scan

The spleen is a difficult organ to evaluate clinically since it is concealed under the left costal margin. Considerable enlargement must occur before it is clinically palpable, and even then clinical assessment of the consistency of the organ is of little diagnostic value. The spleen is most often imaged by a liver/spleen isotope scan using ^{99m}Tc-labeled sulfur colloid, but this merely shows nonspecific space-occupying defects and an approximation of splenic size.

Ultrasound has been used to estimate the volume of the spleen.[1] The introduction of gray-scale techniques, which resulted in the display of the normal tissue consistency, permits small lesions to be defined and their solid or cystic nature differentiated.

The spleen is a difficult organ to scan if it is of normal size; scanning becomes progressively easier as the size increases. The normal-sized spleen must be scanned either obliquely along the 10th intercostal space or in the coronal plane in the midaxillary line. The enlarged spleen may be examined by either technique, but may also be scanned by simple parasagittal scans such as those used for the liver or by simple transverse scanning.

An A-scan through an enlarged spleen shows very low level echoes arising from within the organ; large echoes are seen proximally from the initial pulse and a larger distal echo from the capsule of the spleen, as shown in the figure. It is important not to confuse these appearances with those due to fluid collections, such as a left subphrenic abscess.

Accessory spleens are extremely common and are found in 20–30 percent of autopsies.[2] They are usually found near the tail of the pancreas and may simulate a tumor on ultrasound scanning. Uptake of ^{99m}Tc sulfur colloid allows specific identification of splenic tissue.

Sonographers should also be familiar with the entity referred to as a "wandering spleen." This is the abnormal location of the spleen due to a long pedicle,[3] and occurs especially in pregnant and multiparous women. The entity should be recalled when an abnormal mass is found in the abdomen or pelvis and the spleen is absent from its usual position. Real-time ultrasound examination demonstrates the mobility of the mass with movement of the patient. A ^{99m}Tc sulfur colloid scan allows specific recognition of the position of the organ by splenic uptake.[4]

REFERENCES

1. Kardel T, Holm HH, Rasmussen SN, et al: Ultrasonic determination of liver and spleen volumes. Scand J Clin Lab Invest 27:123–128, 1971
2. Robbins SL: Pathologic Basis of Disease. W.B. Saunders, Philadelphia, 1974
3. Miller EI: Wandering spleen and pregnancy: case report. J Clin Ultrasound 3:281–282, 1975
4. Carswell JW: Wandering spleen: 11 cases from Uganda. Br J Surg 61:495–497, 1974

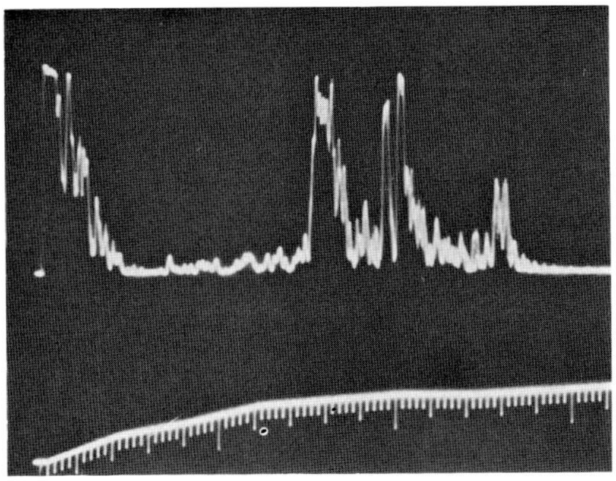

10.2 Oblique Intercostal Scans

For the oblique intercostal scan of the spleen, the patient lies in the right lateral (decubitus) position. It is often helpful to abduct and fully extend the arm, which tends to widen the left intercostal spaces. Occasionally it may be necessary to use a pillow under the right side of the patient to widen the left intercostal spaces further. The costal margin is now identified in the region of the midaxillary line and the plane of the lowest intercostal space is defined. The skin is liberally coated with mineral oil and the transducer placed on the chest wall just anterior to the midaxillary line. The characteristic A-scan through the spleen is shown in Figure 10.1. There are very low level echoes from the splenic consistency and a large distal echo from the capsule.

The position of the transducer is adjusted to allow a scan along the intercostal space. To maintain contact with the skin it may be necessary to angle the transducer cephalad. The spleen is now scanned along the 10th intercostal space (Fig. A). In this position, it will be found that the spleen is surprisingly anterior, lying between the midaxillary line and the left anterior subcostal margin. If the spleen is not satisfactorily imaged in this intercostal space, a higher intercostal space should be used. The advantage of this scan is that the longitudinal axis of the spleen lies along the intercostal space, so that scans of this axis allow us to quantitate splenic size. The resulting scan is shown in Figure B. The alternative to this oblique intercostal scan is the coronal scan.

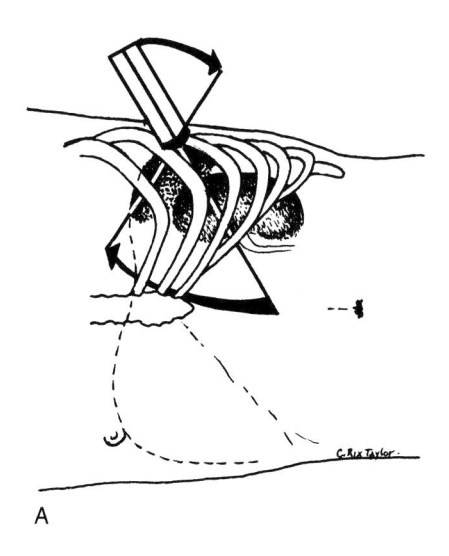

A

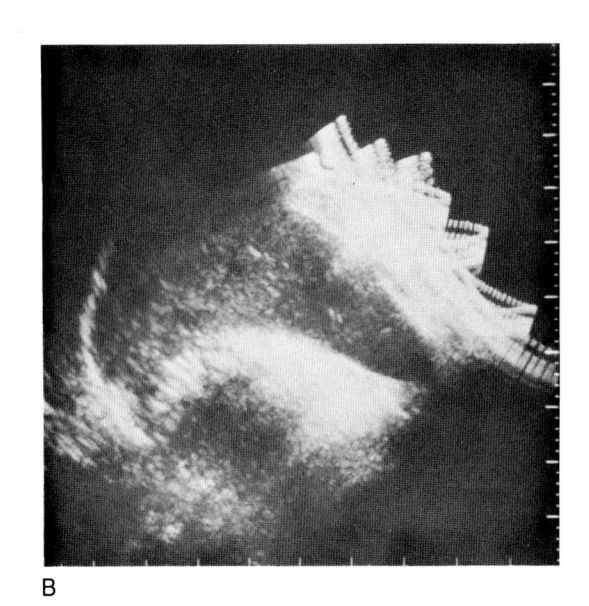

B

10.3 Coronal Scan

Again the patient is scanned in the right lateral (decubitus) position. The transducer is aligned with the patient's body and the lower intercostal spaces are identified in the midaxillary line. The skin is again liberally coated with paraffin oil and small sector scans are made in the lowest intercostal space. These scans are carried out in deep inspiration, since this rotates the lower ribs and increases the size of the intercostal spaces. In very thin patients, there may be difficulty in maintaining skin contact, and a generous quantity of aqueous gel may be valuable as a coupling medium in preference to the cheaper paraffin oil. Extreme rotation of the transducer may be required to record the left hemidiaphragm. This is shown schematically in Figure A. The spleen is seen as a highly homogeneous organ lying between the upper pole of the left kidney and the left hemidiaphragm. A spleen scan obtained by this technique is shown in Figure B. Mechanical sector scanners or sector-phased arrays are most helpful in scanning the left upper quadrant.

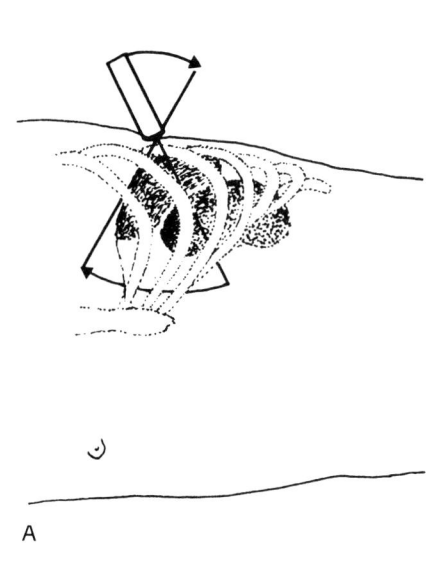

A

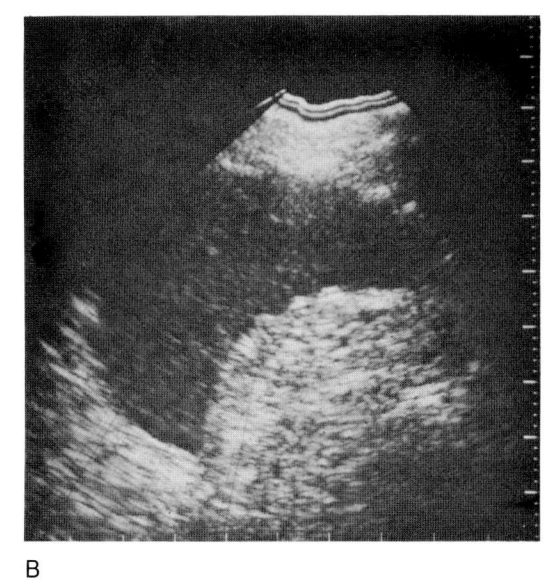

B

10.4 Congenital Cysts

A 29-year-old woman presented with an asymptomatic left upper quadrant mass. There was no history of previous trauma nor of parasitic infestation. Clinical examination disclosed an apparently enlarged spleen and results of laboratory tests were normal. A liver/spleen scan showed an enlarged spleen with multiple filling defects.

A coronal scan of the spleen (Fig. A) showed multiple echo-free, well-circumscribed focal lesions in the spleen consistent with multiple cysts. This was confirmed at surgery which disclosed multiple epithelial-lined cysts of congenital origin (Fig. B).

Bhimji et al. reported the sonographic features of epithelial cysts of the spleen.[1] Splenic cysts may be congenital or acquired (true cysts or pseudocysts resulting from trauma). Worldwide, parasitic cysts are most common almost invariably due to *Echinococcus*. In the United States, pseudocysts are more common, accounting for 80 percent of all splenic cysts. Thus, the epithelial-lined true cyst of the spleen found in this patient is a relatively rare entity.

(This case and figures taken from Dembner AG, Taylor KJW: Grey-scale sonographic diagnosis: multiple congenital splenic cysts. J Clin Ultrasound 6:173–174, 1978. © 1978 John Wiley & Sons, Inc. Reprinted by permission of John Wiley & Sons, Inc.)

REFERENCE

1. Bhimji SD, Cooperberg PL, Naiman S, et al: Ultrasound diagnosis of splenic cysts. Radiology 122:787–789, 1977

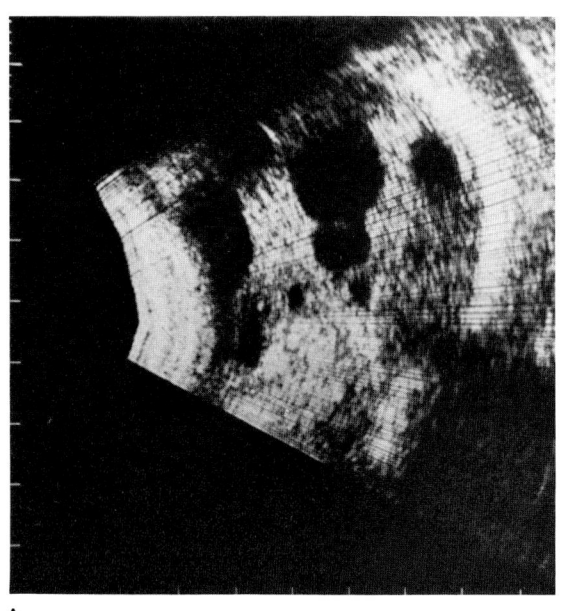

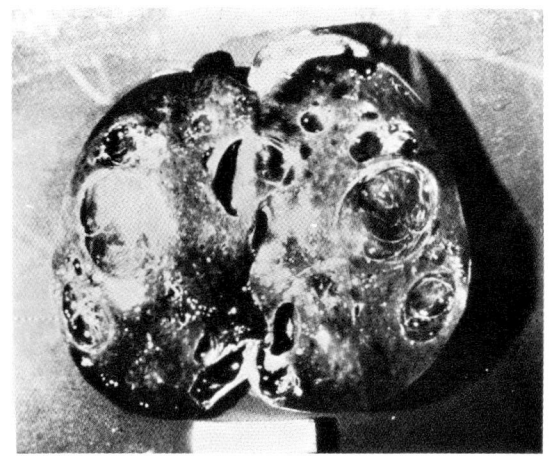

A

B

10.5 Traumatic Hematoma

A 24-year-old pregnant woman was noted to have a left upper quadrant mass when admitted in labor. After delivery the mass was investigated. The transverse sonogram (Fig. A) revealed a mass lying anterior to the spleen but apparently possessing a similar structure to the spleen. The longitudinal sonogram (Fig. B) showed a uniform mass lying between the upper pole of the left kidney and the compressed spleen. The differential diagnosis included a suprarenal tumor, a retroperitoneal lymphoma, and an organizing splenic hematoma. An isotope scan revealed a large splenic defect. Intravenous pyelography showed downward displacement of the left kidney. CT scanning confirmed the presence of a solid left upper quadrant mass. Surgery was delayed for approximately 6 weeks and revealed a splenic cyst with changed blood in its walls, indicating its origin from a hematoma.

There appears to be no doubt that this was an organizing hematoma at the time of the investigation, which resulted in a cyst after further organization of the clot. Undue delay between an ultrasound examination and surgery may result in apparent discrepancies and the skeptical surgeon may not appreciate that change has occurred. Repeat examination immediately before surgery in this patient would have demonstrated the then-fluid contents and modified the surgical incision.

Patients with posttraumatic cysts may not recall the precipitating trauma. They have presented as long as 40 years after the responsible trauma.[1] Propper et al. described two patients with hemorrhagic cysts of the spleen, in whom ultrasound disclosed gravity-dependent layering of two fluids of differing echogenicity.[2] The symptoms are usually those of a slowly enlarging mass, but hypersplenism has also been noted.[3]

McClure and Altemeier recognized that splenic pseudocysts resulted from an encysted hematoma due to intrasplenic injury.[4] The hematoma becomes walled off and organizes to form a cyst; the capsule may calcify. Transformation of the hemorrhage into serous contents may take weeks or years. The possibility of a splenic hemorrhagic cyst should be considered when an intrasplenic mass contains low-level echoes or there is a fluid–fluid level. On a CT scan, the Hounsfield number should allow specific recognition of attenuation by blood.

REFERENCES

1. Fowler RF: Non-parasitic benign cystic tumors of the spleen. Int Abstr Surg 96:209, 1953
2. Propper RA, Weinstein BJ, Skolnick ML, Kisloff B: Ultrasonography of hemorrhagic splenic cysts. J Clin Ultrasound 7:18–20, 1979
3. Janin Y, Strauss R, Katz S, et al: Splenic pseudocyst associated with hypersplenism. Am J Gastroenterol 75:289–293, 1981
4. McClure RD, Altemeier WA: Cysts of the spleen. Ann Surg 116:98–102, 1942

702

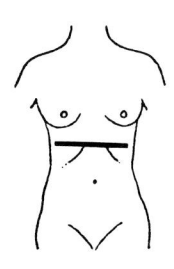

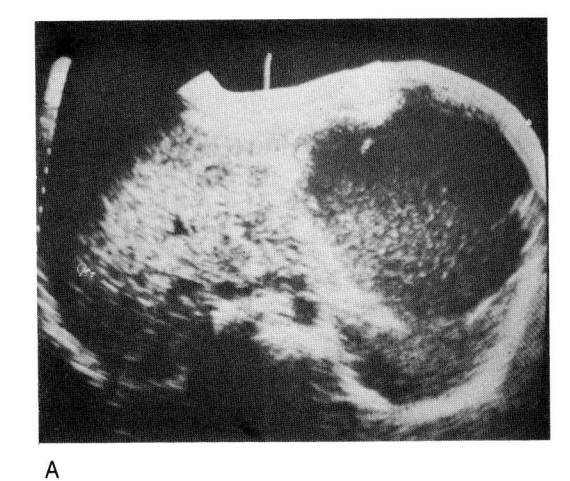

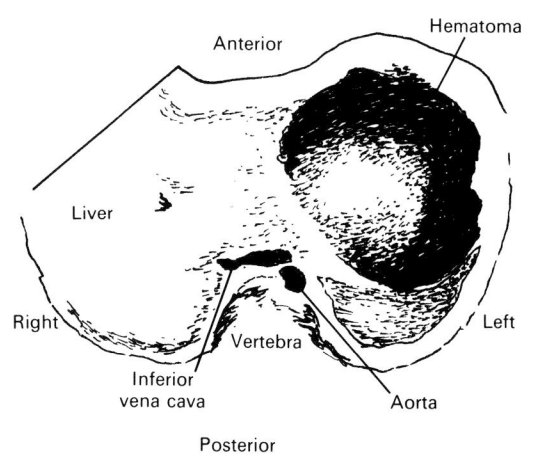

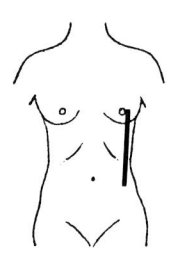

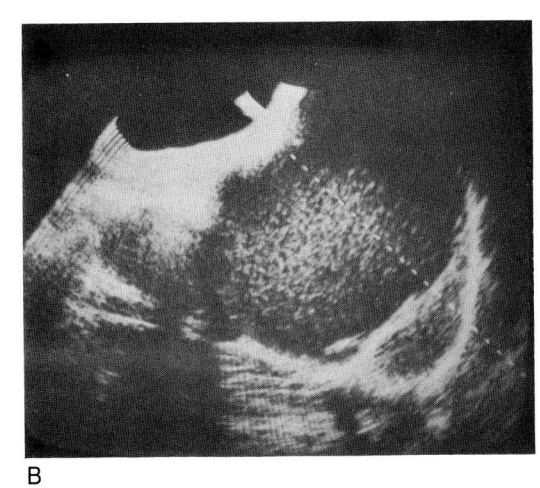

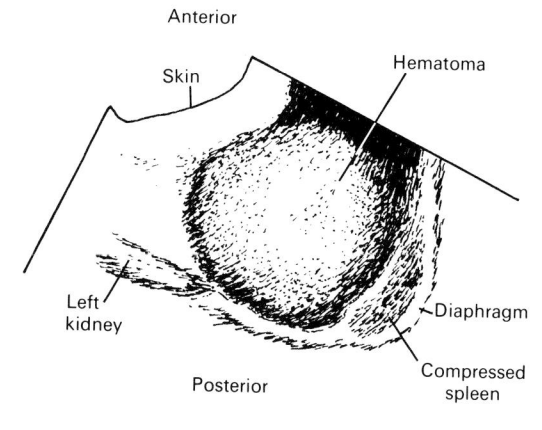

10.6 Pseudocyst

A 12-year-old boy presented with a large palpable left upper quadrant mass and a history of previous injury to the left lower ribs.

A longitudinal scan in the left parasagittal plane (Fig. A) showed a large, echo-free area anterior to the left kidney with a rim of compressed splenic tissue.

These appearances were confirmed on a transverse scan with the patient in the decubitus position (Fig. B). Again, the compressed spleen was seen between the upper pole of the left kidney and the cyst.

Pseudocysts have no true cellular lining as compared with true cysts which have an epithelial lining. In this country, pseudocysts are about four times more common than primary cysts.[1] They are specifically associated with trauma in childhood, whether the trauma is recalled or not. About 70 percent of these patients are asymptomatic.[2] The symptoms are most commonly due to progressive distention. When patients are asymptomatic, the mass may be found incidentally on physical examination.

An extensive differential diagnosis and the imaging modalities available have been considered in the literature.[3] On plain film, calcification may be seen in the cyst wall in about 10 percent of patients, especially if the cyst is echinococcal or posttraumatic in origin. The left hemidiaphragm may be elevated on the chest radiograph. An intravenous urogram demonstrates downward displacement of the left kidney and the stomach is usually displaced medially.

Ultrasound allows a definitive diagnosis of intrasplenic cystic masses which often precludes the need for other imaging modalities. The CT findings are rather repetitive of those seen on ultrasound, although they may be helpful in the diagnosis of a hemorrhagic cyst. If there is any doubt as to the relation of the spleen to the mass, liver/spleen scintigraphy is a valuable and specific way of identifying splenic tissue. Typical appearances have been described for splenic cysts.[4]

REFERENCES

1. Kaufman RA, Silver TM, Wesley JR: Preoperative diagnosis of splenic cysts in children by gray-scale ultrasonography. J Pediatr Surg 14:450–454, 1979
2. Blank E, Campbell JR: Epidermoid cysts of the spleen. Pediatrics 51:75–84, 1973
3. Faer MJ, Lynch RD, Lichtenstein JE, et al: RPC from the AFIP. Radiology 134:371–376, 1980
4. Pearson HA, Touloukian RJ, Spencer RP: The binary spleen: a radioisotopic scan sign of splenic pseudocyst. J Pediatr 77:216–220, 1970

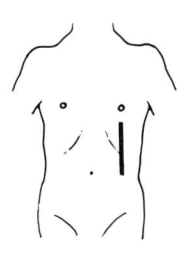

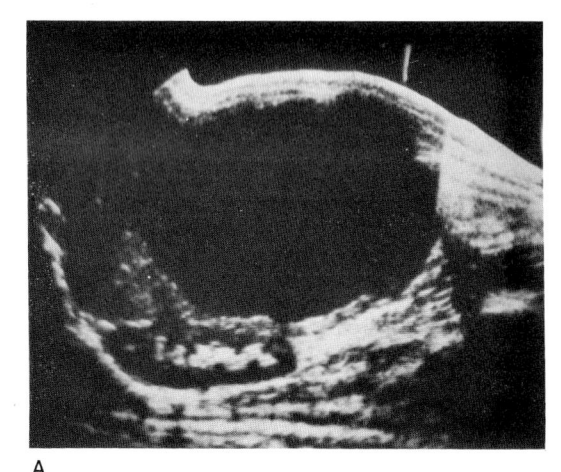

A

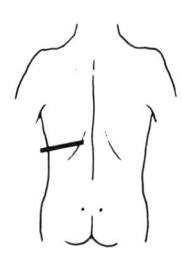

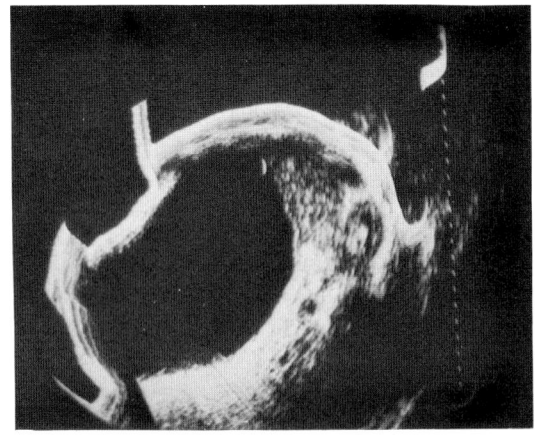

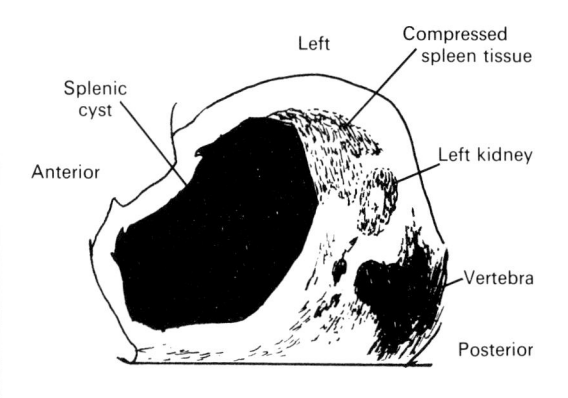

B

Left
Compressed spleen tissue
Splenic cyst
Anterior
Left kidney
Vertebra
Posterior

10.7 Splenic Phlegmon

A 25-year-old white woman presented with a history of 3 days of generalized abdominal pain and 18 hours of vomiting. The pain was constant and periumbilical in location. On examination, her temperature was 102°F and the diagnosis of acute cholecystitis was entertained. Ultrasound examination, however, demonstrated a normal gallbladder without evidence of cholelithiasis. She was therefore taken to the operating room where a ruptured appendix and appendiceal abscess were found. Postoperatively, she remained febrile to 101°F, despite antibiotic therapy. The day after antibiotics were discontinued, her chest radiograph showed a left pleural effusion. A repeat ultrasound scan in the coronal plane, shown in the figure, demonstrated a left pleural effusion and a left subphrenic, perisplenic abscess. The spleen itself was hyperechoic. She was returned to the operating room where a subdiaphragmatic abscess with a splenic phlegmon was found. Splenectomy was performed without complication and the patient subsequently had an uneventful recovery.

This case demonstrates the importance of knowing the patient's clinical history when interpreting sonograms. A subcapsular hematoma presents identical appearances to those of phlegmon,[1] but the clinical history of sepsis, supported by the presence of a sympathetic pleural effusion, indicated the diagnosis. Paresis of the diaphragm may occur, but in our experience this has been an unreliable sign of a subphrenic abscess.

(This case and scan taken from de Graaff CS, Taylor KJW, Jacobson P: Grey scale echography of the spleen. Follow-up in 67 patients. Ultrasound Med Biol 5:13–21, 1979. Pergamon Press, Ltd. Reprinted with permission.)

REFERENCE

1. Johnson MA, Cooperberg PL, Boisvert J, et al: Spontaneous splenic rupture in infectious mononucleosis: Sonographic diagnosis and follow-up. AJR 136:111–114, 1981

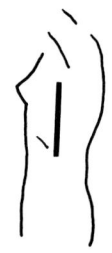

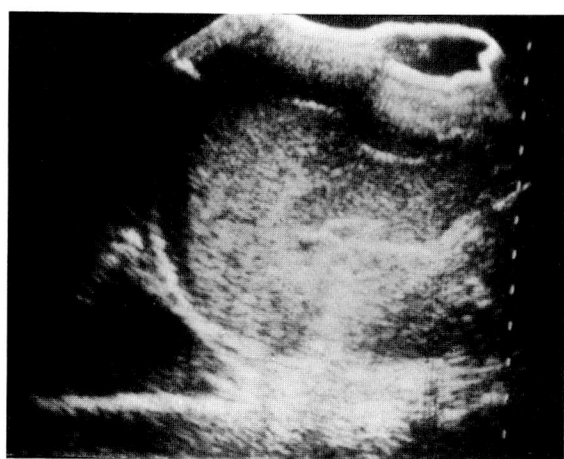

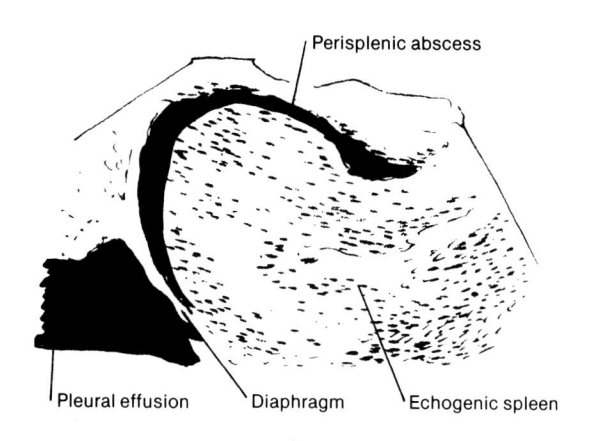

Perisplenic abscess

Pleural effusion   Diaphragm   Echogenic spleen

Abscess (10.8 and 10.9)

10.8 Abscess Related to Drug Abuse

A 23-year-old male drug addict was admitted with fever of unknown origin. Physical examination showed multiple infected needle puncture sites. Echocardiography revealed a fungal vegetation which necessitated mitral valve replacement. Following surgery the patient again presented with fever of unknown origin and was referred for ultrasound evaluation.

A transverse sonogram demonstrated a large hypoechoic region on the lateral aspect of the spleen (Fig. A). This was confirmed on the coronal view (Fig. B). The appearances were those either of a hemorrhagic infarct of the spleen or an intrasplenic abscess. In either case, the patient required long-term antibiotic treatment of his endocarditis and the splenic lesion was treated conservatively. A repeat scan 7 months later demonstrated a significant decrease in the size of the lesion (Fig. C). The lesion had also become better circumscribed. From ultrasound appearances alone, one cannot differentiate between a hemorrhagic infarct and a splenic abscess. In this patient, the clinical history supported the diagnosis of an abscess.

Dubbins described the sonographic appearance of an abscess as a hypoechoic intrasplenic mass.[1] Isolated abscesses of the spleen are rare. Only 10 such patients were reported in 100,000 admissions to the Cleveland Metropolitan Hospital over a 10-year period.[2] However, as intravenous narcotic abuse resulting in endocarditis has increased in recent years, hemorrhagic infarcts of the spleen have become more common. Some of these may progress to abscess formation.

REFERENCES

1. Dubbins PA: Ultrasound in the diagnosis of splenic abscess. Br J Radiol 53:488–489, 1980
2. Chulay JD, Lankerani MR: Splenic abscess. Report of 10 cases and review of the literature. Am J Med 61:513–522, 1976

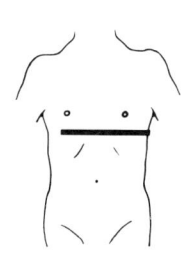

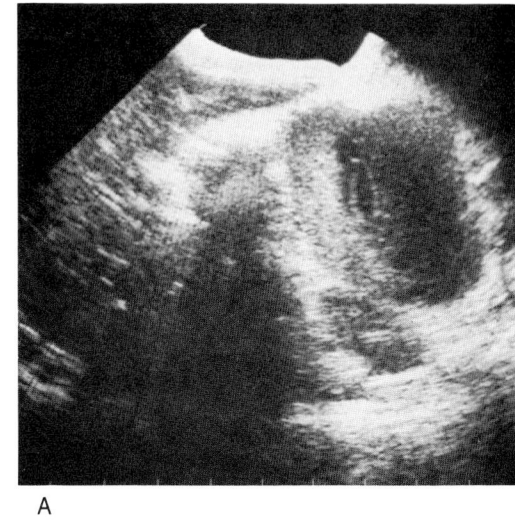

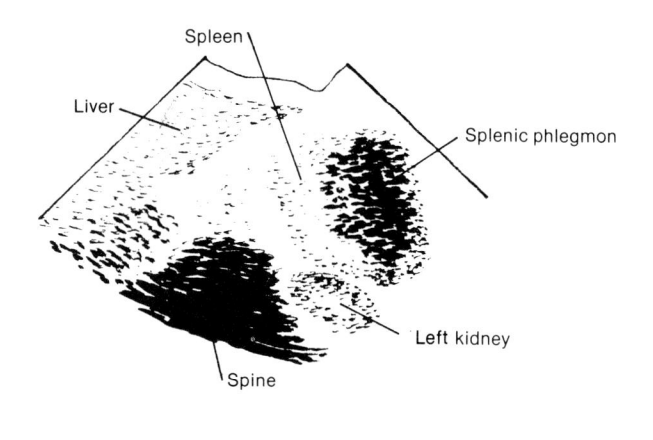

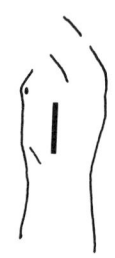

A

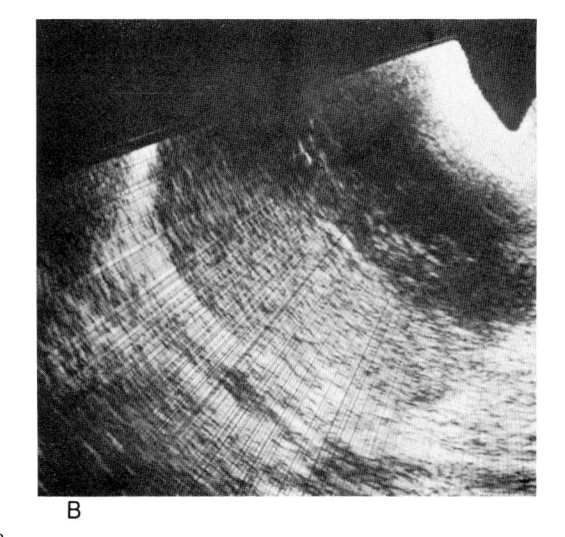

Liver — Spleen
Splenic phlegmon
Left kidney
Spine

B

708

Abscess

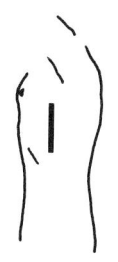

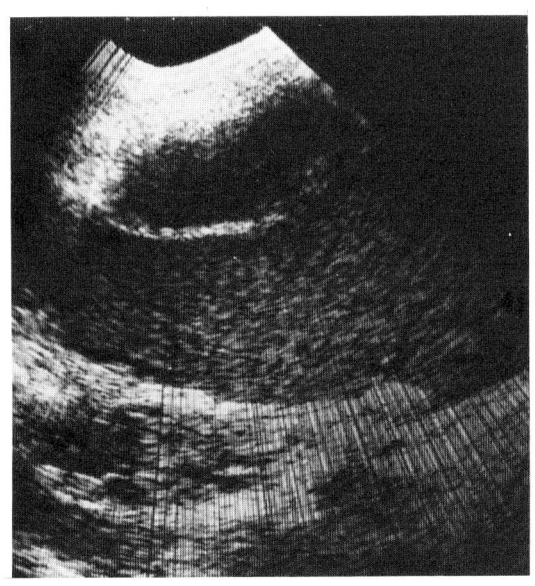

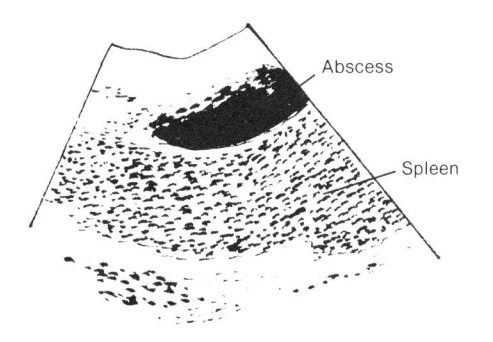

Spleen

C

10.9 Gas-Containing Abscess

A 68-year-old woman was admitted with fevers to 107°F and a history of adenocarcinoma of the cervix. On physical examination, recurrent tumor was noted in the vagina, and an enlarged spleen was also present. A coronal sonogram (Fig. A) demonstrated an ill-defined hypoechoic area within the spleen with a focus of high-intensity reverberating echoes on the surface of the lesion (arrowed). These reverberating echoes indicated air within an otherwise homogeneous lesion. These appearances suggested an intrasplenic abscess.

The same findings were demonstrated and were easier to interpret on the corresponding CT examination (arrowed in Fig. B). A ^{67}gallium scan showed increased uptake in the region of the splenic hilum. At surgery, a tumor mass was found with a fistula into the splenic hilum producing a gas-containing abscess. In view of the recurrent tumor, the ^{67}gallium scan was nonspecific for an inflammatory or a neoplastic mass and was noncontributory to the diagnosis.

The presence of air is suggestive of abscess formation but nitrogen may also be produced by noninfected tissue necrosis. For example, air in a pancreatic phlegmon has been documented without the presence of infection.

Of five splenic abscesses diagnosed by Ralls et al., four were relatively anechoic and one was echogenic due to a gas-containing abscess.[1] Splenic abscesses are very rare and occurred in less than 0.7 percent of a large autopsy series.[2] Forty percent of these were from bacterial endocarditis. Symptoms include left upper quadrant pain, tenderness, and fever, and mortality is high unless effective treatment is instituted.

Sangupta and Mukherjie[3] reported that 75 percent of splenic abscesses were due to hematogenous spread from an infected focus elsewhere. Ten percent were due to local sepsis, for example, carcinoma of the colon, and 15 percent followed trauma to the spleen.[3]

(This case and figures taken from Sommer FG, Gonzalez R, Taylor KJW: Computed tomography and ultrasound findings of a gas-containing splenic abscess. Yale J Biol Med 53:161–163, 1980.)

REFERENCES

1. Ralls PW, Quinn MF, Colletti P, et al: Sonography of pyogenic splenic abscess. AJR 138:523–525, 1982
2. Chun CH, Raff MJ, Contreras L, et al: Splenic abscess. Medicine 59:50–65, 1980
3. Sengupta D, Mukherjee B: Amoebic abscess of the spleen. J Indian Med Assoc 64:45–47, 1975

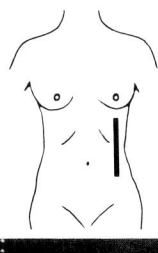

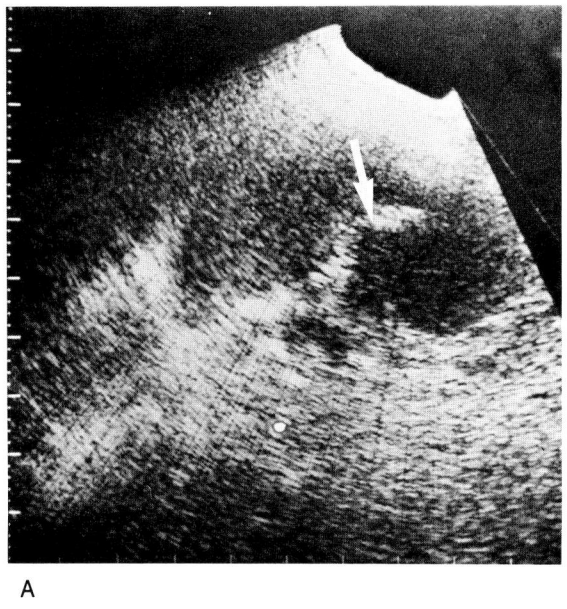

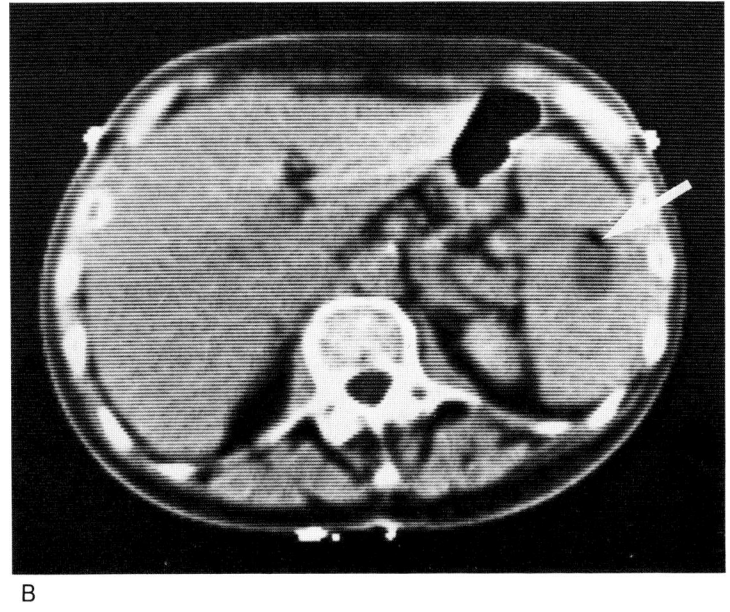

A

B

711

10.10 Infarct

A 22-year-old man with congenital aortic stenosis presented with acute bacterial endocarditis and signs of peripheral emboli. He was referred for ultrasound examination to investigate the possibility of other septic foci.

A longitudinal sonogram through the spleen in the midaxillary line showed definite splenic enlargement with a highly reflective mass just below the left hemidiaphragm, as shown in the figure. These appearances suggested a mass of fibrous tissue and were consistent with a splenic infarct associated with his bacterial endocarditis.

The appearances of a splenic infarct were reported by Itoh et al. in 1978.[1] A wedge-shaped echogenic area was seen which correlated well with the pathologic specimen. Splenic infarcts are common in bacterial endocarditis, myelofibrosis, leukemia, and lupus erythematosus. Repeated infarction in sickle cell anemia may result in autosplenectomy.

REFERENCE

1. Itoh K, Hayashi A, Kawai T, et al: Echography of splenic infarct in a case of systemic lupus erythematosis. J Clin Ultrasound 6: 113–114, 1978

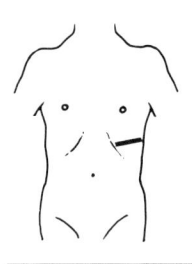

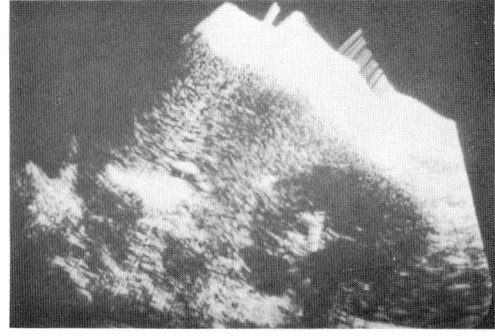

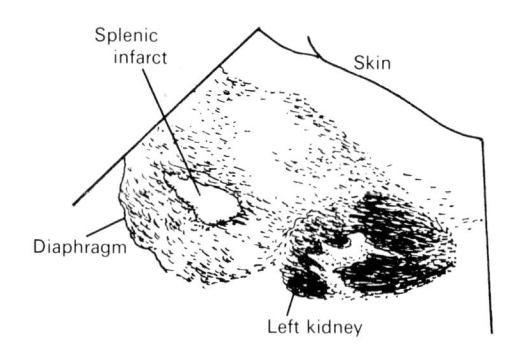

10.11 Autosplenectomy

An 18-year-old black woman had many previous admissions for sickle cell disease. Her brother had died of the disease at the age of 20. She had had multiple previous sickle cell crises since the age of 4 and now required frequent transfusions because of her painful crises. Gallstones had been noted by ultrasound when she was 9.

A liver/spleen scan demonstrated absence of the spleen, which was probably a result of autosplenectomy following multiple splenic infarcts. A coronal sonogram of the splenic fossa demonstrated a small mass containing multiple echogenic nodules, consistent with multiple previous infarcts (arrowed in the figure). In view of the asplenia on the liver/spleen scan, it is apparent that she had no functioning splenic tissue remaining.

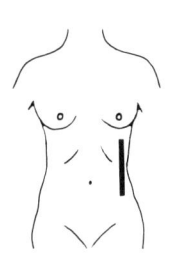

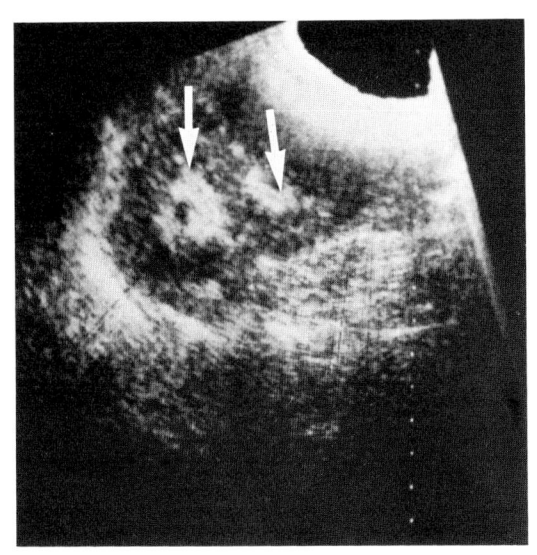

10.12 Rupture

A 14-year-old boy presented with infectious mononucleosis and developed signs of blood loss. His hematocrit dropped from 38 to 27 percent. Marked splenomegaly was present with a longitudinal axis of 20 cm (normal is less than 11 cm) (Fig. A). On a transverse scan, free fluid was seen around the liver, extending down the right flank (Fig. B). In the pelvis, a longitudinal scan showed a large collection lying superior to the bladder and filling the pelvis (Fig. C). This was assumed to be spontaneous rupture of the spleen due to infectious mononucleosis. The radionuclide liver/spleen scan demonstrated no splenic defect. There was considerable discussion about the advisability of surgery but since the patient was stable, a splenectomy was deferred. He underwent a splenic arteriogram to rule out a ruptured spleen. The arteriogram showed an intact spleen and the patient was discharged with a hematocrit of 39 percent.

Miller et al. reported sonographic demonstration of a subcapsular hematoma as a sign of splenic rupture in a patient with infectious mononucleosis.[1] Generally, a ^{99m}Tc sulfur colloid scan is considered to be the initial examination in suspected splenic rupture.[2] However, in this patient, the radionuclide scan was falsely negative. This demonstrates the value of ultrasound under this circumstance to document free peritoneal fluid.

Johnson et al.[3] reported three patients with ruptured spleens due to infectious mononucleosis, which were all diagnosed by ultrasound. Two showed pericapsular collections and one showed free intraperitoneal fluid, as in this patient.

Splenic trauma is common in children and may occur from any blow to the left lower ribs whether there is a fracture or not. This case demonstrates a conservative approach to splenic rupture which has become accepted surgical practice, especially in children. This has resulted from the recognition of the "postsplenectomy syndrome." King and Schumacker noted that fatal sepsis after splenectomy occurred more frequently in children than in adults. A subsequent review demonstrated that the death rate from sepsis was 60 times greater in children following splenectomy than in the normal control cases.[4] Postsplenectomy sepsis consists of rapidly progressive infection, often with meningitis or pneumonia. It is particularly common in infants and occurs most often within the first 1 or 2 years after surgery. In view of this, splenic rupture not leading to exsanguination tends to be treated conservatively with bed rest and transfusion. Should surgery be necessitated, efforts are made to perform a splenic repair (splenorrhaphy).

REFERENCES

1. Miller KB, Kuligowska E, Rich DH: Ultrasonic demonstration of splenic rupture in infectious mononucleosis. J Clin Ultrasound 9:519–520, 1981
2. Shirkhoda A, McCartney WH, Staab EV, et al: Imaging of the spleen: A proposed algorithm. AJR 135:195–198, 1980
3. Johnson MA, Cooperberg PL, Boisvert J, et al: Spontaneous splenic rupture in infectious mononucleosis: Sonographic diagnosis and follow-up. AJR 136:111–114, 1981
4. King H, Schumacker HB, Jr: Splenic studies. I. Susceptibility to infection after splenectomy performed in infancy. Ann Surg 136:239–242, 1952

715

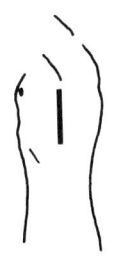

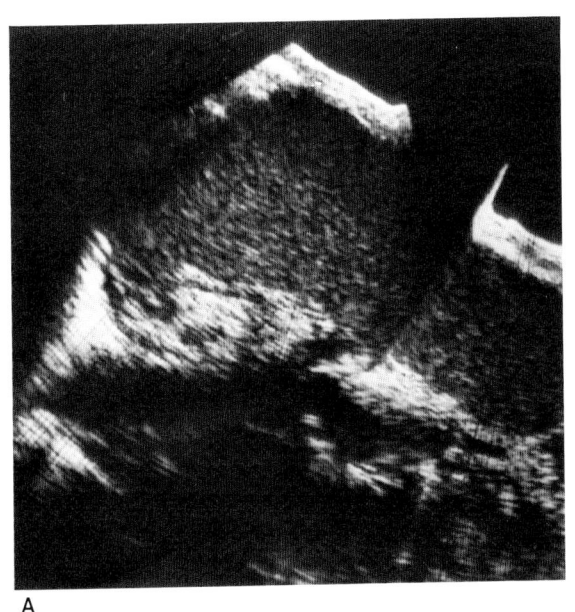

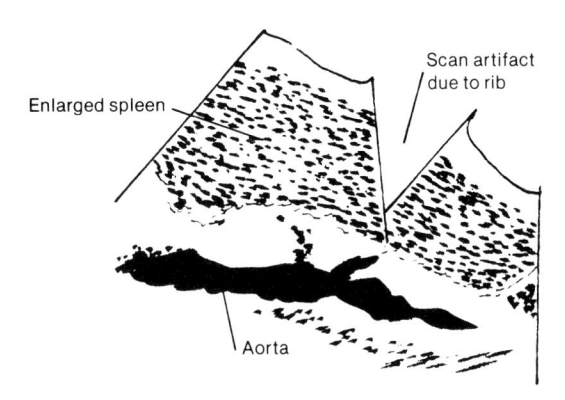

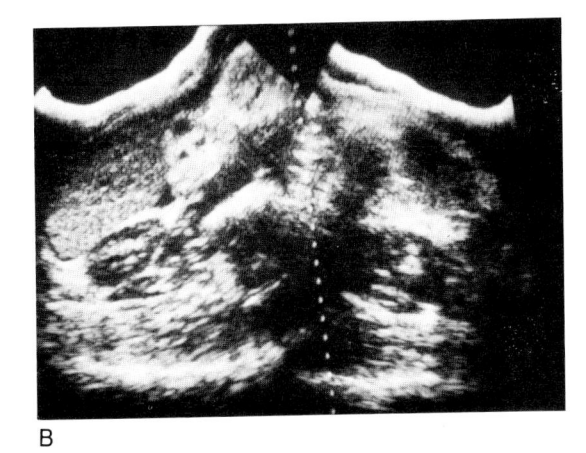

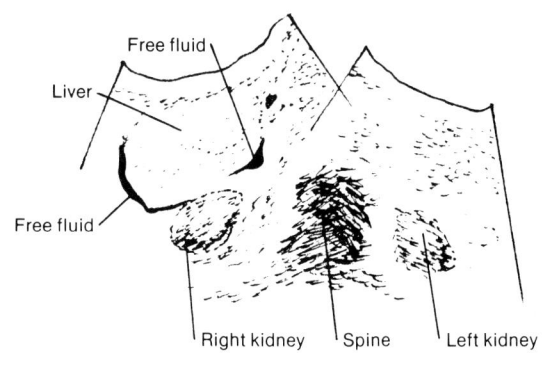

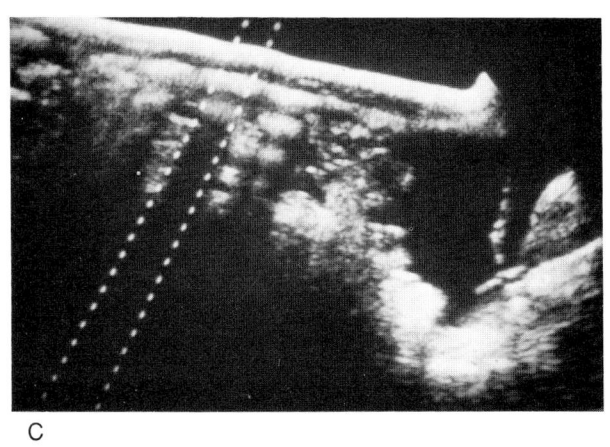

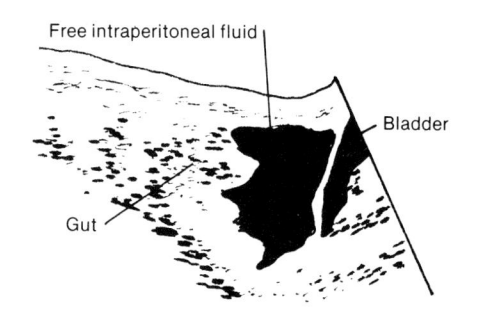

C

10.13 Pseudospleen

A 47-year-old man underwent splenectomy for a ruptured spleen sustained in a motor vehicle accident. He was referred for ultrasound examination because of postoperative fevers.

A coronal sonogram revealed a homogeneous mass in the splenic fossa (Fig. A). A transverse sonogram showed that this mass simulated the appearance of a normal spleen (Fig. B). This was considered to be a hematoma which was possibly infected.

The patient's fevers persisted and he was eventually brought to surgery at which time a left subphrenic abscess due to an infected hematoma was drained.

A postoperative fluid collection may fill the splenic fossa and simulate the appearances of the spleen following splenectomy. This should be differentiated from the later sequelae of splenectomy in which splenic remnants may hypertrophy with time and give rise to functioning splenic tissue, which can be identified by ^{99m}Tc sulfur colloid uptake. This phenomenon has been termed the "born-again spleen."[1]

Lee et al. noted the appearances of different pseudomasses in the splenic fossa.[2] They noted that the stomach and colon fell into the splenic fossa and could simulate a pathologic mass, but this could be differentiated by moving the patient. In contrast, masses due to a subphrenic collection, such as abscesses, did not move with gravity.

REFERENCES

1. Pearson HA, Johnston D, Smith KA, et al: The born-again spleen. Return of splenic function after splenectomy for trauma. N Engl J Med 298:1389–1392, 1978
2. Lee TG, Forsberg FG, Koehler PR: Post-splenectomy: true mass and pseudomass: ultrasound diagnosis. Radiology 134:707–711, 1980

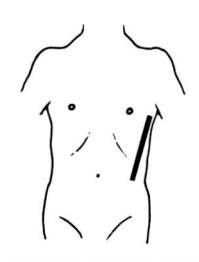

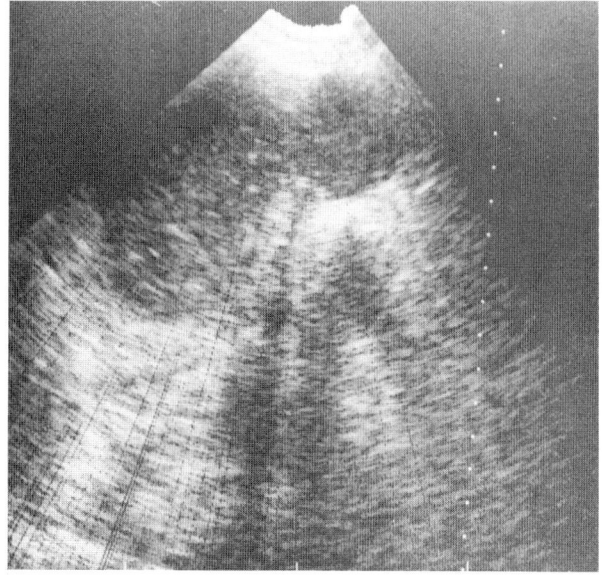

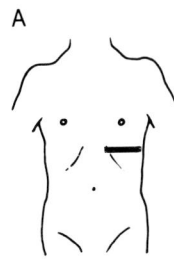

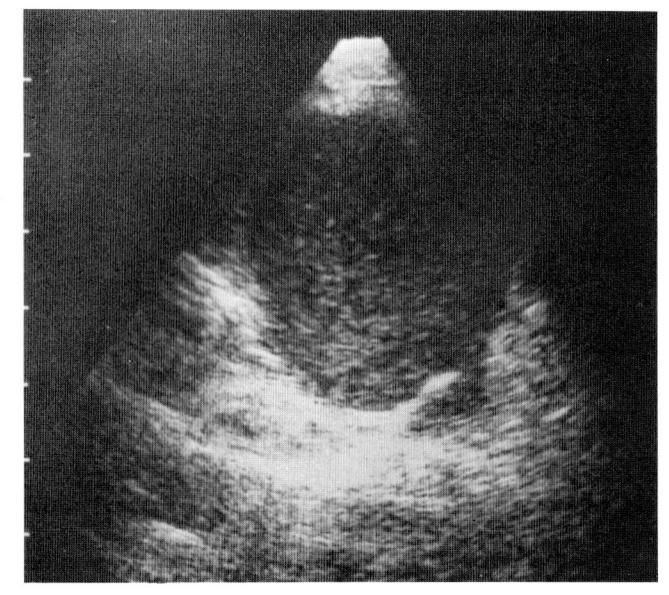

A

B

10.14 Focal Lymphoma

A 14-year-old girl was found to have a large mediastinal mass on routine preschool chest radiography. There was minimal cervical lymphadenopathy. The abdomen was normal, apart from a palpable liver edge. The radiograph showed a large anterior mediastinal mass on the left. Surgery revealed a large, nonresectable mediastinal mass which was biopsied and revealed Hodgkin's disease. A subsequent bone marrow biopsy showed that she had stage IV Hodgkin's disease.

A liver/spleen scan demonstrated large focal defects in the spleen, with focal uptake of ^{67}gallium.

This patient had stage IV nodular sclerosing Hodgkin's disease, treated with MVVPP. A lymphangiogram demonstrated abnormal nodes in both the iliac and paraaortic chain. Laparoscopy and liver biopsy specimens demonstrated no evidence of abdominal or liver involvement.

The sonogram showed a large liver and a palpable mass in the epigastrium due to the enlargement of the pancreas, periaortic nodes and overlying liver. Oblique sections through the spleen (seen in the figure) showed focal defects as well as diffuse enlargement. This patient experienced a progressively downhill course, despite chemotherapy, and died.

At the time of initial staging, about one-third of spleens in patients with Hodgkin's disease show involvement. Increased spleen size is not a reliable predictor of involvement.[1] Focal involvement either by Hodgkin's or non-Hodgkin's lymphoma, is relatively infrequent. When focal lesions are present, they should be detectable by ultrasound, although Sekiya et al. detected only 1 focal lesion of the spleen in 17 found at laparotomy.[2]

REFERENCES

1. Dorfman RJ: Relationship of histology to site in Hodgkin's disease. Cancer Res 31:1786–1793, 1971
2. Sekiya T, Meller ST, Cosgrove DO, McCready VR: Ultrasonography of Hodgkin's disease in the liver and spleen. Clin Radiol 33:635–639, 1982

Spleen

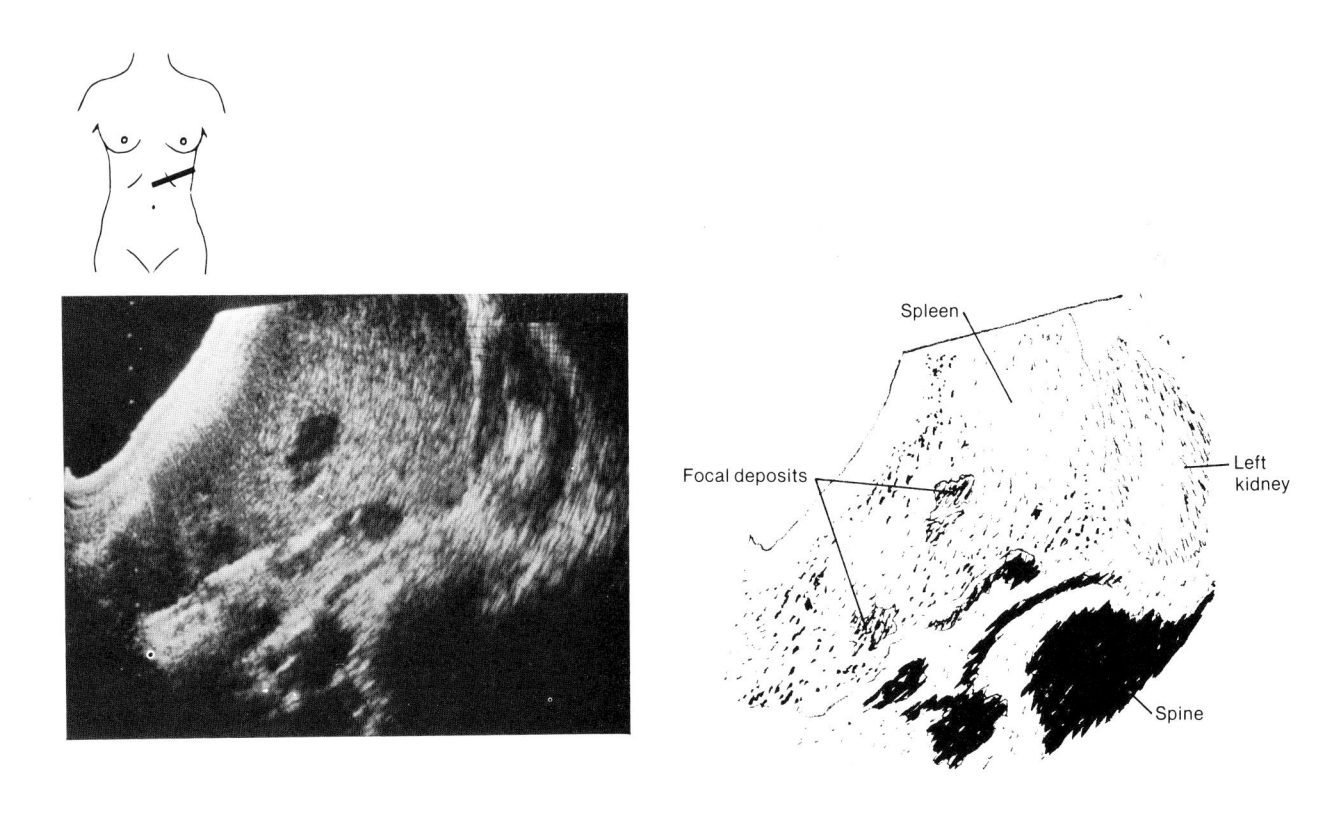

Focal deposits

Left kidney

Spine

10.15 Echogenic Metastases

Metastatic involvement of the spleen is rare but occurred in this elderly man with a carcinoma of the colon and metastatic involvement of the liver on initial presentation. The oblique sonogram along the 10th intercostal space showed enlargement of the spleen and several highly echogenic masses within it, as seen in the figure. The liver metastases were also echogenic. In this patient, metastatic involvement of the spleen from the colonic primary may have been facilitated by the massive liver involvement, producing portal vein obstruction and reversed flow in the portal vein.

Most splenic metastases are sonolucent. Murphy et al. reported five splenic metastases. Two lymphomas and two of three melanomas were sonolucent; one was echogenic.

REFERENCE

1. Murphy JF, Bernardino ME: The sonographic findings of splenic metastases. J Clin Ultrasound 7:195–197, 1979

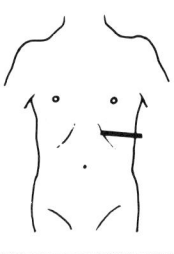

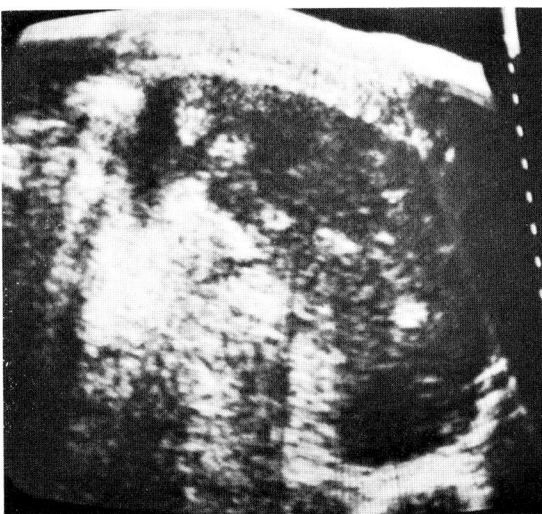

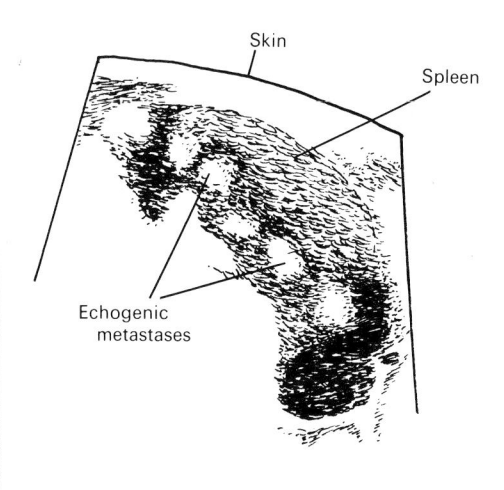

Splenomegaly (10.16 and 10.17)

10.16 Congestive Splenomegaly

A patient was referred for ultrasound examination because of progressive development of jaundice. On ultrasound examination of the liver, obvious cirrhosis was present with enlargement and tortuosity of the portal vein. With the patient in the decubitus position, the longitudinal coronal sonogram showed dilated short gastric veins in the hilum of the spleen, as seen in the figure. The spleen is limited by apposition with the chest wall anteriorly and by the dome of the left hemidiaphragm posteriorly. Splenic consistency is characteristic of congestive splenomegaly and reveals medium-level echoes distributed in a fine and uniform pattern.

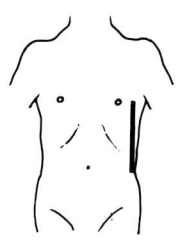

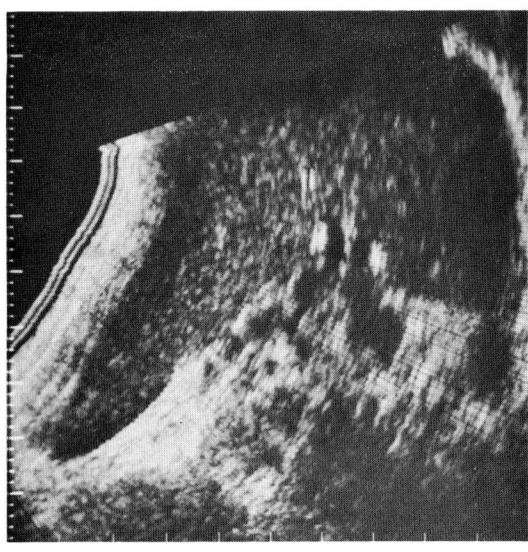

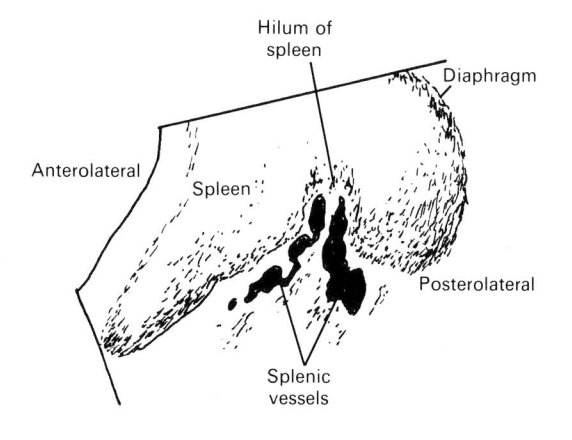

10.17 Inflammatory Splenomegaly

A middle-aged Libyan man presented with malaise and fever. Examination revealed lymphadenopathy and hepatosplenomegaly. The provisional diagnosis was lymphoma. Transverse ultrasound examination, shown in the figure, revealed the tip of the liver, which returned very high level echoes, and marked splenomegaly, also with very high internal echoes. The left and right kidneys and psoas major muscles were seen posteriorly.

High-level echoes are seldom seen in untreated malignancy of the spleen, and untreated lymphomatous infiltration of the liver usually results in very hypoechoic lesions. This examination was therefore at variance with the clinical impression and suggests that the more likely cause of hepatosplenomegaly was a chronic inflammatory state. White nodules were found throughout the spleen at splenectomy; similar findings were apparent on a surgical wedge biopsy specimen of the liver. The eventual histologic diagnosis proved to be tuberculosis and no evidence of any malignancy was found. Subsequently, this patient was successfully treated with antituberculotic therapy.

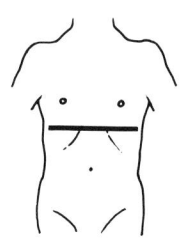

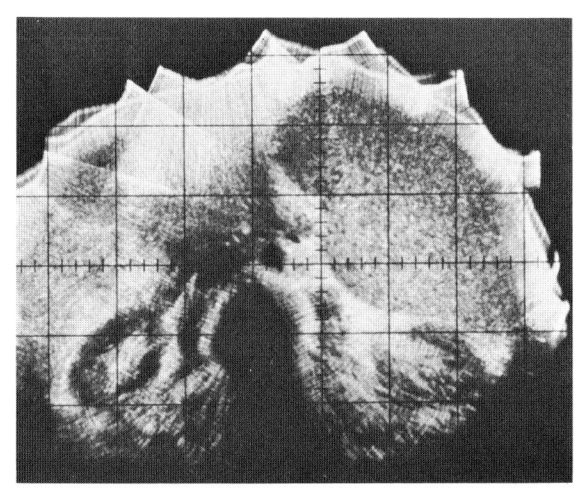

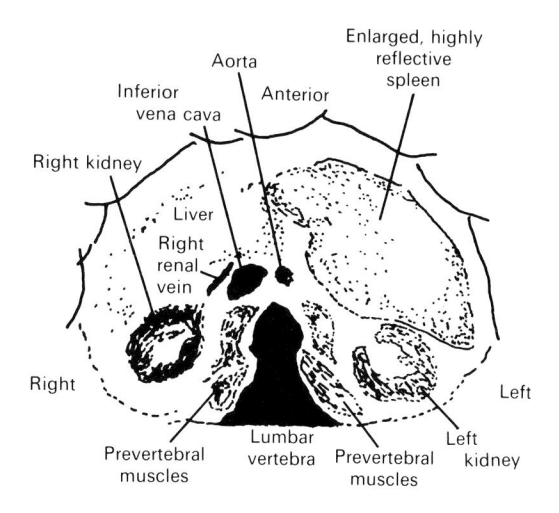

10.18 Chronic Granulomatous Disease

A 60-year-old alcoholic man presented with hepatosplenomegaly. Plain radiography disclosed a calcified mass in the right lobe of the liver. A liver/spleen scan showed a large defect in the right lobe and he was referred for ultrasound. A longitudinal sonogram of the liver showed a markedly enlarged organ with an echogenic, shadowing focus correlating with the calcified mass seen on plain film (Fig. A). A longitudinal section through the spleen showed splenomegaly with a longitudinal axis of 14 cm (normal is less than 11 cm). The parenchyma was homogeneous (Fig B). The liver lesion could be either a hemangioma or calcified granuloma.

In view of the clinical suspicion of a hepatoma, the patient underwent exploratory laparotomy which disclosed a calcified mass in the right dome of the liver, considered to be a hemangioma. Biopsy specimens revealed chronic granulomatous disease with sideroblastic anemia and extramedullary erythropoiesis resulting in hepatosplenomegaly.

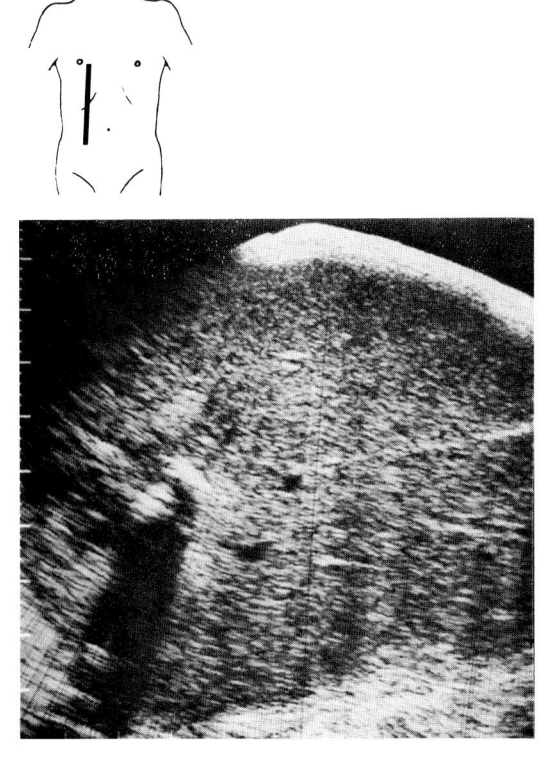

A

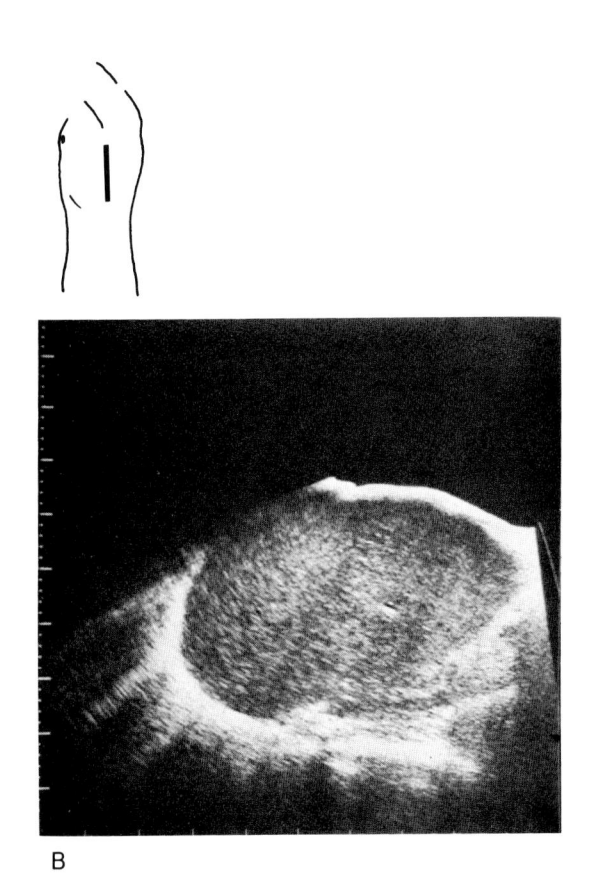

B

10.19 Chronic Myeloid Leukemia

A 66-year-old patient was referred for evaluation of the spleen. She was known to have chronic myeloid leukemia and had been extensively treated for the past 2 years.

A transverse sonogram (Fig. A) using a compound scanning technique to produce an axial tomogram showed a large, highly homogeneous organ which filled the left hypochondrium and extended over the midline into the right hypochondrium. Note that very low level echoes were seen from within this mass, although adjustment of the time gain control (TGC) brought out fine echoes in the deeper parts of this massively enlarged spleen.

A longitudinal sonogram obtained by a simple sector scan in the parasagittal plane again revealed marked enlargement of the spleen, extending inferiorly as far as the umbilicus (Fig. B). Again, the organ was seen to be highly homogeneous although the TGC adjustment brought out a fine echo pattern in the deeper part of the spleen.

The amplitude of the echoes from within the splenic parenchyma varies according to the signal-to-noise ratio of the diagnostic equipment, including the transducer being used. However, under standard conditions it has been noted that malignancy in the spleen tends to return low-level echoes. These appearances may change with prolonged therapy, resulting in high-level echoes. The appearances in congestive splenomegaly are those of intermediate-level echoes, while very high level echoes are found predominantly in chronic inflammatory states.[1] Exceptions certainly occur, however, precluding the use of ultrasound to predict histologic findings with any degree of reliability.[2] Mittelstaedt and Partain noted that the normal echogenicity of the spleen was similar to that of the liver.[3] Similar echogenicity was found in splenomegaly associated with erythropoiesis or congestion.

REFERENCES

1. Taylor KJW, Milan J: Differential diagnosis of chronic splenomegaly by grey scale ultrasonography: clinical observations and digital A-scan analysis. Br J Radiol 49:519–525, 1976
2. Siler J, Hunter TB, Weiss J, et al: Increased echogenicity of the spleen in benign and malignant disease. AJR 134:1011–1014, 1980
3. Mittelstaedt CA, Partain CL: Ultrasonic–pathologic classification of splenic abnormalities: gray scale patterns. Radiology 134:697–705, 1980

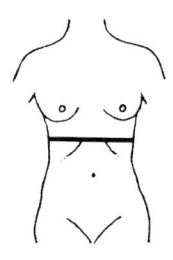

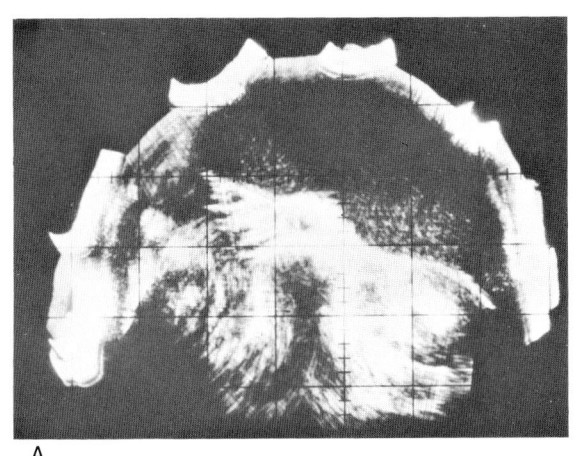

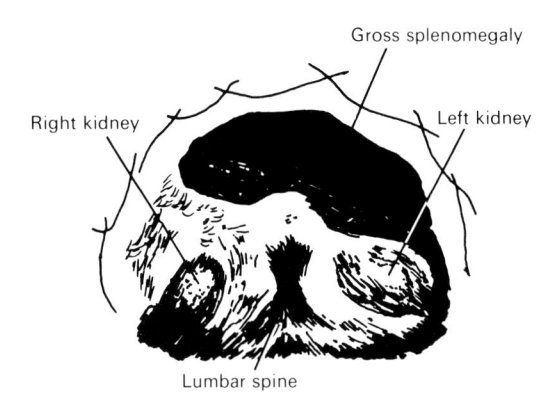

A

Gross splenomegaly
Right kidney
Left kidney
Lumbar spine

B

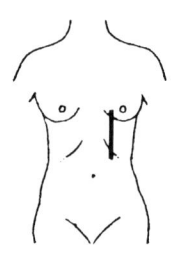

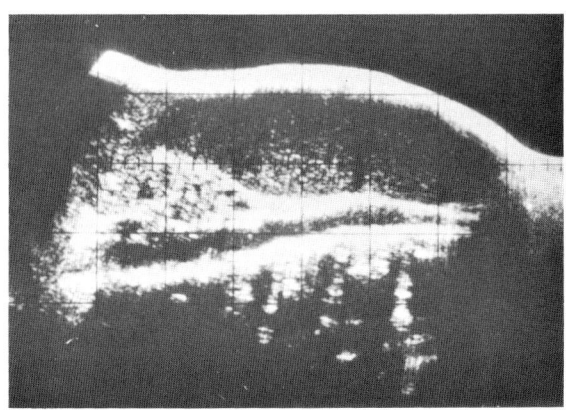

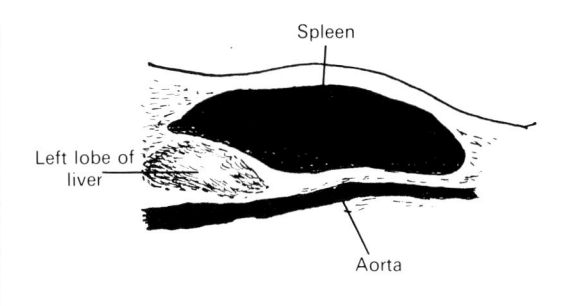

Spleen
Left lobe of liver
Aorta

10.20 Histoplasmosis

Diffuse calcifications within the spleen were an incidental finding on a kidney/ureter/bladder study of a 40-year-old woman. A sonogram of the spleen demonstrated flecks of high-level echoes (arrowed in Fig. A) throughout the spleen. Such appearances are commonly seen due to histoplasmosis. The chest radiograph showed bilateral calcified hilar lymphadenopathy with tiny, calcified foci in the right midlung zone and left apex, consistent with histoplasmosis or tuberculosis (Fig. B).

Histoplasmosis occurs widely throughout the world. The disease is contracted by inhalation of fungal spores, resulting in a primary pulmonary lesion very similar to that of tuberculosis. Occasionally, dissemination of such pulmonary lesions occurs with little clinical evidence, producing calcified lesions in the liver, spleen, nodes, and other viscera. Hepatomegaly, splenomegaly, and generalized lymphadenopathy may be seen.

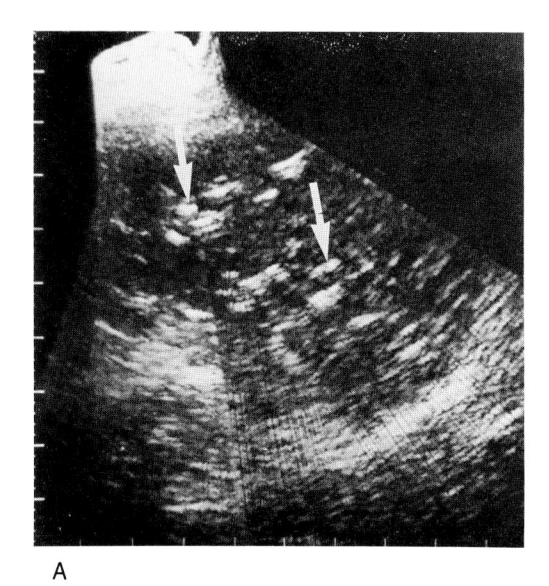

A

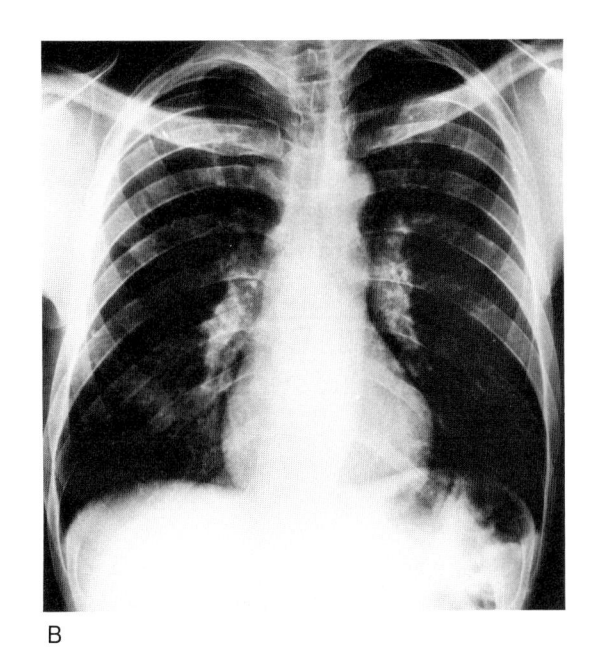

B

10.21 Myelofibrosis

A 70-year-old man presented with anemia and was found to have hepatosplenomegaly. A posterior view of the liver–spleen scan demonstrated hepatosplenomegaly, without evidence of focal defect (Fig. A). A CT scan (Fig. B) also demonstrated diffuse hepatosplenomegaly.

A longitudinal sonogram in the decubitus position demonstrated a markedly enlarged spleen with a uniform parenchymal pattern (Fig. C).

Myelofibrosis or myeloid metaplasia is characterized by extramedullary erythropoiesis with fibrous replacement of the bone marrow. Polycythemia vera and, occasionally, myelogenous leukemia may progress to myelofibrosis or it may also arise as a primary disease. The outcome is variable. Pancytopenia may result in severe anemia and life can only be sustained by repeated blood transfusion. However, in most patients the disease transforms into myelogenous leukemia and the prognosis becomes that of the new disease.

The principle site of extramedullary hematopoiesis is the spleen which is markedly enlarged, as in this patient. It sometimes weighs up to 4,000 g. The cut surface is red and gray, somewhat similar to that seen in myelogenous leukemia. The liver may also be moderately enlarged, again due to extramedullary hematopoiesis.

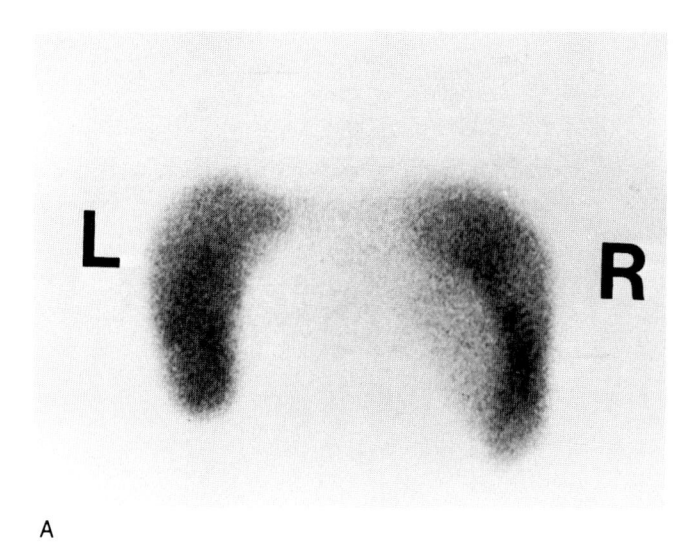

A

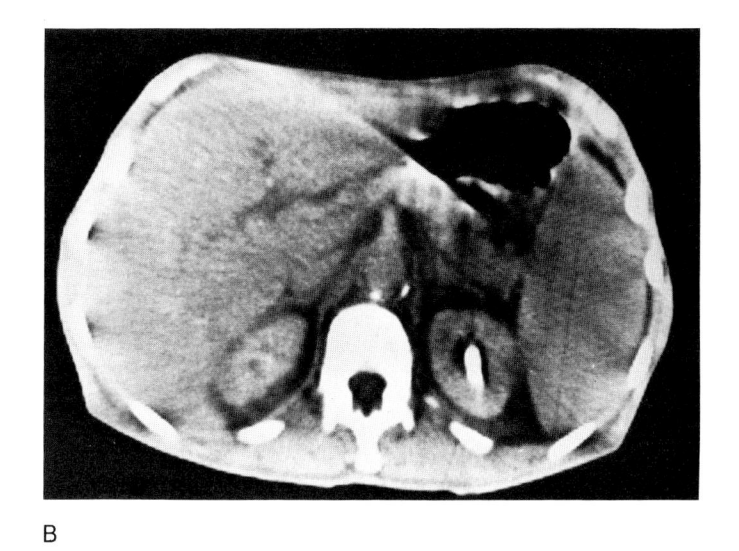

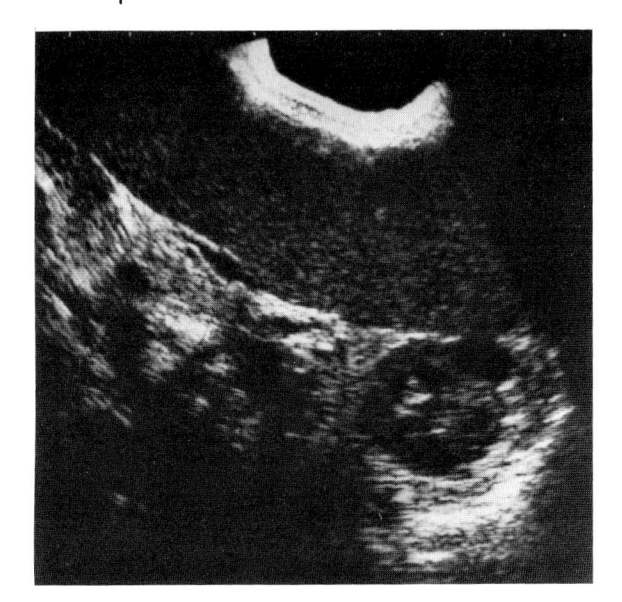

B

C

11 The Urinary Tract

ARTHUR T. ROSENFIELD and TINA RICHMAN

The past few years have witnessed a marked improvement in the ability of imaging techniques to diagnose urinary tract diseases. The kidney has proved to be an excellent target organ for virtually every new abdominal imaging modality and each has had an immediate, lasting impact on the evaluation of the urinary tract. The introduction of angiography permitted specific diagnosis of many renal diseases previously identified only by pathologic examination. Radioisotope scanning provided a modality for the safe evaluation of renal blood flow, the integrity of the renal parenchyma, and renal obstructive disease. Soon after the introduction of computed body tomography (CT), it became apparent that the retroperitoneum was the best region in the abdomen for the application of CT scanning due to the presence of large amounts of fat. The recent application of digital subtraction angiography to the evaluation of renovascular hypertension has provided a relatively safe method for diagnosing this disorder. Interventional radiology in the urinary tract has also become extremely successful. Percutaneous nephrostomies and antegrade pyelograms are now routine. Cyst punctures and apiration of renal masses are easily performed whether guided by sonography, CT, or radiography. Urinary tract tumors can be embolized and percutaneous angioplasties can be used to correct some renal arterial abnormalities.

These major advances, while substantially limiting the indications for excretory urography, have significantly broadened the range of diseases that can be diagnosed by imaging methods or treated by procedures that require an imaging modality for guidance. However, no other technique has approached the impact of ultrasound on urinary tract diagnosis. Even in the early days of bistable ultrasonography, the kidney could be evaluated sonographically for the identification of hydronephrosis and characterization of renal masses. The introduction of gray-scale equipment, combined with the availability of dynamic (real-time) scanners, transrectal and transurethral probes, and machines with pulsed Doppler/sonar devices has led to an expansion in the role of sonography for evaluating the urinary tract. The safety and speed of this modality have made it the technique of choice under appropriate circumstances. Sonograms can be obtained either in the ultrasound laboratory or at the bedside, in the hospital or office. Not only can the kidney be evaluated for anatomic abnormality, but Doppler ultrasound and dynamic scanning also offer the promise of identifying alterations in renal blood flow. Of equal importance, the renal sonogram includes evaluation of all of the adjacent organs including the liver, spleen, gallbladder, and pancreas, so that patients with abdominal symptoms can have many organs evaluated simultaneously. With ultrasound guidance, rapid biopsy of abnormal masses is possible, and fluid collections can be drained when indicated. Since there are many competitive techniques for evaluating the urinary tract, institution of a coherent approach to various renal problems based on the clinical findings and the known advantages and disadvantages of each imaging modality is crucial. Many diseases, however, can be defined only by combining the findings on several imaging studies. For example, the diagnosis of acute focal bacterial nephritis ("lobar nephronia") may require correlation of several imaging studies. This requires physicians familiar with several techniques to provide coordinated imaging and appropriate diagnosis.

The urinary tract is the most common site for congenital abnormalities. It has been estimated that 10 percent of individuals are born with a congenital abnormality of the urinary tract. A duplicated collecting system, renal agenesis, renal fusion, and renal ectopia form the majority of these anomalies. Sonography, which provides outstanding anatomic resolution, especially in children who are thin and require a noninvasive technique, has assumed a major role in identifying these abnormalities.

In our institution, ultrasound is the modality most frequently used for the initial evaluation of patients with suspected renal disease. It is also the most common single imaging modality to be used in the evaluation of the urinary tract. However, since other imaging techniques frequently can provide valuable information about the kidney, and since the technical expertise required for ultrasound is not universally available, its role in renal imaging varies at different institutions. In contrast, ultrasound study of the lower urinary tract and scrotum has provided diagnostic information not previously available from any other technique. Transrectal ultrasonography of the prostate and bladder has defined textural changes useful in the identification and characterization of lesions that previously could be evaluated only by more invasive procedures. Static scans of the scrotum have provided resolution of scrotal structures never approached by any other imaging technique. As discussed in Chapter 15, ultrasound is the technique of choice in the evaluation of scrotal masses and has significant application in the evaluation of acute scrotal abnormalities.

This chapter presents the spectrum of findings to be expected in commonly encountered diseases. No attempt is made to be encyclopedic, and the references have also been limited to a few select articles. Emphasis is placed on findings unique to ultrasound, such as tissue characterization, and on the role of ultrasound in the coordinated imaging of renal diseases.

SUGGESTED READINGS

Resnick MI, Sanders RC (eds): Ultrasound in Urology. Williams & Wilkins, Baltimore, 1979

Rosenfield AT (ed): Genitourinary Ultrasonography. Clinics in Diagnostic Ultrasound, Vol 2. Churchill Livingstone, New York, 1979

Rosenfield AT, Glickman MG, Hodson J (eds): Diagnostic Imaging in Renal Disease. Appleton-Century Crofts, New York, 1979

Wolfman WT, Karstaedt N: Ultrasound anatomy of the kidney. In Resnick MI, Parker MD (eds): Surgical Anatomy of the Kidney. Futura Publishing Company, New York, 1982

Normal Anatomy (11.1 to 11.8)

11.1 Kidney

The normal kidney consists of the renal sinus surrounded by the renal parenchyma. A line that connects the calyceal tips encompasses the renal sinus, which is comprised of blood vessels, fibrous tissue, and fat as well as the collecting system. Everything outside this line represents the parenchyma, which consists of the glomerular-bearing cortex and the medulla. Included in this structure are the septa of Bertin, which are protrusions of cortex toward the renal sinus, and the pyramids (medulla) defined by the renal cortex peripherally, and by the renal sinus centrally.

Figure A is a parasagittal sonogram taken through the right upper quadrant of a normal 5-year-old. The liver parenchyma displays a relatively homogeneous echo pattern. The diaphragm is seen as a curved line of specular, intense echoes. In the central portion of the right kidney, an area of intense echoes is due to the renal sinus. A small amount of urine within the collecting system is seen as an echo-free line in the inferior portion of the renal sinus. The presence of the normal dense central renal sinus excludes hydronephrosis. The echo amplitude of the renal cortex is of a lower level than that of the adjacent liver and the renal sinus. Projections of the cortex (septa of Bertin) are seen radiating toward the renal sinus. The pyramids appear as relatively hypoechoic zones defined by the cortex and renal sinus. Normal pyramids should not be mistaken for cysts or other pathologic changes. The arcuate artery and vein, represented by punctate specular echoes at the corticomedullary junction, are identified in cross- or oblique section.

In the normal adult, the echo amplitude of the parenchymal abdominal organs is, in ascending order: renal medulla, renal cortex, spleen, liver, pancreas, diaphragm, and renal sinus. Alterations in these relationships are used to define diseases. For example, the echogenicity of the renal cortex increases in medical renal disease. However, it must be recalled that in the neonate the echo amplitude of the renal cortex is greater than that of the adjacent liver in normal patients.

Figure B is a limited transverse sonogram taken in the same patient in the supine position. The liver is seen anterior to the right kidney. The scan was taken at the level of the renal hilum, so the renal sinus is seen as a zone of intense echoes in the medial portion of the kidney. The right renal vein and artery are seen entering the renal hilum. Once again, the normal corticomedullary differentiation can be appreciated and the arcuate vessels are seen as punctate echoes at the corticomedullary junction.

SUGGESTED READINGS

Cook JH, III, Rosenfield AT, Taylor KJW: Ultrasonic demonstration of intrarenal anatomy. Am J Roentgenol 129:831–835, 1977

Haller JO, Berdon WE, Friedman AP: Increased renal cortical echogenicity—a normal finding in neonates and infants. Radiology 142:173–174, 1982

Rosenfield AT, Taylor KJW: Grey-scale ultrasound in the imaging of urinary tract disease. Yale J Biol Med 50:335–353, 1977

Rosenfield AT, Taylor KJW: Crade M, et al: Anatomy and pathology of the kidney by grey-scale ultrasound. Radiology 128:737–744, 1978

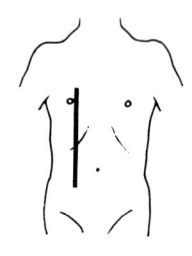

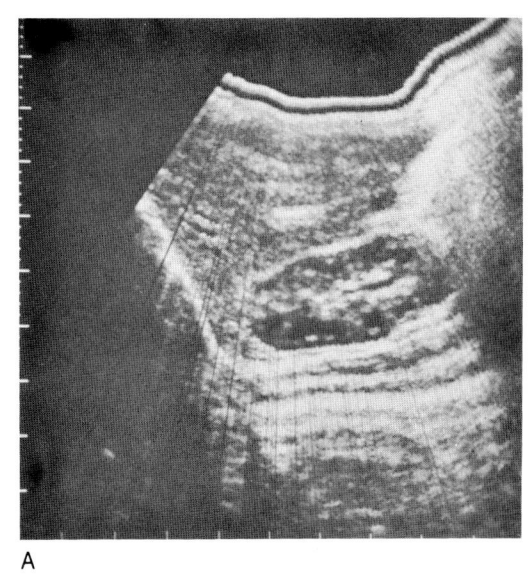

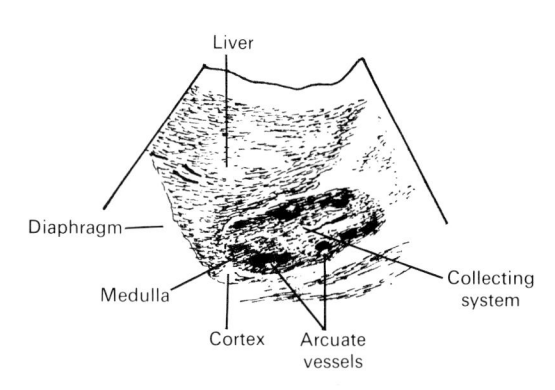

A

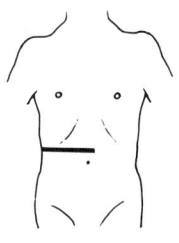

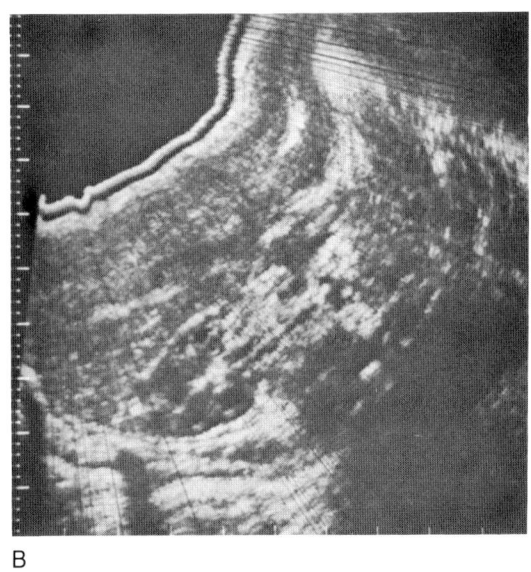

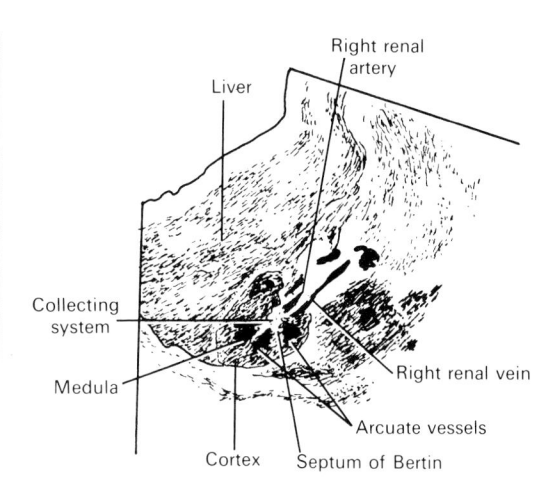

B

11.2 Renal Veins

Figure A shows the right kidney in transverse section, imaged from the anterior aspect through the liver. The right renal vein is seen as a linear, hypoechoic structure (arrowed) running from the right kidney to the inferior vena cava (IVC). The aorta is on the left and is posterior to the IVC. The right renal vein is routinely imaged, and alterations in size can be appreciated both with respiration and transmitted pulsation from the IVC.

Figure B is a transverse sonogram which demonstrates the left renal vein extending from the hilum of the left kidney to the inferior vena cava, running between the aorta and superior mesenteric artery. The diameter of the left renal vein normally is significantly less when situated between the aorta and superior mesenteric artery than when it is proximal to this point. This narrowing of the left renal vein between aorta and superior mesenteric artery, the so called "nutcracker" phenomenon, should not be mistaken for pathologic change. There is often some dilatation of the left renal vein immediately before this narrowing and this must not be mistaken for an aneurysm.

Figure C is a longitudinal sonogram through the aorta, demonstrating the left renal vein in cross-section as it runs between the aorta and superior mesenteric artery. The renal veins should be carefully identified and evaluated in patients suspected of having renal vein thrombosis or renal vein tumor. Tumor can be identified within the vein and thrombus can be identified directly, as well as inferred indirectly, if pulsations from the IVC are not transmitted to the left renal vein.

SUGGESTED READING

Buschi AJ, Harrison RB, Brenbridge ANAG, et al: Distended left renal vein: CT/sonographic normal variant. AJR 135:339–342, 1980

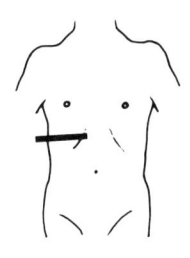

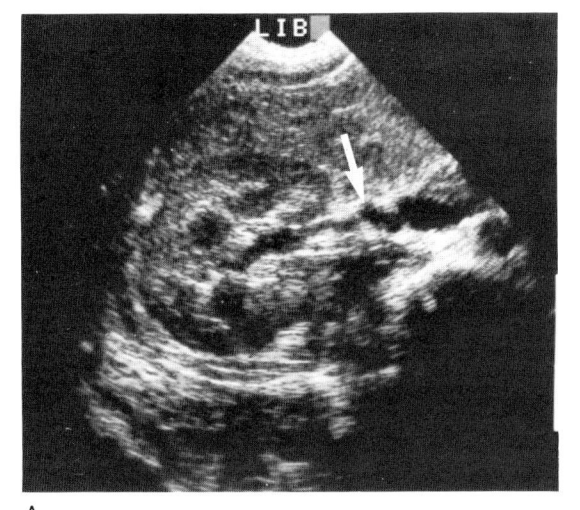

A

B

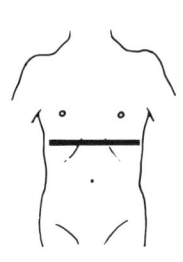

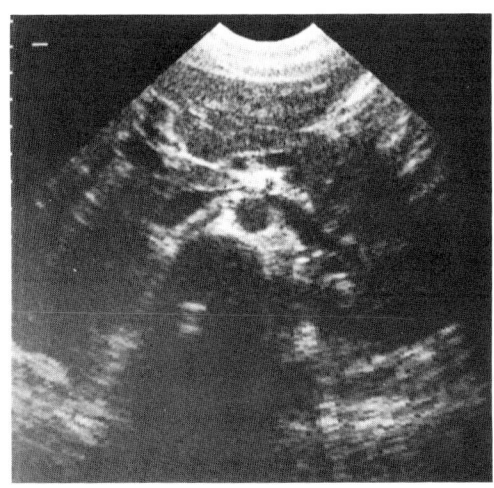

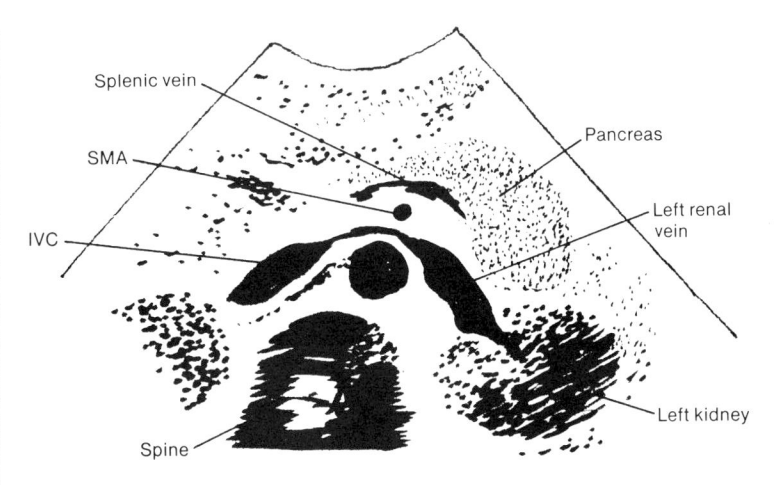

Splenic vein
SMA
IVC
Pancreas
Left renal vein
Left kidney
Spine

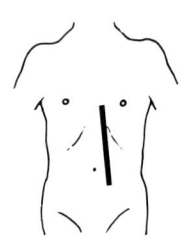

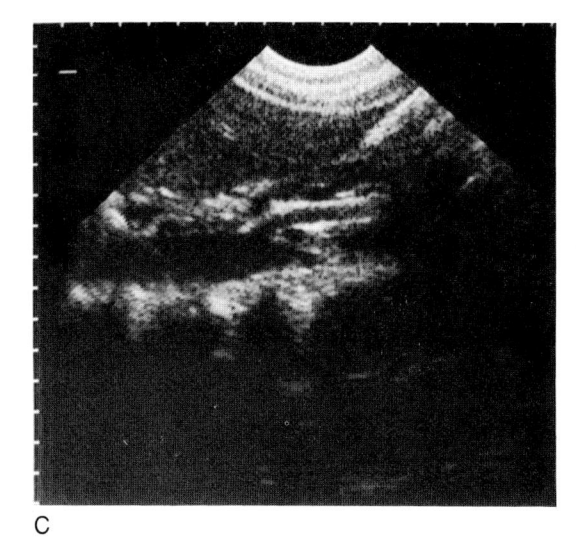

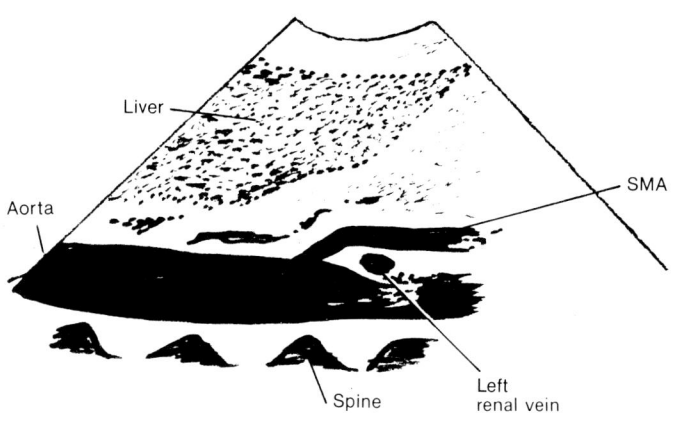

C

11.3 Renal Sinus

Figure A is a coronal sonogram of a supine patient. The kidney contains an incidental renal cyst. The renal sinus is a central region of intense echoes containing a relatively echo-free collecting system. A lower gain than that used to image the renal parenchyma is optimal for evaluating the renal sinus. Note the normal calyceal cup and infundibulum within the upper portion of the renal sinus. The extent to which the fluid-filled collecting system is seen depends upon hydration of the patient, whether there is an intra- or extrarenal pelvis, and the degree of bladder distention. Well-hydrated patients and those with an extrarenal pelvis probably will have a more readily apparent collecting system. However, in other patients, the collecting system may be relatively inapparent, and the central zone contains intense echoes only.

On transverse sonograms through both poles of the kidney, the renal sinus is a central zone of intense echoes. On scans through the renal hilum, the renal sinus exits from the anteromedial portion of the kidney (arrowed in Fig. B). Abnormal position of the renal hilum suggests either a congenital abnormality (such as anterior position of the renal sinus in a horseshoe kidney) or a mass displacing the kidney.

(Fig. B from Wolf B, Rosenfield AT, Taylor KJW, et al: Presymptomatic diagnosis of adult onset polycystic kidney disease by ultrasonography. Clin Genet 14:1–7, 1978. © 1978 Munksgaard International Publishers Ltd., Copenhagen, Denmark.)

SUGGESTED READING

Sanders RC, Conrad MR: The ultrasonic characteristics of the renal pelvocalyceal echo complex. J Clin Ultrasound 5:372–377, 1977

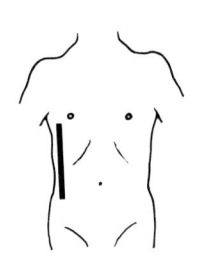

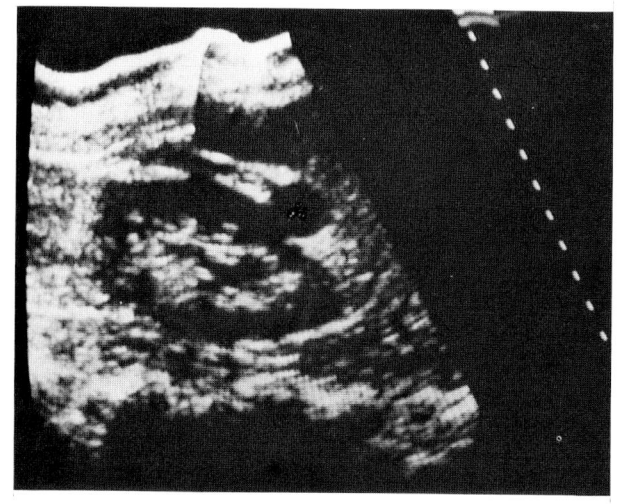

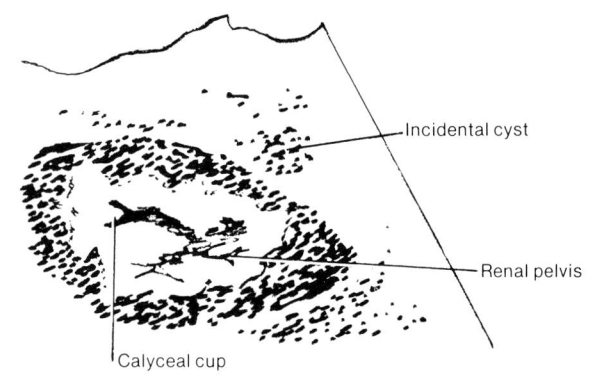

A

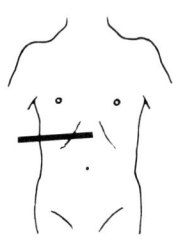

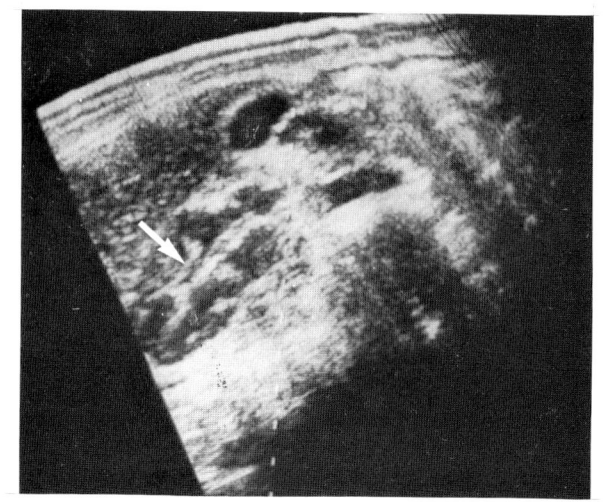

Incidental cyst

Renal pelvis

Calyceal cup

B

11.4 Renal Arteries

The figure shows a transverse sonogram demonstrating both kidneys. The renal arteries extend from the aorta which is just to the left of midline, to the kidneys. Behind the aorta is the spine. The inferior vena cava is collapsed and is not seen.

(Scan from Rosenfield AT, Taylor KJW: Grey-scale nephrosonography: current status. J Urol 117:2–6, 1977. © 1977 The Williams & Wilkins Co., Baltimore.)

SUGGESTED READING

Rosenfield AT, Taylor KJW: Gray scale nephrosonography: current status. J Urol 117:2–6, 1977

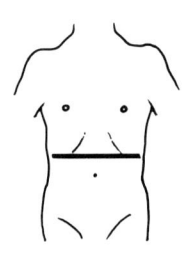

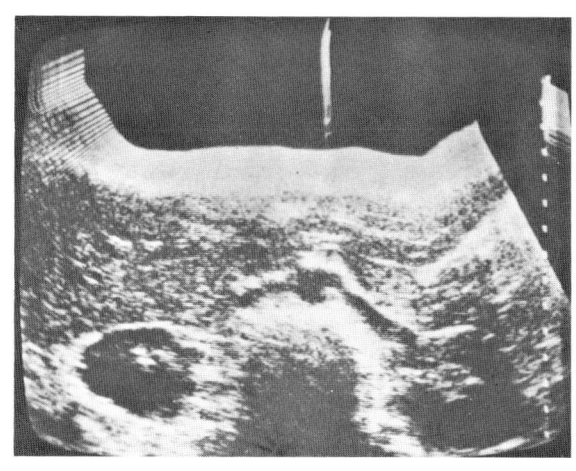

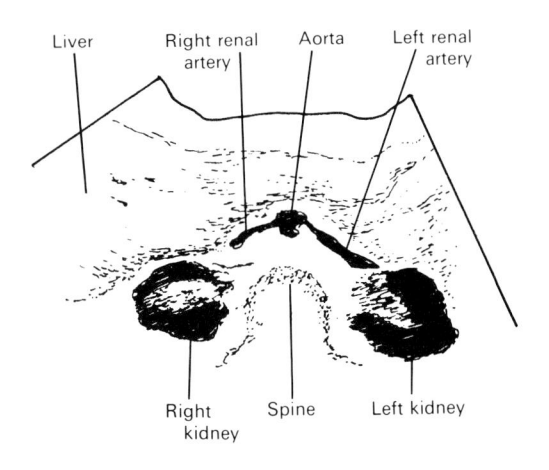

11.5 Neonatal Kidney

Longitudinal (Fig. A) and transverse (Fig. B) sonograms of the right upper quadrant of a normal supine neonate demonstrate a cortex containing homogeneous backscattered echoes and pyramids defined as hypoechoic structures. There is no evidence of hydronephrosis. The echo intensity of the renal cortex is greater than that of the adjacent liver and similar to that of the renal sinus. Although this would be abnormal in adults, it is normal in neonates and infants. Hricik et al.[1] have noted that the glomeruli occupy a greater proportional volume of the cellular compartment of the glomerular tuft, thus leading to increased interfaces and accounting for the increased echogenicity.

SUGGESTED READINGS

Babcock, DS: Medical diseases of the urinary tract and adrenal glands pp. 113–114. In Haller JO, Shkolnik A (eds): Clinics in Diagnostic Ultrasound, Vol. 8. Ultrasound in Pediatrics. Churchill Livingstone, New York, 1981

Haller JO, Berdon WE, Friedman AP: Increased renal cortical echogenicity—a normal finding in neonates and infants. Radiology 142:173–174, 1982

Scheible W, Leopold GR: High-resolution real-time ultrasonography of neonatal kidneys. J Ultrasound Med 1:133–138, 1982

REFERENCE

1. Hricik H, Slovis TL, Callen CW: Neonatal kidneys: sonographic anatomic correlation. Radiology 147:699–702, 1983

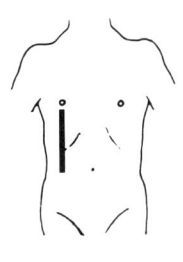

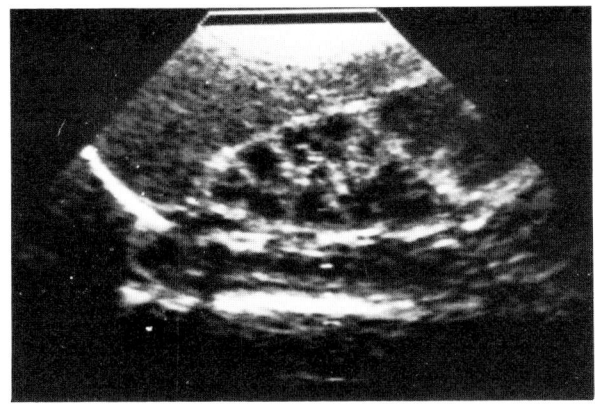

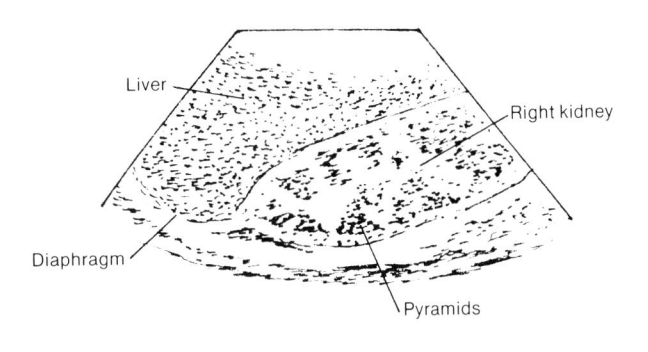

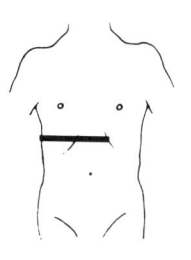

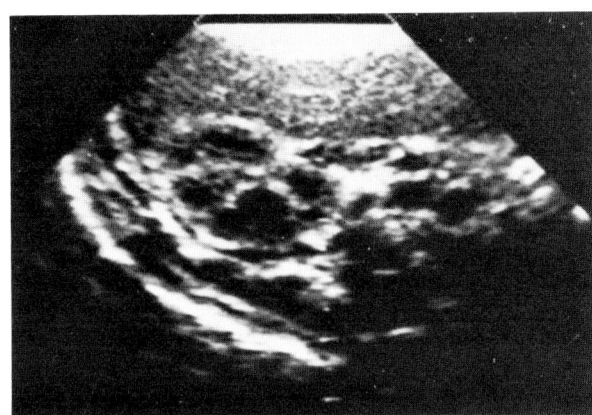

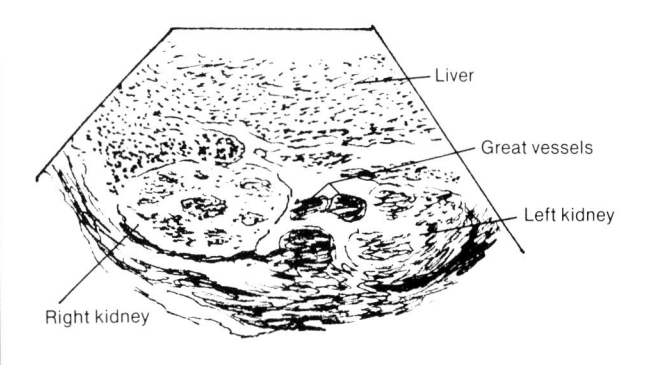

A

B

745

11.6 In Utero

The normal renal anatomy can be appreciated in patients of any age, including the fetus. The figure shows a sonogram through the pregnant uterus, demonstrating one kidney, in cross-section. The cortex contains homogeneous, back-scattered echoes, and the echogenicity of the renal sinus is of similar intensity. The pyramids are relatively echo-free. At the corticomedullary junction, punctate echoes represent the arcuate artery and veins in cross-section. Throughout pregnancy, the normal circumference of the fetal kidney is between 27 and 30 percent of the abdominal circumference.

(Scan from Cook JH III, Rosenfield AT, Taylor KJW: Ultrasonic demonstration of intrarenal anatomy. Am J Roentgenol 129:831–835, 1977. ©1977 Am Roentgen Roy Soc.)

SUGGESTED READINGS

Cook JH III, Rosenfield AT, Taylor KJW: Ultrasonic demonstration of intrarenal anatomy. Am J Roentgenol 129:831–835, 1977

Grannum PAT, Bracken M, Silverman R, et al: Assessment of fetal kidney size in normal gestation by comparison of kidney circumference to abdominal circumference ratio (KC/AC ratio). Am J Obstet Gynecol 136:249, 1980

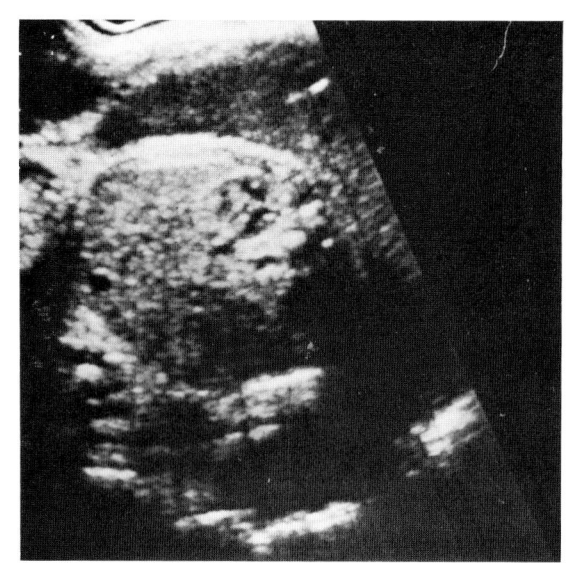

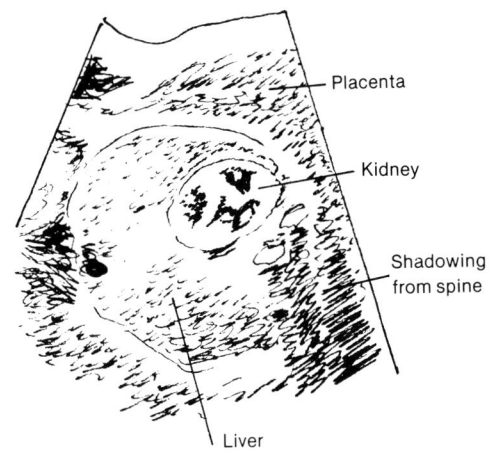

11.7 Juxtarenal Compartments

Figure A is a coronal–transverse section through the left kidney of a patient with no known renal disease. In this patient the perirenal and pararenal fat are both hypoechoic. Gerota's fascia is seen as a reflective line within the fat. (Weill et al.[1] have noted that the hypoechoic pattern is commonly seen in obese patients.) In Figure B the kidney of another patient with no known renal disease is shown in a coronal plane. In this patient the perirenal and pararenal fat is highly reflective. These are the two common appearances of the juxtarenal region.

Two other combinations may be seen in normal patients. In one, the perinephric fat is hypoechoic and the pararenal fat echogenic. When this situation exists, the hypoechoic perirenal fat mimics perinephric fluid. The other uncommon pattern is hypoechoic pararenal fat, which will mimic a pararenal fluid collection. A CT scan of the same region may be necessary to discriminate between fat and lesions such as an abscess or hematoma. The variable echogenicity of perirenal and pararenal fat, as with fat in other areas of the body, is related to a number of factors. These include the physical state of the fat (fluid or solid), and possibly, the amount of water and other substances contained within fatty tissue.

SUGGESTED READINGS

Cunningham JJ: *In vitro* gray scale echography of protein-lipid fluid collections in liver tissue. J Clin Ultrasound 4:255–258, 1976

Davis PL, Filly RA, Goerke J: Investigation of the ultrasonic imaging characteristics of lipids and lipid emulsions. Proceedings of the Annual Meeting of the American Institute of Ultrasound in Medicine. Montreal, Canada, August, 1979

Meyers MA: Dynamic Radiology of the Abdomen. Springer-Verlag, New York, 1976

Rosenfield AT, Taylor KJW, Jaffe CC: Clinical applications of ultrasound tissue characterization. Radiol Clin North Am 18:31–58, 1980

REFERENCE

1. Weill FS, Perriguey G, Rohmer P: Sonographic study of the juxtarenal retroperitoneal components. J Ultrasound Med 1:307–310, 1982

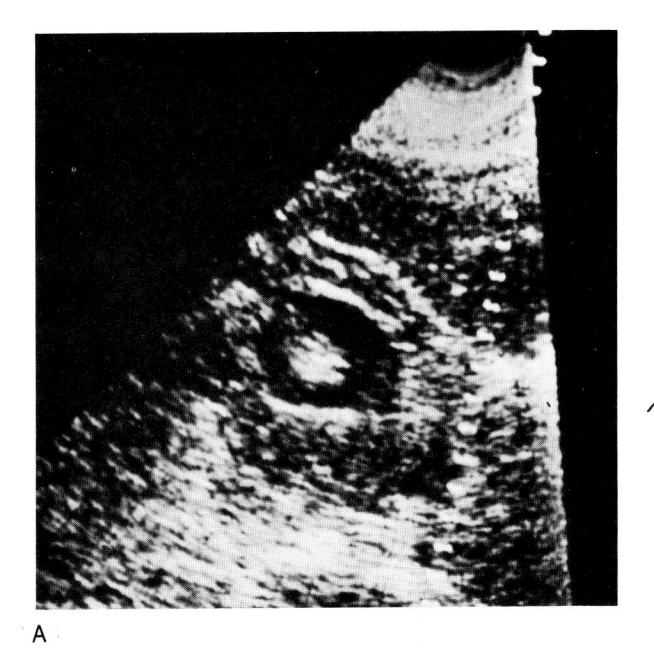

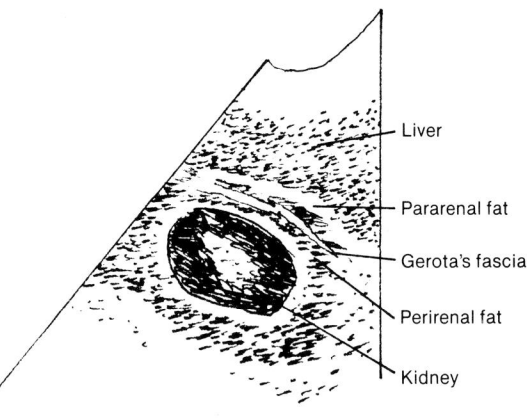

Liver
Pararenal fat
Gerota's fascia
Perirenal fat
Kidney

A

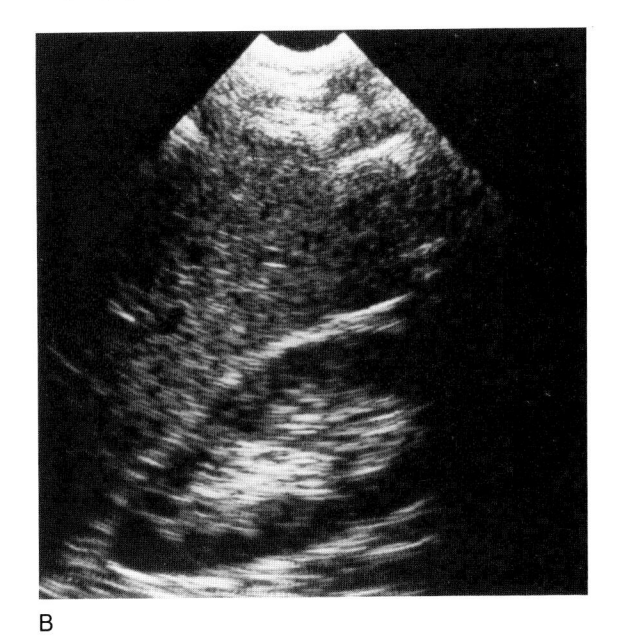

B

748

11.8 The Psoas and Quadratus Lumborum

Figure A shows a longitudinal section through the right upper quadrant demonstrating the liver anterior to the right kidney. Seen behind the right kidney, the quadratus lumborum muscle begins at the 12th rib and extends inferiorly. Because it may be hypoechoic in some patients, this muscle can mimic an abnormal peri- or pararenal mass.

A transverse sonogram of the same patient demonstrates the psoas major muscle medial to the right kidney and the quadratus lumborum muscle posterior to the right kidney (Fig. B). The renal hilum exits medially. Note that the quadratus lumborum and psoas muscles in this patient are relatively hypoechoic. However, this depends upon both the individual patient and the technique used. Particularly in joggers, the psoas major muscle may be very prominent. Once again, it is important not to mistake the quadratus lumborum muscle for a complex fluid collection behind the kidney.

SUGGESTED READING

Callen PW, Filly RA, Marks WM: The quadratus lumborum muscle: a possible source of confusion in sonographic evaluation of the retroperitoneum. J Clin Ultrasound 7:349–352, 1979

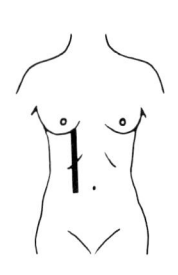

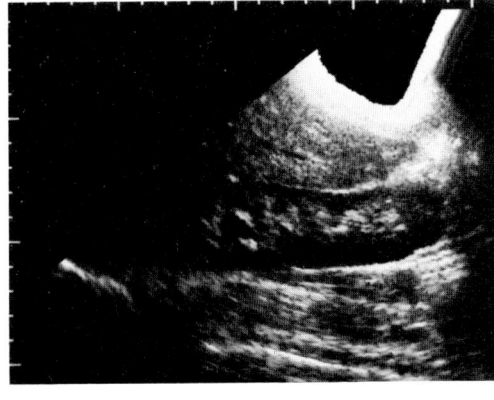

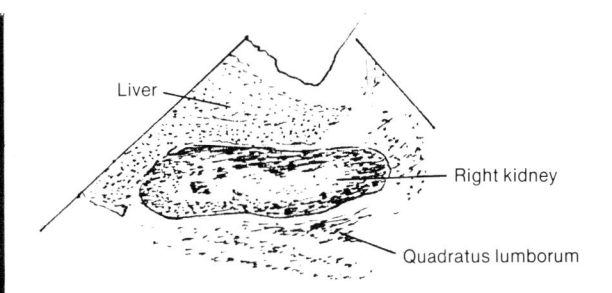

A

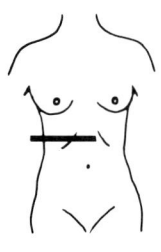

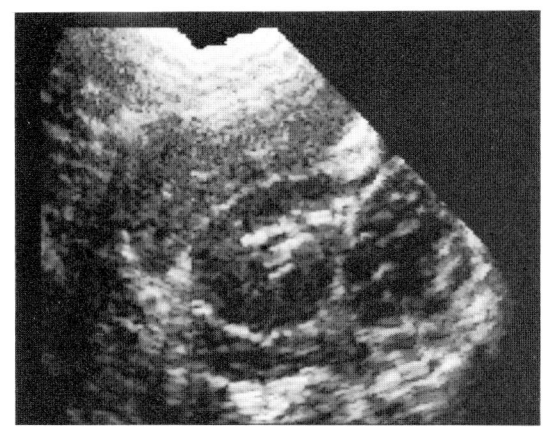

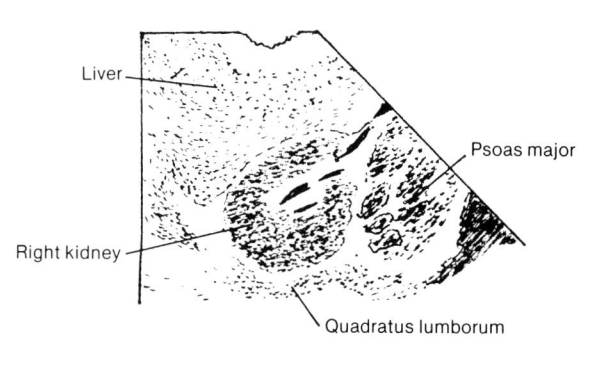

B

11.9 Horseshoe Kidney

A young woman underwent an abdominal sonogram because of left-sided abdominal pain. A longitudinal section through the right upper quadrant demonstrated normal cortex, medulla, and renal sinus (Fig. A). The axis of the kidney, however, was noted to be more vertical than normal. A coronal section through the left renal fossa demonstrated the left kidney to be hydronephrotic (Fig. B). A transverse scan through the abdomen at the level of the inferior renal poles shows the abnormal axis of the right kidney as well as an isthmus running from right kidney to left (Fig. C). These findings are characteristic of horseshoe kidney. Subsequent excretory urography demonstrated the horseshoe kidney. The nephrogram phase is shown in Figure D.

Horseshoe kidney is a common congenital abnormality, found in 0.25 percent of the general population. It is generally asymptomatic but can be associated with hydronephrosis, infection, or calculus formation. Multiple arteries to the kidney are typical. Although the isthmus of the horseshoe kidney can be identified sonographically, bowel gas may preclude visualization of this structure. This can be a particular problem in patients who have an abdominal aortic aneurysm identified sonographically since, if the horseshoe kidney is not clearly appreciated, the surgeon may not be alert to the presence of multiple vessels. Therefore, any patient with a vertical axis to the kidneys shown on the sonogram and in whom the midretroperitoneum is obscured by gas should have a radiographic study such as urography or computed tomography to exclude horseshoe kidney or other abnormalities.

SUGGESTED READINGS

Mindell HJ, Kupic EA: Horseshoe kidney: ultrasonic demonstration. Am J Roentgenol 129:526–527, 1977

Rosenfield AT, Lowman RM, Taylor KJW: Urography in pre-operative evaluation of abdominal aortic aneurysms. Urology 7:652–654, 1976

Trackler RT, Resnick ML, Leopold GR: Pelvic horseshoe kidney: ultrasound findings and case report. J Clin Ultrasound 6:51–52, 1978

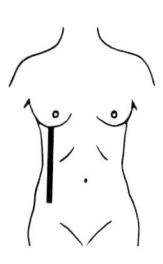

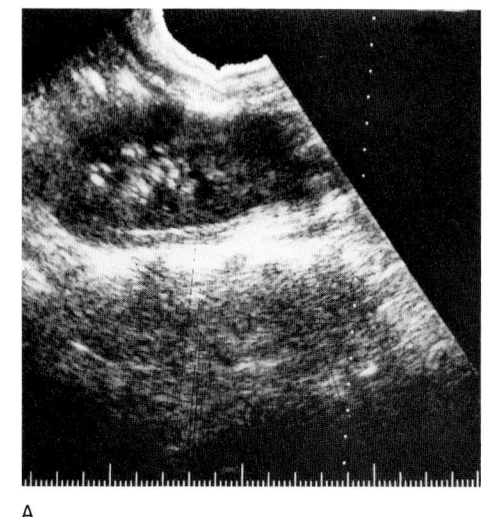

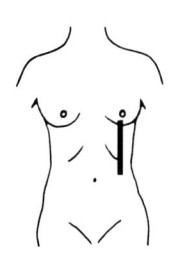

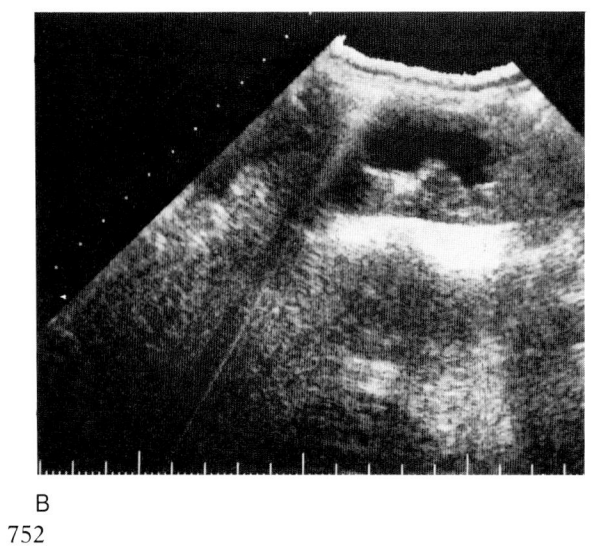

A

B
752

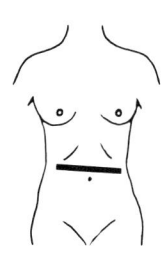

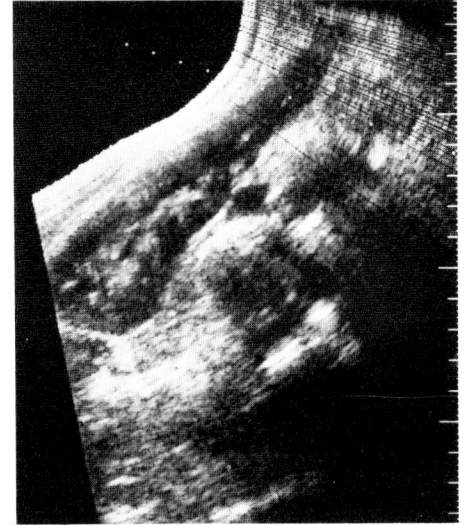

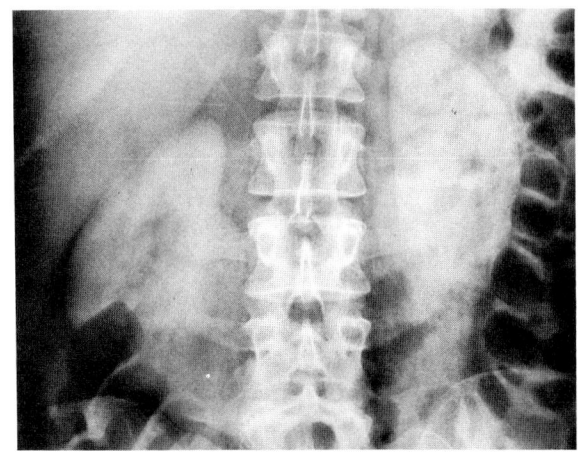

C

D

Renal Masses (11.10 and 11.11)

11.10 Anatomic Splenic Flexure as a Left Renal Impostor

The anatomic splenic flexure is the portion of the colon laterally placed below the tip of the spleen. The normal position of the flexure is considered reliable evidence that there is renal tissue in the left renal fossa. The posterior portion of the left colon lies medial to the stomach in the left renal fossa in cases of renal agenesis or ectopia. In these cases, a pitfall in the ultrasound examination of patients exists. If the splenic flexure is fluid-filled, it may mimic a renal cyst or renal cystic disease. If, however, it is filled with feces, it may mimic a solid mass in the renal fossa.

A 15-year-old boy was admitted with right flank pain. The excretory urogram demonstrates a hypertrophied right kidney and a medial splenic flexure (Fig. A). (The arrows indicate the direction in which barium would flow in a barium enema.) Bistable ultrasound examination of the renal area, done with the patient in the prone position, shows a normal right kidney and a mass with central echoes, suggesting a kidney in the left renal fossa (Fig. B). Identification of the anatomic splenic flexure placed medially in the region of the renal fossa on the urogram indicates that a left kidney is not present, and that the mass seen on ultrasound examination is the anatomic splenic flexure filled with feces. An additional clue on the tranverse sonogram is that the echoes that mimic the left collecting system are laterally placed.

A gray-scale ultrasound examination later shows that the previously noted "kidney" has disappeared (Fig. C). There is no definite structure in the left renal fossa. A fluid-filled stomach is seen anterior to this region.

(Fig. A and Scans B and C from Teele RL, Rosenfield AT, Freedman GS: The anatomic splenic flexure: an ultrasonic renal imposter. Am J Roentgenol 128:115–120, 1977. © 1977 Am Roentgen Ray Soc.)

SUGGESTED READINGS

Meyers MA, Whalen JP, Evans JA, et al: Malposition and displacement of the bowel in renal agenesis and ectopia: new observations. Am J Roentgenol 117:323, 1973

Moscatello V, Lebowitz RL: Malposition of the colon in left renal agenesis and ectopia. Radiology 120:371–376, 1976

Teele RL, Rosenfield AT, Freedman GS: The anatomic splenic flexure: an ultrasonic renal imposter. Am J Roentgenol 128:115–120, 1977

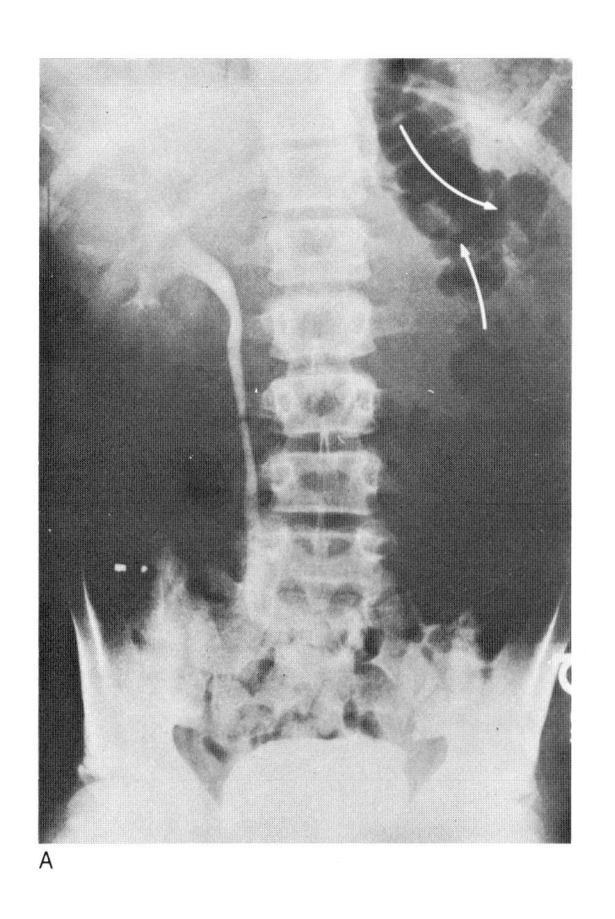

A

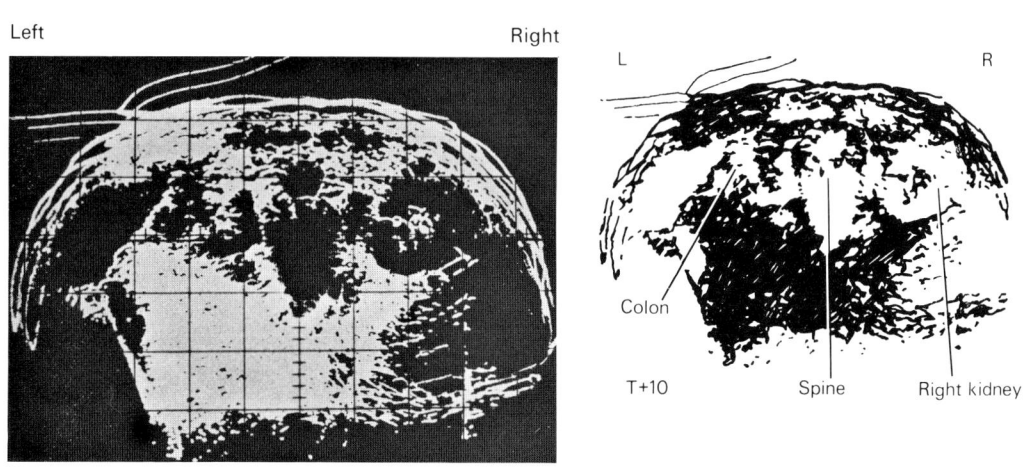

Left   Right

L   R

Colon

T+10   Spine   Right kidney

B

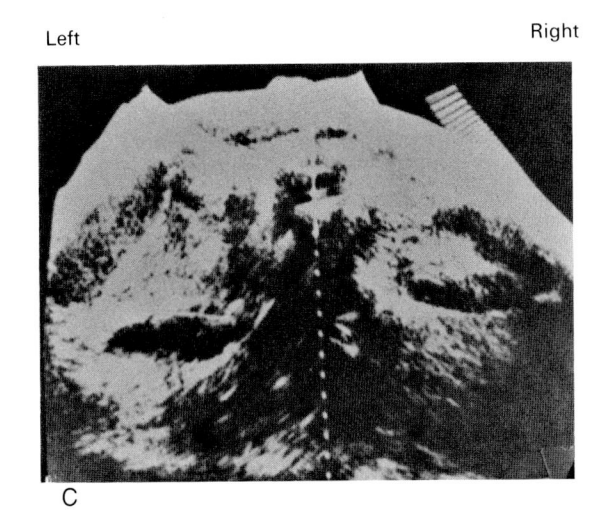

Left Right

C

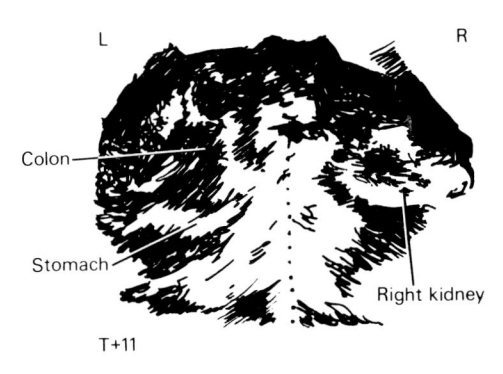

L R

Colon
Stomach
Right kidney

T+11

11.11 Anatomic Hepatic Flexure as Right Renal Imposter

A 4-year-old boy presented with a history of anuria and convulsions. A palpable left upper quadrant mass was noted at physical examination. A longitudinal coronal scan of the left upper quadrant showed the mass to be a hydronephrotic left kidney (Fig. A). Sonography through the right upper quadrant showed multiple fluid-filled structures in the right renal fossa. (Fig. B is a longitudinal study with the patient supine.) A subsequent sonogram demonstrated echogenic bowel in the right renal fossa as well as the left hydronephrosis. Figure C is performed with the patient prone, K is the left kidney, S the spine, P is the dilated renal pelvis.

Curtis et al.[1] reported that in right renal agenesis and ectopia the descending duodenum and lucent jejunum may be positioned in the right renal fossa. As with the left renal fossa, bowel may mimic a mass or even normal kidney.

(Figs. A-C from Rosenfield AT, Berg GR, Taylor KJW: Anuria and palpable left upper quadrant mass in a four-year-old. pp. 249–250. In Rosenfield AT (ed.): Genitourinary Ultrasonography. Clinics in Diagnostic Ultrasound, Vol 2. Churchill Livingstone, New York, 1979.)

SUGGESTED READINGS

Meyers MA, Whalen JP, Evans JA, et al: Malposition and displacement of bowel in renal agenesis and ectopia: new observations. Am J Roentgenol 117:323–333, 1973

Rosenfield AT, Berg GR, Taylor KJW: Anuria and palpable left upper quadrant mass in a four-year-old. pp. 249–250. In Rosenfield AT (ed): Genitourinary Ultrasonography. Clinics in Diagnostic Ultrasound, Vol 2. Churchill Livingstone, New York, 1979

Teele RL, Rosenfield AT, Freedman GS: The anatomic splenic flexure: an ultrasonic renal impostor. Am J Roentgenol 128:115–120, 1977

REFERENCE

1. Curtis JA, Sudhu V, Steiner RM: Malposition of the colon in right renal agenesis, ectopia, and anterior nephrectomy. Am J Roentgenol 129:845–850, 1977

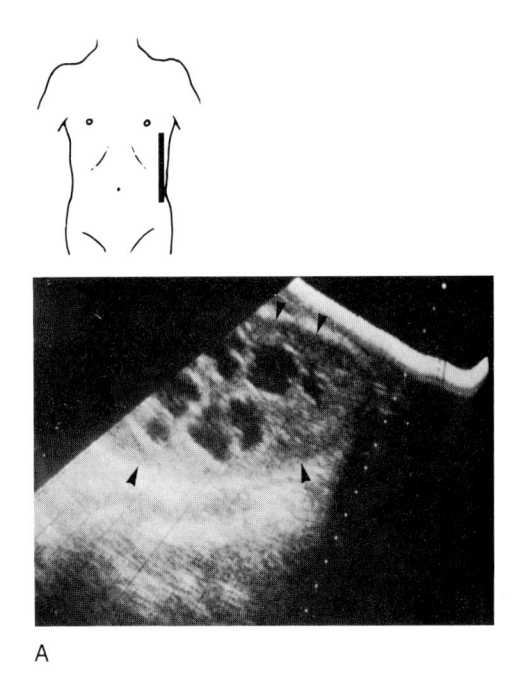

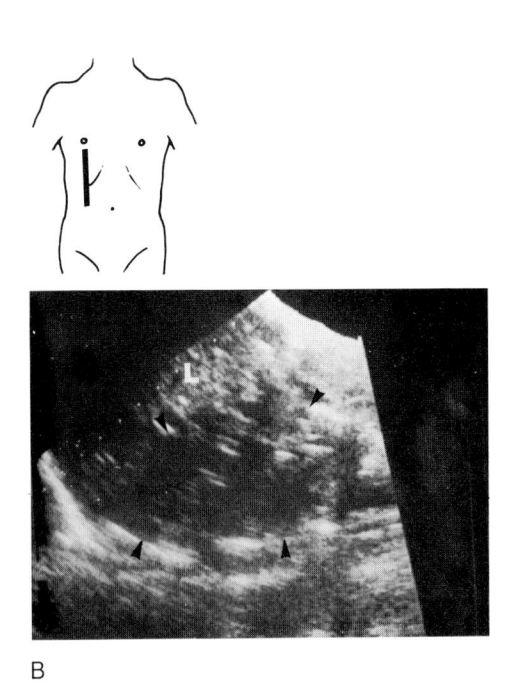

A

B

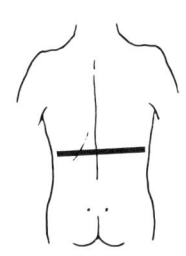

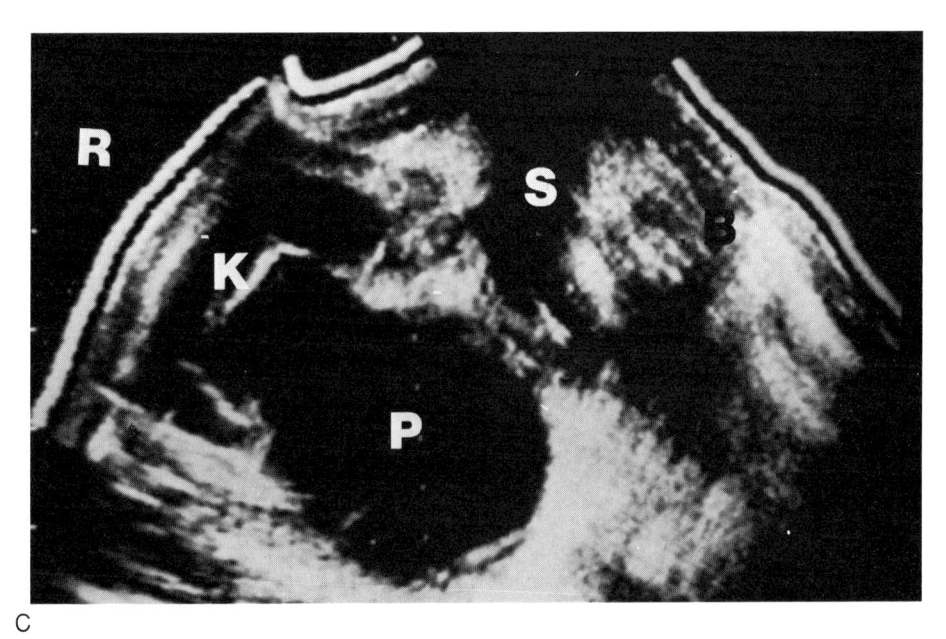

C

11.12 Duplication of the Collecting System

Sonography was performed on a newborn girl because hydronephrosis on the right side was identified in utero. Sections through the right kidney (Fig. A) demonstrate fluid-filled masses throughout; exiting from the kidney are two ovoid fluid-filled structures consistent with dilated ureters (Fig. B). A longitudinal sonogram taken through the right true pelvis shows one of these two distended ureters coursing behind the bladder and ending in a ureterocele (Fig. C). Transverse sonograms through the pelvis once again show the dilated right ureter and the ureterocele in the bladder. The second dilated ureter emerging from the right kidney terminates at the level of the true pelvis on the sonogram (Fig. B). Excretory urography (Fig. D) demonstrates the lower pole ureter, which is narrowed (arrowed) in the true pelvis by the dilated upper pole ureter which does not fill with contrast medium. Surgery revealed a duplicated collecting system on the right side with an ectopic ureterocele related to the upper pole moiety.

Duplication of the urinary tract is a common congenital abnormality. The upper pole ureter is malpositioned and may be obstructed, leading to an ectopic ureterocele. The lower pole system also may be dilated due to vesicoureteral reflux or obstruction from the upper pole system, as in this patient. If the obstructed upper pole system does not function and if the moiety is small, its identification at excretory urography may be difficult. Sonography, which is independent of renal function, permits ready localization of the upper half of the kidney and identification of the ureterocele within the bladder. Ultrasound may also be used to guide percutaneous puncture for antegrade pyelography where this is indicated to identify the termination of an ectopic ureter.

SUGGESTED READINGS

Bird K: Duplicated collecting system with pyohydronephrosis of the lower pole system. pp. 249–250. In Rosenfield AT (ed): Genitourinary Ultrasound. Clinics in Diagnostic Ultrasound, Vol 2. Churchill Livingstone, New York, 1979

Mascatello VJ, Smith EH, Carrera GF, et al: Ultrasound evaluation of the obstructed duplex kidney. Am J Roentgenol 129:113, 1977

Rose JS, McCarthy J, Yeh HC: Ultrasound diagnosis of ectopic ureterocele. Pediatr Radiol 8:17–20, 1979

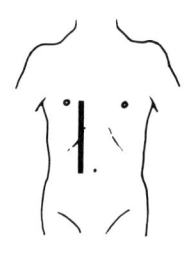

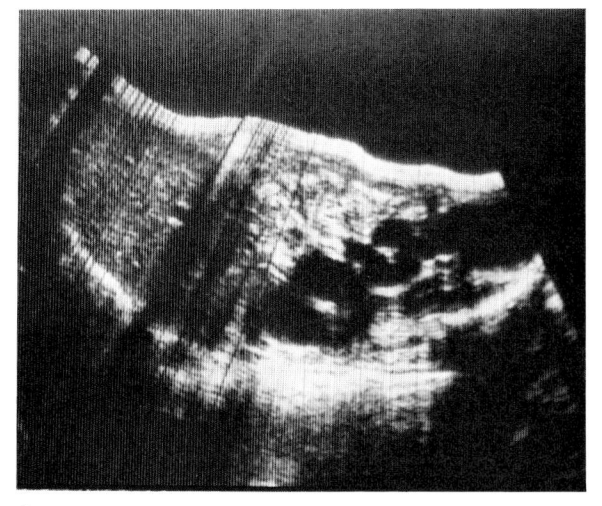

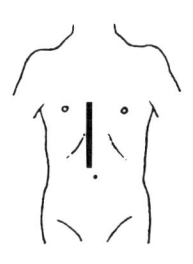

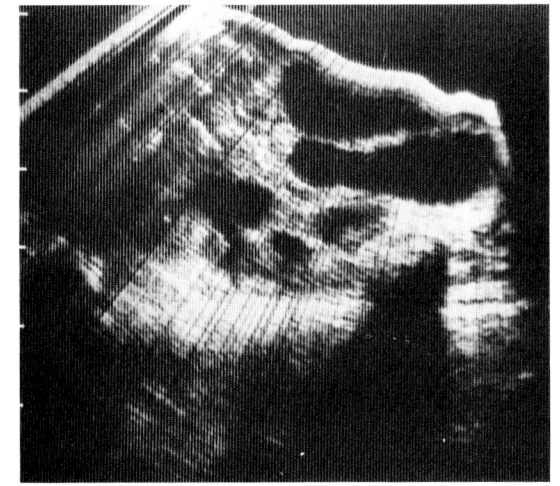

A

B

761

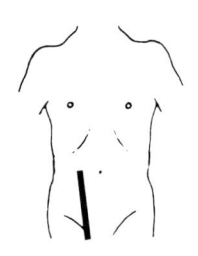

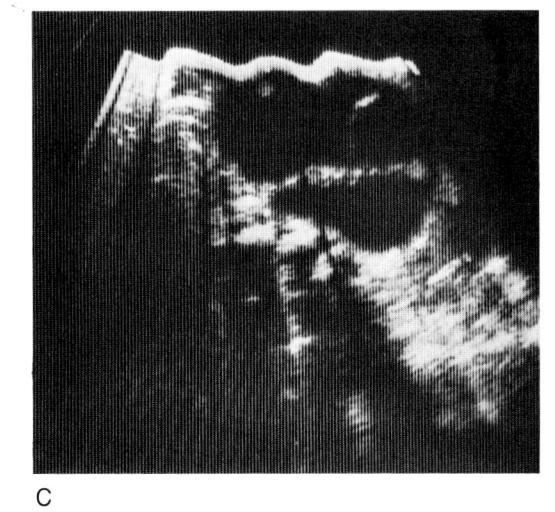

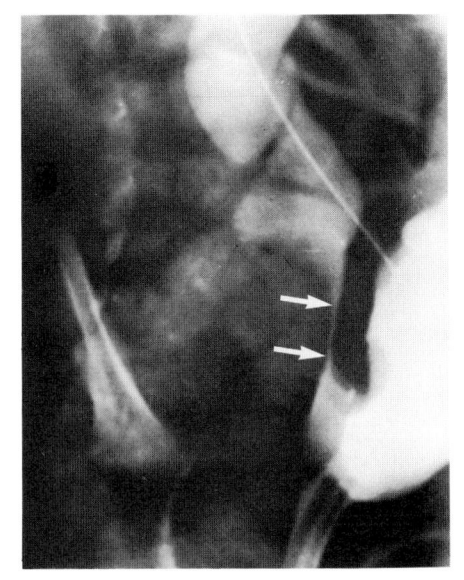

C

D

11.13 Malrotation

Longitudinal and transverse coronal sonograms through the left upper quadrant of a middle-aged woman with a pelvic mass are shown in Figures A and B. The renal sinus is seen to exit laterally on both projections. This finding is typical of malrotation of the kidney. This phenomenon should not be mistaken for pathologic change.

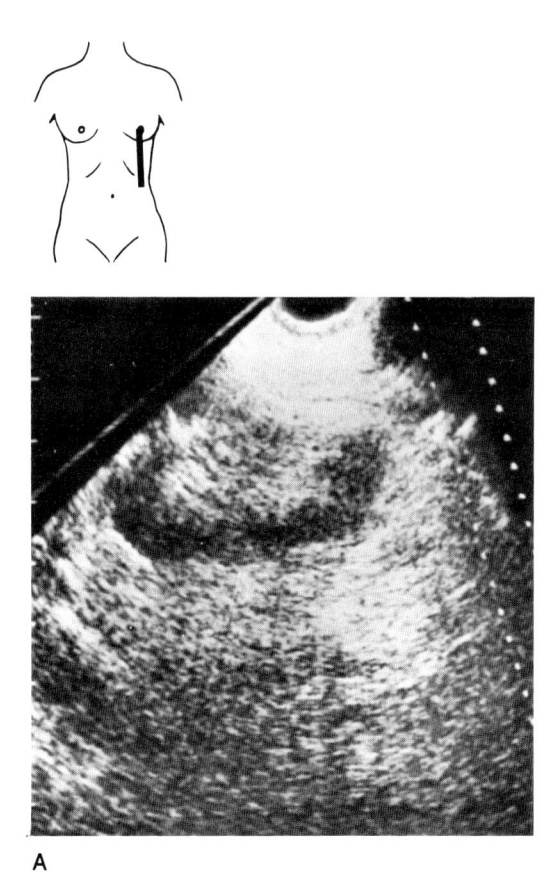

A

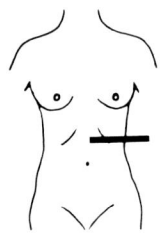

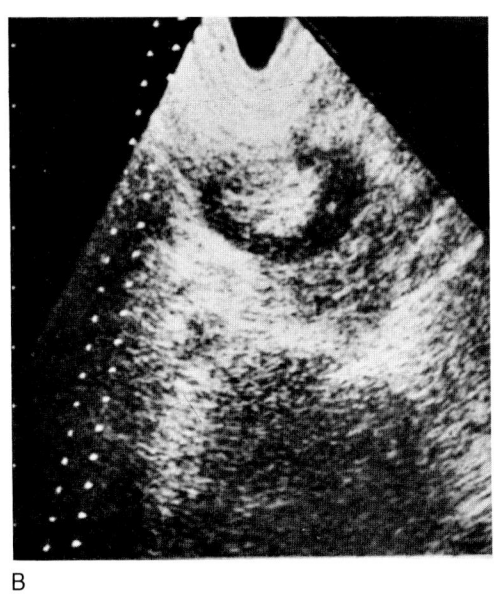

B

11.14 Pelvic Kidney

A longitudinal sonogram was taken through the bladder of a young woman who presented with a palpable left pelvic mass. The sonogram showed the mass to be an ectopic kidney. The ability of ultrasound to identify normal renal anatomy in the pelvic kidney permitted the correct diagnosis and excluded hydronephrosis and masses, thereby eliminating the need for excretory urography.

(Scan from Rosenfield AT, Taylor KJW, Crade M: Renal ultrasound 1979: gray scale, real time, Doppler pp. 1–23. In Rosenfield AT (ed): Genitourinary Ultrasonography. Clinics in Diagnostic Ultrasound, Vol. 2. Churchill Livingstone, New York, 1979.)

SUGGESTED READING

Trackler RT, Resnick ML, Leopold GR: Pelvic horseshoe kidney: ultrasound findings and case report. J Clin Ultrasound 6:51–52, 1978

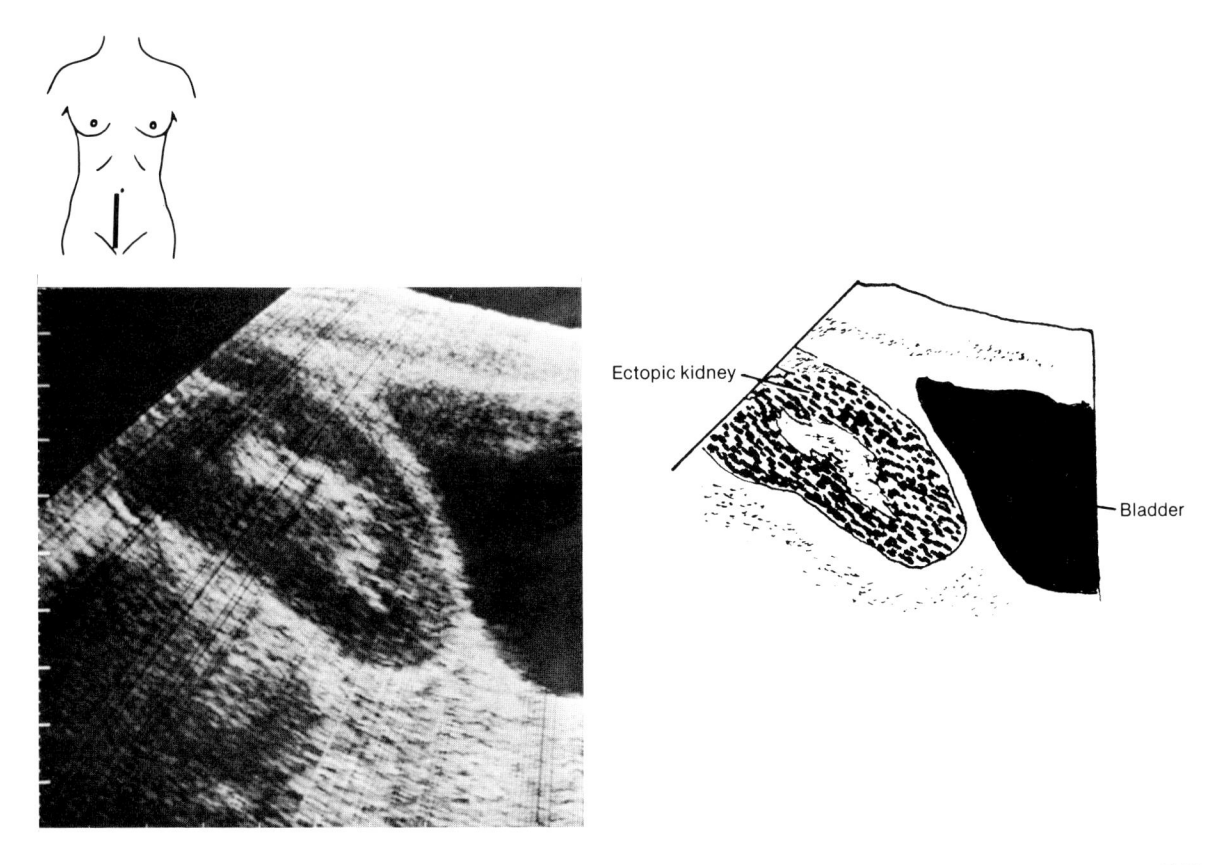

11.15 Renal Failure and the Nonfunctioning Kidney

The ability to diagnose or exclude hydronephrosis by sonography without employing ionizing radiation or contrast media has led to the use of ultrasound as the initial study in evaluating patients in renal failure. The following section on the renal sinus includes a discussion of the uses of ultrasound in evaluating the kidneys for urinary tract dilatation as well as some of the pitfalls of ultrasound diagnosis. Ultrasound has also proved useful for tissue characterization and can play a role in defining medical renal disease. The section on the renal parenchyma describes the findings encountered in bilateral medical renal disease and renal vascular occlusion.

Major acute insults to the kidney may lead to apparent nonfunction on excretory urography. The two principal causes are renal trauma and urinary tract infection. These are discussed in the appropriate sections.

The evaluation of the patient with renal failure and/or a nonfunctioning kidney must be individualized. In most instances, ultrasound will be the initial examination but other techniques may sometimes be more desirable. If indicated, ultrasound can also be used to guide percutaneous puncture for antegrade pyelography, or percutaneous nephrostomy.

The renal transplant patient presents a special situation in which acute or chronic transplant rejection, lymphocele or urinoma formation, acute tubular necrosis, and obstruction are all major considerations. The section on renal transplantation discusses these entities.

SUGGESTED READINGS

Behan M, Wisxon D, Kazam E: Sonographic evaluation of the non-functioning kidney. J Clin Ultrasound 7:449–548, 1979

McClennan: Current approaches to the azotemic patient. Radiol Clin North Am 17:197–211, 1979

Rosenfield, AT: Ultrasound evaluation of renal parenchymal disease and hydronephrosis. Urol Radiol 4:125–133, 1982

Rosenfield AT, Taylor KJW, Dembner AG, et al: Ultrasound of the renal sinus: new observations. AJR 133:441–448, 1979

Sanders RC, Bearman S: B-scan ultrasound in the diagnosis of hydronephrosis. Radiology 108:375–382, 1973

Renal Sinus (11.16 and 11.17)

11.16 Abnormal Sinus

The most common application of ultrasound to the renal sinus is the exclusion of hydronephrosis. Identification of a normal renal sinus is generally thought to be a reliable indicator that obstruction is not present. The ultrasound findings with respect to the size of the collecting system correlate well with the findings on excretory urography. However, the excretory urogram is performed during osmotic diuresis, secondary to the contrast medium, which challenges the kidney with fluid. Ultrasound generally is not performed under these conditions. In chronic renal failure, the major cause of a false-negative ultrasound study is retroperitoneal fibrosis, which is known to be associated in some patients with inapparent obstruction. In acute renal failure, an intrarenal collecting system may not be obviously dilated in the first few hours following obstruction. False-positive sonograms for hydronephrosis are common and/are related mainly to an extrarenal collecting system, overhydration, or fluid-filled masses such as parapelvic cysts, calyceal diverticula, or renal artery aneurysms mimicking a dilated collecting system. Also, hydronephrosis is not equivalent to obstruction, since other causes of urinary tract dilatation including infection, vesicoureteral reflux, and postobstructive changes, can be responsible. Tables 11-1 and 11-2, modified from Amis et al.,[1] summarize the causes of false-negative and false-positive sonograms for urinary tract obstruction.

Other lesions of the renal sinus, including nephrolithiasis and tumor also can be evaluated by ultrasound and are discussed below.

Table 11-1. Causes of False-Negative Ultrasound for Obstruction

Acute Renal Obstruction
  Early: system not dilated
  Decompression secondary to ruptured calyx
  Partial obstruction
  Intermittent obstruction
Chronic Obstruction
  Retroperitoneal fibrosis
  Partial obstruction
  Intermittent obstruction
Technical Factors
  Staghorn calculus: stone obscures hydronephrosis
  Dehydrated patient (partial obstruction or retroperitoneal fibrosis)

(Modified from Amis ES, Cronan JJ, Pfister RC, et al: Ultrasonic inaccuracies in diagnosis of renal obstruction. Urology 19:101–105, 1982.)

Table 11-2. Causes of False-Positive Ultrasound for Obstruction

Normal System
  Extrarenal pelvis
  Full bladder (especially infants)
  High flow rate
    Diabetes insipidus
    Medication (e.g., diuretics)
    Overhydration
  Nonobstructive dilatation in pyelonephritis
  Vesicoureteral reflux
Blunted Calyces: No Obstruction
  Papillary necrosis
  Congenital megacalyces
  Reflux nephropathy
Renal Sinus Structures Mimicking Hydronephrosis
  Parapelvic cyst
  Calyceal diverticulum
  Renal artery aneurysm
  Arteriovenous malformation

(Modified from Amis ES, Cronan JJ, Pfister RC, et al: Ultrasonic inaccuracies in diagnosis of renal obstruction. Urology 19:101–105, 1982.)

SUGGESTED READINGS

Amis ES, Cronan JJ, Pfister RC, et al: Ultrasonic inaccuracies in diagnosis of renal obstruction. Urology 19:101–105, 1982

Cronan JJ, Amis ES, Yoder IC, et al: Peripelvic cysts: an impostor of sonographic hydronephrosis. J Ultrasound Med 1:229–236, 1982

Ellenbogen PH, Scheible FW, Talner LB, et al: Sensitivity of gray scale ultrasound in detecting urinary tract obstruction. AJR 130:731–733, 1978

Hasch E: Ultrasound scanning for monitoring childhood hydronephrosis. J Clin Ultrasound 6:156–159, 1978

Rosenfield AT, Taylor KJW, Dembner AG, et al: Ultrasound of the renal sinus: new observations. AJR 133:441–448, 1979

Sanders RC, Bearman S: B-scan ultrasound in the diagnosis of hydronephrosis. Radiology 108:375–382, 1973

Sanders RC, Conrad MR: The ultrasonic characteristics of the renal pelvocalyceal echo complex. J Clin Ultrasound 5:372–377, 1977

Talner LB, Scheible WF, Ellenbogen PH, et al: Ultrasound diagnosis of hydronephrosis in azotemic patients. Urol Radiol 3:1–6, 1981

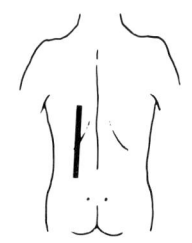

11.17 Normal: Variation with Hydration

Figure A is a longitudinal sonogram through the left kidney with the patient prone. Note the normal renal sinus, identified as a zone of intense echoes. Fluid within the collecting system is not seen in this patient who has been fasting for 12 hours.

Figure B is a similar scan of the same patient following ingestion of a fluid load immediately after the scan obtained in Figure A. Note that the central portion of the collecting system is somewhat dilated. The state of the collecting system varies with the degree of hydration. When findings are similar to those in Figure A, hydronephrosis can be excluded, except in cases such as those discussed in the following pages.

SUGGESTED READINGS

Hasch E: Changes in renal pelvic size in children after fluid intake demonstrated by ultrasound. Ultrasound Med Biol 2:287–290, 1977

Hasch E: Ultrasound scanning for monitoring childhood hydronephrosis. J Clin Ultrasound 6:156–159, 1978

Rosenfield AT, Taylor KJW, Dembner AG, et al: Ultrasound of the renal sinus: new observations. AJR 133:441–448, 1979

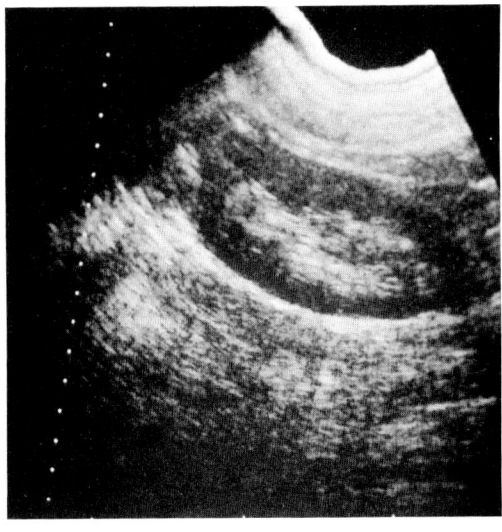

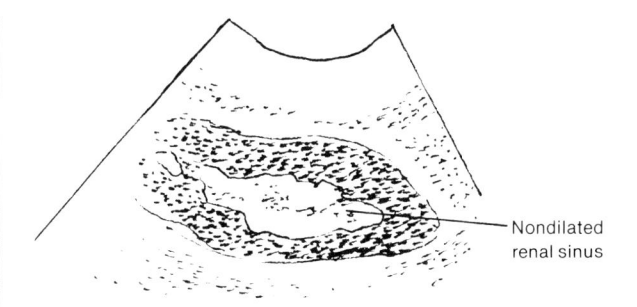

A

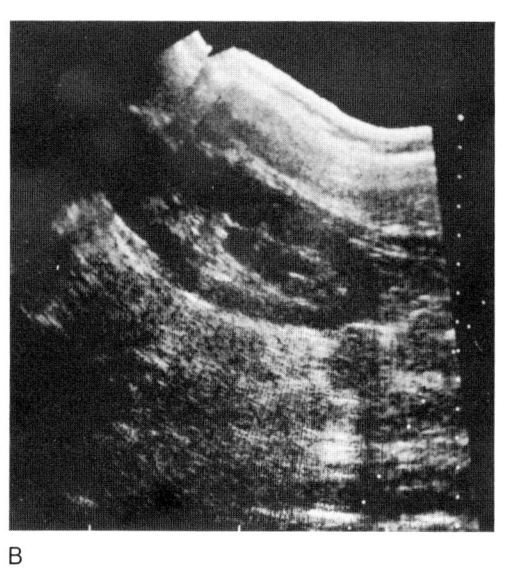

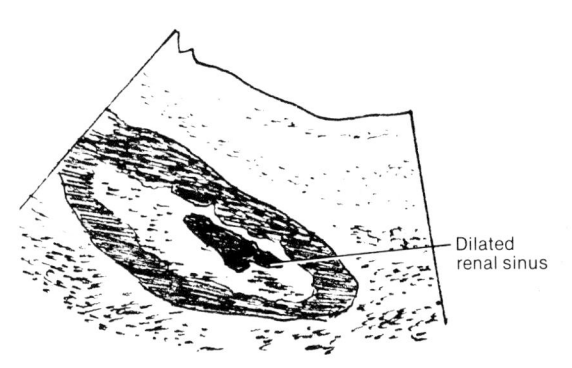

B

Dilated renal sinus

Hydronephrosis (11.18 to 11.25)

11.18 Incidence and Appearance

Obstructive uropathy is the most common cause of dilatation of the collecting system. The earliest finding is separation of the collecting system walls by anechoic fluid seen on a transverse sonogram in Figure A and on a longitudinal scan in Figure B. When more distended, the dilated pelvis appears as an ovoid or figure-8 structure (Fig. C). The dilated calyces are blunted, fluid-filled structures which can be traced into the pelvis (Fig. D). The final result of obstructive uropathy is the formation of a hydronephrotic sac with little or no renal parenchyma (Fig. E). Although no statement can be made about renal function from the sonographic findings, the thickness of the remaining parenchyma can be estimated and the cause of the hydronephrosis may be apparent. In the presence of established hydronephrosis, the brightness of the parenchyma of the kidney may be more intense. In Figure E the brightness of the parenchyma of the kidney is greater than that of the liver, a reversal of the normal relationship. This increased echogenicity is due both to compressed parenchyma and to the deposition of collagen.

SUGGESTED READINGS

Amis ES, Cronan JJ, Pfister RC, et al: Ultrasonic inaccuracies in diagnosis of renal obstruction. Urology 19:101–105, 1982

Lee JKT, Baron RL, Melson L, et al: Can real-time ultrasonography replace static B-scanning in the diagnosis of renal obstruction? Radiology 139:161–165, 1981

Rosenfield AT: Ultrasound evaluation of renal parenchymal disease and hydronephrosis. Urol Radiol 4:125–133, 1982

Sanders RC, Bearman S: B-scan ultrasound in the diagnosis of hydronephrosis. Radiology 108:375–382, 1973

Sanders RC, Conrad MR: The ultrasonic characteristics of the renal pelvocalyceal echo complex. J Clin Ultrasound 5:372–377, 1977

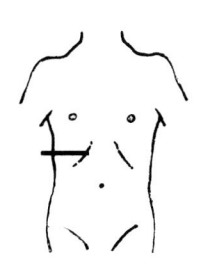

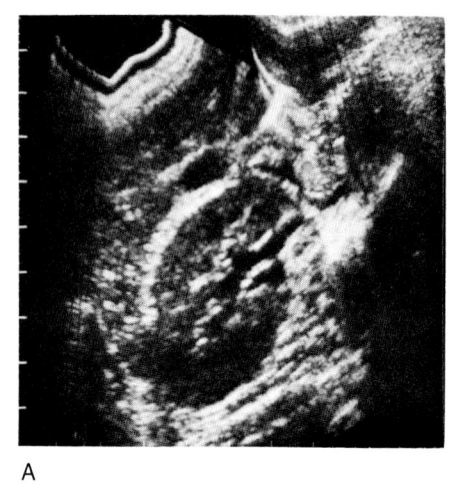

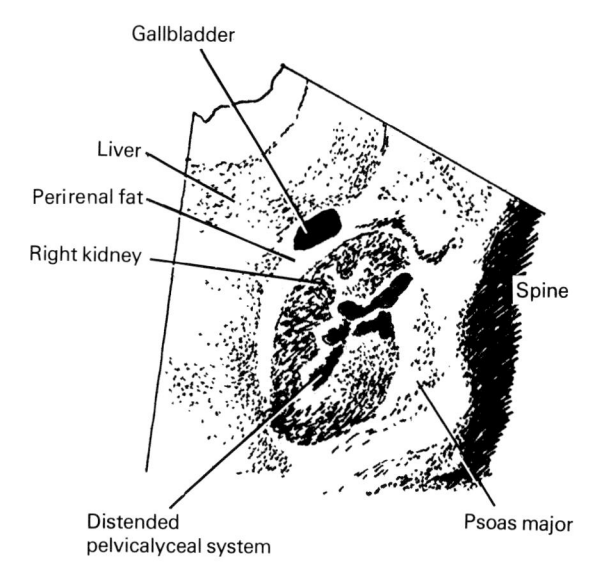

A

- Gallbladder
- Liver
- Perirenal fat
- Right kidney
- Distended pelvicalyceal system
- Spine
- Psoas major

B

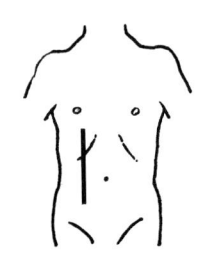

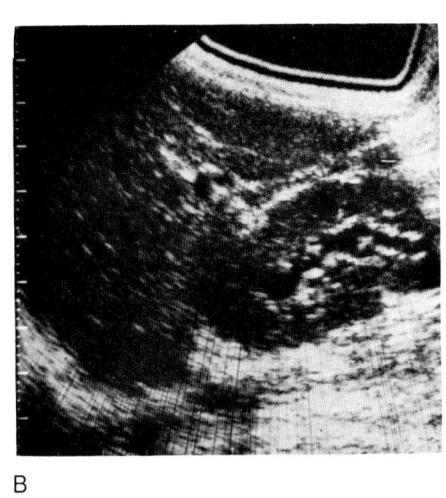

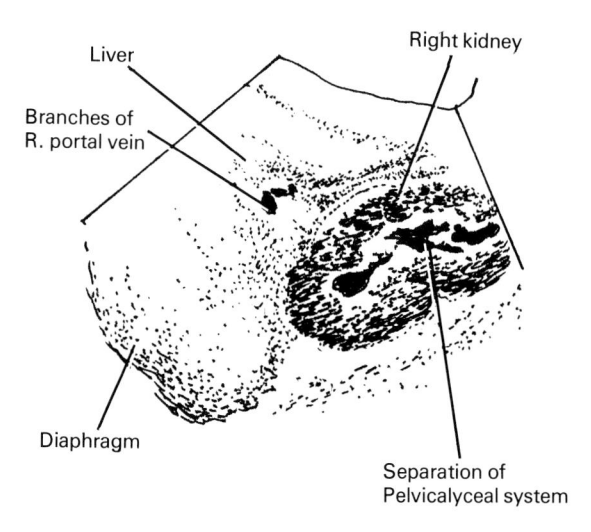

- Liver
- Branches of R. portal vein
- Right kidney
- Diaphragm
- Separation of Pelvicalyceal system

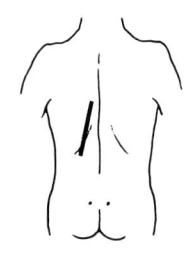

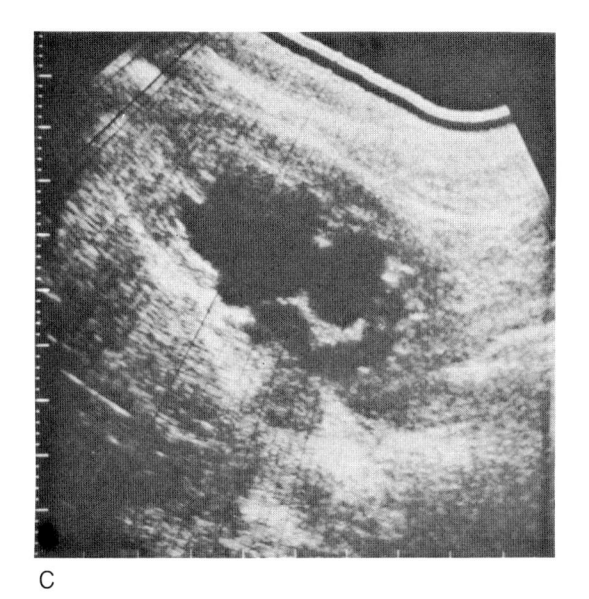

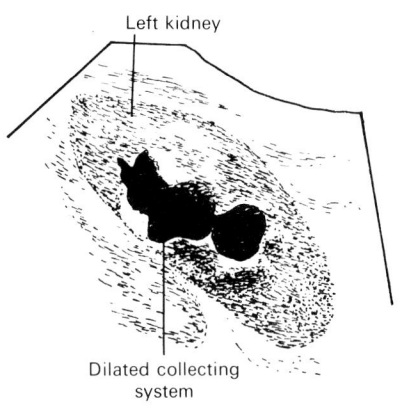

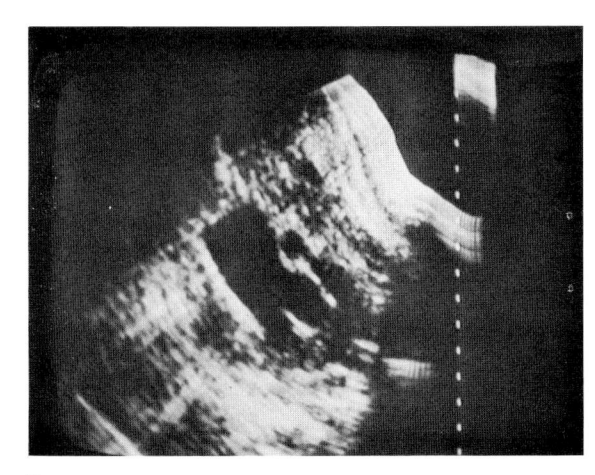

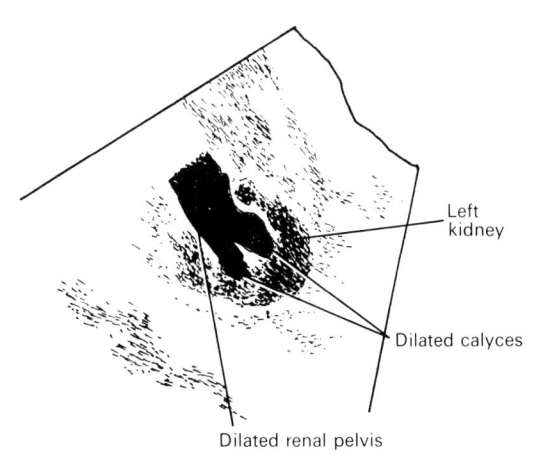

C

D

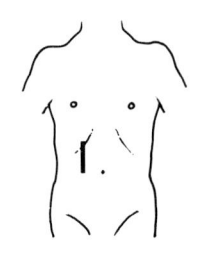

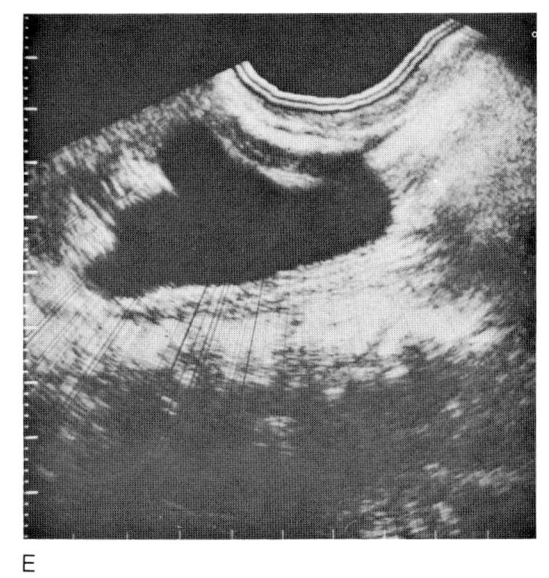

E

11.19 Neonatal: Ureteropelvic Junction Obstruction

The figure shows a coronal section through the upper abdomen of a young neonate in renal failure with the patient in left-side-down decubitus position. The sonogram demonstrates dilated fluid-filled masses (r and l) replacing the normal renal sinus and parenchyma. The distention is more marked on the right side. Note the normal Liver (L) and spleen (S). Bilateral ureteropelvic junction obstruction was relieved by surgery. The failure to identify a dilated ureter on the ultrasound study is a strong indicator that the obstruction is at the ureteropelvic junction.

(This case and figure taken from Rosenfield AT, Taylor KJW, Crade M: Renal ultrasound 1979: Gray scale, real time, Doppler. pp 1–23. In Rosenfield AT (ed): Clinics in Diagnostic Ultrasound, Vol 2. Genitourinary Ultrasonography. Churchill Livingstone, New York, 1979.)

SUGGESTED READINGS

Chop RA, Teele R: Hydronephrosis: narrowing the differential diagnosis with ultrasound. J Clin Ultrasound 8:473–478, 1980

Rosenfield AT, Taylor KJW, Crade M: Renal ultrasound 1979: gray scale, real time, Doppler. pp. 1–23. In Rosenfield AT (ed): Clinics in Diagnostic Ultrasound, Vol 2. Genitourinary Ultrasonography. Churchill Livingstone, New York, 1979

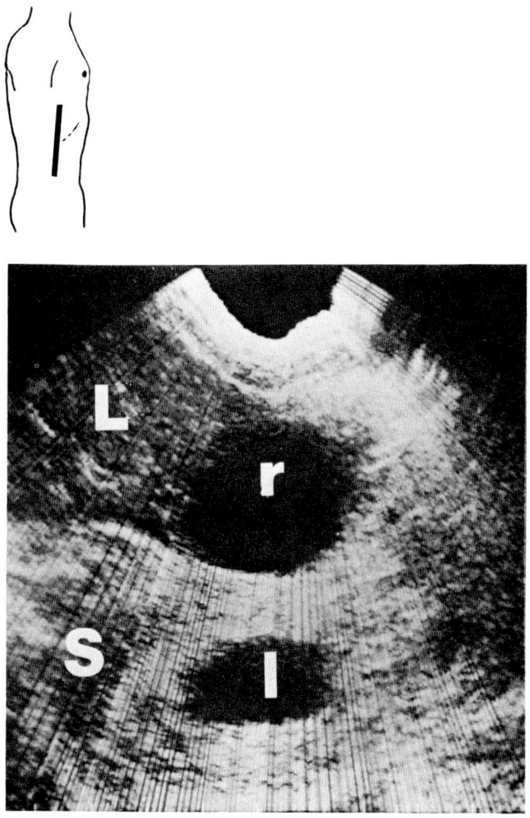
L
r
S
I

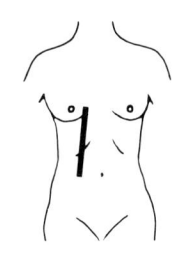

11.20 Partial Obstruction: The Ultrasound "Whittaker Test"

The identification of partial obstruction may require a fluid challenge to the kidney, initially described by Whittaker. Antegrade pyelography was performed by him and saline infused at varying flow rates. Failure of the pressure to rise with flow rates of 10 ml/minute was considered indicative of a nonobstructed system. The "Whittaker test" has found extensive application not only in partial obstruction but also in evaluating the dilated collecting system. If dilation is due to obstruction, the pressure rises during the Whittaker test whereas dilatation not due to obstruction, such as postobstructive changes or dilatation due to reflux, will not cause a rise in pressure. The principle of increasing the flow rate and following the appearances of the collecting system has also been applied to routine excretory urography, radioisotope studies, and ultrasound. Increased flow rate can be induced by ingestion of a large amount of fluid or a diuretic and may lead to dilatation.

A longitudinal sonogram (Fig. A) was performed through the right upper quadrant in a patient who had right flank pain following ingestion of a large amount of beer. The initial study performed on this patient before drinking demonstrated no dilatation of the collecting system although there was a questionable fullness of the upper pole. The patient was asked to ingest enough beer to reproduce her symptoms. A second sonogram was then taken, which demonstrated definite hydronephrosis in the upper pole moiety (arrows, Fig. B). At surgery, partial obstruction to the upper pole collecting system was confirmed.

(Figs. A & B from Rosenfield AT, Taylor, KJW, Dembner AG, et al: Ultrasound of the renal sinus: new observations. AJR 133:441–448, 1979, © 1979 Am Roentgen Ray Society.)

SUGGESTED READINGS

Hasch E: Ultrasound scanning for monitoring childhood hydronephrosis. J Clin Ultrasound 6:156–159, 1978

Rosenfield, AT, Hodson CJ: Excretory urography and nephrotomography. pp. 3–20. In Rosenfield AT, Glickman MG, Hodson J (eds): Diagnostic Imaging in Renal Disease. Appleton-Century Crofts, New York, 1979

Rosenfield AT, Taylor KJW, Dembner AG, et al: Ultrasound of the renal sinus: new observations. AJR 133:441–448, 1979

Whittaker RH: Methods of assessing obstruction in dilated ureters. Br J Urol 45:15–22, 1973

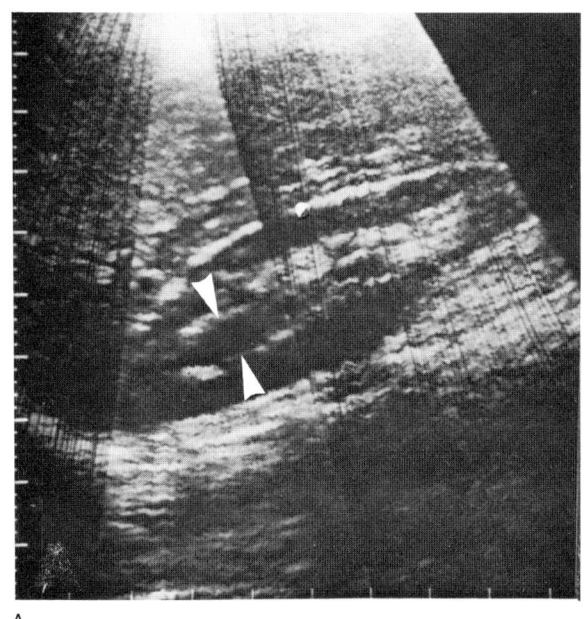

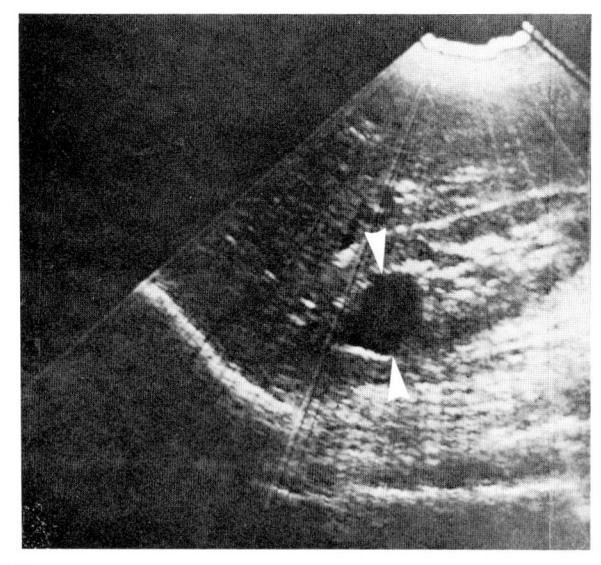

A

B

11.21 Hydronephrosis of Pregnancy

Hydronephrosis during pregnancy is a common finding, particularly during the third trimester. In one series there was hydronephrosis in 70 percent of pregnant woman in the right kidney and in 30 percent in the left during the third trimester compared to nonpregnant controls. There is also a higher incidence of urinary tract infection during pregnancy. Excretory urography is not desirable for routine screening during pregnancy because of irradiation to the fetus. Ultrasound examination of the urinary tract is a safe method of imaging which can diagnose anatomic abnormalities without using ionizing radiation. Hydronephrosis during pregnancy can be recognized by the separation of the normal central pelvicalyceal echoes. The kidneys may be more difficult to image in the pregnant woman, but the use of sector scanning will generally permit an adequate examination.

A 24-year-old pregnant woman presented with right upper quadrant pain. The clinical impression was of likely right-sided urinary tract disease. The longitudinal sonogram through the right lobe of the liver and gravid uterus demonstrates the entire medical picture (see Fig. 11-22B). The uterus is seen and there is a fundal placenta with the fetal head in vertex presentation. In addition, the mother's right kidney is well-seen; there is separation of the central pelvicalyceal echoes, characteristic of hydronephrosis. The gallbladder is anterior to the right kidney. There are gallstones within the gallbladder, with attenuation of the beam behind the gallstones creating a "shadow" which obscures a portion of the kidney. The gallstones were believed to be responsible for the patient's symptoms, and no radiologic procedures were required for further diagnosis.

SUGGESTED READING

Erickson LM, Nicholson SF, Lewall DB, et al: Ultrasound evaluation of hydronephrosis of pregnancy. J Clin Ultrasound 7:128–132, 1979

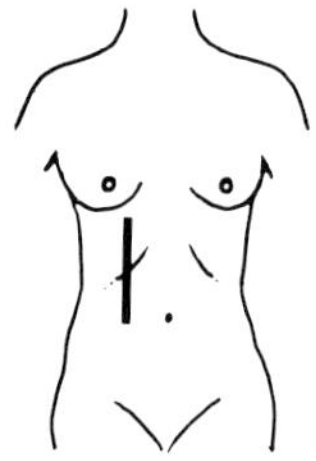

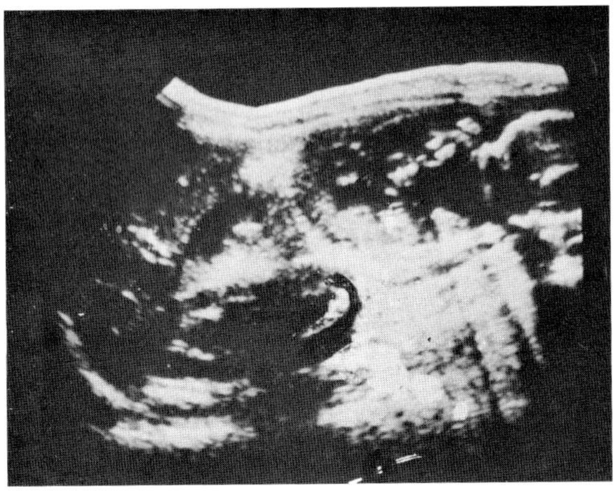

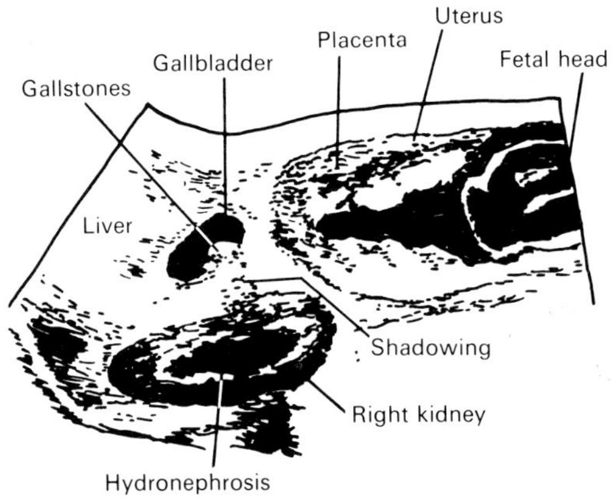
Uterus
Placenta
Fetal head
Gallbladder
Gallstones
Liver
Shadowing
Right kidney
Hydronephrosis

11.22 Secondary to Adenopathy

An adult with lymphoma underwent ultrasound examination of the right upper quadrant. The transverse sonogram (Fig. A) demonstrates right-sided hydronephrosis secondary to retroperitoneal adenopathy. In the right kidney, the pelvis was dilated and distended calyces were seen leading into the pelvis. Adenopathy is identified as lobulated masses which obscure the aorta and inferior vena cava. A longitudinal sonogram through the right upper quadrant (Fig. B) demonstrated the inferior vena cava displaced anteriorly by the adenopathy.

(Scans A & B from Rosenfield, AT: Renal and adrenal ultrasonography. pp. 28–58. In Filly RA, ed. Syllabus for the Categorical Course in Ultrasonography, Annual Meeting of the American Roentgen Ray Society, March 22–27th, 1982. © 1982 Am Roentgen Ray Soc.)

SUGGESTED READING

Chop RA, Teele R: Hydronephrosis: narrowing the differential diagnosis with ultrasound. J Clin Ultrasound 8:473–478, 1980

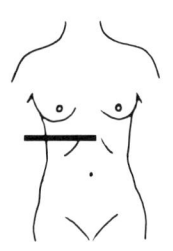

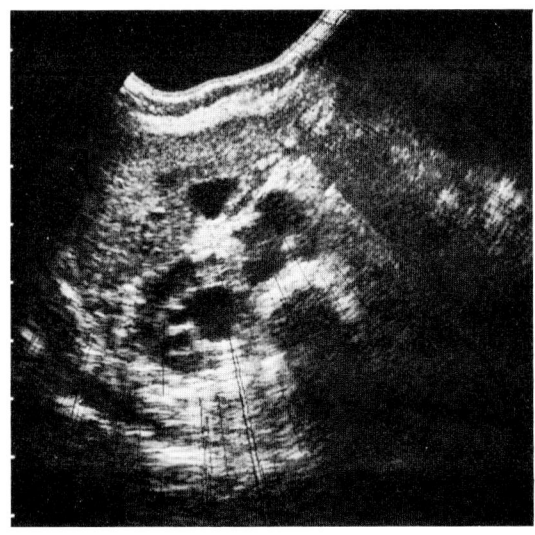

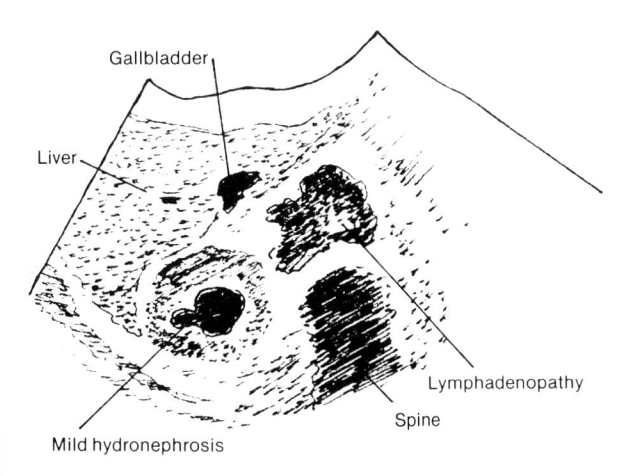

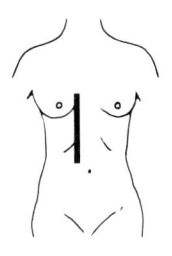

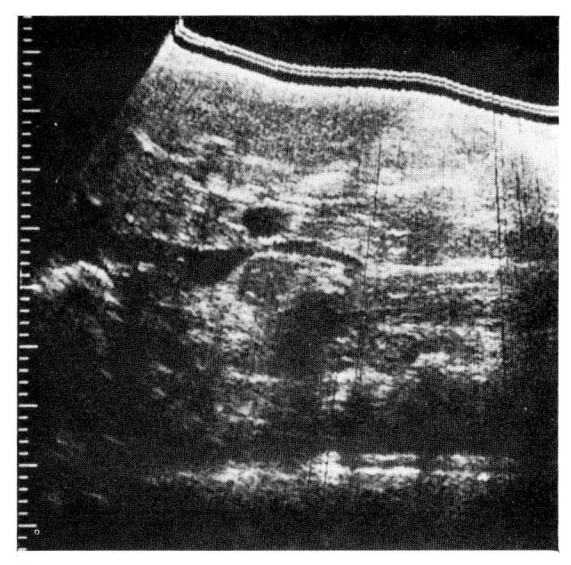

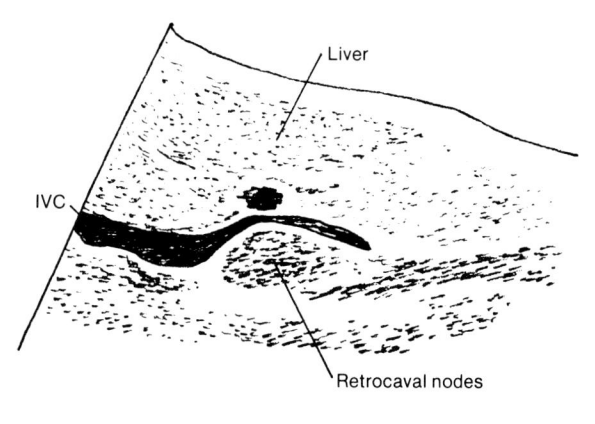

B

11.23 The Prune Belly Syndrome

A 6-year-old boy presented with the classic findings of prune belly syndrome: abdominal musculature deficiency, cryptorchidism, and urinary tract abnormality.[1] In this syndrome, the prognosis is dependent upon the degree of underlying renal dysplasia. The characteristic sonographic appearances are elongated, tortuous ureters without proportionate dilatation of the intrarenal collecting system. This is due to an intrinsic abnormality of the ureter with fibrous replacement of smooth muscle. A longitudinal sonogram through the right upper quadrant (Fig. A) showed no significant intrarenal collecting system dilatation and massive dilatation of the ureter. A transverse sonogram through the right kidney (Fig. B) again showed massive dilatation of the extrarenal pelvis and ureter, but minimal intrarenal change. A longitudinal sonogram through the midleft abdomen demonstrated a portion of the elongated tortuous left ureter. Figure C shows the corresponding excretory urogram. Note again the tortuous, disproportionately dilated ureters. Ultrasound also can be used to identify the undescended testes present in the syndrome if they are below the inguinal ring. A urachal process from the bladder dome or patent urachus may also be present and can be demonstrated sonographically.

Garris et al.[2] have categorized the sonographic findings in the upper urinary tract into three groups. In one group, a fluid-filled mass representing the hydronephrotic collecting system is seen in the renal fossae. Little parenchyma is visible. These findings are characteristic of dysplastic kidneys. Our case is typical of a second group of patients who have marked dilatation of the ureter with little or no dilatation of the renal pelvis and calyces. The final category includes patients with mild ureterectasis or normal findings on diagnostic studies.

REFERENCES

1. Buckett JE Jr: The prune belly syndrome. pp. 615–635. In Kulalis PP, King LR (eds): Clinical Pediatric Urology. W.B. Saunders, Philadelphia, 1976
2. Garris J, Kangarloo H, Sarti D, et al: The ultrasound spectrum of prune belly syndrome. J Clin Ultrasound 8:117–120, 1980

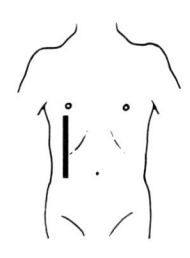

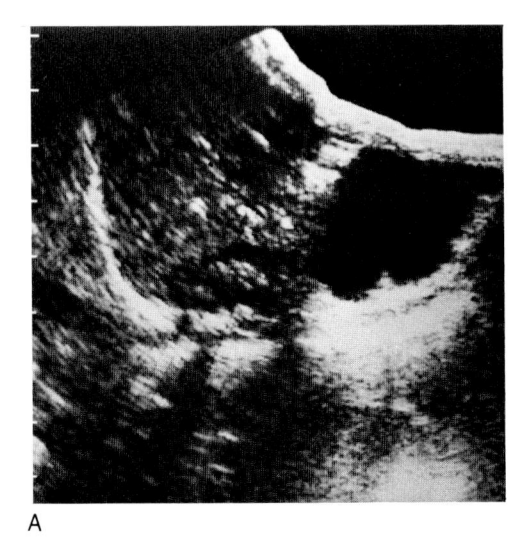

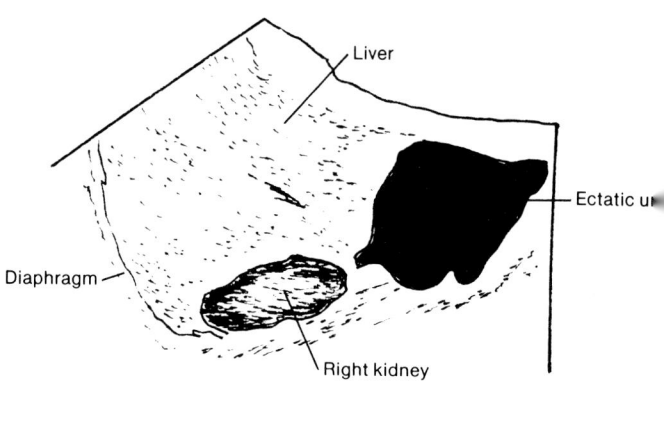

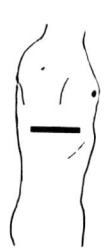

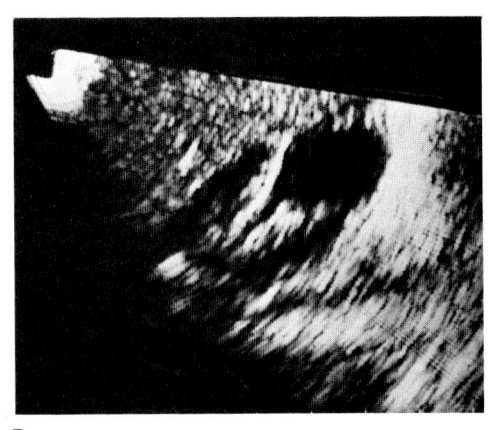

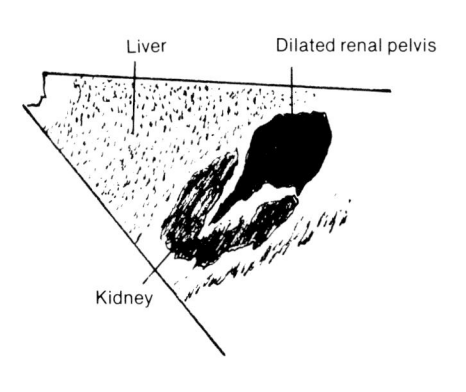

A

B

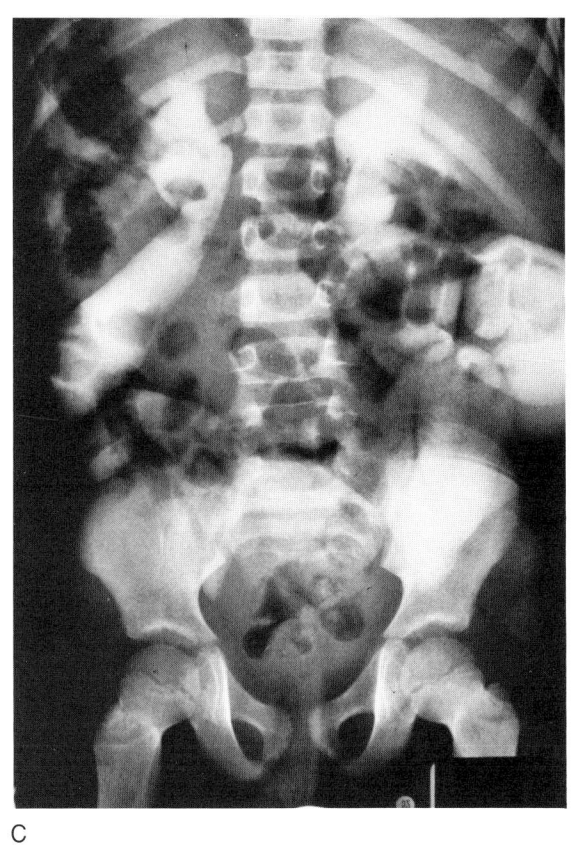

C

11.24 Staghorn Calculus with Secondary Hydronephrosis

An elderly woman had similar findings in both kidneys. In the right kidney (Fig. A) a fluid-filled structure occupies most of the kidney. In addition, in the medial aspect of the kidney there is a collection of high-level echoes with shadowing behind it. This combination of hydronephrosis and high-level echoes with shadowing is typical of a calculus obstructing the renal pelvis. The presence of high-level echoes and shadowing associated with the calculus is not dependent upon the presence of calcium within the stone.

Excretory urography verifies the presence of bilateral staghorn calculi in this patient (Fig. B).

Renal failure secondary to obstructive uropathy may be present without evidence of hydronephrosis on the ultrasound study when staghorn calculi are within the collecting system. It is, therefore, important to search carefully for an acoustic shadow behind the renal sinus in the evaluation of chronic renal failure. We have also noted that when retroperitoneal fibrosis is the cause of chronic renal failure, a false-negative sonogram may occur. With most other causes of chronic renal failure, ultrasound evidence of dilatation of the collecting system will be present. In its absence, hydronephrosis is excluded.

SUGGESTED READINGS

Rosenfield AT, Taylor KJW, Dembner AG, et al: Ultrasound of the renal sinus: new observations. AJR 133:441–448, 1979

Talner LB, Scheible W, Ellenbogan PH, et al: How accurate is ultrasonography in detecting hydronephrosis in azotemic patients? Urol Radiol 3:1–6, 1981

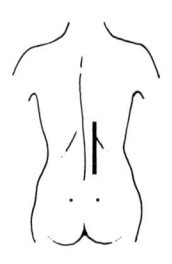

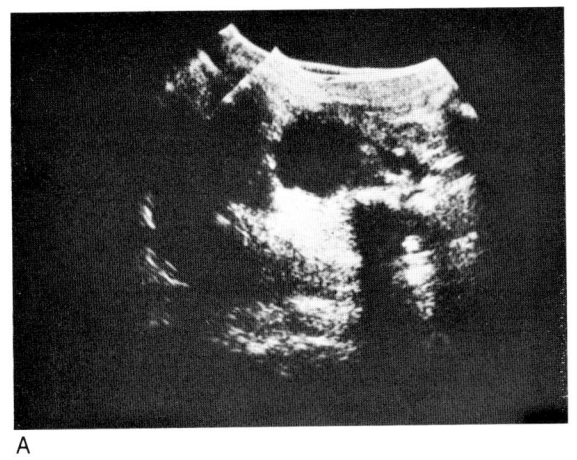

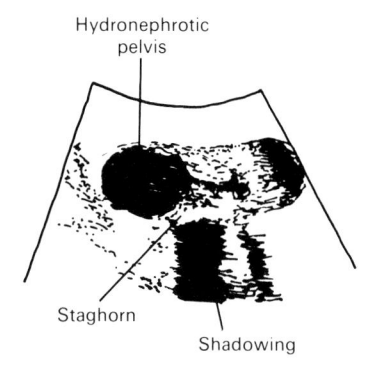

A

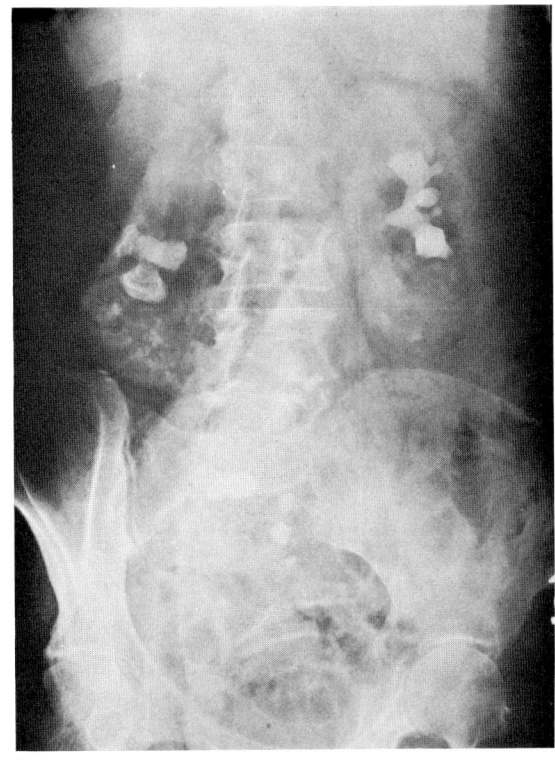

Hydronephrotic pelvis

Staghorn Shadowing

B

787

11.25 Hydronephrosis–Pyonephrosis

A 22-year-old woman presented with a history of recurrent right-sided pain of unknown etiology. An appendectomy had been performed at another institution. Six weeks after the surgery, the patient developed fever and right upper quadrant abdominal pain. Clinically, this was believed to be a right upper quadrant abscess, and ultrasound examination was performed to evaluate the patient further.

Both longitudinal (Fig. A) and transverse (Fig. B) sonograms through the right kidney demonstrate marked hydronephrosis. In addition to the hydronephrosis, however, ill-defined echoes were noted within the dilated collecting system, representing cellular debris. These are most consistent with the diagnosis of pyonephrosis, presumably associated with an underlying long-standing obstructive uropathy.

Subsequent excretory urography confirms the gross hydronephrosis (Fig. C). Retrograde examination demonstrates a partial obstruction of the ureteropelvic junction (Fig. D). At nephrectomy, the presence of pyonephrosis and ureteropelvic junction obstruction was confirmed.

The finding of debris within a dilated collecting system is seen in two situations: (1) when infection is superimposed on hydronephrosis (bacterial, tuberculous, or fungal pyonephrosis) and (2) when blood is present within the collecting system (see Fig. 11-28A). The clinical findings generally permit differentiation between these two situations, although aspiration of the collecting system may be needed for firm diagnosis. Sonography also can be used to guide percutaneous nephrostomy placement.

SUGGESTED READINGS

Coleman BG, Arger PH, Mulhern CB, et al: Pyonephrosis: sonography in the diagnosis and management. AJR 137:939–943, 1981

Pollack HM, Arger PH, Goldberg BB, et al: Ultrasonic detection of nonopaque renal calculi. Radiology 127:233–237, 1978

Rosenfield AT, Taylor KJW, Dembner AG, et al: Ultrasound of the renal sinus: new observations. AJR 133:441–448, 1979

Stuck KJ, Silver TM, Jaffe MH, et al: Sonographic demonstration of renal fungus balls. Radiology 142:473–474, 1981

Subramanyam BR, Raghavendra BN, Bosniak MA, et al: Sonography of pyonephrosis: a prospective study. AJR 140:991–993, 1983

Yoder IC, Pfister RC, Lindfors KK, et al: Pyonephrosis: imaging and intervention. AJR 141:735–740, 1983

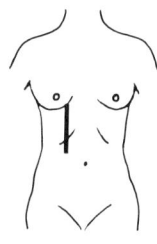

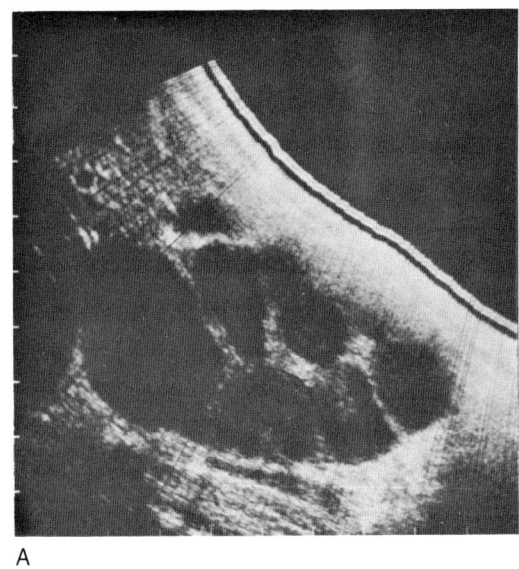

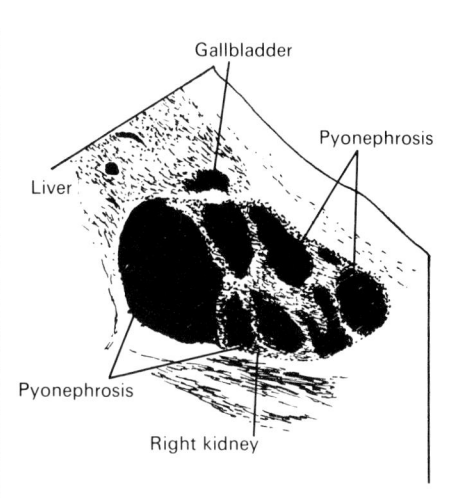

A

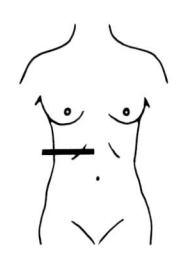

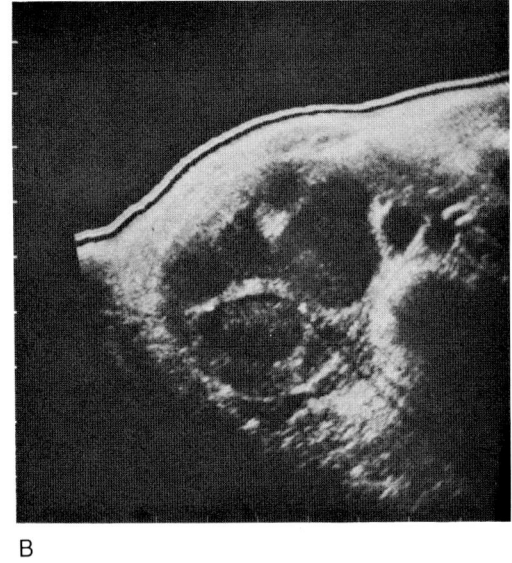

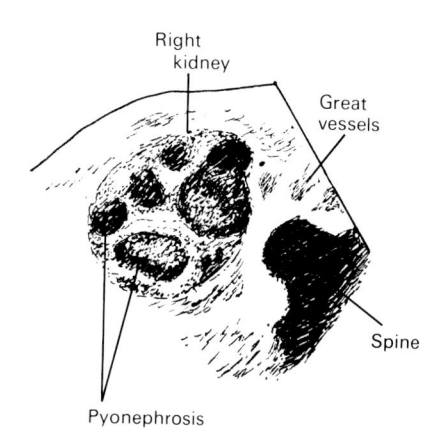

B

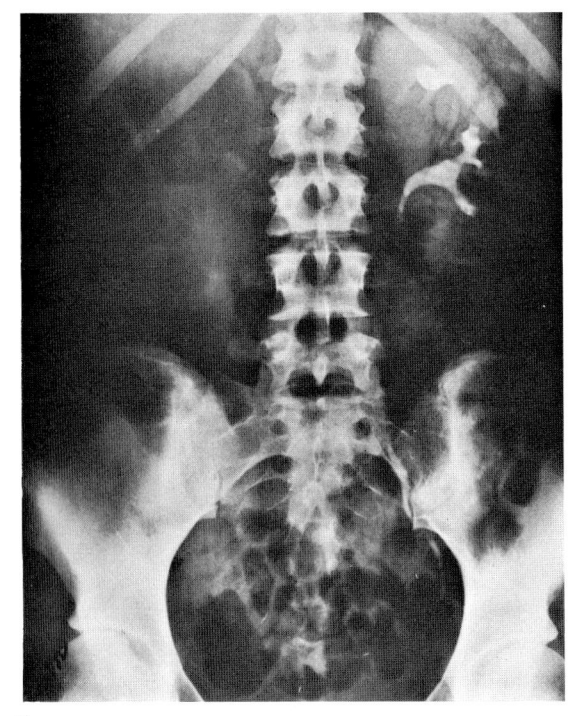

Right kidney
Great vessels
Spine
Pyonephrosis

C

790

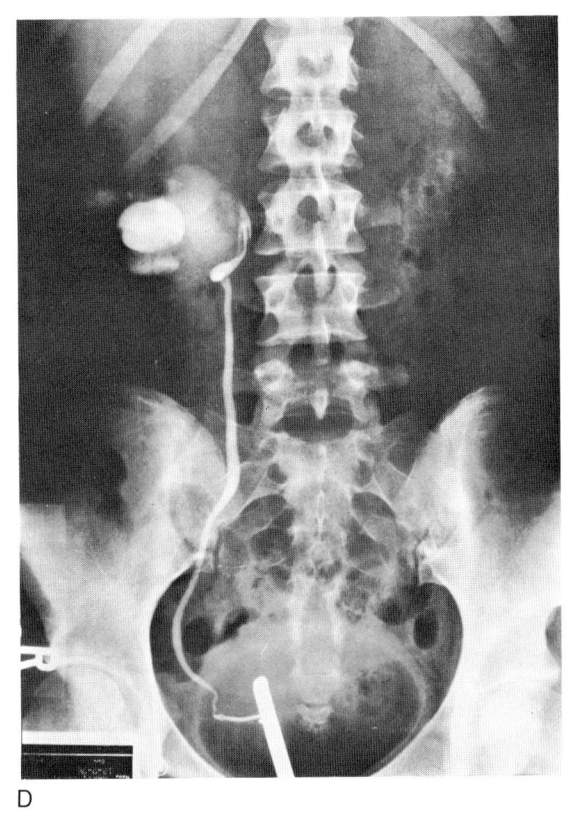

D

11.26 Retroperitoneal Fibrosis

A 68-year-old hypertensive woman was admitted with a cholesteatoma to undergo elective left radical mastoidectomy. Routine analysis disclosed elevated blood urea nitrogen and creatinine levels. Ultrasound examination revealed moderate hydronephrosis of the left kidney (Fig. A) but failed to demonstrate a right kidney. A hypoechoic mass was seen surrounding the aorta (A) at the level of the midlumbar spine (Fig. B). A CT scan verified the presence of a mass around the aorta (arrowed, Fig. C). A radioisotope renal scan was performed, revealing either absence or nonfunction of the right kidney and impaired function of the left kidney. A percutaneous nephrostomy was performed and antegrade pyelography showed a long stricture of the left ureter (arrowed, Fig. D). However, contrast material flowed freely into the urinary bladder from the kidney. A guidewire was passed into the bladder and a catheter placed for drainage prior to surgery. At surgery, a biopsy specimen of the left periureteral tissue revealed fibrosis and fat necrosis but no evidence of tumor. The patient's history was remarkable in that she had had a translumbar aortogram for evaluation of peripheral vascular disease.

Retroperitoneal fibrosis may be idiopathic or may be secondary to drugs, inflammatory processes, or due to desmoplastic response to retroperitoneal tumor. The diagnosis is of particular importance since in renal failure due to retroperitoneal fibrosis the degree of dilatation may be minimal compared with the degree of renal failure. If retroperitoneal fibrosis of any cause is suspected in a patient with renal failure, it is important to stress the patient with a large fluid volume or a diuretic to avoid missing this diagnosis. The differential diagnosis for a mass in the area of the great vessels is between retroperitoneal fibrosis and retroperitoneal adenopathy. Both these entities can produce retroperitoneal masses which are visible adjacent to the aorta and inferior vena cava on ultrasound and CT studies. Adenopathy typically envelops the structures and may elevate them while retroperitoneal fibrosis tends not to cause a significant mass posterior to the great vessels.

SUGGESTED READINGS

Lalli AF: Retroperitoneal fibrosis and inapparent obstructive uropathy. Radiology 122:339–342, 1977

Sanders RC, Duffy T, McLoughlin MG, et al: Sonography in the diagnosis of retroperitoneal fibrosis. J Urol 118:944–946, 1977

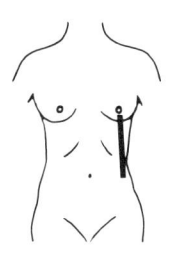

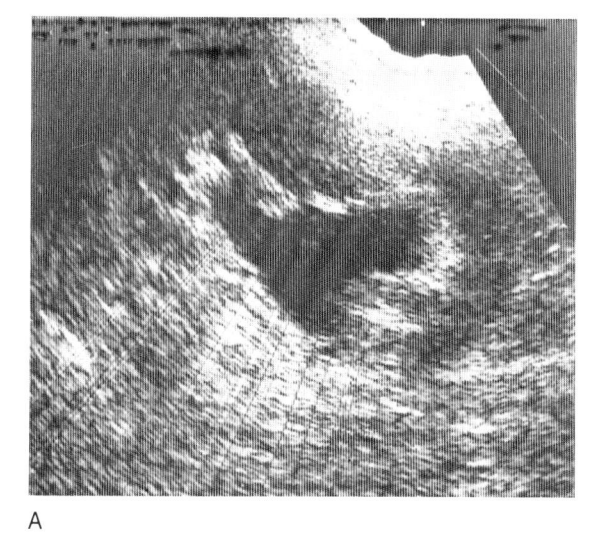

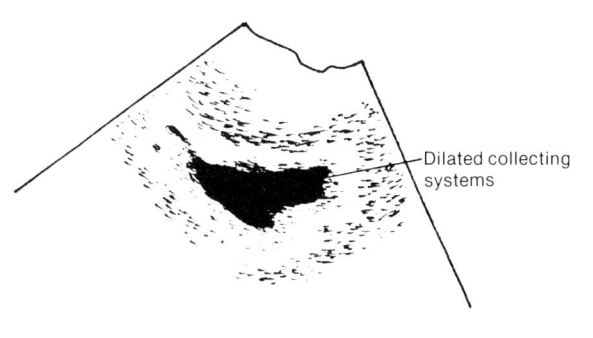

A

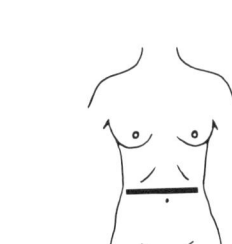

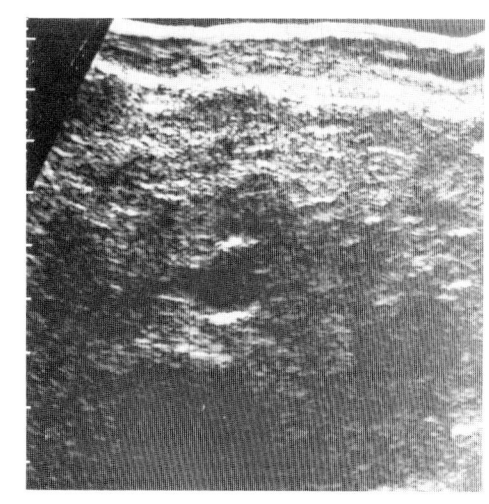

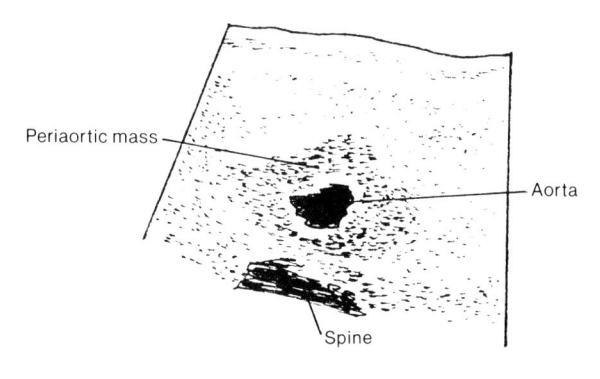

B

Dilated collecting systems

Periaortic mass

Aorta

Spine

793

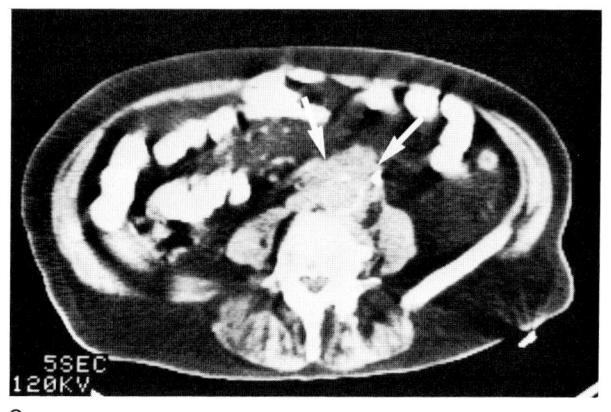

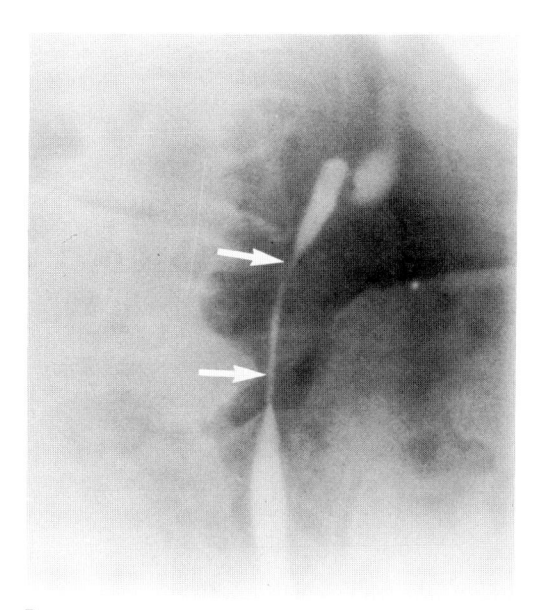

C

D

794

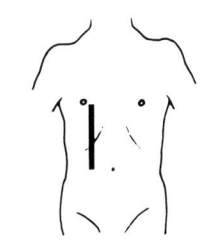

11.27 Nephrolithiasis

Nephrolithiasis typically appears as a zone of intense echoes within the renal sinus (Fig. A). An acoustic shadow distal to this zone may occur due to the significant attenuation of the beam by the stone. Since the high-level, specular echoes of the renal sinus are compressed by current signal processing, the intense echoes of the renal stone may be difficult to differentiate from the surrounding renal sinus when severe hydronephrosis is not present (arrow, Fig. A). The acoustic shadow is therefore crucial to the diagnosis, and optimal technique is required when nephrolithiasis is suspected. The same factors of correct gain and position of the stone in the focal zone of the transducer apply to elicit shadowing as discussed for gallstones (arrow, Fig. B). A stone within the ureter or bladder also may be recognized as a zone of intense echoes with an acoustic shadow(s).

Tumor within the renal sinus presents as a mass but does not cause a significant acoustic shadow. Therefore, it has been suggested that ultrasound be used to distinguish a uric acid stone from tumor when a nonopaque filling defect is identified within the collecting system on excretory urography. However, if a uric acid stone is strongly suspected, computed tomography (CT) is a more accurate modality for identifying this entity. Although uric acid stones are not opaque on standard radiographs, they are significantly more opaque than soft tissue on the CT scan.

(Figs. A & B from Rosenfield AT, Taylor KJW, Crade M: Renal ultrasound 1979: gray scale, real time, Doppler. pp. 1–23. In Rosenfield AT (ed): Genitourinary Ultrasonography. Clinics in Diagnostic Ultrasound Vol. 2. Churchill Livingstone, New York, 1979.)

SUGGESTED READINGS

Edell S, Zegel H: Ultrasonic evaluation of renal calculi. AJR 130:261–263, 1978

Pollack HM, Arger PH, Goldberg BB, et al: Ultrasonic detection of nonopaque renal calculi. Radiology 127:235–237, 1978

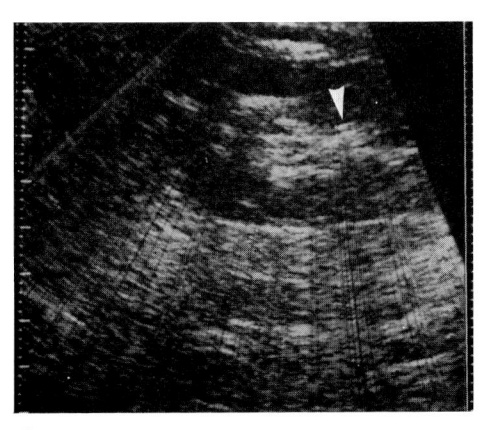

A

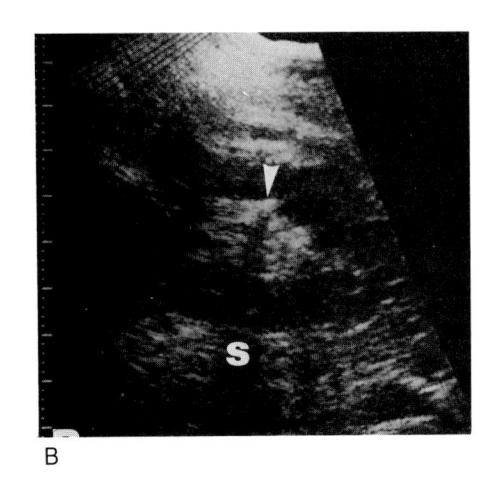

B

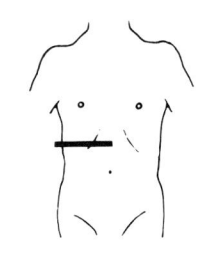

11.28 Blood Clot within the Renal Sinus

A transverse scan was taken through the right upper quadrant in this patient with hematuria (Fig. A). A mass containing low-level echoes separates the walls of the collecting system and is consistent with transitional cell carcinoma, mycetoma, or blood clot. When these ultrasound findings are identified, it is advantageous to delay excretory urography to see if the ultrasound findings return to normal. Three days later (Fig. B), the abnormality previously identified is no longer present. The change in appearances is typical of blood clot. By performing the excretory urogram at this time, an optimal search of the collecting system can be made.

(Figs. A & B from Rosenfield, AT, Taylor, KJW, Crade M: Renal ultrasound 1979: gray scale, real time, Doppler. pp. 1–23. In Rosenfield AT (ed); Clinics in Diagnostic Ultrasound, Vol 2. Churchill Livingstone, New York, 1979.)

SUGGESTED READING

Rosenfield AT, Taylor KJW, Dembner AG, et al: Ultrasound of the renal sinus: new observations. AJR 133:441–448, 1979

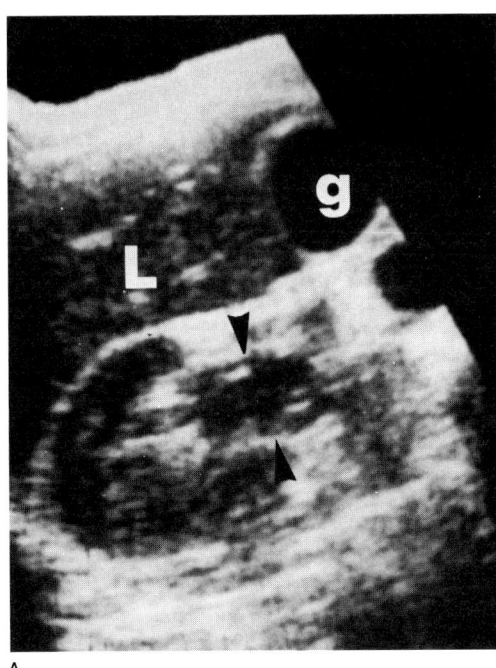

A

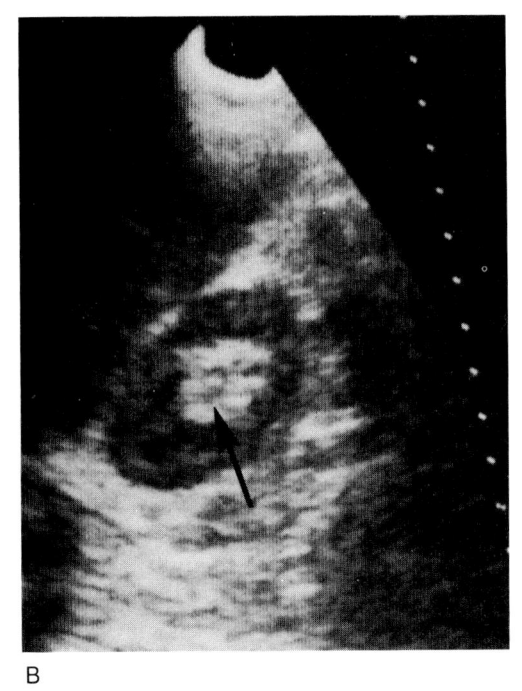

B

11.29 Renal Parenchymal Disease

A variety of benign and neoplastic diseases affect the renal parenchyma. These diseases can be divided into two major categories: those that accentuate cortical echoes with preservation of the relatively hypoechoic appearance of the medulla (Type I), and those that distort normal anatomy, including the elimination of corticomedullary definition, in a focal or diffuse manner (Type II). Type I diseases include a variety of bilateral medical renal diseases, both acute and chronic. Leukemia is the only malignancy to produce these findings in the kidney. In the early stage of medical renal disease, the kidneys typically enlarge, whereas in the late stage they become relatively small. End-stage kidneys are small with diffusely echogenic parenchyma and loss of corticomedullary definition. Preservation of corticomedullary definition with intense echoes in the cortex, when unilateral, is typically seen in renal vein thrombosis in the subacute stage. This generally occurs about 10 days to 2 weeks after the acute onset. Occasionally, acute infection gives a similar pattern.

The other renal parenchymal diseases can be classified according to whether (1) there is a diffuse or focal abnormality in the kidney, (2) the abnormality is bilateral or unilateral, (3) there is an increase or decrease in size of the kidney, or (4) there is focal mass or scar. By combining these descriptive findings with the clinical picture, which includes whether the symptoms are acute, a relatively narrow differential diagnosis can be reached. For example, in a patient with acute symptoms, a unilaterally enlarged kidney, with global loss of corticomedullary definition resulting from diffusely decreased cortical echogenicity, the differential diagnosis includes acute renal vein thrombosis, acute pyelonephritis, or acute renal infarction. Similarly, a focal mass with echogenicity greater than normal has a relatively narrow differential diagnosis which can be limited further by looking for other ultrasound findings. The most likely diagnosis for this type of mass is renal cell carcinoma or, in children, a Wilms' tumor. Angiomyolipoma, a relatively rare benign tumor of the kidney usually has high-amplitude echoes due to fat. If the lesion has enough fat, the slow speed of sound in fat compared to adjacent tissue may lead to artifactual alteration in the position of structures behind the mass. Intense echoes may be seen in some mimicking an abscess which may appear solid. Identification of a refractive shadow at the junction of the abscess and solid tissue usually permits the correct diagnosis.

Demonstration of renal parenchymal anatomy requires a meticulous technique. Longitudinal (Fig. A) and transverse (Fig. B) sonograms are best obtained using the liver as a window so that the kidney is within the focal zone of the transducer. Renal cortex, medulla, and arcuate vessels generally can be identified. Similarly, using the spleen as a window, coronal scans through the left kidney (Fig. C) permit identification of cortex, medulla, and arcuate vessels. When medical renal disease is present, the gain must be lowered to permit identification of corticomedullary definition. Our basic approach to nephrosonography is summarized in Figure D.

The cases that follow demonstrate the sonographic findings in the common renal parenchymal diseases. These entities may present as renal failure, nonfunctioning kidney, or focal renal lesions. Other medical renal diseases such as acute focal bacterial nephritis (lobar nephronia), chronic atrophic pyelonephritis, complications of renal transplantation, and renal masses are discussed in other sections.

(Figs. A–C from Rosenfield AT, Taylor KJW, Crade M: Renal ultrasound 1979: gray scale, real time, Doppler. pp. 1–23. In Rosenfield AT (ed): Genitourinary Ultrasonography. Clinics in Diagnostic Ultrasound, Vol 2. Churchill Livingstone, New York, 1979.)

(Fig. D from Rosenfield AT, Taylor KJW, Crade M, et al: Anatomy and pathology of the kidney by gray-scale ultrasound. Radiology 128:737–744, 1978.)

SUGGESTED READINGS

Cook JH, Rosenfield AT, Taylor KJW: Ultrasonic demonstration of intrarenal anatomy. Am J Roentgenol 129:831–835, 1977

Hricak H, Cruz C, Romanski R: Renal parenchymal disease: sonographic-histologic correlation. Radiology 144: 141–147, 1982

Rosenfield AT, Segal N: Renal parenchymal disease: histopathologic-sonographic correlation. AJR 137:793–798, 1981

Rosenfield AT, Taylor KJW, Crade M, et al: Anatomy and pathology of the kidney by gray scale ultrasound. Radiology 128:737–744, 1978

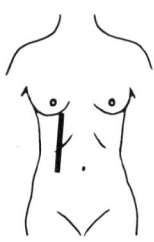

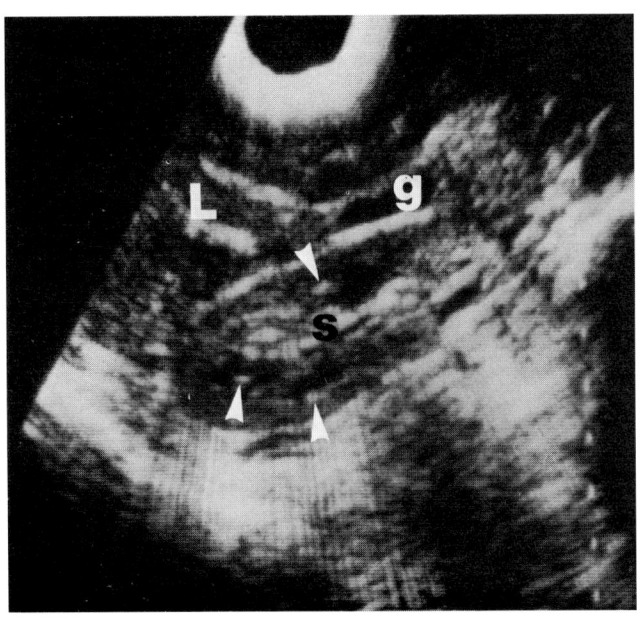

A

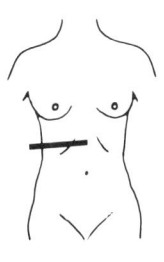

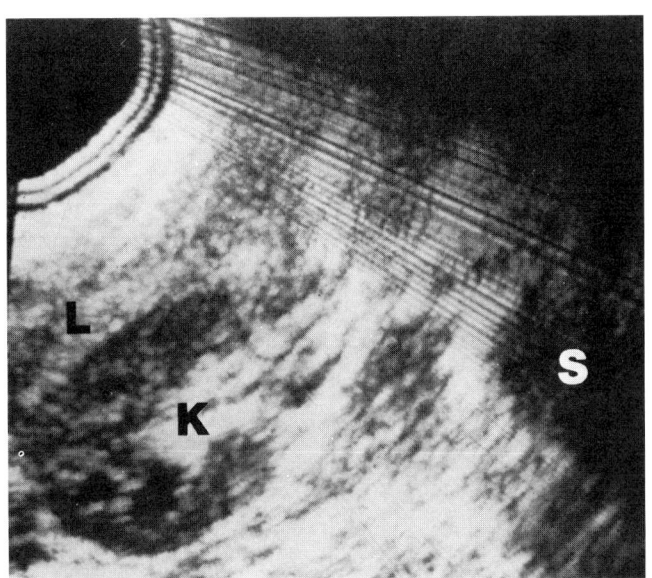

B

802

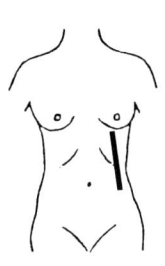

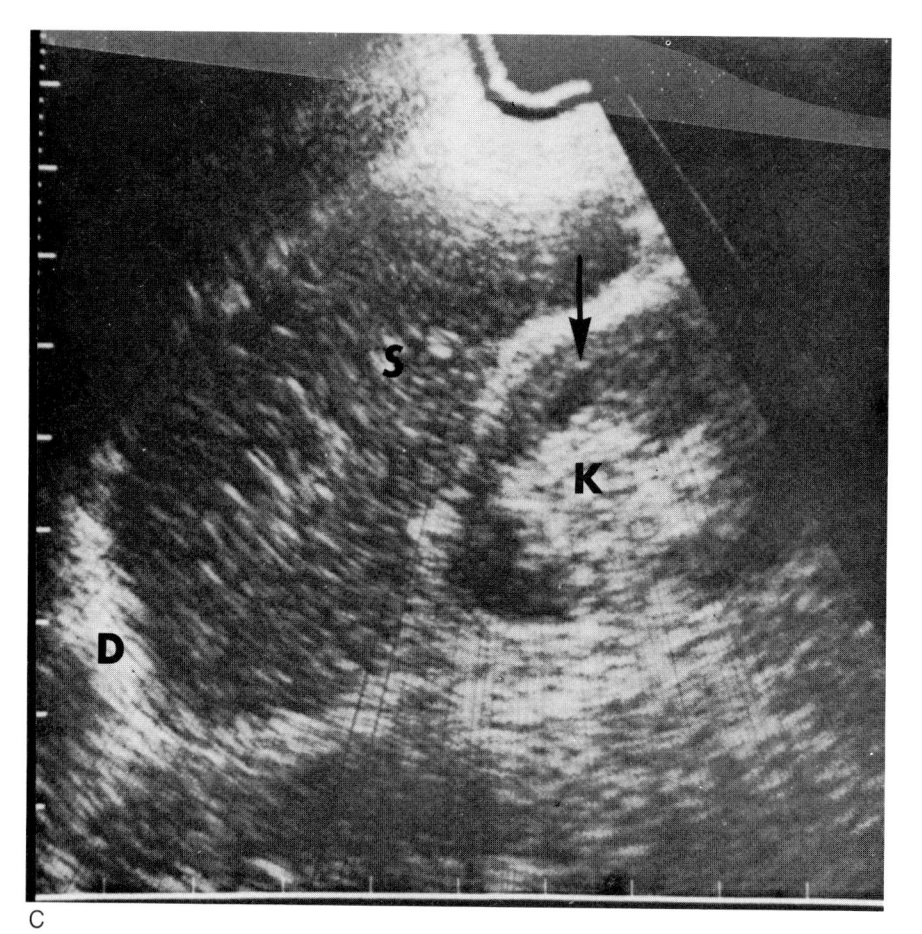

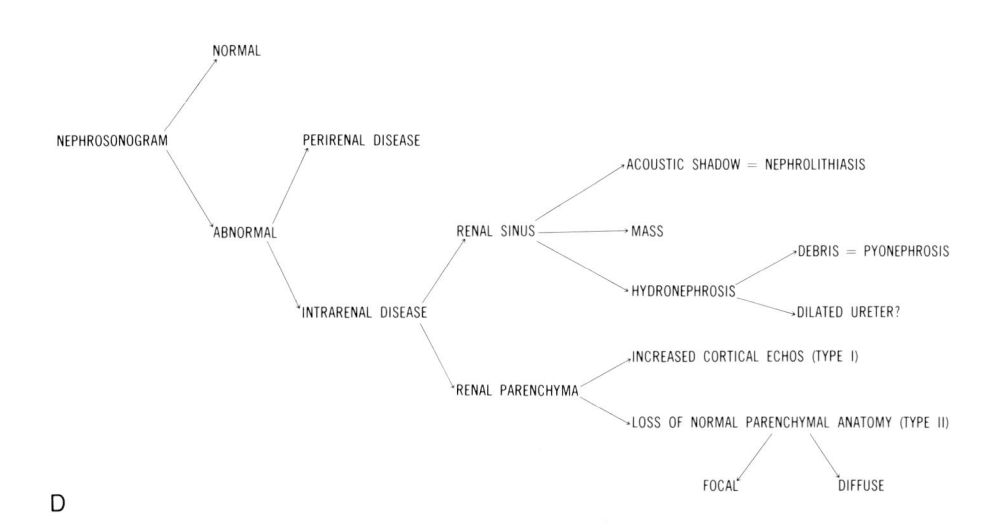

```
NEPHROSONOGRAM ─→ NORMAL
               └─→ ABNORMAL ─→ PERIRENAL DISEASE
                            └─→ INTRARENAL DISEASE ─→ RENAL SINUS ─→ ACOUSTIC SHADOW = NEPHROLITHIASIS
                                                                 ├─→ MASS
                                                                 └─→ HYDRONEPHROSIS ─→ DEBRIS = PYONEPHROSIS
                                                                                    └─→ DILATED URETER?
                                                  └─→ RENAL PARENCHYMA ─→ INCREASED CORTICAL ECHOS (TYPE I)
                                                                       └─→ LOSS OF NORMAL PARENCHYMAL ANATOMY (TYPE II) ─→ FOCAL
                                                                                                                        └─→ DIFFUSE
```

D

Medical Renal Disease (11.30 and 11.31)

11.30 Acute Disease

Figure A shows a longitudinal sonogram taken through the right upper quadrant in a 6-year-old boy whose foot was crushed. Acute renal failure developed secondary to myoglobinuria. Nephromegaly is visible and cortical echogenicity is increased with preservation of corticomedullary definition. In a normal kidney, the echogenicity of the cortex would be less than that of the liver, spleen, or renal sinus. In this patient, there was a slight increase in echogenicity; the right kidney was minimally more echogenic than the liver and markedly less echogenic than the renal sinus. Since nephromegaly was present bilaterally, the findings are typical of acute renal insult.

Figure B demonstrates the right kidney (arrowed) in a child with acute glomerulonephritis who was scanned supine. Figure C shows the right kidney (arrowed) with the patient prone. The cortex of the right kidney is much more echogenic than the adjacent liver and equal in echogenicity to the renal sinus. The pyramids are vaguely seen as echo-poor areas.

Three types of disease process can produce an increase in cortical echogenicity with preservation of corticomedullary definition bilaterally (Type I pattern). The first is acute or chronic medical renal disease. Entities such as acute glomerulonephritis, chronic glomerulonephritis, lupus nephritis, and Alport's disease are in this group. Our work has indicated no correlation between the intensity of the cortical echoes and the nature or severity of the glomerular process. However, the type of interstitial process does correlate with the echo amplitude. Focal interstitial disease increases echogenicity slightly. Diffuse scarring produces a greater increase in echogenicity, while active interstitial infiltrate causes the greatest increase. Thus, while ultrasound cannot be used to diagnose the type of disease affecting the kidney, it can be used in place of serial biopsies to look for improvement. The echogenicity increases proportionally to the severity of pathologic changes in the interstitial areas. Hricak et al.[1] have shown some correlation between cortical echogenicity and biopsy findings but concluded that it is not currently feasible to distinguish different types of medical renal disorders using ultrasound.

The second class of disease to increase cortical echoes with preservation of corticomedullary definition includes infiltrative processes such as leukemia and amyloidosis. Leukemic infiltration typically produces nephromegaly with this pattern. In amyloidosis, nephromegaly is seen early, but as the disease progresses the kidneys become small.

The third group of diseases that cause the Type I pattern includes disorders that lead to cortical nephrocalcinosis. While the late stage of cortical nephrocalcinosis produces a highly echogenic parenchyma with sufficient attenuation to cause acoustic shadowing, the earlier ultrasound appearance is simply one of increased cortical echoes. This appearance may be identified prior to visualization of calcification of the cortex on the radiograph. Diseases that form this group are chronic glomerulonephritis, Alport's disease, the early stage of oxalosis, some cases of transplant rejection, and the subacute and chronic stages of renal cortical necrosis.

(Figs. B and C from Rosenfield AT, Taylor KJW, Crade M, et al: Anatomy and pathology of the kidney by gray scale ultrasound. Radiology 128:737–744, 1978.)

SUGGESTED READINGS

Babcock DS: Medical diseases of the urinary tract and adrenal glands. pp 113–134. In Haller JO, Shkolnik A (eds): Ultrasound in Pediatrics. Clinics in Diagnostic Ultrasound, Vol 8. New York, Churchill-Livingstone, 1981

Brennan JN, Diwan RS, Makker SP, et al: Ultrasonic diagnosis of primary hyperoxaluria in infancy. Radiology 145:147–148, 1982

Cook JH, Rosenfield AT, Taylor KJW: Ultrasonic demonstration of intrarenal anatomy. Am J Roentgenol 129:831–835, 1977

Finberg AJ, Hillman B, Smith EH: Ultrasound in the evaluation of the non-functioning kidney. pp. 105–124. In Rosenfield AT (ed): Genitourinary Ultrasonography. Clinics in Diagnostic Ultrasound, Vol. 2. New York, Churchill-Livingstone, 1979

Goh TS, LeQuesne GW, Wong KY: Severe infiltration of the kidneys with abnormalities in acute lymphoblastic leukemia. Am J Dis Child 132:1204–1205, 1978

Hricak H, Toledo-Pereyra LH, Eyler WR, et al: Evaluation of acute post-transplant renal failure by ultrasound. Radiology 133:443–447, 1979

Kay C, Rosenfield AT, Armm M: Ultrasound evaluation or renal trauma. AJR 134:461–466, 1980

LeQuesne GW: Assessment of glomerulonephritis in children by ultrasound. pp. 205–207. In White D, Lyons EA (eds): Ultrasound in Medicine, Vol 4. Plenum Press, New York, 1978

Rosenfield AT: Ultrasound evaluation of renal parenchymal disease and hydronephrosis. Urol Radiol 4:125–133, 1982

Rosenfield AT, Segal NJ: Renal parenchymal disease: histopathologic-sonographic correlation. AJR 137:793–798, 1981

Rosenfield AT, Taylor KJW, Crade M, DeGraaff: Anatomy and pathology of the kidney by gray scale ultrasound. Radiology 128:737–744, 1978

Sanders RC: Examination of kidneys not seen at excretion urography. pp. 146–169. In Resnick MI, Sanders RC (eds): Ultrasound in Urology. Williams & Wilkins, Baltimore, 1979

REFERENCE

1. Hricak H, Cruz C, Romanski R: Renal parenchymal disease: sonographic–histologic correlation. Radiology 144:141–147, 1982

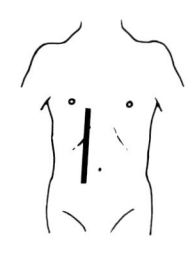

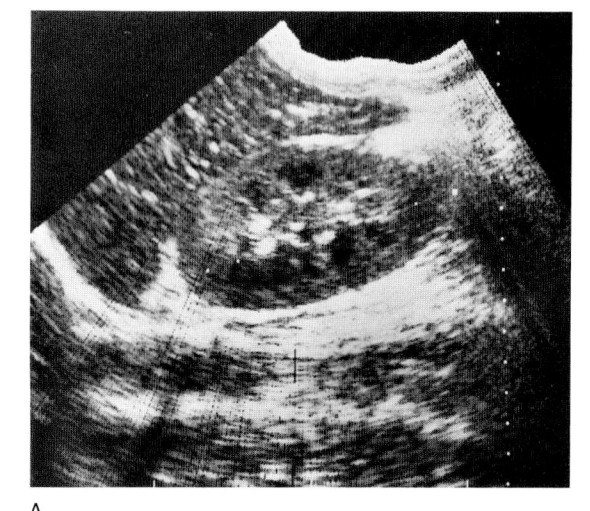

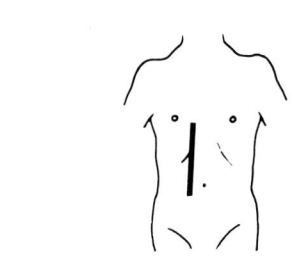

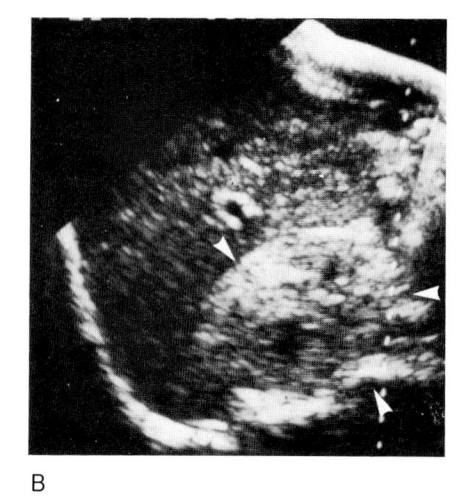

A

B

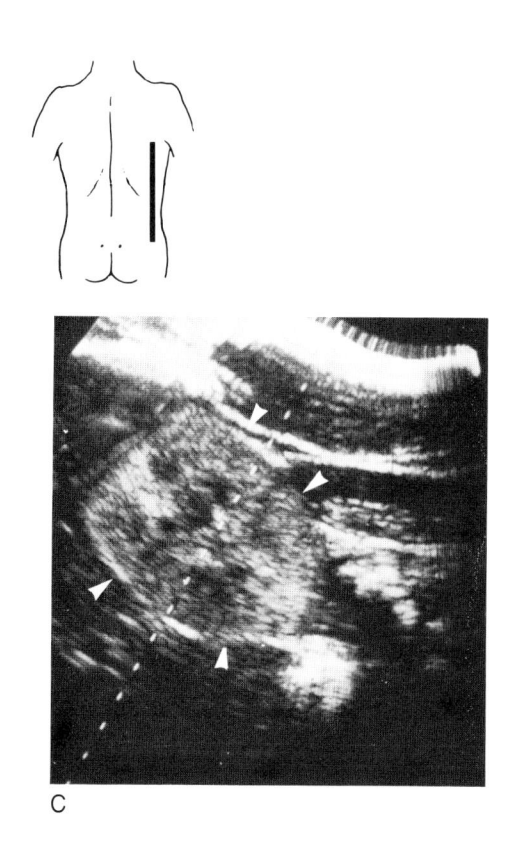

C

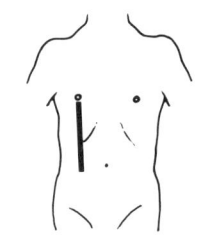

11.31 Histogram Analysis

Right parasagittal sections in this patient with leukemic infiltration demonstrated the echogenicity of the cortex of the kidney to be greater than that of the adjacent liver. This can be quantified by histogram analysis. The area of interest is indicated by the squares in the figures and the range of echo intensities are plotted. Figure A shows the echogenicity of the liver and Figure B that the echogenicity is greater in the cortex. The X axis demonstrates the gray scale in ascending order of brightness while the Y axis represents the number of echoes for each echo intensity. For this technique, it is essential that areas compared are at the same distance from the transducer and at identical time gain control and gain settings.

(Figs. A & B from Rosenfield AT, Taylor KJW, Jaffe CC: Clinical applications of ultrasound tissue characterization. Radiol Clin North Am 18:31–56, 1980.)

SUGGESTED READINGS

Rosenfield AT, Segal NJ: Renal parenchymal disease: histopathologic-sonographic correlation. AJR 137:793–798, 1981

Rosenfield AT, Taylor KJW, Jaffe CC: Clinical applications of ultrasound tissue characterization. Radiol Clin North Am 18:31–56, 1980

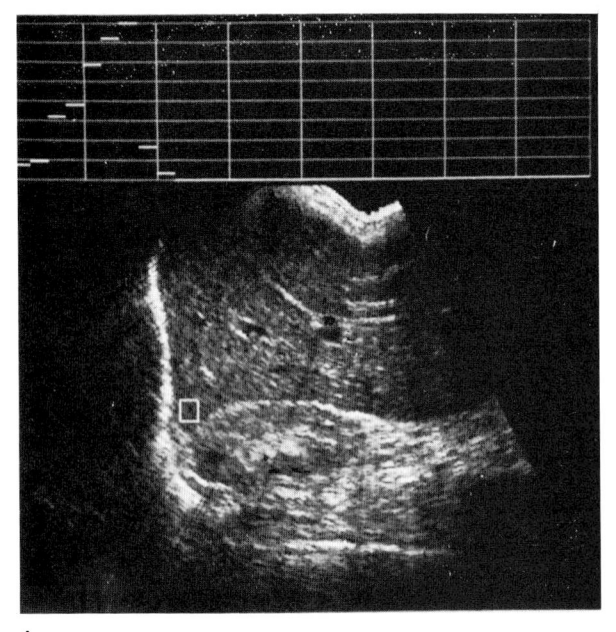

A

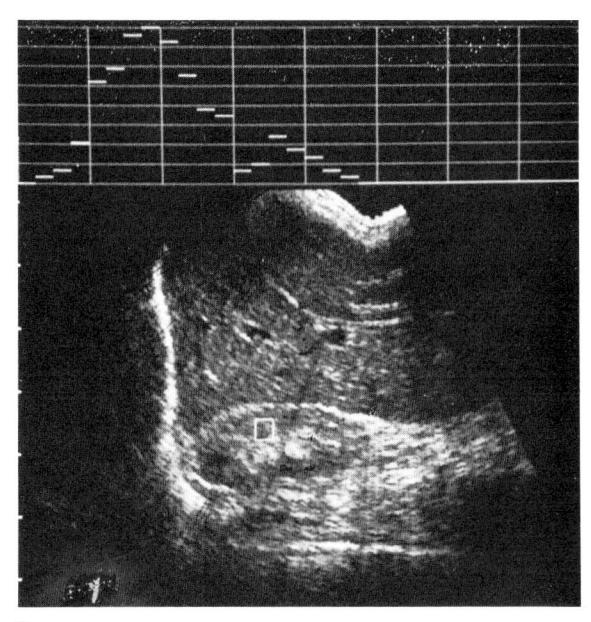

B

11.32 Chronic Renal Failure

A longitudinal section through the right upper quadrant in a patient with chronic renal failure demonstrated a small right kidney, shown in the figure. An increase in cortical echogenicity was appreciated. The echoes were more intense than those of the adjacent liver but lower than those of the renal sinus. The left kidney was similar. These appearances were typical of chronic medical renal disease. In time, the pyramids become more echogenic and corticomedullary definition is lost as the size of the kidney decreases.

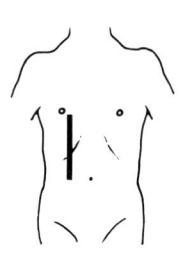

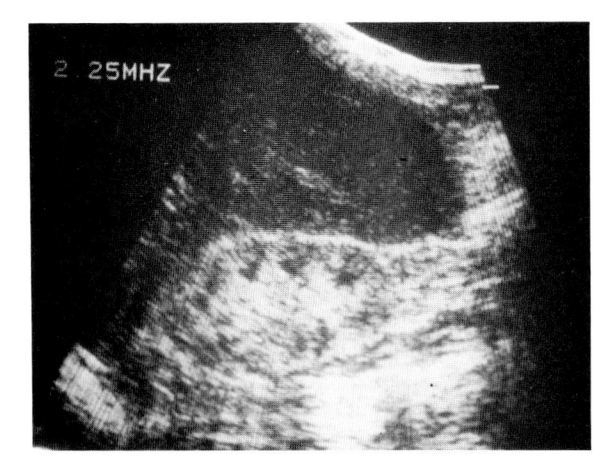

Renal Vein Thrombosis (11.33 and 11.34)

11.33 Acute Thrombosis

A transverse sonogram through the upper abdomen of a patient who had left flank pain of 12 hours' duration demonstrates nephromegaly (arrowed in the figure) with a decrease in cortical echoes. This pattern is typical of acute renal vein thrombosis during the first few days after the insult. In a patient with acute symptoms, the differential diagnosis for this pattern includes acute pyelonephritis and acute renal infarction. Pulsed Doppler ultrasound of the left renal vein demonstrated no flow. Subsequent follow-up Doppler examinations demonstrated a return of flow.

(This case and figure taken from Rosenfield AT, Zeman RK, Cronan JJ, et al: Ultrasound in experimental and clinical renal vein thrombosis. Radiology 137:735–741, 1980.)

SUGGESTED READINGS

Braun B, Weilemann LS, Weigand W: Ultrasonic demonstration of renal vein thrombosis. Radiology 138:157–158, 1981

Hricak H, Sandler MA, Madrazo BL, et al: Sonographic manifestations of acute renal vein thrombosis: an experimental study. Invest Radiol 1:30–35, 1981

Rosenfield AT, Zeman RK, Cronan JJ, et al: Ultrasound in experimental and clinical renal vein thrombosis. Radiology 137:735–741, 1980

Taylor KJW, Atkinson P, de Graaff CS, et al: Clinical evaluation of pulse-Doppler device linked to gray scale B-scan equipment. Radiology 129:745–749, 1978

812

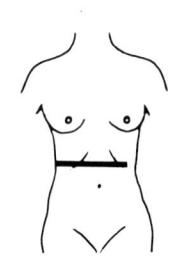

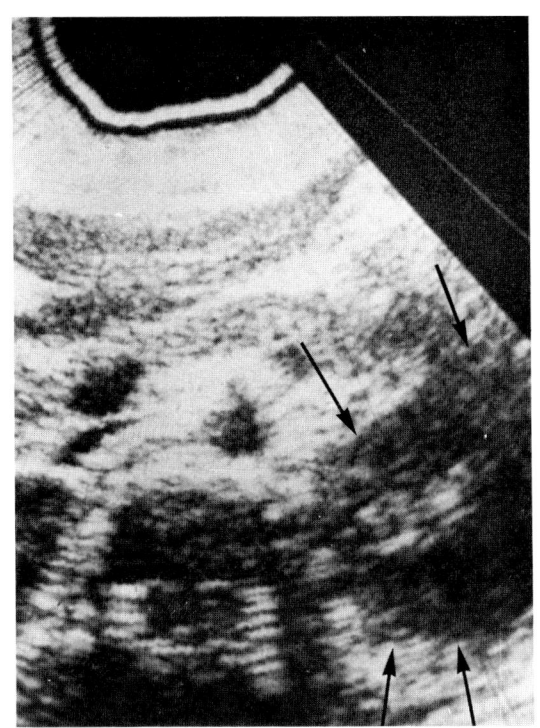

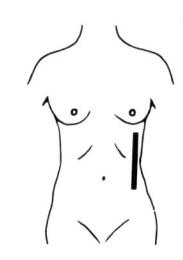

11.34 Subacute Thrombosis

A coronal sonogram was taken through the left upper quadrant of a woman who had had left flank pain of 10 days' duration following a difficult delivery (Fig. A). The left kidney (K) was seen to contain intense echoes with preservation of corticomedullary definition (arrowed). The right kidney was normal. A unilateral increase in cortical echoes with preservation of corticomedullary definition is typically seen in renal vein thrombosis after 7–10 days. Obstruction of the renal vein was verified on venography.

Two years later the patient was seen in the ultrasound laboratory for other problems. A coronal sonogram through the left upper quadrant at this time (Fig. B) demonstrated a much smaller left kidney (K) with a slight increase in parenchymal echoes and loss of corticomedullary definition. This pattern is typical of chronic renal vein thrombosis. The renal parenchymal findings in renal vein thrombosis are summarized in Table 11-3.

Table 11-3 Parenchymal Findings in Renal Vein Thrombosis

Static	
Immediate:	Decreased cortical echoes
	Nephromegaly
Approx. 2 weeks:	Markedly increased cortical echoes
	Preservation of corticomedullary definition
	Variable renal size
Late:	Increased parenchymal echoes
	Loss of corticomedullary definition
	Decreased renal size
Real Time	
	Absence of normally transmitted venous pulsations
Doppler	
	No venous flow

(Rosenfield AT, Zeman RK, Cronan JJ, et al: Ultrasound in experimental and clinical renal vein thrombosis. Radiology 137:735–741, 1980.)

(This case and figures from Rosenfield AT, Zeman RK, Cronan JJ, et al: Ultrasound in experimental and clinical renal vein thrombosis. Radiology 137:735–741, 1980.)

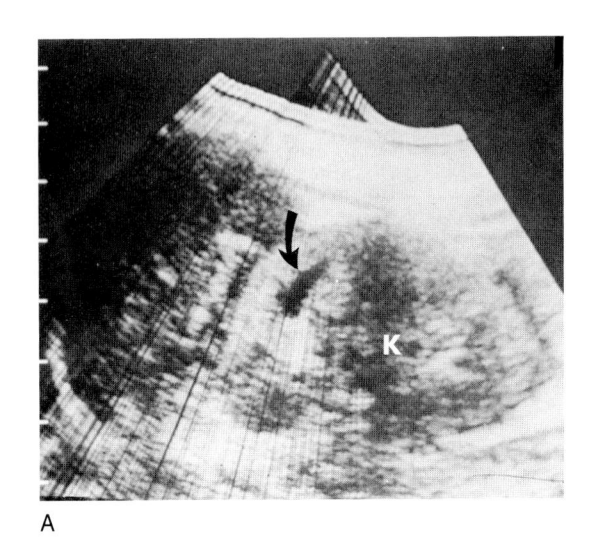

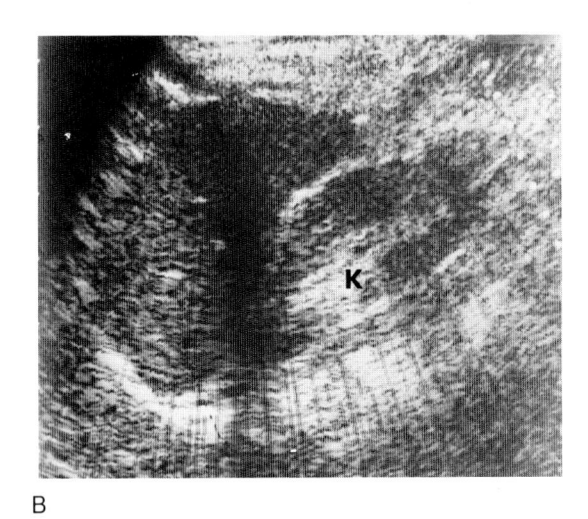

A

B

814

11.35 Reflux Nephropathy (Chronic Atrophic Pyelonephritis)

A focal scar with a blunted calyx opposite it is a typical finding in reflux nephropathy, an entity which has previously been termed "chronic atrophic pyelonephritis." Work by Hodson[1] and others has demonstrated that reflux of infected urine from the bladder into the collecting system and subsequently into the parenchyma of the kidney can cause this lesion. The ultrasound findings parallel those seen on the urogram. A longitudinal sonogram of the right kidney with the patient in the prone position reveals a small, scarred kidney (Fig. A). A focal loss of parenchyma with associated scarring (arrowed) is indicated by the renal sinuses being adjacent to the margin of the kidney. The corresponding findings on the urogram are shown in Figure B.

Sonographically, a similar pattern may be seen with other entities such as renal infarction, although on urography the calyx is blunted with reflux nephropathy but not with renal infarction. Hydration or ureteric compression can permit distention of the collecting system during the sonographic study to allow evaluation for the calyceal clubbing. Alternatively, if indicated, excretory urography permits a definitive diagnosis.

(This case and figures from Kay CJ, Rosenfield AT, Taylor KJW, et al: Ultrasound gray-scale characteristics of chronic atrophic pyelonephritis. AJR 132:683–685, 1979. ©1979 Am Roentgen Ray Soc.)

SUGGESTED READING

Kay CJ, Rosenfield AT, Taylor KJW, et al: Ultrasound gray-scale characteristics of chronic atrophic pyelonephritis. AJR 132:683–685, 1979

REFERENCE

1. Hodson CJ: Reflux nephropathy: a personal historical review. AJR 137:451–462, 1981

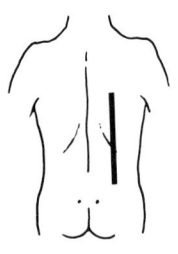

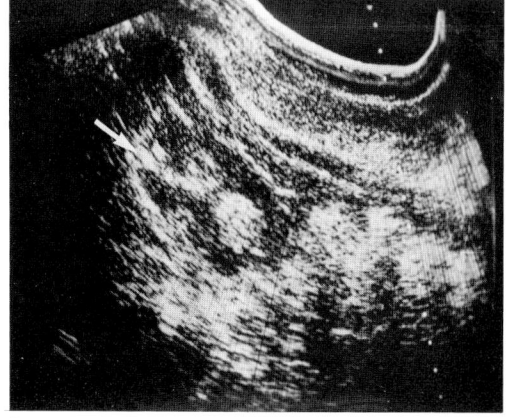

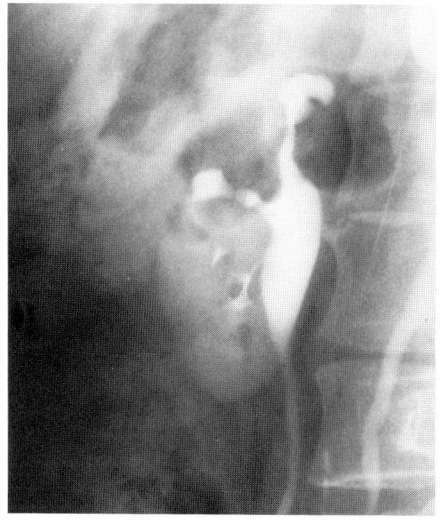

A

B

816

Nephrocalcinosis (11.36 and 11.37)

11.36 Medullary

Diffuse calcification of the kidney may exist in the pyramids (medullary nephrocalcinosis) or cortex (cortical nephrocalcinosis). The medullary nephrocalcinosis is typically seen with diseases that cause hypercalcemia and/or hypercalcuria. These include hyperparathyroidism, milk alkali syndrome, renal tubular acidosis, widespread malignancy with or without bony involvement, hypervitaminosis D, idiopathic hypercalcuria, idiopathic hypercalcemia of infancy, Cushing's disease and syndrome, and patients at bedrest particularly those with underlying disorders such as Paget's disease. Medullary sponge kidney may be associated with stone formation in the distal collecting tubules, leading to an identical appearance. In this entity the calcification may be limited to a single kidney or even a single pyramid.

The typical ultrasound appearance of advanced medullary nephrocalcinosis is echogenic pyramids (arrowed in the figure). This is a reversal of the normal echo pattern of hypoechoic pyramids compared with the adjacent cortex. Acoustic shadowing due to attenuation of the ultrasound beam by the calcifications may be identified behind the dense pyramids. Medullary nephrocalcinosis may be identified sonographically before it becomes apparent radiographically. In this situation, the pyramids are echogenic without evidence of acoustic shadowing.

Thus, ultrasound may be used to screen patients with current nephrolithiasis but no radiographic evidence for medullary nephrocalcinosis. The pattern of reversal of normal corticomedullary echogenicity with pyramids more echogenic than the cortex has also been reported in some cases of the renal tubular ectasia disorders (infantile polycystic kidney disease) and congenital hepatic fibrosis with tubular ectasia (isolated renal tubular ectasia). As indicated, excretory urography can be used to differentiate between these entities (medullary nephrocalcinosis and renal tubular ectasia) since the tubular ectasia should be readily apparent on the urogram.

(Fig. from Rosenfield AT: Ultrasound evaluation of renal parenchymal disease and hydronephrosis. Urol Radiol 4:125–133, 1982.)

SUGGESTED READINGS

Cacciarelli AA, Young N, Levine AJ: Gray-scale ultrasonic demonstration of nephrocalcinosis. Radiology 128:459–460, 1978

Glazer GM, Callen PW, Filly RA: Medullary nephrocalcinosis: sonographic evaluation. AJR 138:55–57, 1982

Manz F, Jaschke W, van Kaick G, et al: Nephrocalcinosis in radiographs, computed tomography, sonography and histology. Pediatr Radiol 9:19–26, 1980

818

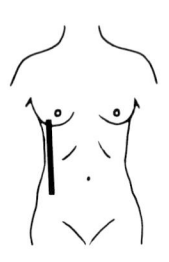

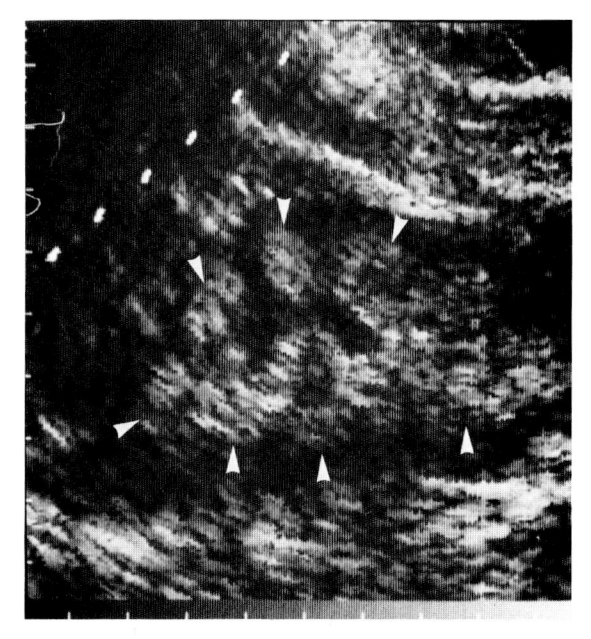

11.37 Cortical

Calcification of the cortex occurs in several renal parenchymal diseases particularly chronic glomerulonephritis, renal cortical necrosis in the subacute and chronic stages, Alport's disease, acute renal transplant rejection, and some cases of oxalosis. In other cases of oxalosis the cortex and medulla may calcify. The early ultrasound appearance of cortical nephrocalcinosis is high-level echoes in the cortex with preservation of corticomedullary definition identical to the pattern seen in any medical renal disease (Fig. A). With time, the echogenicity of the cortex increases significantly. The echogenicity of the pyramids also increases in some cases due to both technical factors and fibrotic changes in the pyramids. Eventually the kidney is seen as a highly reflective structure which attenuates the ultrasound beam sufficiently to produce an acoustic shadow. This patient has known chronic glomerulonephritis and has already required renal transplantation. The corresponding plain film demonstrating calcification of the cortex is shown in Figure B.

SUGGESTED READINGS

Brennan JN, Diwan RV, Makker SP, et al: Ultrasonic diagnosis of primary hyperoxaluria in infancy. Radiology 145:147–148, 1982

Shuman WP, Mack LA, Rogers IV: Diffuse nephrocalcinosis: hyperechoic sonographic appearance. AJR 136:830–832, 1981

Wilson DA, Wenzel JE, Altshuler GP: Ultrasound demonstration of diffuse cortical nephrocalcinosis in a case of primary hyperoxaluria. AJR 132:659–661, 1979

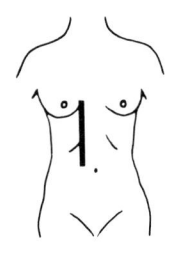

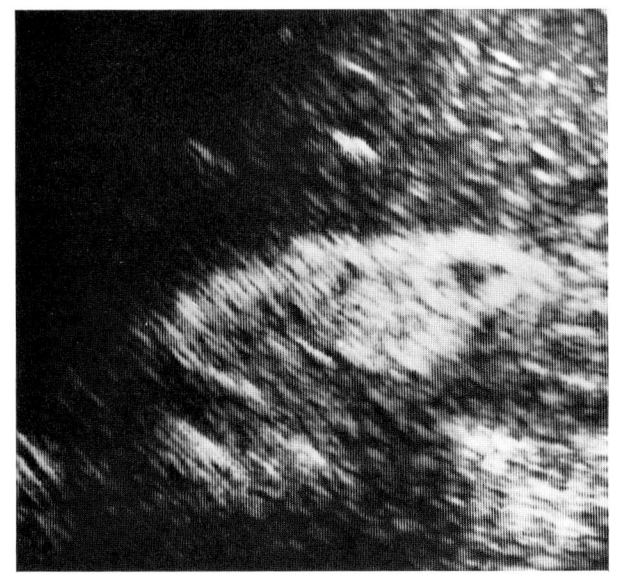

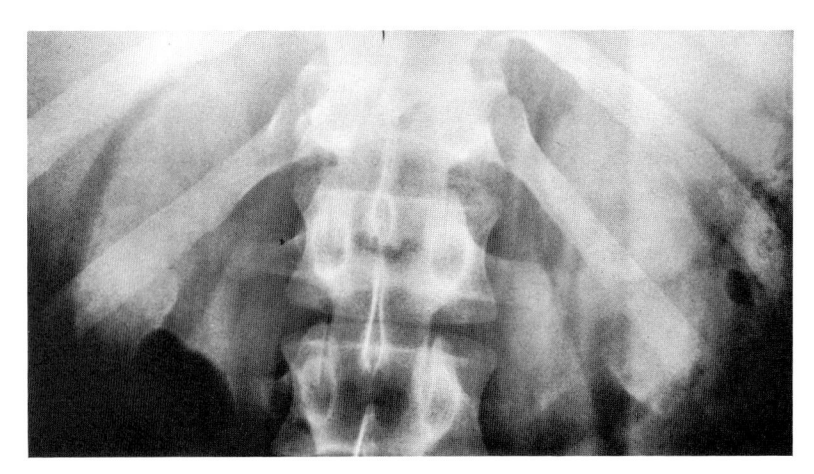

A

B

Renal Transplanation (11.38 to 11.45)

11.38 Evaluation

Ultrasound has become a routine part of the evaluation of the renal transplant for complications. The primary role of sonography in this setting is to identify or exclude hydronephrosis and to identify extrarenal masses such as abscesses, lymphoceles, or hematomas. Sonography and radioisotope scanning are generally performed simultaneously in the evaluation of transplant patients with acute renal failure; the former provides excellent anatomical detail whereas the latter is used for physiological information. In patients suspected of having an abscess, computed tomography can be of great value as an additional study.

11.39 Acute Rejection

The most common ultrasound appearances of acute renal transplant rejection are those of medical renal disease: high-level echoes in the cortex with preservation of corticomedullary definition. There is also an increase in the size of the pyramids. As demonstrated in the figure, this leads to a kidney consisting of highly reflective parenchyma and large hypoechoic pyramids. Other findings that have been described in renal transplant rejection include: a decrease in prominence of the renal sinus echoes, focal areas of decreased echogenicity in the parenchyma due to renal infarcts, and in some cases poor definition between cortex and medulla. The arcuate vessels are frequently difficult to identify in the highly reflective parenchyma. In the absence of hydronephrosis, the major differential diagnosis for renal failure is rejection and acute tubular necrosis. The latter causes only a minimal increase in cortical echoes while rejection causes a major increase in echogenicity. Ultrasound therefore offers promise to be of use in this distinction.

(This case and figure taken from Rosenfield AT, Taylor KJW, Dembner AG, et al: Ultrasound of the renal sinus: new observations. AJR 133:441–448, 1979. ©1979 Am Roentgen Ray Soc.)

SUGGESTED READINGS

Conrad MR, Dickerman R, Love IL: New observations in renal transplants using ultrasound. AJR 131:851–855, 1978

Hillman BJ, Birnholz JC, Busch GJ: Correlation of echographic and histologic findings in suspected renal allograft rejection. Radiology 132:673–676, 1979

Hricak H, Cruz C, Eyler WR: Acute post-transplantation renal failure: differential diagnosis by ultrasound. Radiology 139:441–449, 1981

Hricak H, Toledo-Pereyra LH, Eyler WR: The role of ultrasound in the diagnosis of kidney allograft rejection. Radiology 132:667–672, 1979

Leopold GR: Renal transplant size measured by reflected ultrasound. Radiology 95:687–689, 1970

Maklad NF, Wright CH, Rosenthal SJ: Gray scale ultrasonic appearances of renal transplant rejection. Radiology 131:711–717, 1979

Rosenfield AT, Taylor KJW, Dembner AG, et al: Ultrasound of the renal sinus: new observations. AJR 133:441–448, 1979

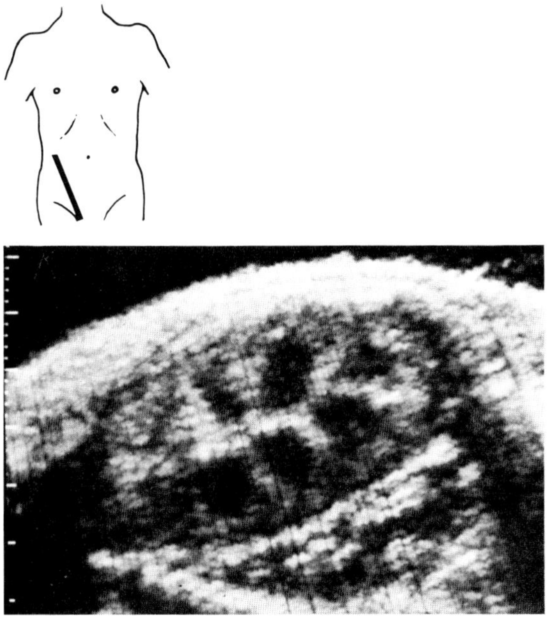

11.40 Chronic Rejection

An 8-year-old girl had received two renal transplants. In her right true pelvis was a recent renal transplant which was normal (Fig. A). Note the reflective renal sinus, the normal cortical echogenicity, and the normal-sized pyramids (arrowed) which were easily identified. In the left true pelvis, a chronically rejecting kidney had not been removed (Fig. B). The kidney demonstrated a highly reflective cortex, similar to that seen in the renal sinus. Pyramids (arrowed) in this case were still identifiable. Note the bladder (b) adjacent to the kidney.

The ultrasound appearances in chronic transplant rejection initially show an increase in cortical echogenicity as well as a decrease in renal size. Eventually the pyramids become echogenic as well and the kidney is identical to that seen in any case of end-stage renal failure with no differentiation possible between cortex and medulla.

(Figs. A & B from Rosenfield AT, Ultrasound of renal parenchymal disease and hydronephrosis. Urol Radiol 4:125–133, 1982.)

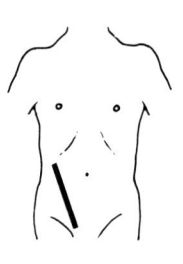

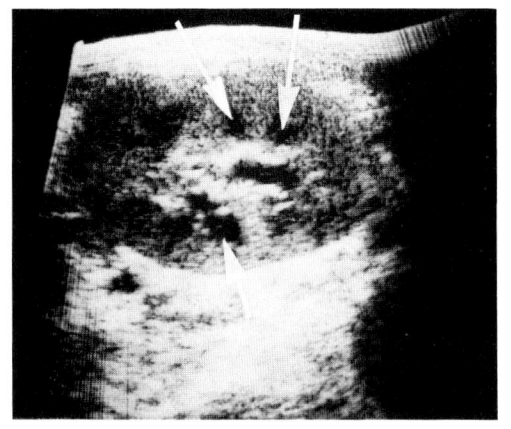

A

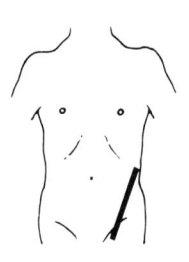

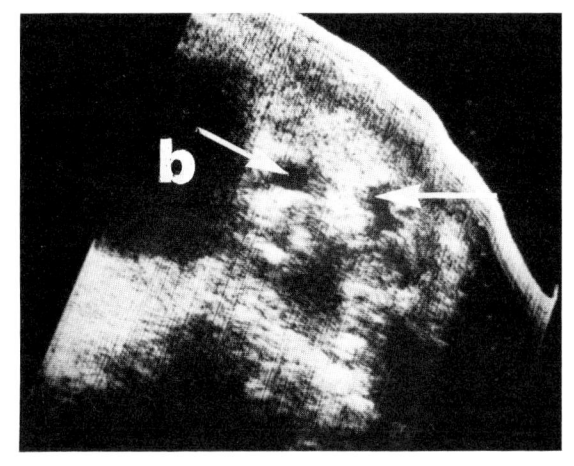

B

11.41 Obstructive Uropathy

A 7-year-old boy received a renal transplant for renal failure due to long-standing obstructive uropathy. Postoperatively the patient was noted to have decreased urine output. Radionuclide evaluation was performed 4 days postoperatively, and showed normal perfusion but delayed excretion, as well as a dilated pelvocalyceal system. Since an adult kidney had been transplanted, it was possible that the large renal pelvis might reflect the discrepancy in size between the transplanted kidney and the small patient. Ultrasound was therefore performed on the 5th postoperative day to clarify the radionclide findings.

In Figure A the collecting system of the transplanted kidney is grossly dilated, consistent with obstruction, but no dilated ureter is appreciated and no extrarenal fluid collection is visible.

Subsequent excretory urography confirms the presence of obstruction to the urinary tract (Fig. B)

A repeat ultrasound examination on the 10th day demonstrates continued dilatation of the urinary system (Fig. C). Repeat ultrasound (Fig. D) on the 19th hospital day shows a marked decrease in the pyelocaliectasis.

This case demonstrates the value of ultrasound in initially diagnosing obstructive uropathy in the transplanted kidney when such a diagnosis may be more difficult to make using excretory urography or radioisotope studies, since both require adequate renal perfusion and function. Ultrasound also provides a means of evaluating these patients serially without exposing them to additional ionizing radiation or discomfort. As shown in Figures 11-43A and B, when a mass is present, such as a lymphocele or urinoma, it can be identified. Thus ultrasound has a potential to identify the nature of the obstruction or, equally significantly, to rule out an extrinsic mass as the cause of the obstructive uropathy.

(Scans A, C, and D and Fig. B from Rosenfield AT, Taylor KJW: Obstructed uropathy in the transplanted kidney: evaluation by grey-scale sonography. J Urol 116:101–102, 1976. © 1976 The Williams & Wilkins Co., Baltimore.)

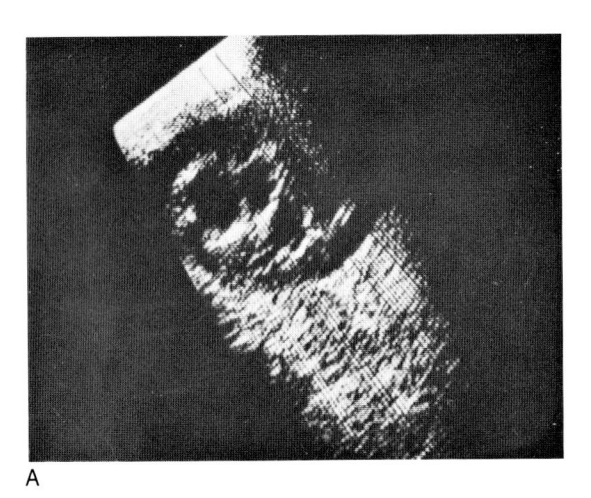

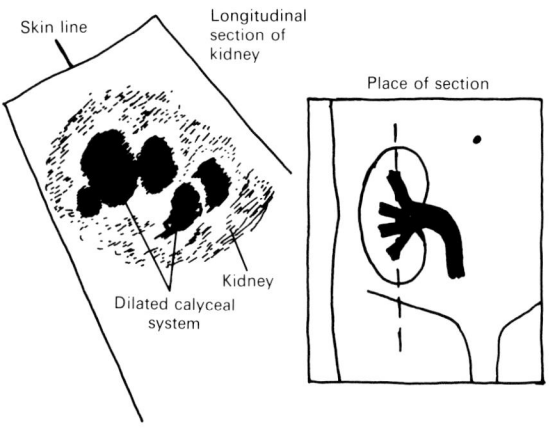

A

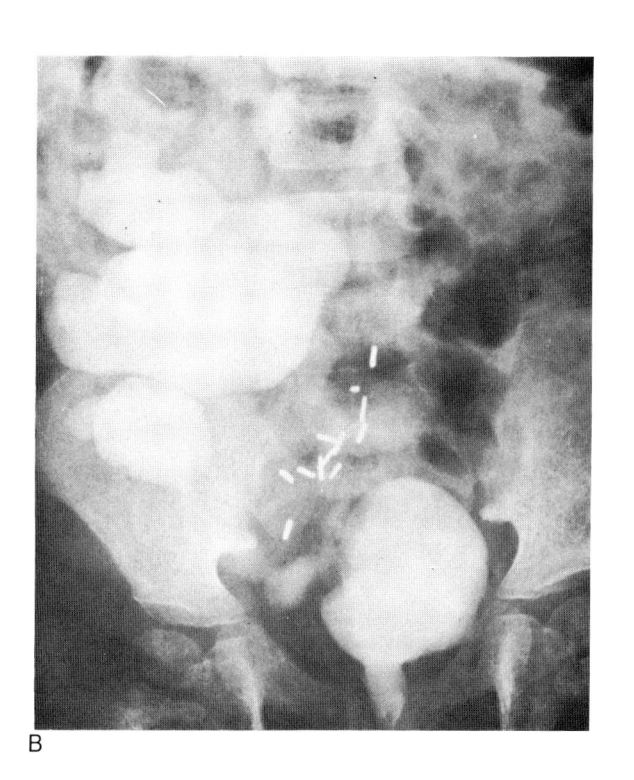

B

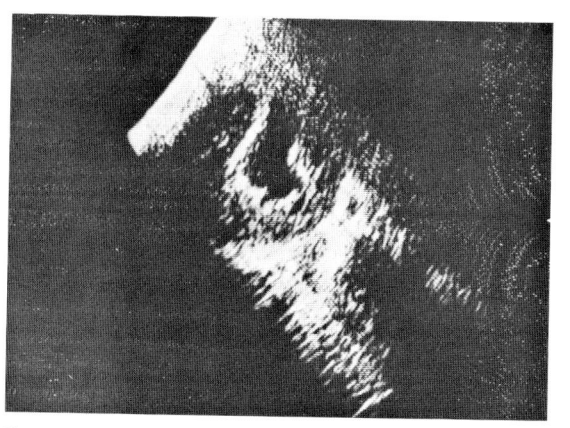

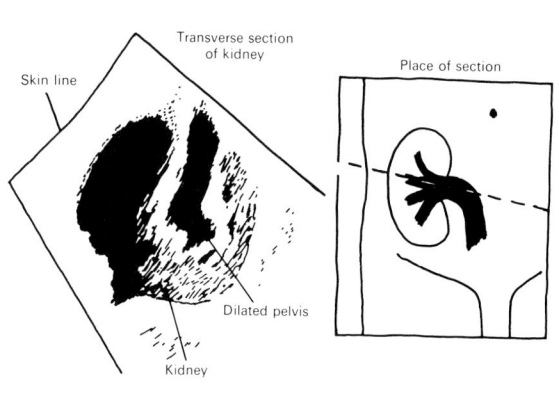

C

Transverse section of kidney

Skin line

Dilated pelvis

Kidney

Place of section

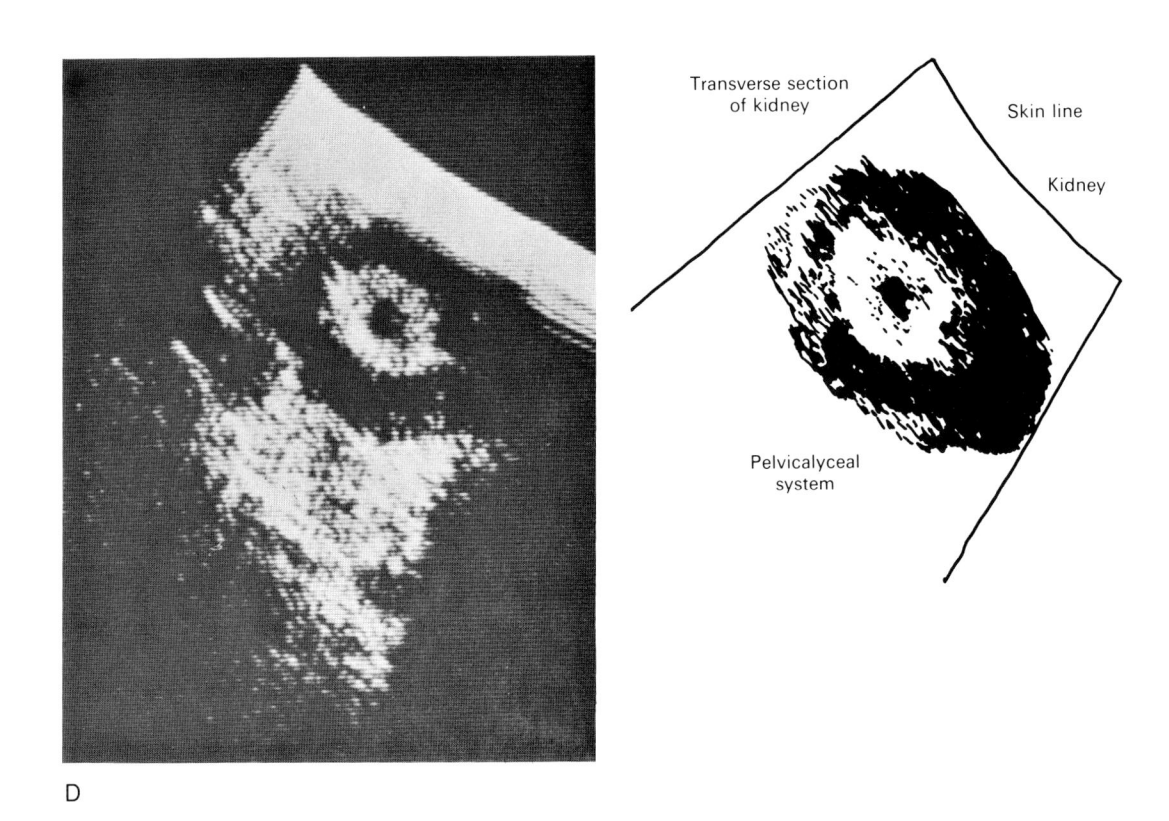

D

Transverse section of kidney

Skin line

Kidney

Pelvicalyceal system

11.42 Antegrade Pyelography and Whittaker Test in the Evaluation of Hydronephrosis

A 21-year-old man had received a renal transplant from a related donor at another institution 10 years prior to admission. During the next 6 years, repeated urologic complications developed, primarily involving the allograft ureter and the ureterovesical anastomosis. When this patient was initially seen at our institution approximately 4 years after the last operative procedure, his serum creatinine level had increased during a 3-month period to 6.7 mg %. Ultrasound demonstrated hydronephrosis in the graft (Fig. A). An antegrade pyelogram was performed to determine whether hydronephrosis was obstructive or nonobstructive. Figure B demonstrates the needle placed within the collecting system under ultrasound guidance. A continuous recording of intrapelvic pressure and perfusion rates from 0 to 2 ml/minute was obtained (Fig. C). Note the rapid rise in pressure at 1 ml/minute. For comparison, normal results of Whittaker flow study are demonstrated (Fig. D).

It is well-accepted that a dilated, nonrefluxing collecting system is not necessarily obstructed. Whittaker pioneered the use of pressure studies following antegrade puncture of the collecting system. These pressure evaluations are performed at increasing flow rates. At flow rates of up to 10 ml/minute, pressure should not rise in the normal system. More recently, it has been suggested that flow rates greater than 10 ml/minute can be accepted by a normal kidney. Ultrasound provides an excellent technique to guide the antegrade puncture for the Whittaker test.

Hydronephrosis may be obstructive or nonobstructive. In both the normotopic and transplanted kidney, antegrade pyelography combined with the Whittaker test can be used to make this distinction.

(Figs. A–D from Schiff M, Rosenfield AT, McGuire EJ: The use of percutaneous antegrade renal perfusion in kidney transplant recipients. J Urol 122:246–248, 1979. © 1979 The Williams & Wilkins Co., Baltimore.)

SUGGESTED READINGS

Schiff M, Rosenfield AT, McGuire EJ: The use of percutaneous antegrade renal perfusion in kidney transplant recipients. J Urol 122:246–248, 1979

Whittaker RH: Methods of assessing obstruction in dilated ureters. Br J Urol 45:15–22, 1973

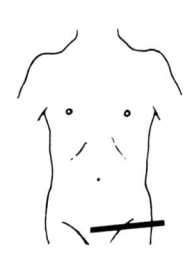

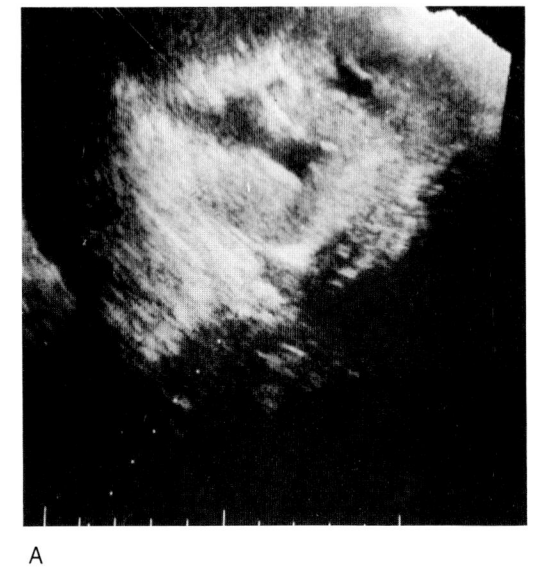

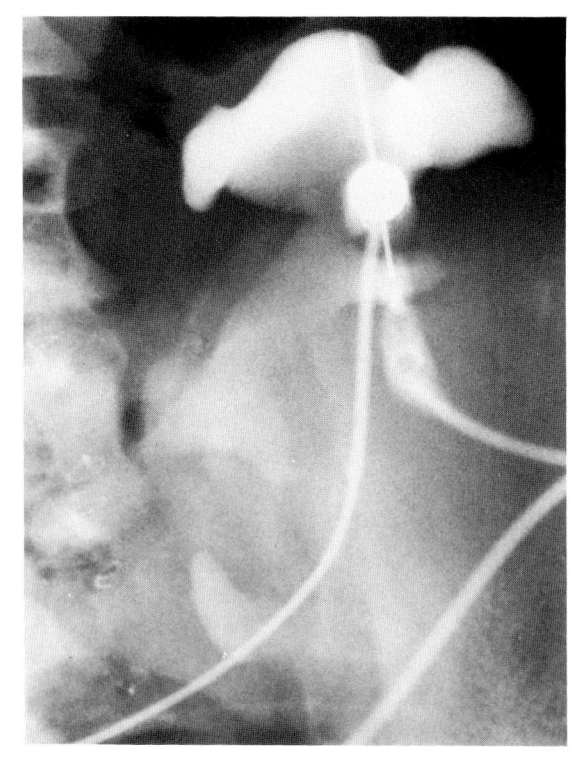

A

B

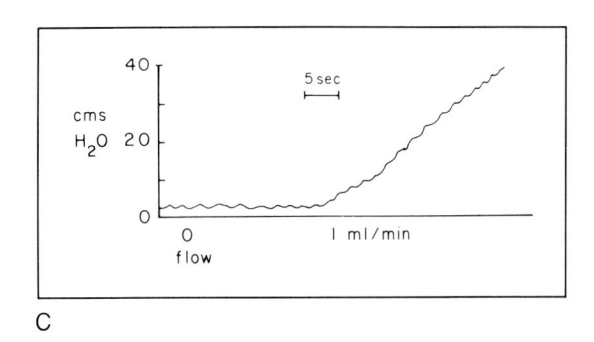

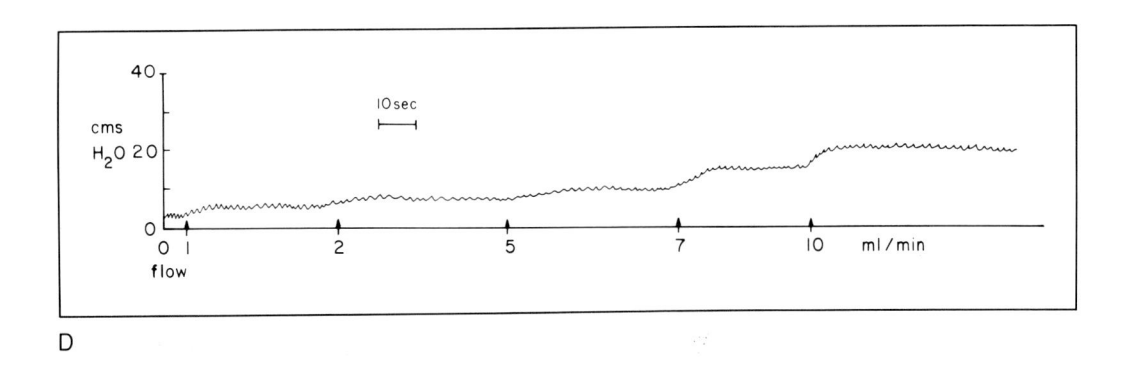

C

D

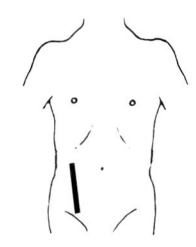

11.43 Lymphocele

Two longitudinal scans (Figs. A and B) demonstrated a septate fluid-filled mass contiguous with a transplanted kidney. The bladder could be identified as a separate fluid-filled structure on other scans. Aspiration of this mass produced fluid consistent with a lymphocele.

Lymphoceles appear as fluid-filled masses that may have septa. If it is unclear whether a fluid-filled mass is a lymphocele or the bladder itself, a postvoid sonogram can be taken to see whether the structure changes in size. The differential diagnosis for a fluid-filled extrarenal structure includes lymphocele, urinoma, hematoma, and abscess. Aspiration will generally permit differentiation among these possibilities. Drainage of the structure may also be used therapeutically to relieve associated hydronephrosis or prevent infection.

SUGGESTED READINGS

Gomes AS, Scholl D, Feinberg S, et al: Lymphangiography and ultrasound in management of lymphoceles. Urology 13:104–108, 1979

Koehler PR, Kanemoto HH, Maxwell GJ: Ultrasonic "B" scanning in the diagnosis of complications in renal transplant patients. Radiology 119:661–664, 1976

Phillips JF, Neiman HL, Brown TL: Ultrasound diagnosis of postransplant renal lymphocele. Am J Roentgenol 126:1194–1196, 1976

Silver TM, Campbell D, Wicks JD, et al: Peritransplant fluid collections. Radiology 138:145–151, 1981

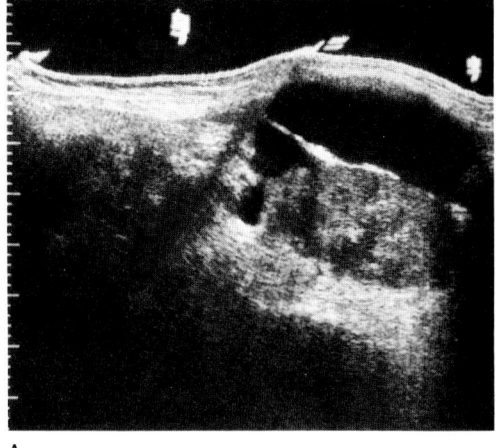

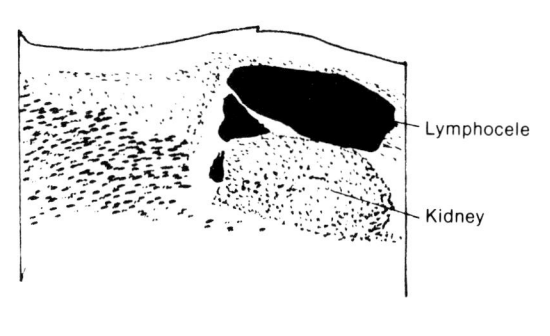

A

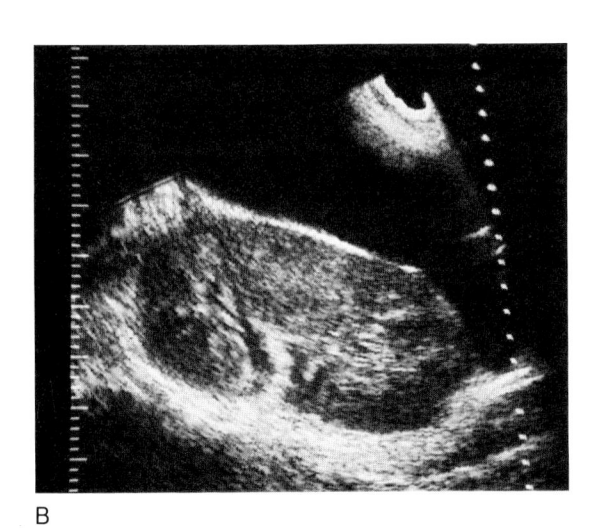

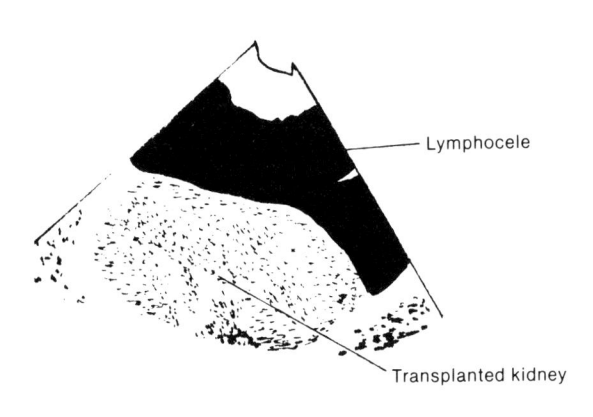

B

Lymphocele

Transplanted kidney

11.44 Hematoma

A longitudinal scan beneath the incision of a patient who had undergone renal transplantation 7 days prior to the study demonstrates a cystic mass 11.3 cm long and of mixed echogenicity. This proved to be a posttransplant hematoma. Sonographically, hematomas can appear echo-free, echogenic, or mixed, as in this case.

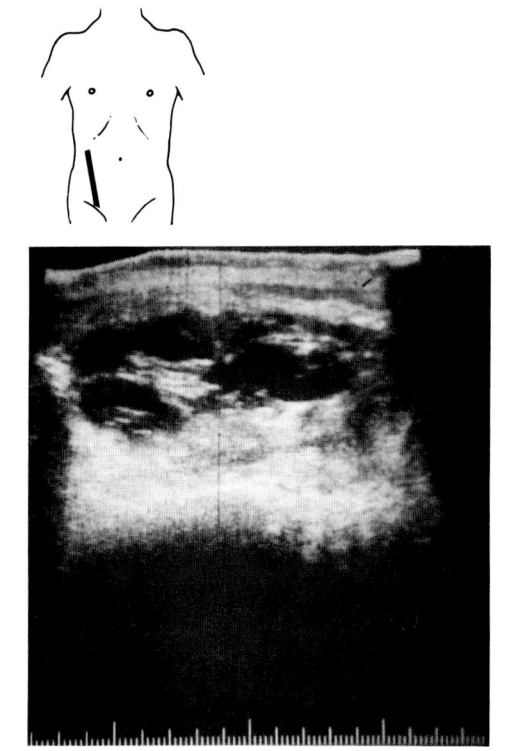

11.45 Blood Clot in the Renal Pelvis Secondary to Rejection

A 19-year-old man was seen 2 years after renal transplantation with anuria of several hours' duration. On the evening prior to admission he had developed pain in the region of the transplant and gross hematuria. The sonogram taken at admission (Fig. A) demonstrates high-level echoes in the cortex with preservation of corticomedullary definition consistent with acute transplant rejection. In the renal sinus there is a debris/fluid level with a few scattered low-level echoes seen in the fluid above the debris. This finding is consistent with either blood or pus within the collecting system. In view of the history of hematuria, this was considered to represent blood within the collecting system. Figure B shows the excretory urogram 3 months prior to admission, which was normal. Figure C is the excretory urogram at admission, demonstrating the blood clot forming the cast of the collecting system. At surgery 3 days later, a kidney undergoing acute rejection was removed. There was old blood within the collecting system.

(Scans A–C from Rosenfield AT, Taylor KJW, Dembner AG, et al: Ultrasound of the renal sinus: new observations. AJR 133:441–448, 1979. ©1979 Roentgen Roy Soc.)

SUGGESTED READING

Rosenfield AT, Taylor KJW, Dembner AG, et al: Ultrasound of the renal sinus: new observations. AJR 133:441–448, 1979

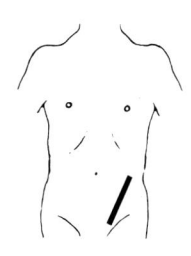

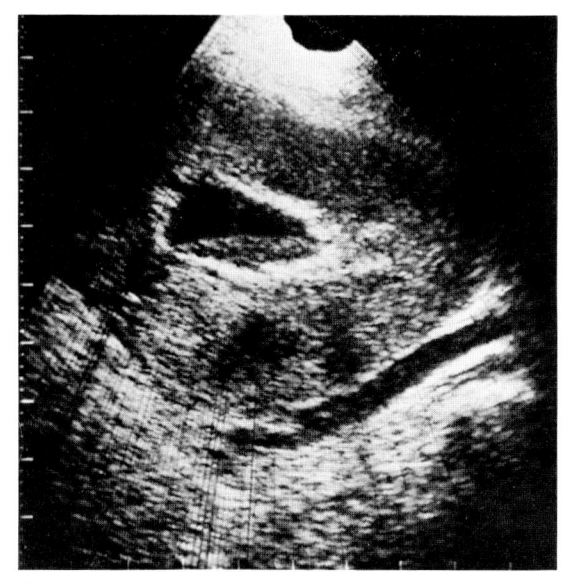

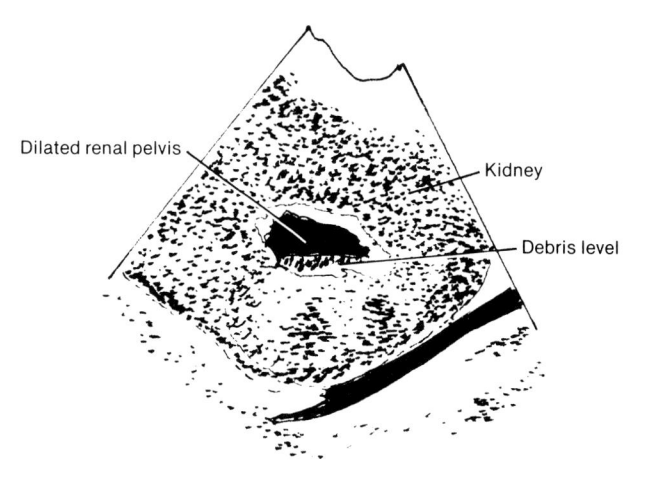

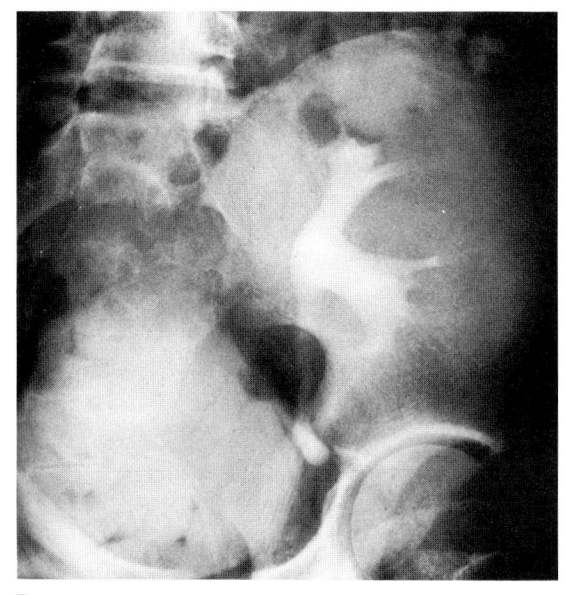

A

B

836

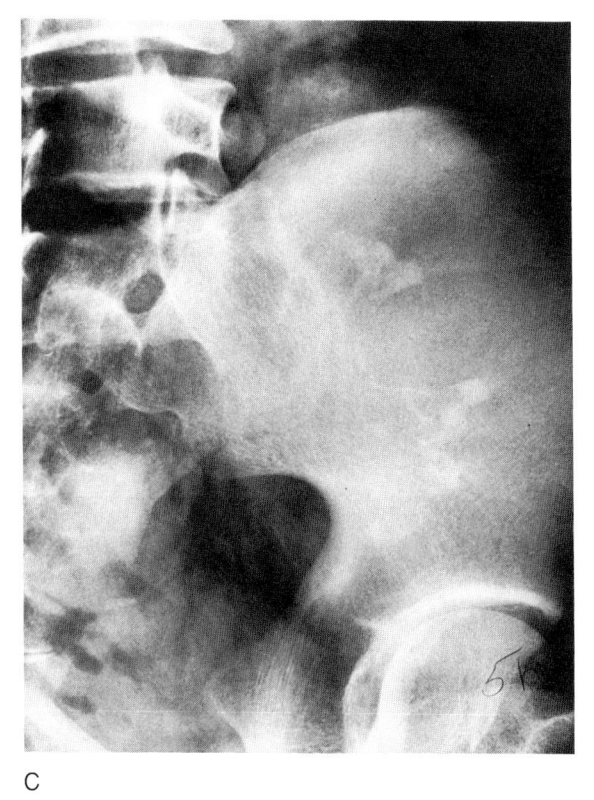

C

12 Renal Masses, Cystic Disease, Trauma, and Disorders of the Bladder and Prostate

ARTHUR T. ROSENFIELD and TINA RICHMAN

12.1 Introduction

The diagnostic work-up of renal masses has changed rapidly as new techniques have become available. The role of imaging in the evaluation of renal masses is to distinguish those that require no therapy, primarily those comprised of normal renal tissue and those representing simple renal cysts, from masses requiring surgery. A coordinated approach to the diagnosis of renal lesions is essential. In general, tests that are simple should be utilized before those that are more complicated or have a greater morbidity and mortality.

A secondary but major role for imaging renal masses is the staging of neoplastic disease. Our experience has been similar to that reported by others: computed tomography is the optimal technique for staging renal cell carcinoma and determining adjacent organ invasion, lymph node metastases, and venous extension. However, when computed tomography is not available, ultrasound is often the most useful alternative to angiography for preoperative tumor assessment.

Most renal masses are initially identified on the excretory urogram. We use the excretory urogram to determine which tests should be done next. If a mass is identified that may be normal functioning tissue such as a "pseudotumor," a radioisotope scan is the safest technique to use. Any mass over 2 cm in diameter that does not contain functioning renal tissue will be seen as a photon-deficient area on the isotope study. A mass containing functioning renal tissue such as a pseudotumor, has normal or increased activity on scanning with a renal parenchymal agent. A diagnosis of "pseudotumor" can be made on an anatomical basis, using ultrasound, by identifying normal cortex and medulla within the mass. However, the functional information available from an isotope study makes this the technique of choice for this purpose.

When the mass identified on the excretory urogram is considered most likely to be a simple renal cyst, ultrasonography is the technique of choice to verify this diagnosis. If all of the features of a simple renal cyst are present, cyst puncture is generally not indicated. However, cyst puncture should be performed on young patients (below the age of 40 years), on patients who are symptomatic (pain, hematuria), on patients with obstructive uropathy secondary to the lesion, or if there is any suspicious finding on the ultrasound study. Similarly, if a mass is indeterminate on the excretory urogram, ultrasound is the ideal technique for differentiating a cystic from a solid mass.

As indicated above, computed tomography is the optimal technique for staging renal masses. Since computed tomography is comparable to ultrasound in its ability to distinguish cystic from solid lesions, computed tomography can simultaneously stage and determine the nature of the mass. Our approach to renal masses is summarized in the figure.

SUGGESTED READINGS

Cronan JJ, Zeman RK, Rosenfield AT: Comparison of computed tomography, ultrasound and angiography in staging renal cell carcinoma. J Urol 127:712–714, 1982

Green B: Renal masses. pp. 273–298. In Rosenfield AT, Glickman MG, Hodson J (eds): Diagnostic Imaging in Renal Disease. Appleton-Century-Crofts, New York, 1979

Pollack HM, Banner MP, Arger PH, et al: Comparison of computed tomography and ultrasound in the diagnosis of renal masses. pp. 25–72. In Rosenfield AT (ed): Clinics in Diagnostic Ultrasound, vol 2. Churchill Livingstone, New York, 1979

Pollack HM, Edell S, Morales JO: Radionuclide imaging in renal pseudotumors. Radiology 111:639–644, 1974

Zeman RK, Cronan JJ, Viscomi GN, et al: Coordinated imaging in the detection and characterization of renal masses. CRC Crit Rev Diagn Imaging 15:273–318, 1981

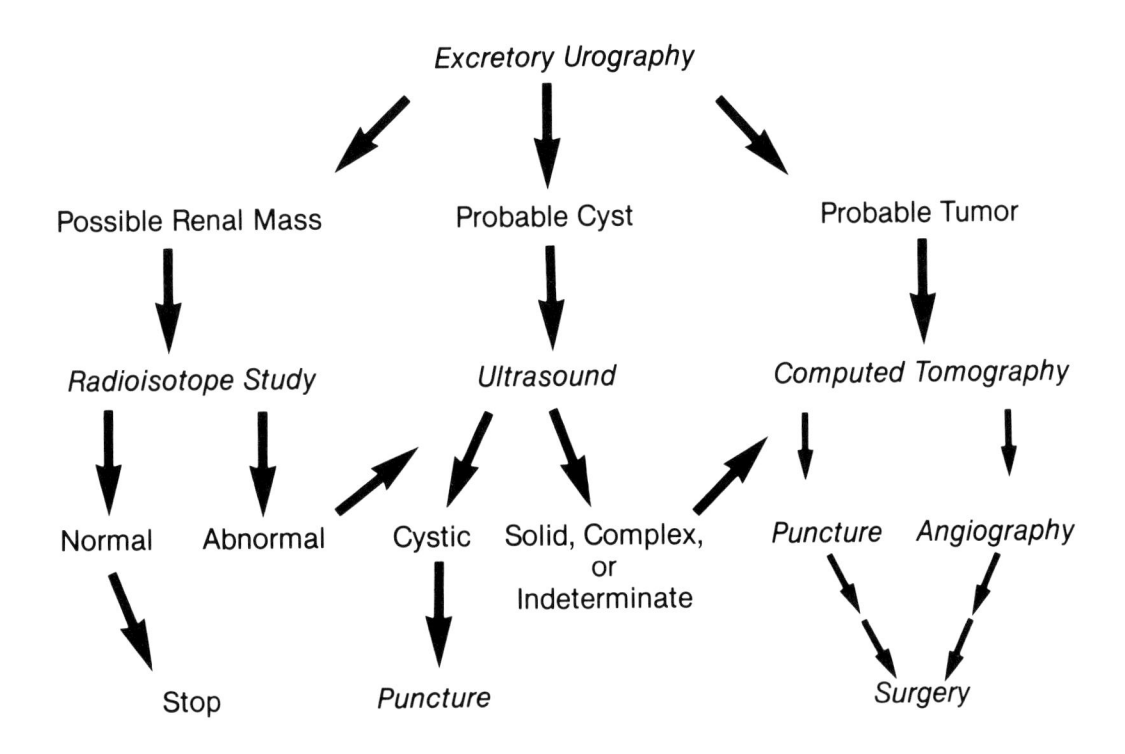

```
                        Excretory Urography
                   ↙          ↓          ↘
        Possible Renal Mass  Probable Cyst   Probable Tumor
                ↓               ↓                ↓
         Radioisotope Study   Ultrasound    Computed Tomography
              ↓     ↓        ↗  ↓    ↘       ↗   ↓         ↓
          Normal  Abnormal  Cystic  Solid, Complex,  Puncture  Angiography
            ↓                 ↓     or Indeterminate    ↘       ↙
           Stop            Puncture                      Surgery
```

12.2 Septum of Bertin

A 58-year-old man with malignant hypertension was admitted in acute renal failure. Ultrasound examination was performed to rule out hydronephrosis. A mass measuring 1.8 cm in diameter which impinged on the renal sinus anteriorly was identified (arrowed in Fig. A). The mass had a consistency identical to that of normal renal tissue. Correlation with subsequent intravenous nephrotomography confirmed that the mass was identical in texture to the remainder of the cortex (Fig. B).

Ultrasound is not the technique of choice to evaluate psuedotumors, both because it is a tomographic technique and because it provides no physiological information. While radioisotope parenchymal scanning remains the technique of choice for this purpose, other imaging techniques including urography with nephrotomography, computed tomography, and angiography are capable of making this diagnosis.

SUGGESTED READINGS

Hodson CJ, Mariani S: Large cloisons. AJR 139:327–332, 1982

Pollack HM, Edell S, Morales JO: Radionuclide imaging in renal pseudotumors. Radiology 111: 639–644, 1974

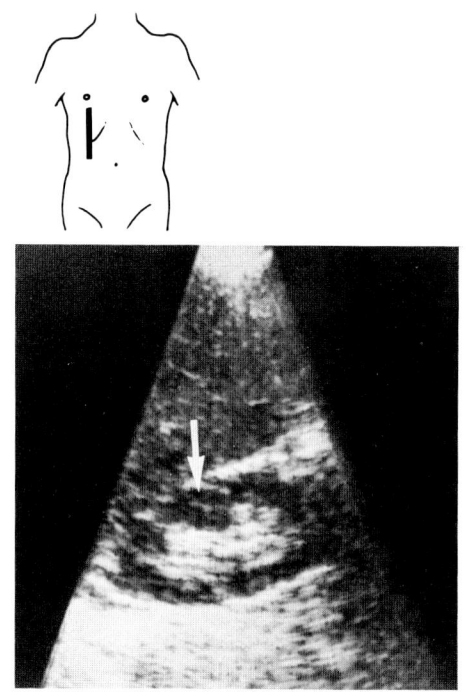

A

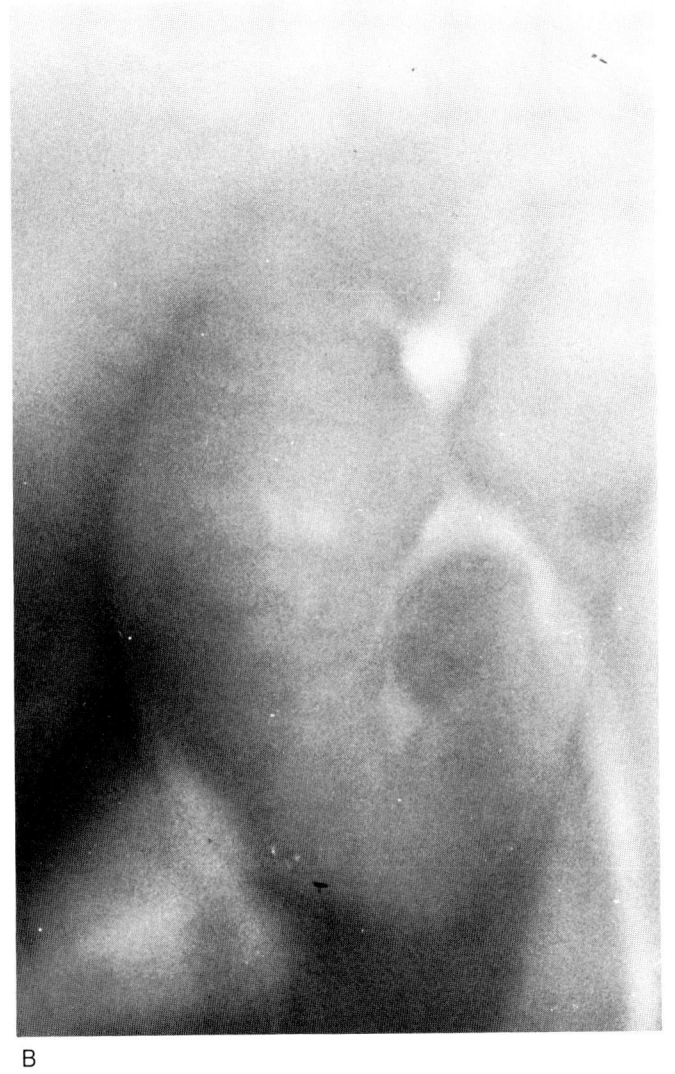

B

Renal Cysts (12.3 and 12.4)

12.3 Simple Cyst

An elderly man presented with hematuria and a mass in the upper pole of the right kidney which was demonstrated on excretory urography. A longitudinal parasagittal section through the kidney (Fig. A) demonstrated that the lower pole was normal but that a 6.5-cm mass protruded from the upper pole. The scale on the scan shows 1-cm intervals.

A simple renal cyst must meet three major criteria:

1. The cyst must be echo free, except for artifactual echoes such as reverberation artifact.
2. The cyst must demonstrate good through-transmission, so that the amplitude of echoes behind the cyst is greater than that behind equivalent solid tissue.
3. There should be a smooth distal wall (Table 12-1)

The mass shown in Figure A meets all three of these major criteria.

In Figure B, which is the A-mode sonogram of the patient in Figure A, the major criteria are once again met. The back wall of the lesion has a greater echo amplitude than the front wall due to the good transmission through the cyst in a situation in which the time gain control has been set for solid tissue. There are a few very low-level echoes in the anterior portion of the cyst, which represent reverberation artifact. These should not be mistaken for true internal echoes.

Figure C demonstrates an intrarenal cyst of the kidney with all the major criteria fulfilled. Note also the shadows (arrowed) from the edges of the renal cyst. Due to refraction of the ultrasound beam, these artifacts are minor criteria for simple renal cysts, and are extremely useful when a complicated cyst is present. For example, a mass containing internal echoes which demonstrates these refractive shadows is most likely to be a complicated cyst such as abscess or hemorrhagic cyst.

Figure D demonstrates a cyst protruding from the lateral aspect of the left kidney. Internal echoes (arrowed) are seen in the anterior aspect of this cyst. These echoes are reverberation echoes from the anterior abdominal wall. This artifact should not be mistaken for true internal echoes. Changing the scanning plane demonstrates that these echoes are not actually within the cyst.

The position of the cyst within the beam width is important with respect to its echogenicity. Due to beam-width artifact, small cysts may appear echo-free only in the focal zone of the transducer. Similarly, the finding of distal ultrasound enhancement depends on technical factors. Distal sonic enhancement occurs because the time gain control is set for attenuation through solid tissues. Because of the low attenuation in a cyst, the echoes distal to it are amplified inappropriately. Since increasing acoustic frequency leads to increasing tissue attenuation, the TGC slope must be increased when the frequency is increased. For this reason, sonic enhancement is best identified with the highest-frequency transducer that can penetrate the area in question.

Table 12-1. Criteria for Simple Renal Cyst

Major
  Echo-free mass
  Good transmission
  Smooth wall
Minor
  Refraction artifact
  Reverberation artifact

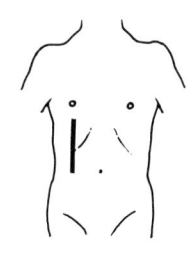

SUGGESTED READINGS

Jaffe CC, Rosenfield AT, Sommer G, et al: Technical factors influencing the imaging of small anechoic cysts by B-scan ultrasound. Radiology 135:429–433, 1980

Leopold GR, Talner LB, Asher WM, et al: Renal ultrasonography: an updated approach to the diagnosis of the renal cyst. Radiology 109:671–678, 1973

Pollack HM, Goldberg BB, Morales JO, et al: A systemized approach to the differential diagnosis of renal masses. Radiology 113:653–659, 1974

Rosenfield AT, Taylor KJW, Jaffe CJ: Clinical applications of tissue characterization. Radiol Clin North Am 18:31–58, 1980

Sommer FG, Filly RA, Minton MJ: Acoustic shadowing due to refractive and reflective effects. AJR 132:973–977, 1979

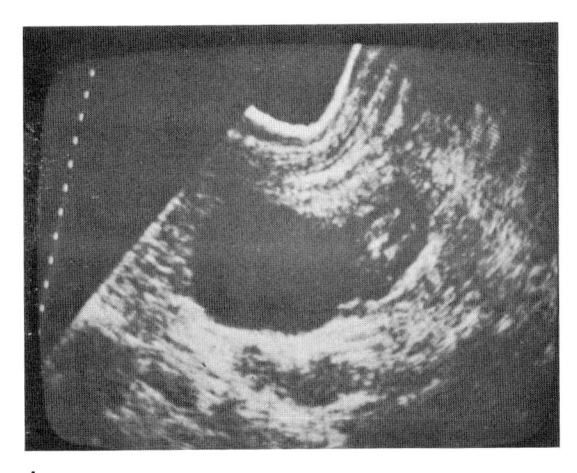

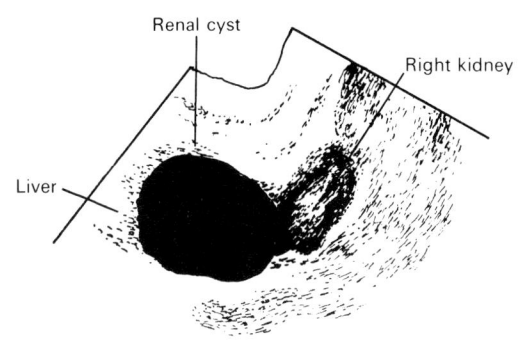

A

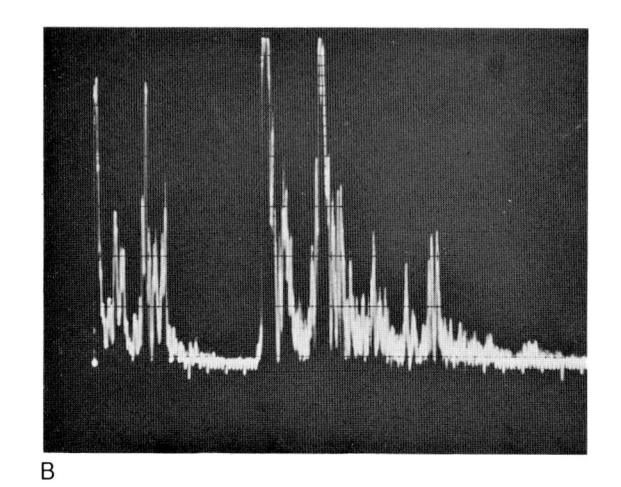

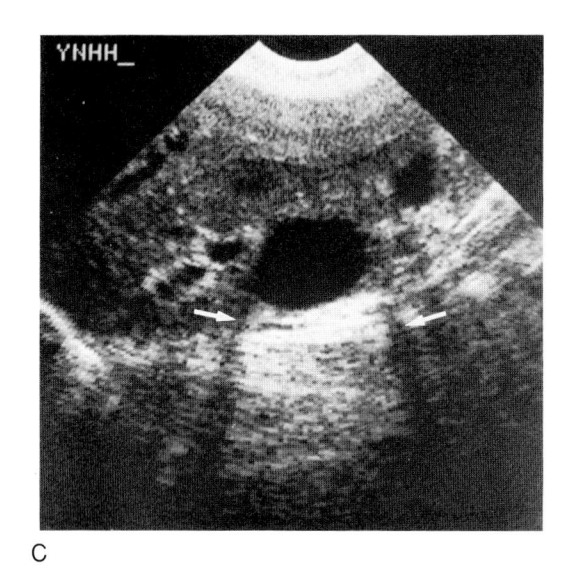

B

C

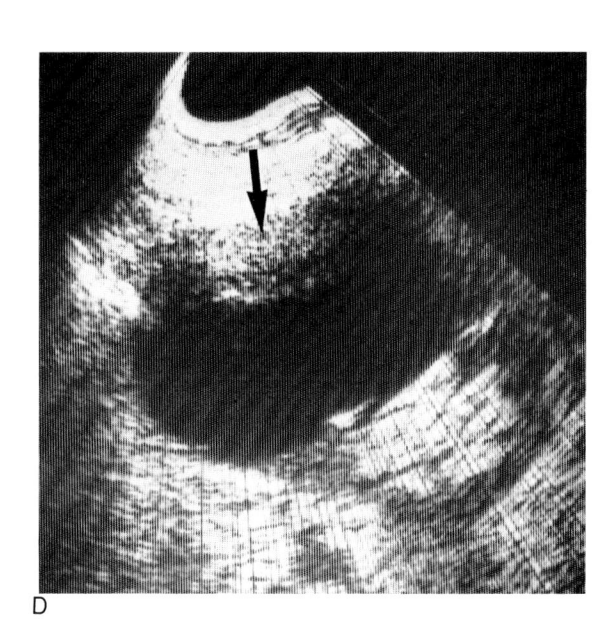

D

12.4 Aspiration

A renal cyst is aspirated with the patient in the prone position under local anesthesia. The cyst may be localized using ultrasound, computed tomography, or fluoroscopy following an intravenous injection of contrast material. The type and incidence of complications are similar for either fluoroscopy or ultrasound-guided aspiration. Sonography permits the depth of the lesion to be gauged, and does not require injection of contrast medium. The expected findings in a suspected renal cyst upon puncture are summarized in Table 12-2. A renal cyst should contain clear or straw-colored fluid. Bloody fluid does not necessarily indicate a renal tumor, but only that one is not dealing with a simple renal cyst. For example, there may be hemorrhage into a renal cyst. Fluid should be withdrawn for cytologic study to exclude a renal tumor. If pus is obtained, it should be cultured. In addition, the lactic dehydrogenase (LDH) level in a simple renal cyst is typically less than that of blood and renal cysts do not contain fat. Although contrast is frequently injected into renal cysts to evaluate their contour under subsequent fluoroscopy, we do not believe this to be essential. We think that contrast administration can lead to false-positive diagnoses under some circumstances. However, if a mass identified on excretory urography is subsequently punctured under ultrasound guidance, injection of a small amount of contrast medium and a subsequent kidney/ureter/bladder study can be extremely helpful in verifying that the lesion identified and punctured under ultrasound guidance was the same as that seen on IVP. Sonography is capable of detecting renal cysts that are not identified on urography, but since it is a tomographic technique, the actual area of interest may, in theory, be missed.

Although cyst puncture is considered a relatively definitive approach to renal masses (with an accuracy approaching 100 percent) there has been a dramatic decline in the use of cyst puncture for diagnosis. Since in autopsy series at least 50 percent of patients over age 50 years have a solitary renal cyst, and since renal cysts are now routinely identified on ultrasound and computed tomographic studies performed for other reasons, it is no longer considered cost-effective to puncture these lesions routinely. Asymptomatic lesions meeting the major criteria for cysts on either ultrasonography or computed tomography need not be punctured. Figures A and B are B-scan sonograms of cysts before and after puncture, respectively. Note that although enough fluid has been withdrawn for evaluation, it is not necessary to aspirate the entire cyst. However, should a renal cyst be causing symptoms because of its size, it should be aspirated completely.

The recent availability of real-time ultrasound transducers that permit guided aspiration allows extremely accurate needle placement. An alternative method of renal cyst puncture under ultrasound guidance involves initial static scanning for localization of the lesion with cyst puncture performed from the posterior aspect, and the patient prone. Scanning from the lateral aspect of the patient can be performed during the procedure to identify the needle, as shown in Figures C–E. In Figure C the needle has not yet entered the cyst. In Figure D, the needle is at the

Table 12-2 Findings in Puncture of Suspected Renal Cyst

Fluid:	Clear
Cytologic analysis	Negative
Lactic dehydrogenase:	Less than blood level
Fat:	None

cyst wall. In Figure E, the needle is seen in the cyst. The size of the cyst can be observed by ultrasound as it is aspirated.

Puncturing the mass after initially determining the angle and depth using standard scanning techniques is the approach generally used in most centers. It provides a rapid, safe, and efficacious way to puncture cysts as well as solid lesions.

SUGGESTED READINGS

Holm HH, Pedersen JF, Kristensen JK, et al: Ultrasonically guided percutaneous puncture. Radiol Clin North Am 13:493–503, 1975

Lang EK: The differential diagnosis of renal cysts and tumors: Cyst puncture, aspiration and analysis of cyst content for fat as diagnostic criteria for renal cysts. Radiology 87:883–888, 1966

Lang EK: Renal cyst puncture and aspiration: a survey of complications. Am J Roentgenol 128:723–727, 1977

Lindgren PG: Ultrasonically guided punctures. Radiology 137:235–237, 1980

McClellen BL, Stanley RJ, Melson GL, et al: CT of the renal cyst: is cyst aspiration necessary? AJR 133:671–675, 1979

Zegel HG, Pollack HM, Banner MP, et al: Percutaneous nephrostomy: comparison of sonographic and fluoroscopic guidance. AJR 137:925–927, 1981

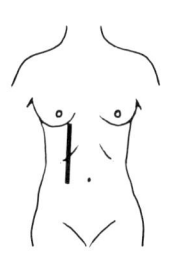

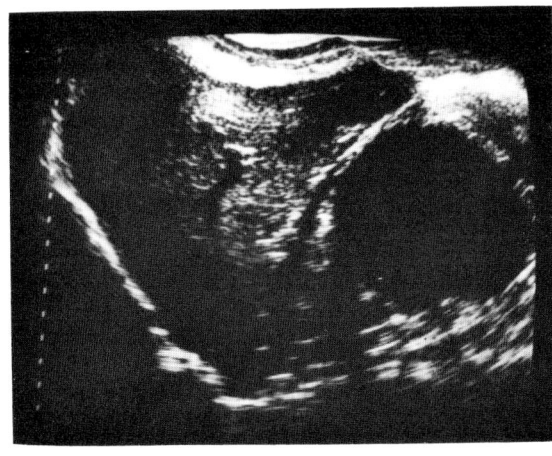

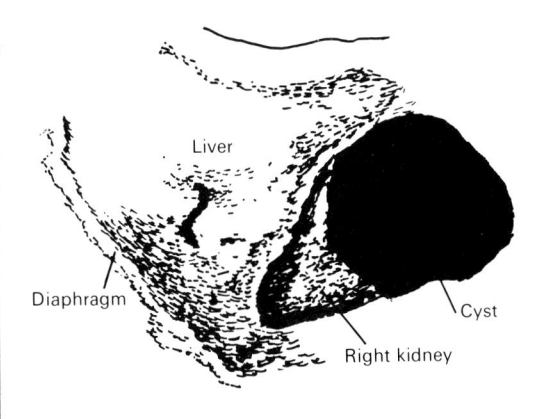

A

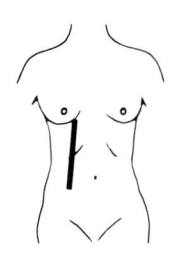

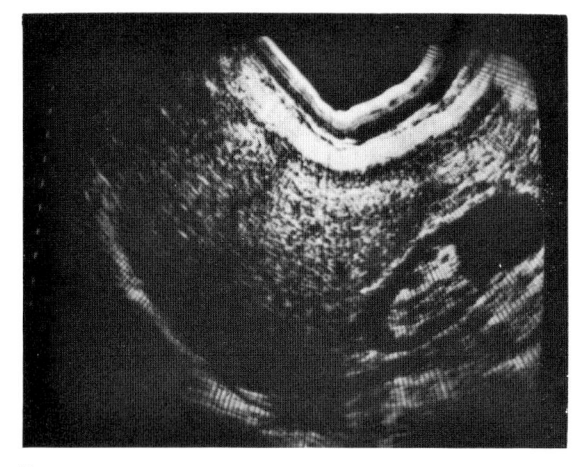

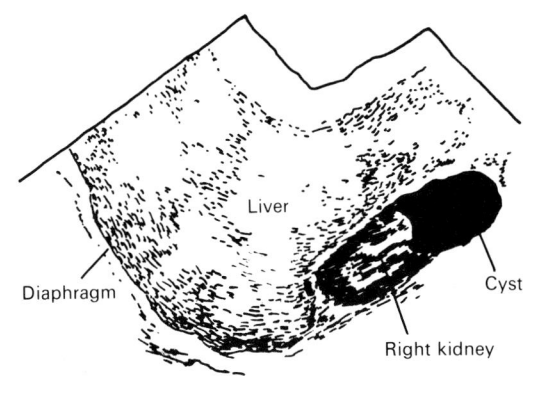

B

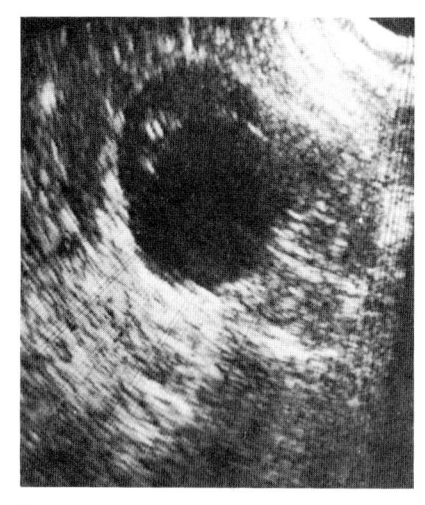

Diaphragm | Liver | Cyst | Right kidney

C

850

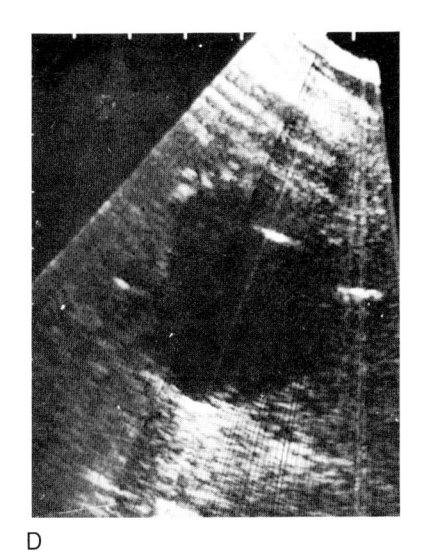

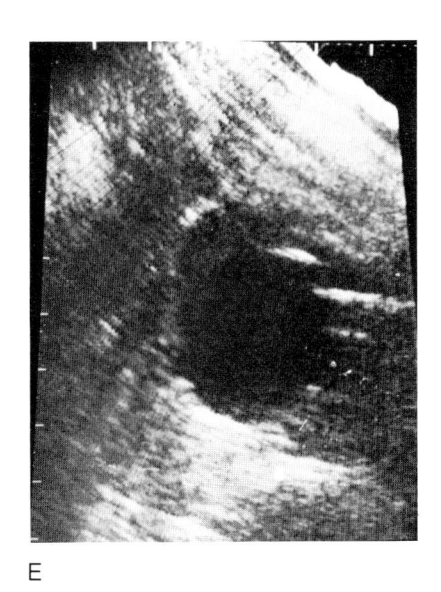

D

E

Renal Cell Carcinoma (12.5 to 12.8)

12.5 Solid Renal Mass

Longitudinal (Fig. A) and transverse (Fig. B) ultrasound examination of the right kidney demonstrates an 11-cm mass extending from the lower pole of the kidney. The mass is clearly solid and contains internal echoes. Small focal zones are echo-free, possibly representing tumor necrosis. In addition, on the transverse scan some localized calyceal dilatation can be seen. The border between the mass and the kidney is poorly defined, which is consistent with tumor. At surgery a hypernephroma was found.

SUGGESTED READINGS

Coleman BG, Arger PH, Mulhern CB, Jr, et al: Gray-scale sonographic spectrum of hypernephromas. Radiology 137:757–765, 1980

Cronan JS, Zeman RK, Rosenfield AT: Comparison of computed tomography, ultrasound, and angiography in staging renal cell carcinoma. J Urol 127:712–714, 1983

Gore RM, Callen PW, Filly RA: Displaced retroperitoneal fat: sonographic guide to right upper quadrant mass localization. Radiology 142:701–705, 1982

Pollack HM, Banner MP, Arger PH, et al: Comparison of computed tomography and ultrasound in the diagnosis of renal masses. pp. 25–72. In Rosenfield AT (ed): Clinics in Diagnostic Ultrasound, vol 2. Churchill Livingstone, New York, 1979

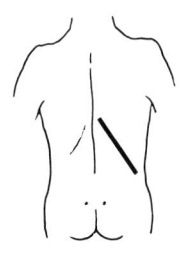

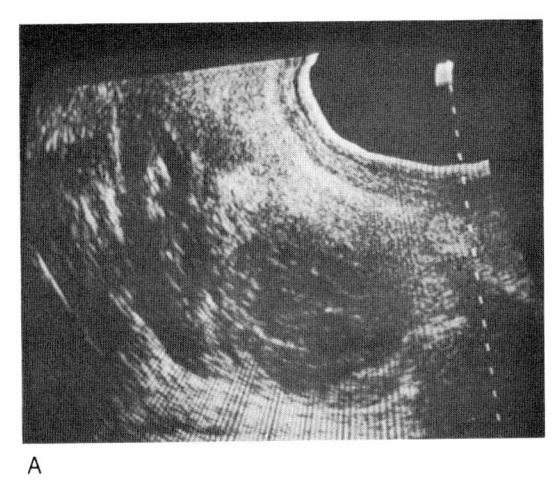

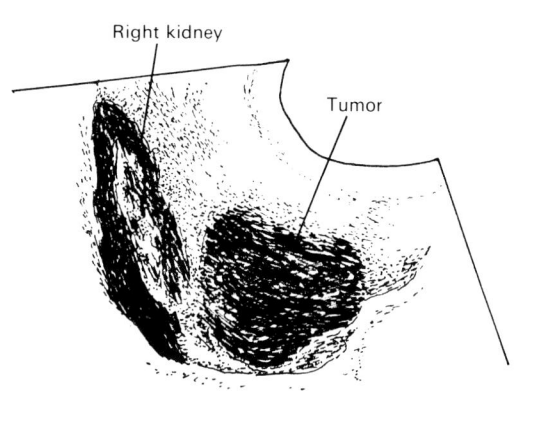

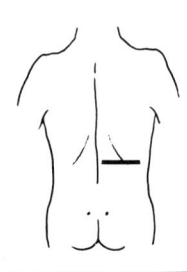

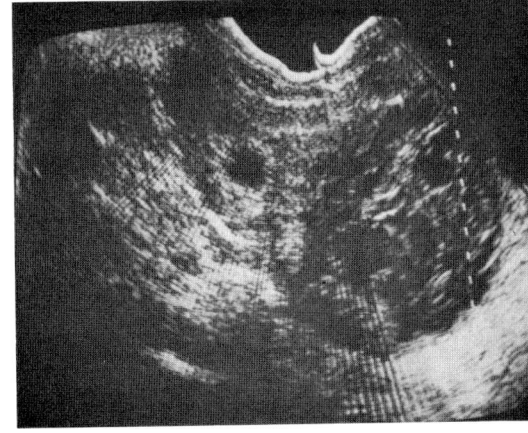

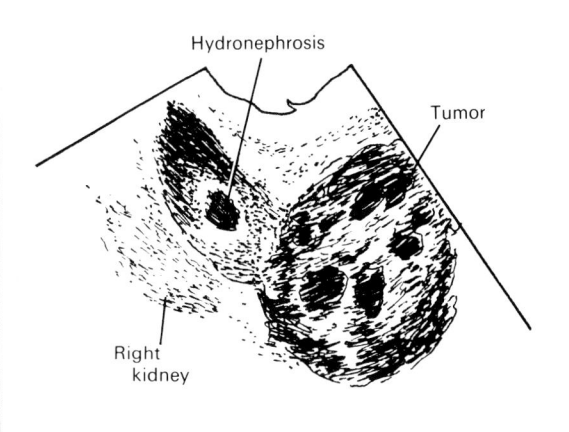

A

B

12.6 Carcinoma with Tissue Necrosis

A middle-aged man presented with hematuria. A longitudinal sonogram (Fig. A) demonstrated a solid mass (arrowed) in the upper pole of the right kidney. The lower pole was unremarkable. Figure B demonstrated the same mass in transverse section. There is necrosis in the central portion of the mass, as represented by an echo-free zone. Note the reflective perirenal fat between the renal mass and the liver. The presence of this fat line indicates that the mass is extrahepatic. If the fat line is identified in continuity (best seen in Fig. B), direct invasion of the liver by the mass is excluded. The nephrographic phase of an arteriogram (Fig. C) confirms the presence of the mass. Surgery disclosed a renal cell carcinoma.

Renal cell carcinoma may be more, as, or less echogenic than the adjacent renal parenchyma. As in this case, tissue necrosis may be present as suggested by the central echo-free region. While the echogenicity of renal cell carcinoma has been related to the vascularity of the lesion as well as to the presence of fat within it, no consistent single parameter correlates well with tumor echogenicity. Whenever a solid renal mass is identified, examination of the liver, retroperitoneum, renal vein, and inferior vena cava should automatically be performed to search for tumor spread. Other renal masses may contain internal echoes; these include complicated cysts, angiomyolipomas, hematomas, oncocytomas, and lesions of the renal capsule such as fibromas.

SUGGESTED READINGS

Coleman BG, Arger PH, Mulhern CB, Jr, et al: Grayscale sonographic spectrum of hypernephromas. Radiology 137:757–765, 1980

Cronan JS, Zeman RK, Rosenfield AT: Comparison of computed tomography, ultrasound, and angiography in staging renal cell carcinoma. J Urol 127:712–714, 1983

Gore RM, Callen PW, Filly RA: Displaced retroperitoneal fat: sonographic guide to right upper quadrant mass localization. Radiology 142:701–705, 1982

Pollack HM, Banner MP, Arger PH, et al: Comparison of computed tomography and ultrasound in the diagnosis of renal masses. pp. 25–72. In Rosenfield AT (ed): Clinics in Diagnostic Ultrasound, vol 2. Churchill Livingstone, New York, 1979

Pollack HM, Goldberg BB, Morales JO, et al: A systematized approach to the differential diagnosis of renal masses. Radiology 113:653–659, 1974

Zeman RK, Cronan JJ, Viscomi GN, et al: Coordinated imaging in the detection and characterization of renal masses. CRC Crit Rev Radiology 15:273–281, 1981

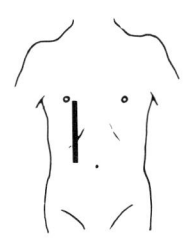

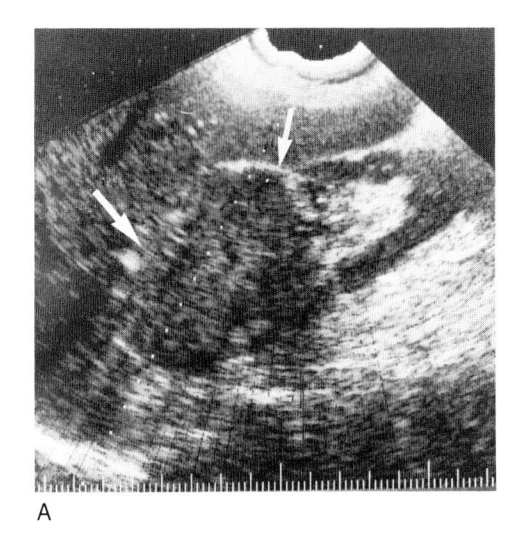

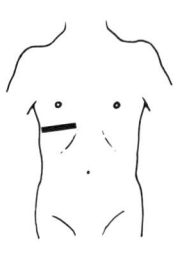

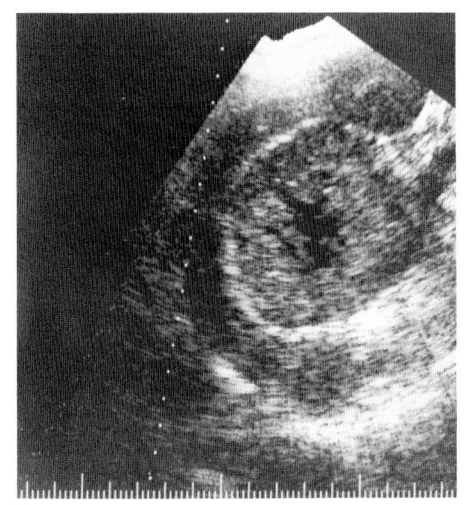

A

B

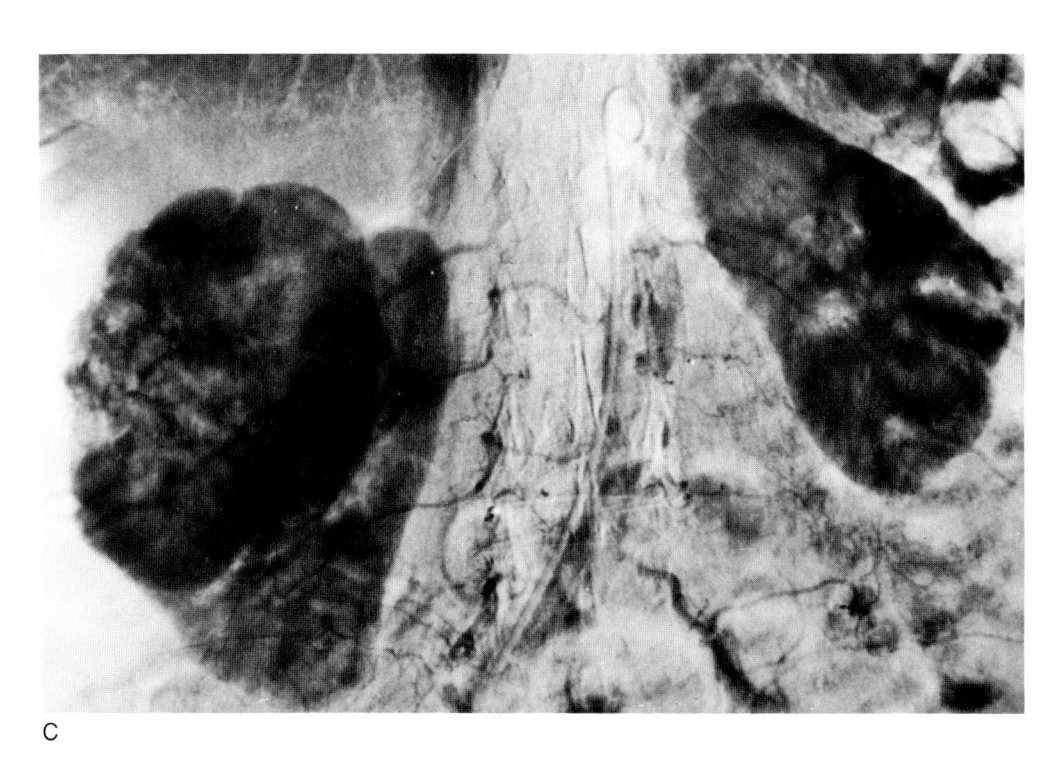

C

12.7 Carcinoma with Involvement of the Right Renal Vein and Inferior Vena Cava

A 74-year-old white man presented with right leg pain and swelling. He had experienced intermittent episodes of gross hematuria during the previous year. Sonography revealed a solid mass (arrowed) in the upper pole of the right kidney (Fig. A) and thrombus within the inferior vena cava (IVC) (arrowed in Fig. B). Computed tomography demonstrated tumor within the IVC (arrowed in Fig. C).

Inferior vena caval involvement with tumor from the kidney occurs in approximately 5 percent of patients with renal cell carcinoma. Ultrasound is capable of identifying tumor in the renal vein, inferior vena cava, as well as extension to the right atrium. A widened inferior vena cava with internal echoes or visualization of tumor thrombus in a patient with a renal mass is characteristic of this entity.

SUGGESTED READINGS

Azimi F, Marangola JP, Kirch KH: Ultrasonic diagnosis of tumor thrombosis of the right renal vein. Urology 12:106–107, 1978

Goldstein HM, Green B, Weaver RM: Ultrasonic detection of renal tumor extension into the inferior vena cava. AJR 130:1083–1085, 1978

Gosink BB: The inferior vena cava: mass effects. AJR 130:533–536, 1978

Greene D, Steinbach HL: Ultrasonic diagnosis of hypernephroma extending into the inferior vena cava. Radiology 115:679–680, 1975

Pollack HM, Banner MP, Arger PH, et al: Comparison of computed tomography and ultrasound in the diagnosis of renal masses. pp. 25–72. In Rosenfield AT (ed): Clinics in Diagnostic Ultrasound, vol 2. Churchill Livingstone, New York, 1979.

Slovis TL, Philippart AI, Cushing B, et al: Evaluation of the inferior vena cava by sonography and venography in children with renal and hepatic tumors. Radiology 140:767–772, 1981

Zeman RK, Cronan JJ, Viscomi GN, et al: Coordinated imaging of renal masses. CRC Crit Rev Diagn Imaging 15:273–318, 1981

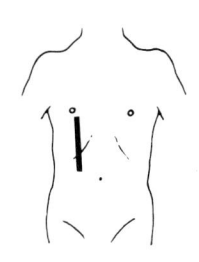

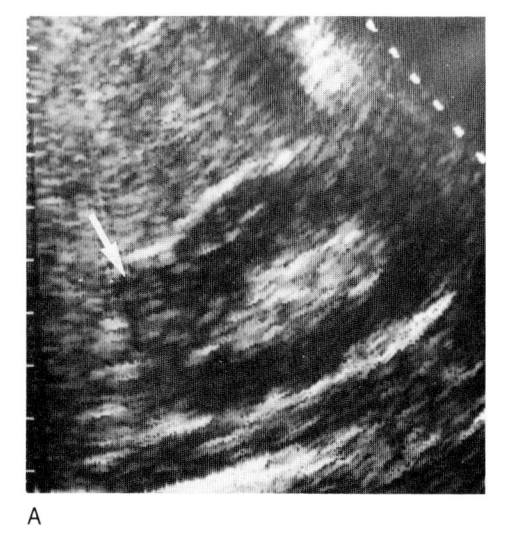

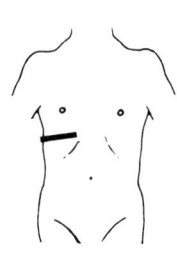

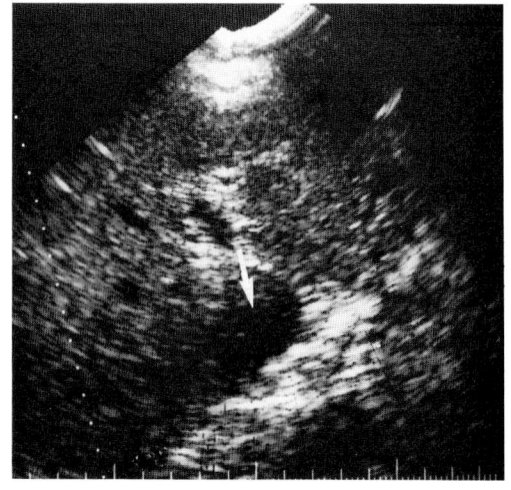

A

B

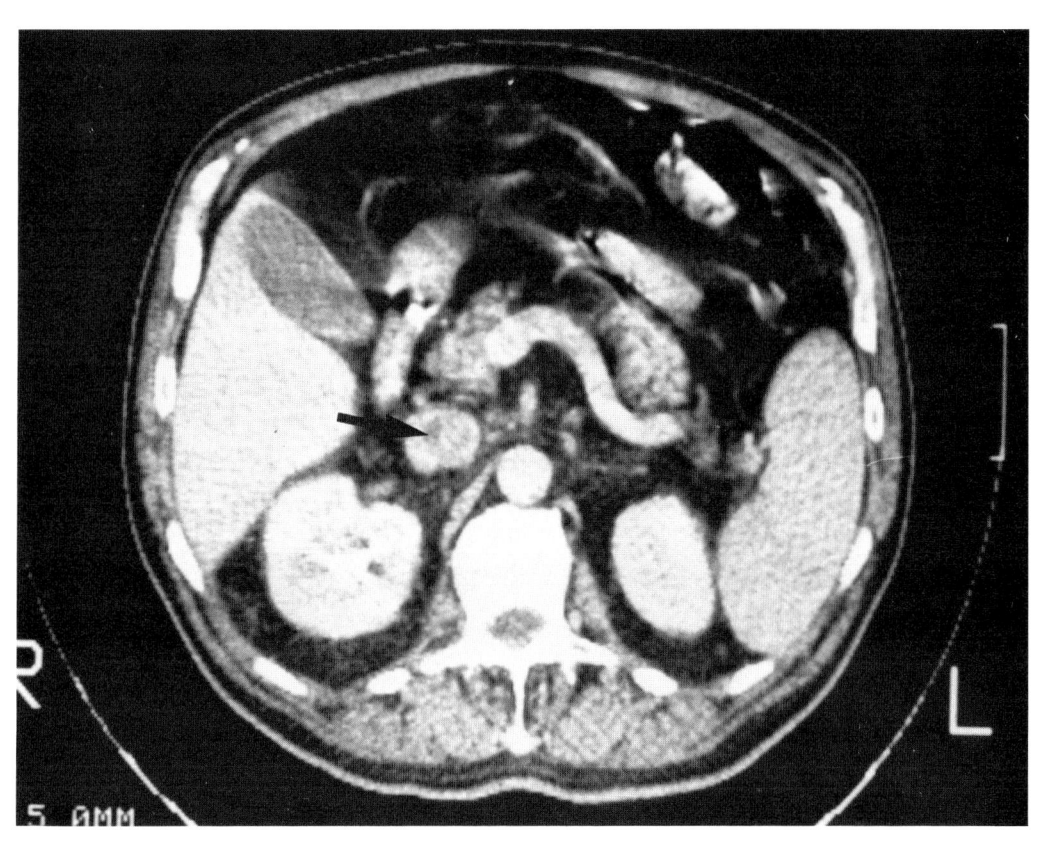

C

12.8 Left Renal Cell Carcinoma with Tumor in the Left Renal Vein and Inferior Vena Cava

A 52-year-old woman with congestive heart failure had microscopic hematuria noted on routine urinalysis. Ultrasonography, which was the first study performed, demonstrated a mass (M) in the left kidney (K) (Fig. A) with scattered low-level internal echoes. A transverse sonogram at the level of the renal hilum (Fig. B) demonstrated widening of the left renal vein with internal echogenicity extending from the origin of the kidney into the left half of the inferior vena cava (c). There is also tumor in the periaortic region displacing the left renal vein anteriorly. These findings are typical of renal cell carcinoma with venous and retroperitoneal extension. Renal biopsy specimens disclosed renal cell carcinoma and subsequent computed tomography also demonstrated tumor in the IVC (c) (Fig. C). The liver (L) and spleen (S) are marked as is the left renal vein (arrow). In the presence of any renal tumor, careful examination of the retroperitoneum, renal vein, inferior vena cava, and liver should be performed.

(Figs. A–C from Gonzalez-Gomez R, Richman AH, Taylor KJW, et al: Urinary tract ultrasonography. pp. 29–54. In Finberg HJ (ed): Case Studies in Diagnostic Ultrasound, Clinics in Diagnostic Ultrasound, vol 9. Churchill Livingstone, New York, 1981.)

SUGGESTED READINGS

Azimi F, Marangola JP, Kirch KH: Ultrasonic diagnosis of tumor thrombosis of the right renal vein. Urology 12:106–107, 1978

Goldstein HM, Green B, Weaver RM: Ultrasonic detection of renal tumor extension into the inferior vena cava. AJR 130:1083–1085, 1978

Gosink BB: The inferior vena cava: mass effects. AJR 130:533–536, 1978

Greene D, Steinbach HL: Ultrasonic diagnosis of hypernephroma extending into the inferior vena cava. Radiology 115:679–680, 1975

Pollack HM, Banner MP, Arger PH, et al: Comparison of computed tomography and ultrasound in the diagnosis of renal masses. pp. 25–72. In Rosenfield AT (ed): Clinics in Diagnostic Ultrasound, vol 2. Churchill Livingstone, New York, 1979

Slovis TL, Philippart AI, Cushing B, et al: Evaluation of the inferior vena cava by sonography and venography in children with renal and hepatic tumors. Radiology 140:767–772, 1981

Zeman RK, Cronan JJ, Viscomi GN, et al: Coordinated imaging of renal masses. CRC Crit Rev. Diagn Imaging 15:273–318, 1981

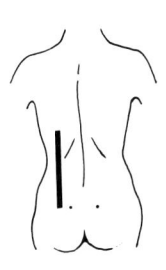

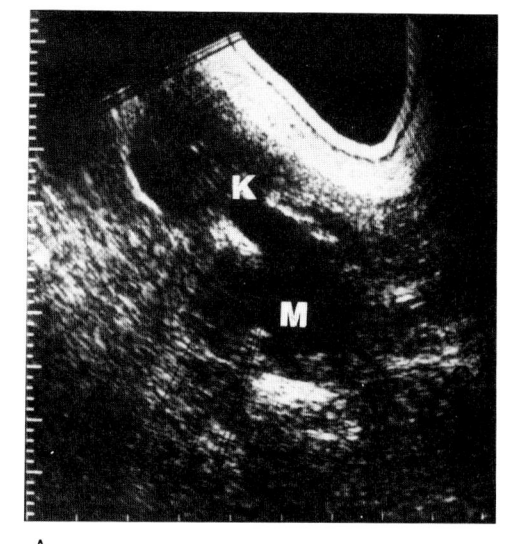

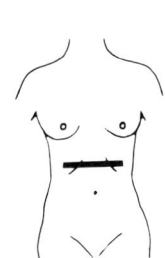

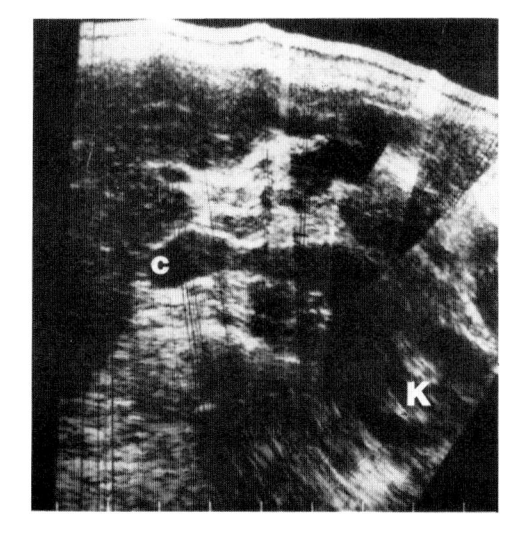

A

B

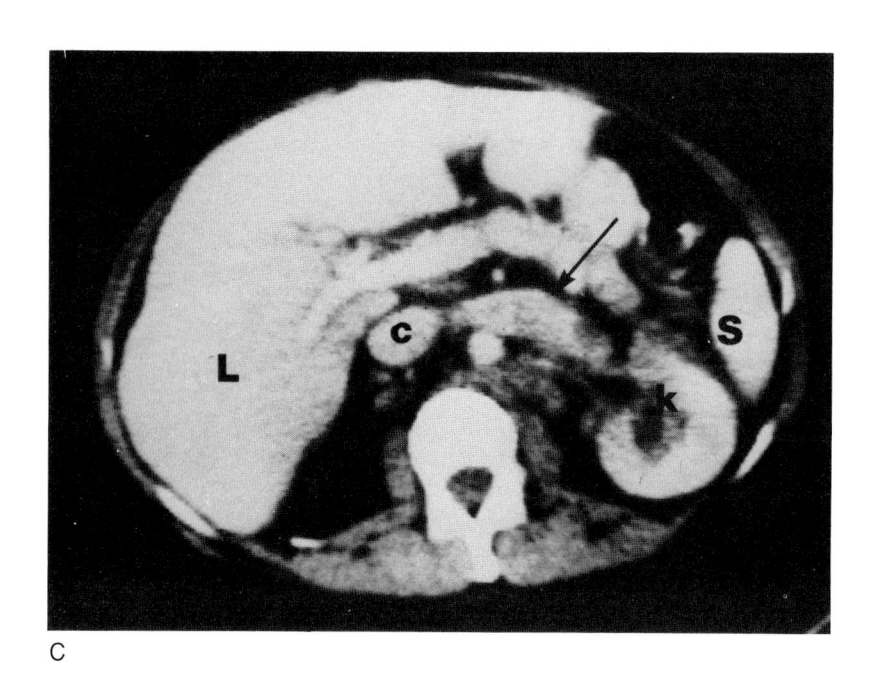

C

12.9 Transitional Cell Carcinoma

An elderly man presented with hematuria and left flank pain. Excretory urography (Fig. A) shows poor excretion of the contrast medium from the left kidney and a suggestion of a filling defect in the collecting system of the left kidney. An incidental right renal cyst is also noted. The sonogram demonstrates invasion of the walls of the renal pelvis by a mass containing low-level echoes (arrowed, Fig. B). A transverse scan through the kidney once again shows the full renal pelvis with an ill-defined solid mass indicated by the cursors in Figure C. Subsequent computed tomography (Fig. D) shows a solid mass as a filling defect within the renal pelvis.

Transitional cell carcinoma is the most common tumor of the renal pelvis. Sonographically, it presents as a mass in the renal pelvis containing low-level echoes. The differential diagnosis for such a mass includes other tumors of the renal pelvis such as squamous cell or adenocarcinoma, which are rare, as well as blood clot (the appearance will change on sequential examinations) and a fungal ball. When the diagnosis is in question, needle aspiration can be performed to obtain specimens for cytologic study or culture. Unlike nephrolithiasis, there is no significant distal acoustic shadow associated with transitional cell carcinoma.

SUGGESTED READINGS

Arger PH, Mulhern CB, Pollack HM, et al: Ultrasonic assessment of renal transitional cell carcinoma: preliminary report. AJR 132:407–411, 1979

Cunningham JJ: Ulreasonic demonstration of renal collecting system invasion by transitional cell cancer. J Clin Ultrasound 10:339–341, 1982

Mulholland SG, Arger PH, Goldberg BB, et al: Ultrasonic differentiation of renal pelvic filling defects. J Urol 122:14–16, 1979

Subramanyam BR, Raghavendra N, Madamba MR: Renal transitional cell carcinoma: sonographic and pathologic correlation. J Clin Ultrasound 10:203–210, 1982

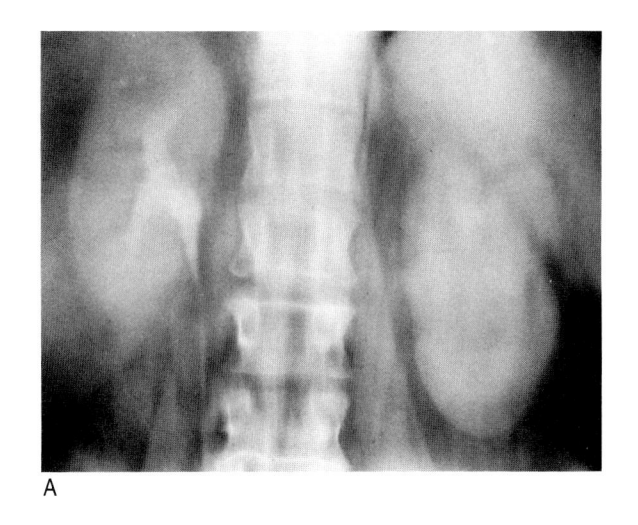

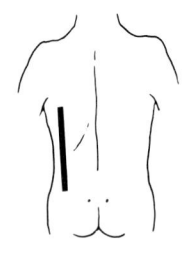

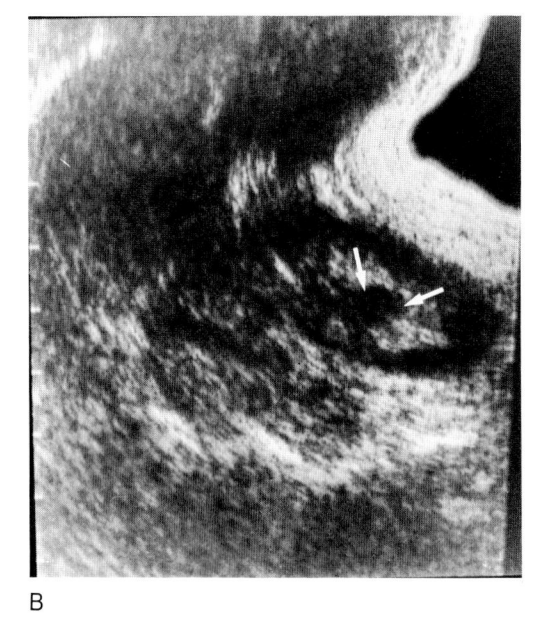

A

B

864

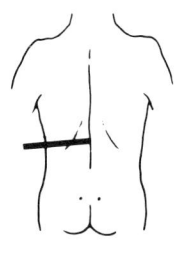

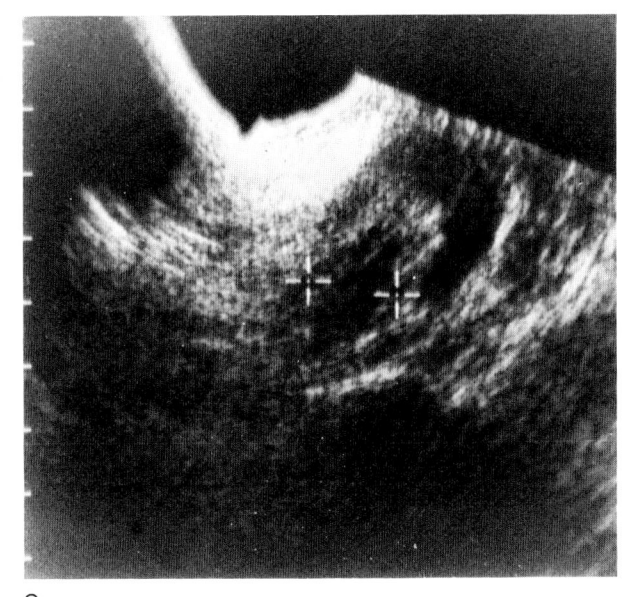

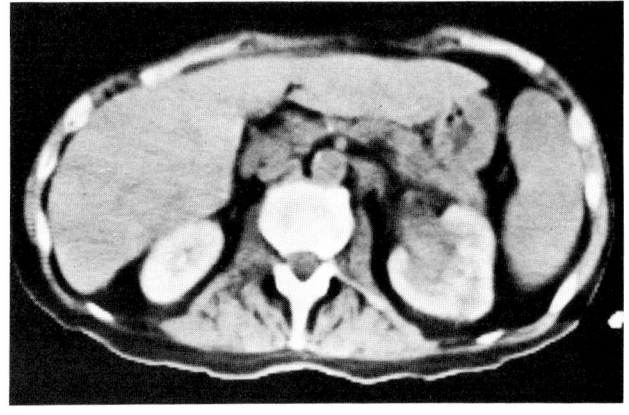

C

D

12.10 Renal Mass: Lymphoma

A 60-year-old man with known lymphoma presented with a nonfunctioning right kidney. The figure is a transverse sonogram with the patient supine, demonstrating that the left kidney is replaced by a mass containing low-level echoes. The typical appearance of lymphoma in any portion of the abdomen is low-level internal echoes, as seen in this case. Lymphoma of the kidney may present with diffuse involvement, as in this instance, or with focal disease. A single lesion may be identified in the region of the kidney, or at times both kidneys may have multiple focal lesions. This pattern on imaging studies may be confused with adult (dominant) polycystic kidney disease.

(Scan from Rosenfield AT, Taylor KJW: Greyscale ultrasound in the imaging of urinary tract disease. Yale J Biol Med 50:335–354, 1977.)

SUGGESTED READINGS

Gregory A, Behan M: Lymphoma of the kidneys: unusual ultrasound appearance due to infiltration of the renal sinus. J Clin Ultrasound 9:343–345, 1981

Heiken JP, Gold RP, Schnur MJ, et al: Computed tomography of renal lymphoma with ultrasound correlation. J Comput Assist Tomography 7:245–250, 1983

Kaude JV, Lacy GD: Ultrasonography in renal lymphoma. J Clin Ultrasound 6:295–382, 1978

Shirkhoda A, Staab EV, Mittelstaedt CA: Renal lymphoma imaged by ultrasound and ^{67}gallium citrate. Radiology 137:175–180, 1980

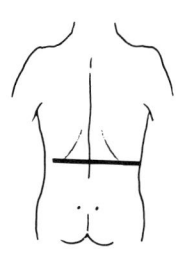

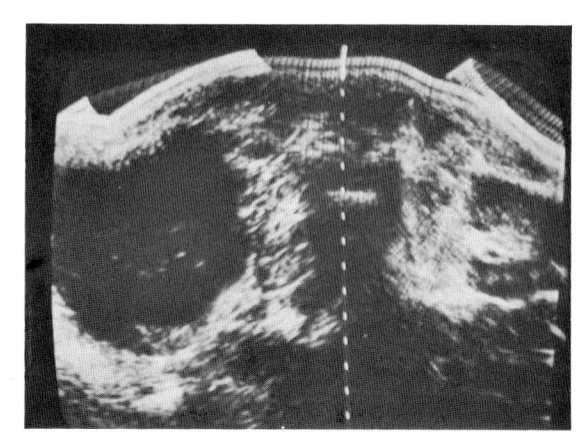

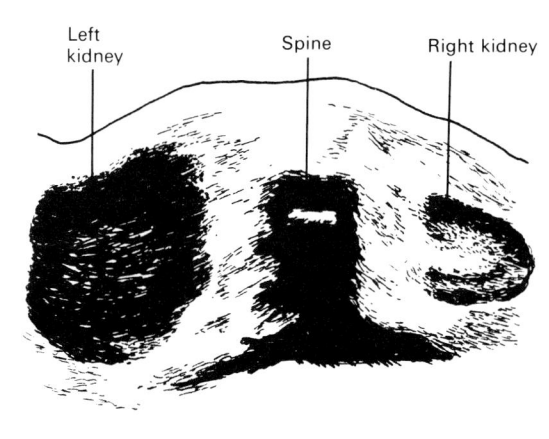

12.11 Wilms' Tumor (Nephroblastoma)

A 3-year-old white boy developed abdominal pain and fever which increased in intensity during the day prior to admission. Because of the presumptive diagnosis of acute appendicitis, an appendectomy was performed. However, fever continued postoperatively.

A sonogram demonstrated a solid mass in the upper portion of the right kidney with some lucency consistent with central necrosis (Fig. A). Subsequent urography (Fig. B) confirmed the presence of this mass (arrow). At surgery, a Wilms' tumor was found.

In a review of a series of patients undergoing ultrasound study of Wilms' tumors these tumors were large, predominantly solid, and well circumscribed. They show variable echogenicity ranging from less than that of the kidney to greater than that of the liver. Small anechoic areas may be seen within the masses, representing necrosis. Calcification may be seen in Wilms' tumor though it is much less common than in neuroblastoma. A solid intrarenal mass in children is presumed to be a Wilms' tumor until proven otherwise. Nephroblastomatosis consisting of small nodules or sheets of primitive metanephric epithelium is present in 1:200–400 autopsy specimens from infants younger than 4 months. These nodules, when they persist, may be precursors for a Wilms' tumor. Although the nodules of nephroblastomatosis may occasionally be large, most of them are quite small, and in our experience are difficult to identify sonographically.

SUGGESTED READINGS

Bowen A, Dominguez R, Young LW: Diagnostic ultrasound. Current pediatric applications. Am J Dis Child 135:954–964, 1981

Jaffe MH, White SJ, Silver TM, et al: Wilms' tumor: Ultrasonic features, pathologic correlation, and diagnostic pitfalls. Radiology 140:147–152, 1981

Rosenfield NS, Shimkin P, Berdon W, et al: Wilms' tumor arising from spontaneously regressing nephroblastomatosis. AJR 135:381–384, 1980

Slovis TL, Perlmutter AD: Recent advances in pediatric urological ultrasound. J Urol 123:613–620, 1980

Teele RL: Ultrasonography of the genitourinary tract in children. Radiol Clin North Am 15:109–128, 1977

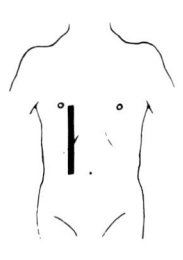

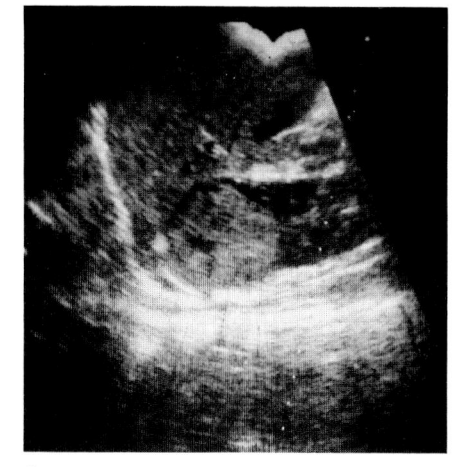

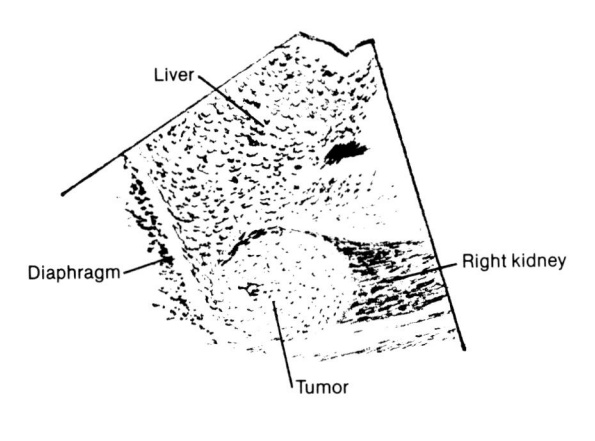

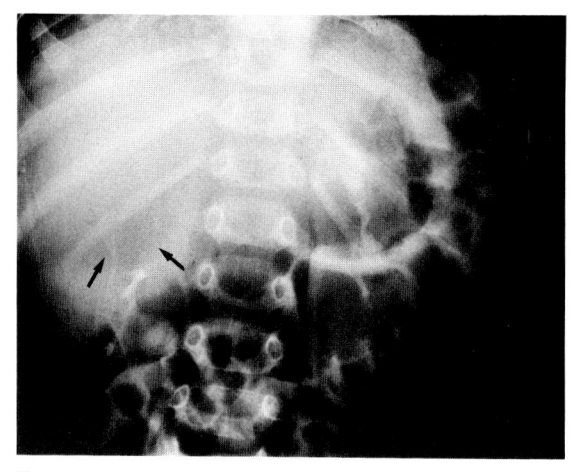

A

B

12.12 Angiomyolipoma

A 30-year-old woman presented with hematuria. Investigation disclosed multiple masses in both kidneys. A longitudinal scan of the right kidney (Fig. A) demonstrated several highly reflective masses. A transverse sonogram confirmed this (Fig. B). Computed tomography (Fig. C) demonstrated low attenuation masses indicating the presence of fat typically seen in angiomyolipomas.

CT is the technique of choice to verify the diagnosis of angiomyolipoma. A highly reflective renal mass on ultrasonography is strongly suggestive of an angiomyolipoma. If there is evidence for slow propagation of sound within the mass, this is characteristic of a fatty lesion. Similarly, the demonstration of fat within the lesion on the CT scan is characteristic. However, some angiomyolipomas do not contain significant amounts of fat and are not echogenic.

Angiomyolipomas of the kidney are commonly found in young patients with tuberous sclerosis, in which case they are frequently multiple. Solitary angiomyolipomas have a higher incidence in middle-aged women. More recently, small angiomyolipomas of the kidney have been described as incidental findings at sonography and CT. In the pathology literature, small nodules of tissue in the renal parenchyma containing adipose tissue and smooth muscle are present in approximately 11 percent of kidneys.

SUGGESTED READINGS

Bosniak MA: Angiomyolipoma (hamartoma of the kidney): a preoperative diagnosis is possible in virtually every case. Urol Radiol 3:135–142, 1981

Hartman DS, Goldman SM, Friedman AC, et al: Angiomyolipoma: ultrasonic–pathologic correlation. Radiology 139:451–458, 1981

Lee TG, Henderson SC, Freeny PC, et al: Ultrasound findings of renal angiomyolipoma. J Clin Ultrasound 6:150–155, 1977

Raghavendra BN, Bosniak MA, Megibow AJ: Small angiomyolipoma of the kidney: sonographic CT evaluation. AJR 141:575–578, 1983

Scheible W, Ellenbogen PH, Leopold GR, et al: Lipomatous tumors of the kidney and adrenal: apparent echogenic specificity. Radiology 129:153–156, 1978

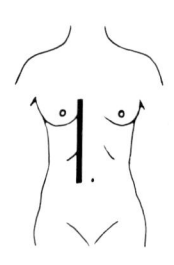

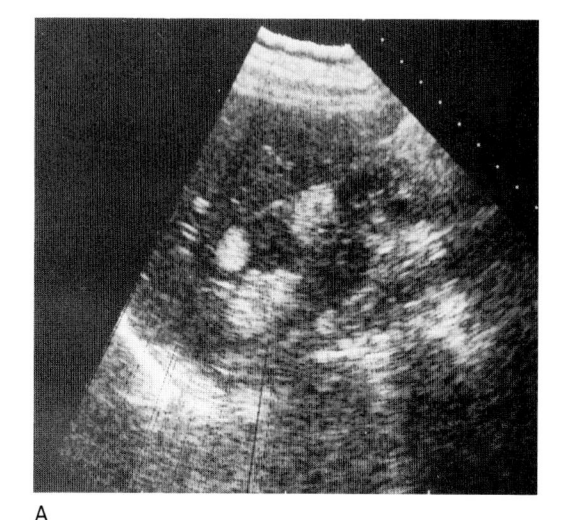

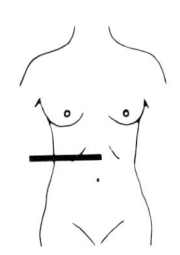

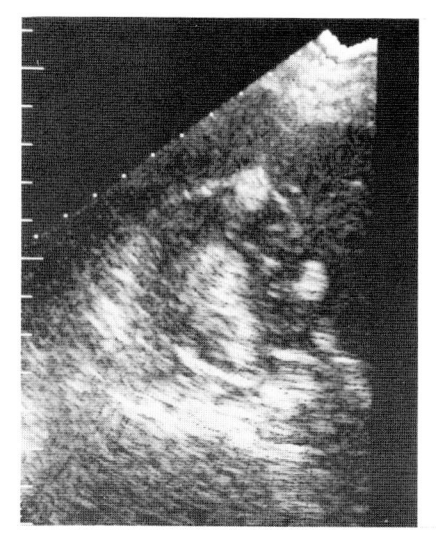

A

B

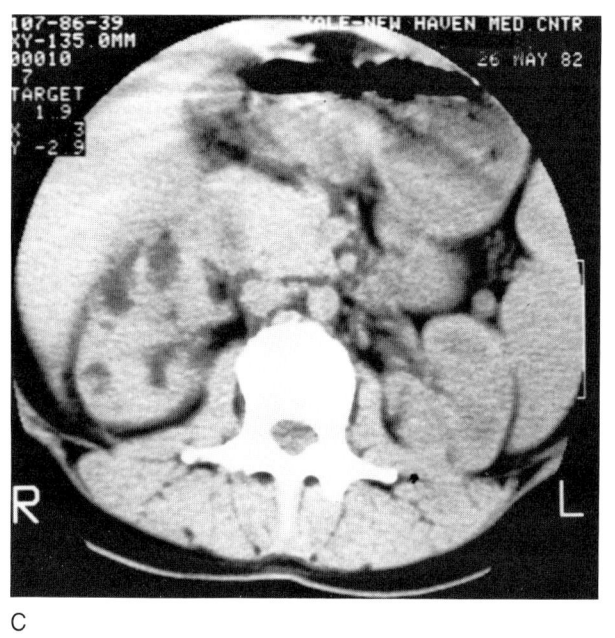

C

12.13 Hydatid Cyst

A 32-year-old Israeli man had undergone a right nephrectomy because of traumatic injury 6 months prior to admission. He presented with fever and a mass in the right renal fossa. A longitudinal sonogram through the right upper quadrant demonstrates a mass composed of multiple cystic structures. At surgery, this was found to be an echinococcal cyst with blood within it.

Hydatid cysts result from human infection by either *Echinococcus granulosis* or *Echinococcus multilocularis* sheep tapeworms. Cysts are typically multilocular, may calcify, and can appear in several organs including the liver, lung, and kidney.

(Case and figure courtesy of Dr. Yackov Itzchak, Dept. Radiology, Chaim-Sheba Medical School, Tel-Hashomer, Israel.)

SUGGESTED READINGS

Hadidi A: Ultrasound findings in liver hydatid cysts. J Clin Ultrasound 7:365–368, 1979

Itzchak Y, Rubinstein Z, Heyman Z, et al: Role of ultrasound in the diagnosis of abdominal hydatid disease. J Clin Ultrasound 8:341–345, 1980

Itzchak Y, Rubinstein Z, Shilo R: Ultrasound in tropical diseases. pp. 69–93. In Sanders RC, Hill M (eds): Ultrasound Annual, 1983. Raven Press, New York, 1983

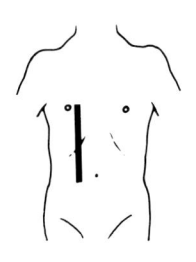

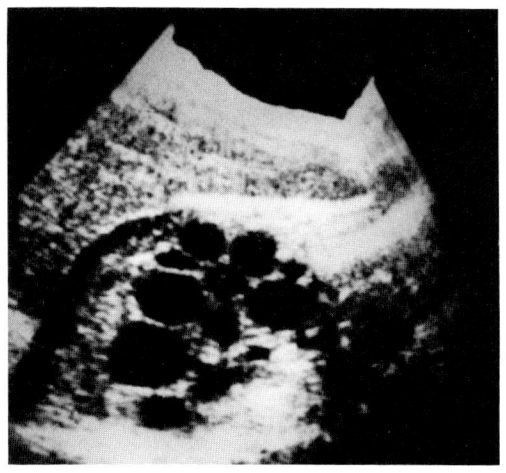

Renal Infection (12.14 and 12.15)

12.14 Acute Pyelonephritis

A middle-aged diabetic patient presented with fever, left flank pain, and pyuria. Longitudinal sonograms of the left (Fig. A) and right (Fig. B) kidneys show the left kidney to be significantly larger than the right with global decrease in echogenicity and loss of corticomedullary definition. The differential diagnosis for this pattern when seen in a patient with acute symtoms includes acute pyelonephritis, acute renal vein thrombosis, or renal infarction secondary to arterial occlusion. The patient's history is typical of acute pyelonephritis and *E. coli* was subsequently cultured from the urine. Following appropriate therapy, the patient's symptoms resolved.

(Figs. A & B from Gonzalez-Gomez R, Richman AH, Taylor KJW, et al: Urinary tract ultrasonography. pp. 29–52. In Finberg HJ, (ed): Case Studies in Diagnostic Ultrasound. Clinics in Diagnostic Ultrasound, vol 9. Churchill Livingstone, New York, 1981.)

SUGGESTED READINGS

Edell SL, Bonavita JA: The sonographic appearance of acute pyelonephritis. Radiology 132:683–685, 1979

Gonzalez-Gomez R. Richman AH, Taylor KJW, et al: Urinary tract ultrasonography. pp. 29–52. In Finberg HJ (ed): Case Studies in Diagnostic Ultrasound. Clinics in Diagnostic Ultrasound, vol 9. Churchill Livingstone, New York, 1981

Rosenfield AT, Glickman MG, Taylor KJW: Focal bacterial nephritis (acute lobar nephronia). Radiology 132:553–561, 1979.

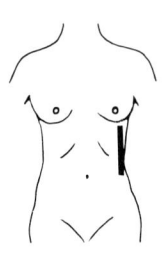

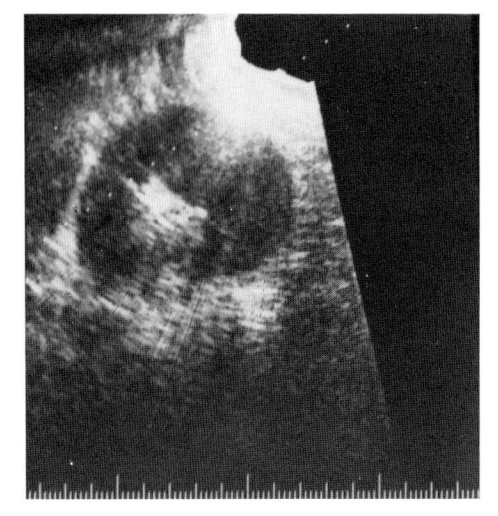

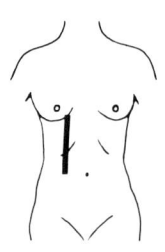

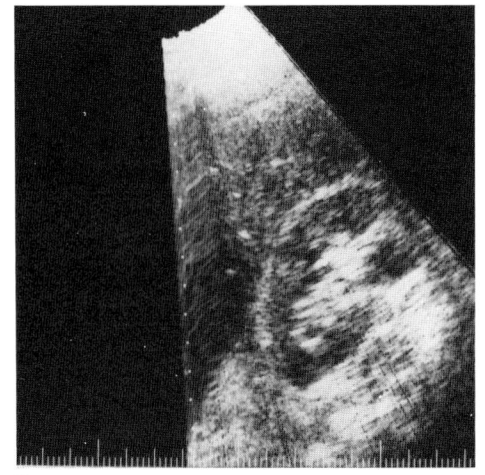

A

B

12.15 Acute Focal Bacterial Nephritis (Acute Lobar Nephronia)

A 60-year-old woman with a history of several previous urinary tract infections presented with fever and right flank pain. The sonogram (Fig. A) performed at admission shows a mass (arrowed) in the lateral aspect of the right kidney extending posteriorly, which has lower echogenicity than the contiguous renal cortex. A ^{67}gallium scan demonstrated areas of abnormal gallium activity in the region of the right kidney (arrowed, Fig. B). The patient was treated conservatively with antibiotics, resulting in cessation of symptoms. Two weeks later, urography and ultrasonography showed resolution of the mass. Normal cortex, corticomedullary definition, and cortical echogenicity in the region of the previous mass were found (Fig. C).

These findings are typical of acute focal bacterial nephritis (acute lobar nephronia). The entity consists of focal infection without liquefaction and leads to a mass which can mimic either a tumor or an abscess on imaging studies. The 45 cases of acute lobar nephronia we have studied all had an echogenicity equal to or less than the adjacent renal parenchyma although we have observed exceptions to this rule. If the echogenicity in the renal mass is greater than normal parenchyma in a patient with symptoms of renal infection, the lesion is either an abscess or a renal tumor (with signs and symptoms of infection due to another cause).

Coordinated imaging in acute focal bacterial nephritis frequently permits the correct diagnosis based on these findings:

1. A focal mass with echogenicity equal to or less than that of the normal renal parenchyma
2. Abnormal ^{67}gallium activity within the mass (there frequently may be abnormal gallium activity in the remainder of the ipsilateral kidney or in the contralateral kidney as well)
3. A solid mass on some imaging studies such as excretory urography or computed tomography

The mass on nephrotomography or CT generally has a decreased nephrographic pattern but, unlike a simple renal cyst or an abscess, it is not composed of a well-defined rounded lucent zone in the kidney. Recently, two basic CT patterns have been described. One is a triangular defect in the nephrogram on the CT scan which is probably the most common finding in acute focal bacterial nephritis. The other is a solid mass with multiple low-attenuation nephrographic defects. The latter appearance is more common in diabetic patients.

Sonography is a valuable initial screening technique to evaluate patients with fever and flank pain. An abscess, whether intrarenal or perinephric, can be identified and hydronephrosis, pyelonephrosis, or nephrolithiasis may also be diagnosed. If the findings are typical of acute focal bacterial nephritis, the patient should be treated with appropriate antibiotics and the studies repeated to verify that the mass has resolved. This is important since other entities, particularly lymphoma, might present with similar imaging findings.

Angiographic findings in acute focal bacterial nephritis may be confusing. The arteriogram typically shows displaced vessels throughout the mass. However, the venogram shows irregular tortuous vessels within the mass which may mimic malignancy. The abnormality is also more extensive on the epinephrine venogram than on the arteriogram.

SUGGESTED READINGS

Lee JKL, McClellan BL, Melson GL, et al: Acute focal bacterial nephritis: emphasis on gray scale sonography and computed tomography. AJR 135:87–92, 1980

Rauschkolb EN, Sandler CM, Patel S, et al: Computed tomography of renal inflammatory disease. J Comput Assist Tomogr 6:502–506, 1982

Rosenfield AT, Glickman MC, Taylor KJW, et al: Acute focal bacterial nephritis (acute lobar nephronia). Radiology 132:552–561, 1979

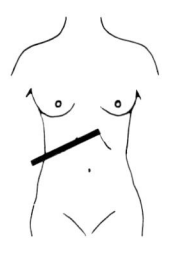

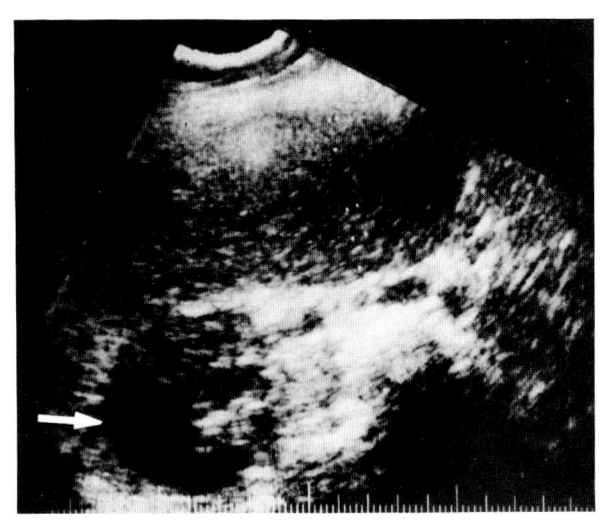

A

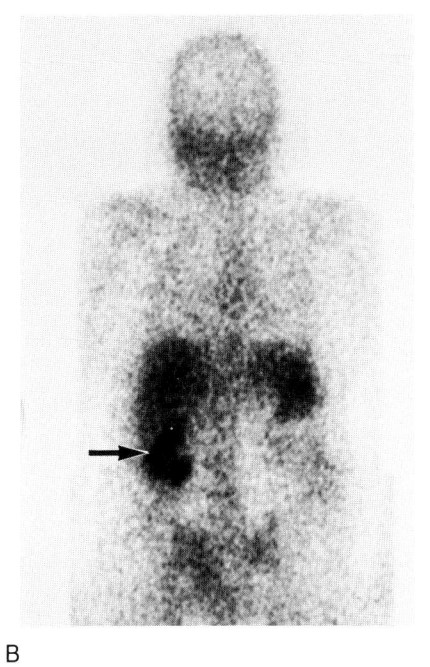

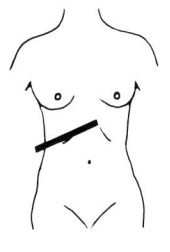

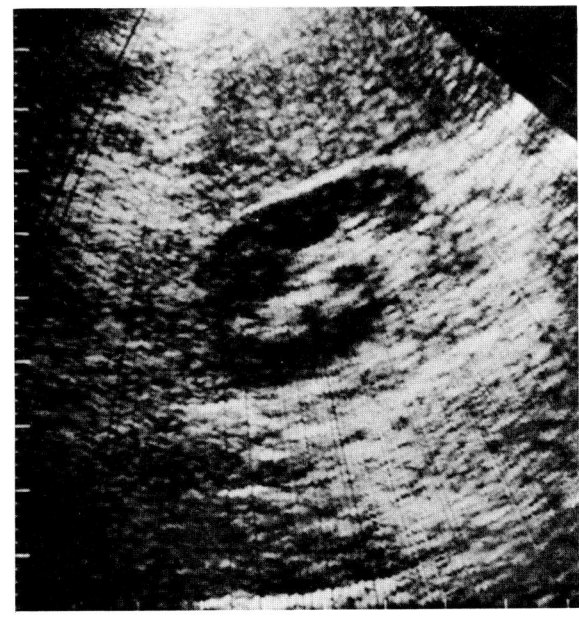

B

C

Renal Cystic Disease (12.16 to 12.20)

12.16 Adult (Dominant) Polycystic Disease

A 55-year-old man with known adult (dominant) polycystic kidney disease (APKD) was admitted with epigastric pain. Ultrasound examination through the right kidney (Fig. A) demonstrated multiple cysts in the right kidney and liver. A coronal scan through the left kidney (Fig. B) demonstrated multiple cysts in the left kidney. Note the considerable irregularity of the cyst walls; this does not conflict with the diagnosis of APKD.

Dominant APKD is characterized by nephromegaly and bilateral renal cystic disease. Hepatic cysts occur in at least one-third of patients in most series. Cysts may be seen in other organs as well, including the spleen and pancreas. Ultrasound can be used to identify the cysts in APKD in both the kidneys and other organs. In addition, ultrasonography can be used to evaluate patients with known APKD and fever to search for an infected cyst. The infected cyst, whether in the kidney or other abdominal organ, generally has internal echoes and may have a debris/fluid level. Aspiration of this cyst under ultrasound guidance can be performed to confirm the diagnosis. Drainage of the lesion may also be performed percutaneously under ultrasound guidance. Ultrasonography is the technique of choice to evaluate the patient in renal failure for evidence of APKD, although computed tomography is also capable of identifying the pathologic changes.

APKD is a genetic disease inherited as an autosomal dominant trait. The disease typically leads to progressive renal failure but usually does not present with symptoms until middle age. Our initial experience with 36 presymptomatic children indicated that cysts from adult polycystic kidney disease appear in childhood prior to the development of symptoms. Our work also indicated that ultrasound alone is sufficient to screen asymptomatic progeny for APKD. Subsequent work using multiple modalities for screening suggests that if a cyst has not appeared by age 19, it is extremely unlikely that the patient is affected. Thus, ultrasound can be used for genetic counseling. These longitudinal studies are showing the natural history of adult polycystic kidney disease.

SUGGESTED READING

Kelsey JA, Bowie JD: Gray-scale ultrasonography in the diagnosis of polycystic kidney disease. Radiology 122:791–795, 1977

Lawson TL, McClennan BL, Shirkhoda A: Adult polycystic kidney disease: ultrasonographic and computed tomographic appearance. J Clin Ultrasound 6:297–302, 1978

Lufkin EG, Alfrey AC, Trucksess ME, et al: Polycystic kidney disease: earlier diagnosis using ultrasound. Urology 4:5–12, 1974

Milutinovic J, Philips LA, Bryant JI, et al: Autosomal dominant polycystic kidney disease: early diagnosis and data for genetic counselling. Lancet 1:1203–1205, 1980

Ralls PW, Esensten ML, Boger D, et al: Severe hydronephrosis and severe renal cystic disease: Ultrasonic differentiation. AJR 134:473–475, 1980

Rosenfield AT, Curtis A McB, Putman CE, et al: Gray scale ultrasonography, computerized tomography, and nephrotomography in evaluation of polycystic kidney and liver disease. Urology 9:436–438, 1977

Rosenfield AT, Lipson MH, Wolf B, et al: Ultrasonography and nephrotomography in the presymptomatic diagnosis of dominantly inherited (adult-onset) polycystic kidney disease. Radiology 135:423–427, 1980

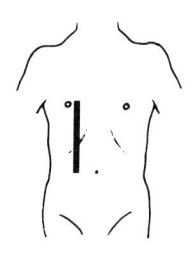

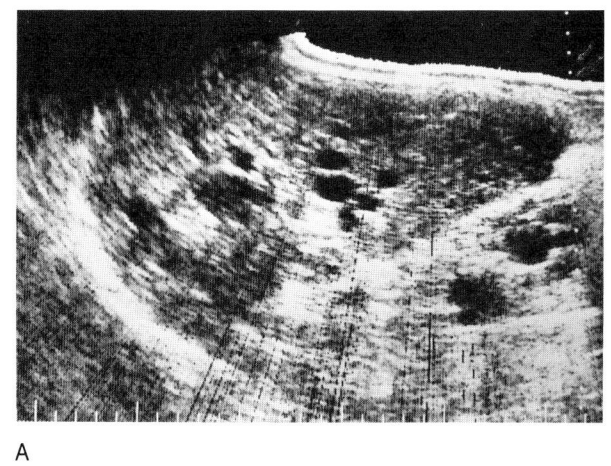

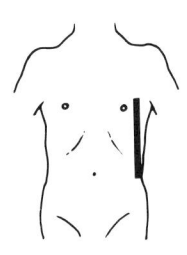

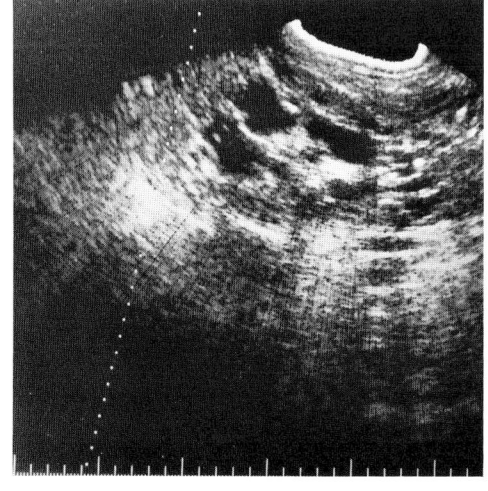

A

B

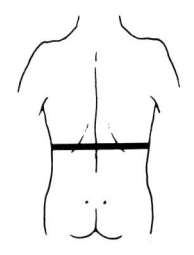

12.17 Medullary Cystic Disease

A 19-year-old man presented in chronic renal failure. Figures A and B are transverse scans of the right and left kidneys, respectively, with the patient prone. Multiple cysts (c) are noted at the corticomedullary junction and do not significantly alter the outline of the kidneys. The scan showed other similar renal cysts. There was no evidence of cysts in the liver, spleen, or pancreas. The finding of medullary and corticomedullary cysts in small kidneys in a young adult is typical of medullary cystic disease.

Medullary cystic disease is inherited as an autosomal recessive trait. Patients with this disease typically present as young adults with renal failure. By the time of presentation, renal function is frequently very poor, since the typical associated findings such as hypertension and proteinuria are not present in this entity. Nephropathy, however, is a prominent feature of this disease. Ultrasonography is a safe technique for identifying medullary and corticomedullary cysts in small kidneys, permitting the correct diagnosis. Although nephrotomography can sometimes demonstrate the renal cysts, this study is often equivocal due to poor renal function. Sonography is far more desirable for this purpose.

SUGGESTED READING

Rosenfield AT, Siegel NJ, Kappelman NB, et al: Gray scale ultrasonography in medullary cystic disease of the kidney and congenital hepatic fibrosis with tubular ectasia: new observations. Am J Roentgenol 129:297–303, 1977

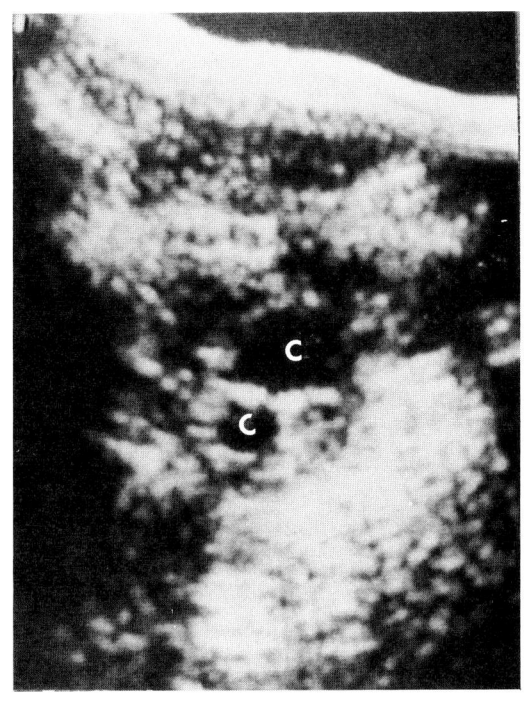

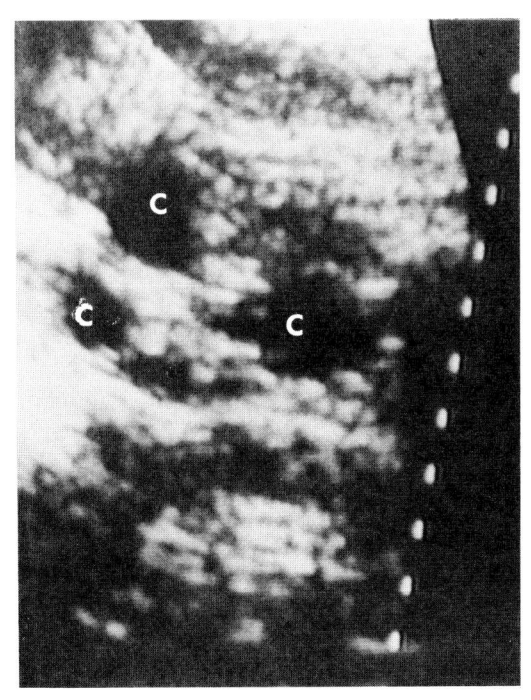

A

B

12.18 Congenital Hepatic Fibrosis with Tubular Ectasia

A 4-year-old child presented with nephromegaly. A longitudinal scan through the right kidney (Fig. A) with the patient prone shows an enlarged kidney (arrowed). There is a generalized increase in parenchymal echogenicity causing the loss of demarcation between the renal sinus and adjacent structures. However, there is a thin rim of decreased echogenicity peripherally. A longitudinal section through the right upper quadrant (Fig. B) shows increased parenchymal echoes in the liver (L) consistent with diffuse hepatocellular disease. The gallbladder (GB) is seen. The right kidney (K) is seen in this scan. The left kidney showed similar findings.

The findings in this patient are typical of those in renal tubular ectasia. This pattern consists of increased echogenicity of the kidney, frequently with loss of distinction between renal parenchyma and renal sinus, and a rim of less echogenic tissue in the periphery of the cortex. The entities presenting with renal tubular ectasia include congenital hepatic fibrosis with tubular ectasia, infantile polycystic kidney disease, and isolated renal tubular ectasia. The high-level echoes in the liver are consistent with hepatic fibrosis. This patient had no evidence of renal failure, making the likely diagnosis congenital hepatic fibrosis with tubular ectasia.

Progressive hepatic fibrosis occurs in congenital hepatic fibrosis with tubular ectasia. The associated renal tubular ectasia, although it may be dramatic on imaging studies, does not generally lead to renal failure. Patients' prognoses are dependent on the extent of the liver disease. Portal hypertension frequently develops and must be treated with shunting. There is controversy in the literature as to whether congenital hepatic fibrosis with tubular ectasia is a variant of infantile polycystic kidney disease or an entirely different entity.

SUGGESTED READING

Rosenfield AT, Siegel NJ, Kappelman NB, et al: Gray scale ultrasound in medullary cystic disease of the kidney and congenital hepatic fibrosis with tubular ectasia: new observations. Am J Roentgenol 129:297–303, 1977

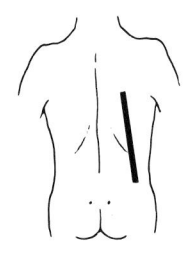

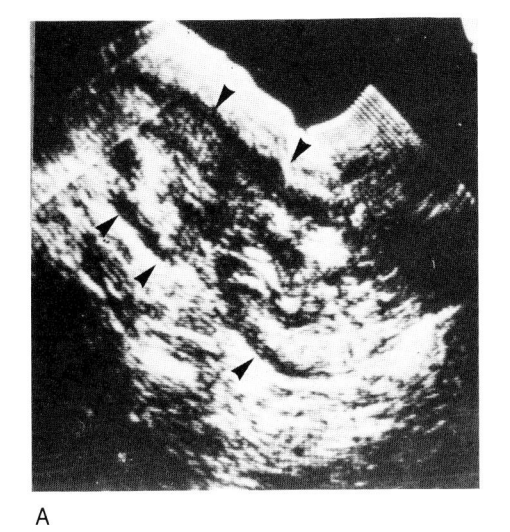

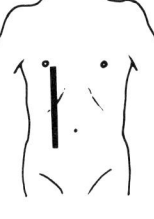

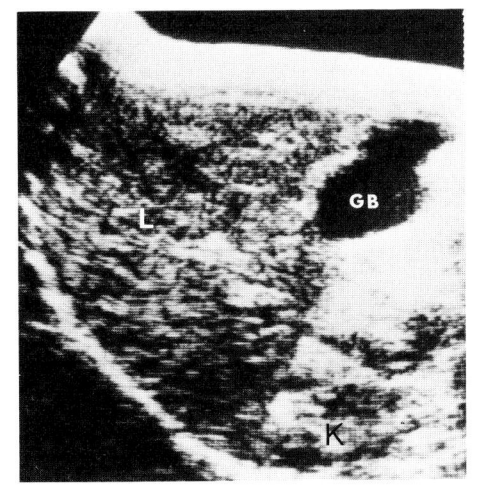

A

B

12.19 Infantile Polycystic Disease

A longitudinal scan through the gravid uterus demonstrates two abnormally large kidneys with the aorta between them. Note that the echo pattern of the kidneys is diffusely increased echogenicity with loss of corticomedullary definition but with a thin rim of decreased echoes at the periphery. These findings are typical of renal tubular ectasia. The patient's mother had had a previous child with infantile polycystic kidney disease and this diagnosis was made in utero.

Infantile polycystic kidney disease (IPKD) is inherited as an autosomal recessive trait. Thus, patients who have one child with this condition have a 25 percent chance of having another child with this disease, which is generally fatal. Ultrasound allows prenatal diagnosis. The circumference of the kidneys in the normal fetus is between 27 and 30 percent of the abdominal circumference. In the fetus with IPKD, this ratio is usually more than twice normal. The abnormal parenchymal pattern is also seen.

Very small cysts are present in IPKD. They are too small to be seen using current diagnostic ultrasound equipment. Therefore, individual cysts are generally not seen in the kidney, although they may occasionally be. Hepatic cysts and fibrosis may both be seen in IPKD, so the liver should also be carefully examined. As with the renal tubular ectasias in general, two basic parenchymal patterns may be seen in the kidneys. The common pattern is one of increased parenchymal echogenicity, loss of corticomedullary definition, and loss of demarcation between the renal sinus and the parenchyma, but well-defined cysts may be seen. A less common pattern is increased echoes in the pyramids of the kidney.

SUGGESTED READINGS

Boal DK, Teele RL: Sonography of infantile polycystic kidney disease. AJR 135:575–580, 1980

Habif DV, Berdon WE, Yeh MN: Infantile polycystic kidney disease: in utero sonographic diagnosis. Radiology 142:475–477, 1982

Rosenfield AT, Hobbins JC, Taylor KJW, et al: Renal ultrasound. pp. 21–50. In Rosenfield AT, Glickman MG, Hodson J (eds): Diagnostic Imaging in Renal Disease. Appleton-Century Crofts, New York, 1979

Stapleton FB, Magill HL, Kelly DR: Infantile polycystic kidney disease: an imaging dilemma. Urol Radiol 5:89–94, 1983

Thomas JL, Sumner TE, Crowe JE: Neonatal detection and evaluation of infantile polycystic disease by gray scale echography. J Clin Ultrasound 6:343–344, 1978

Common iliac arteries

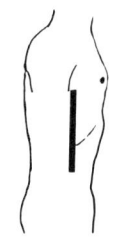

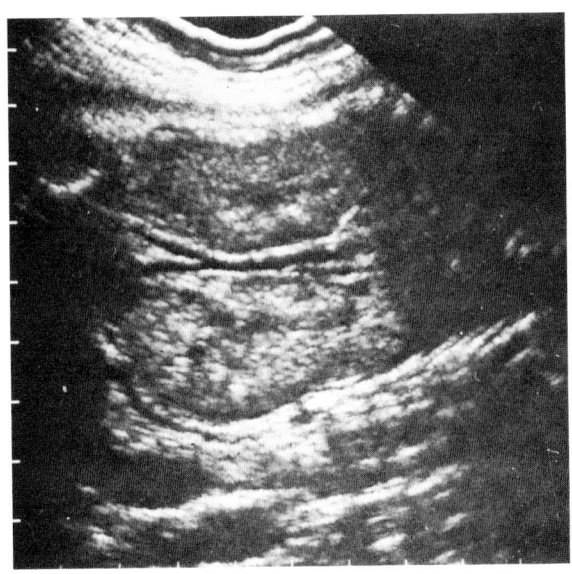

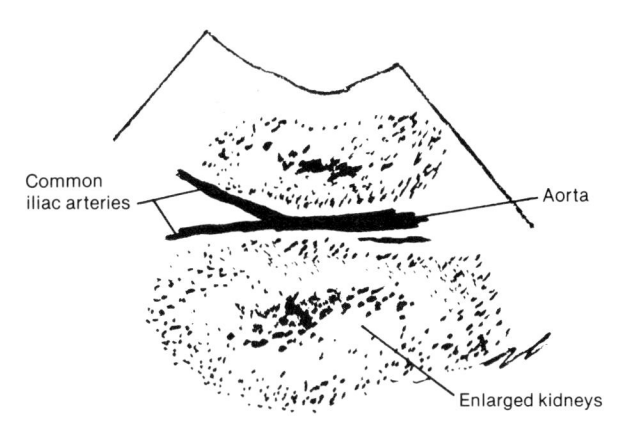

Aorta

Enlarged kidneys

12.20 Multicystic Dysplastic Kidney

A newborn infant presented with a palpable right-sided renal mass. Sonography showed that the mass consisted of multiple cysts and solid tissue. A longitudinal scan is shown in the figure. Radioisotope scans showed no flow to the affected kidney. At surgery, a multicystic dysplastic kidney was found. The contralateral kidney was normal.

Multicystic dysplastic kidney is a congenital abnormality. Although this dysplasia does not have a definite cause, there has been speculation that it is related to pelvoinfundibular atresia in utero. Typically, no identifiable pelvis or collecting system is seen. The renal artery and ipsilateral ureter may be atretic. There is also an association with hydronephrosis due to ureteropelvic junction obstruction in the contralateral kidney. Multicystic dysplastic kidney is one of the two most common causes of a palpable renal mass in the neonate, the other being congenital hydronephrosis.

The ultrasound appearance of unilateral multicystic dysplastic kidney is multiple cysts separated by linear echoes or solid tissue. Although a pelvis is not identified in the common variety, a hydropelvis may be present when a lesion is the "hydronephrotic" form of multicystic dysplastic kidney, atresia of the ureter being the main lesion.

SUGGESTED READINGS

Bearman SB, Hine PL, Sanders RC: Multicystic kidney: a sonographic pattern. Radiology 118:685–688, 1976

Felson B, Cussen LJ: The hydronephrotic type of unilateral congenital multicystic disease of the kidney. Semin Roentgenol 10:113, 1975

Griscom NT, Vawter GF, Fellers FX: Pelvo infundibular atresia: the usual form of multicystic kidney: 44 unilateral and two bilateral cases. Semin Roentgenol 10:125, 1975

Summer T, Friedland GW, Parker B: Preoperative diagnosis of unilateral multicystic kidney with hydropelvis. Urology 11:521–522, 1978

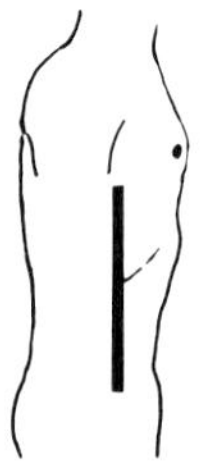

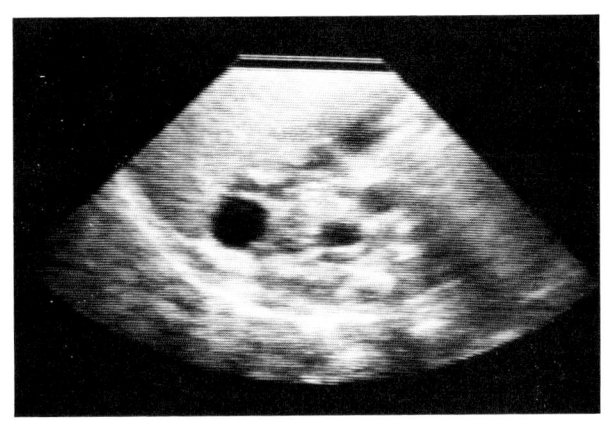

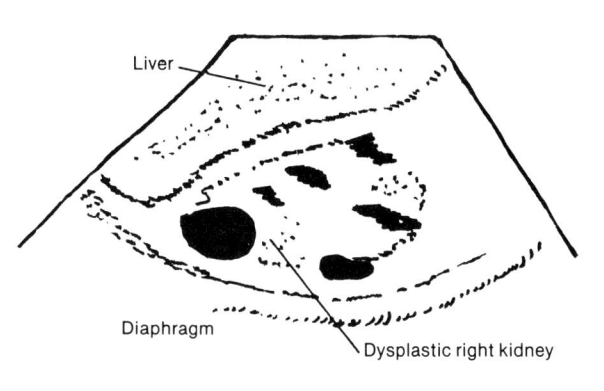

Liver

Diaphragm

Dysplastic right kidney

The Bladder (12.21 to 12.27)

12.21 Anatomy

To be visualized within the pelvis, the normal bladder must be at least partially filled. A longitudinal scan through the pelvis of a man demonstrates a fluid-filled bladder as an echo-free mass within the pelvis (Fig. A). The prostate can be demonstrated as a solid mass (arrowed) about 2.5 cm in diameter below the bladder neck. Note the echogenic linear central zone representing the urethra and periurethral glands. Figure B is a transverse scan of the same patient. Once again note that, except for reverberation artifact, the bladder is echo-free. The prostate is a rounded mass.

At normal gain, urine is echo-free. Internal echoes may be seen in the anterior portion of the bladder due to the reverberation artifact (arrowed, Fig. C). When debris is seen lying in the posterior portion of the bladder, purulent cystitis should be considered (Fig. D).

(Fig. D from Morley P: The bladder. p. 147. In Rosenfield AT (ed): Genitourinary Ultrasonography. Clinics in Diagnostic Ultrasound, vol 2. Churchill Livingstone, New York, 1979.)

SUGGESTED READING

Morley P: The bladder. p. 147. In Rosenfield AT ed: Genitourinary Ultrasonography. Clinics in Diagnostic Ultrasound, vol. 2. Churchill Livingstone, New York, 1979

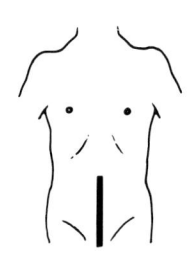

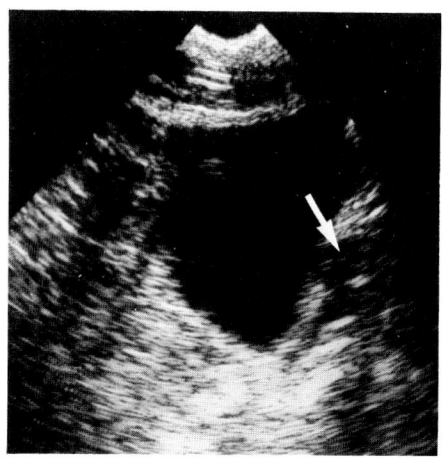

A

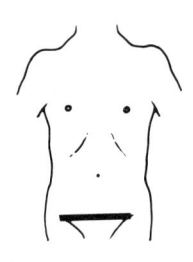

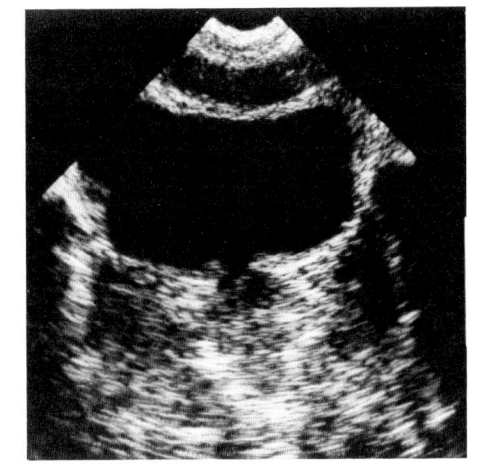

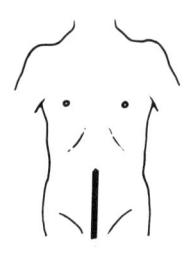

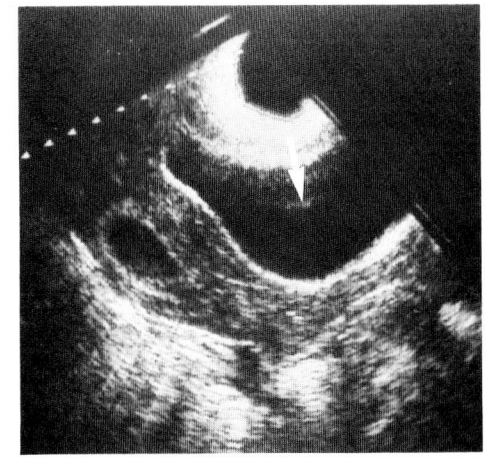

B

C

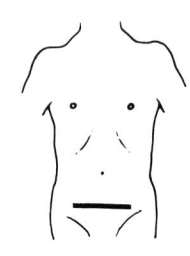

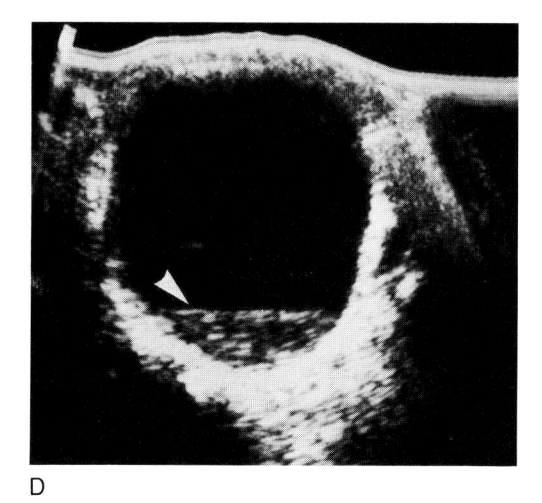

D

890

12.22 Cytoxan (Cyclophosphamide) Cystitis

Ultrasound examination was performed on an 8-year-old boy with Burkitt's lymphoma whose therapy included cyclophosphamide. A longitudinal scan (Fig. A) and the transverse scan (Fig. B) demonstrate mucosal thickening; the bladder mucosa measured 9 mm at its maximum diameter. The upper limits of normal for the mucosa of the bladder is 2 mm. In view of the history, these findings are typical of Cytoxan cystitis. Cystitis due to other causes, including infections secondary to gram-negative bacteria, tuberculosis, schistosomiasis, or radiation can lead to a similar phenomenon.

Development of sterile hemorrhagic cystitis in patients receiving Cytoxan therapy is a well-recognized occurrence. Early in the course of therapy (within 48 hours) hemorrhagic cystitis may ensue which is reversible with cessation of therapy. A second chronic form may also occur approximately 3 months following cessation of therapy in which there is a fibrotic reaction in the bladder. This form is not reversible. However, there is significant overlap between these two forms. Cytoxan cystitis is believed to be due to the effect of the metabolities of cyclophosphamide in the urine on the wall of the bladder.

SUGGESTED READING

Renert WA, Berdon WE, Baker DH: Hemorrhagic cystitis and vesicoureteral reflux secondary to cytotoxic therapy for childhood malignancies. Am J Roentgenol 117:664–668, 1973

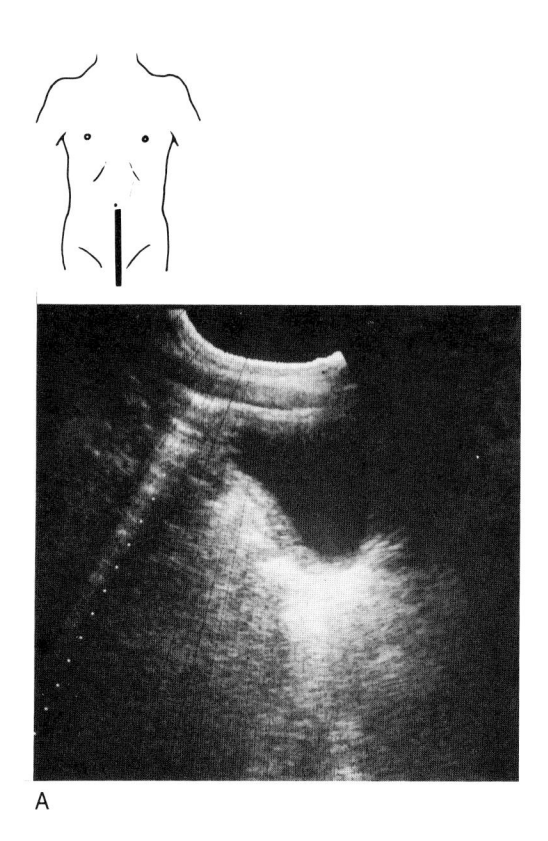

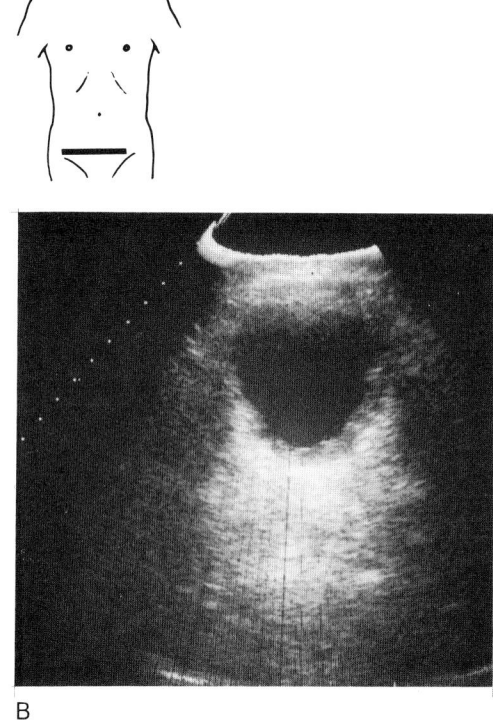

A

B

12.23 Duplication

A 25-year-old pregnant woman was referred for ultrasound evaluation of gestational maturity. A transverse sonogram scan reveals a duplicated bladder (B), as well as a double uterus (U), cervix, and vagina. Review of the patient's medical record indicated that the patient had multiple congenital anomalies. In addition to those mentioned above, the patient had two clitori and two urethrae. The kidneys and ureters, as well as the fallopian tubes and ovaries, were normal in number. A transverse scan demonstrated the duplicated, noncommunicating bladders.

Complete reduplication of the urinary bladder is rare: only 40 cases have been reported in the surgical literature. The pattern of complete reduplication seen here consists of two separate bladders, each with its own mucosa and muscularis, lying side by side, separated by a peritoneal fold. Each bladder receives an ipsilateral ureter and empties into a separate urethra through its own external meatus. Common associations include reduplication of the genital and gastrointestinal systems and, less commonly, reduplication or fusion of the lower spine. Anorectal atresia, stenosis, ectopia, and other abnormalities of cloacal development frequently occur. Anomalies of the upper urinary tract may occur. Complete reduplication of the bladder alone is usually asymptomatic. However, in association with other congenital anomalies, complications may occur.

(Figure from Richman TS, Taylor KJW: Sonographic demonstration of bladder duplication. AJR 139:604–605, 1982. ©1982 Am Roentgen Ray Soc.)

SUGGESTED READINGS

Abrahamson J: Double bladder and related anomalies: clinical and embryological aspects and a case report. Br J Urol 33:195–212, 1961

Esham W, Holt H: Complete duplication of bladder and urethra: a case report. J Urol 123:773–775, 1980

Richman TS, Taylor KJW: Sonographic demonstration of bladder duplication. AJR 139:604–605, 1982

894

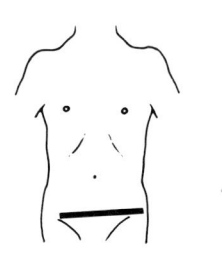

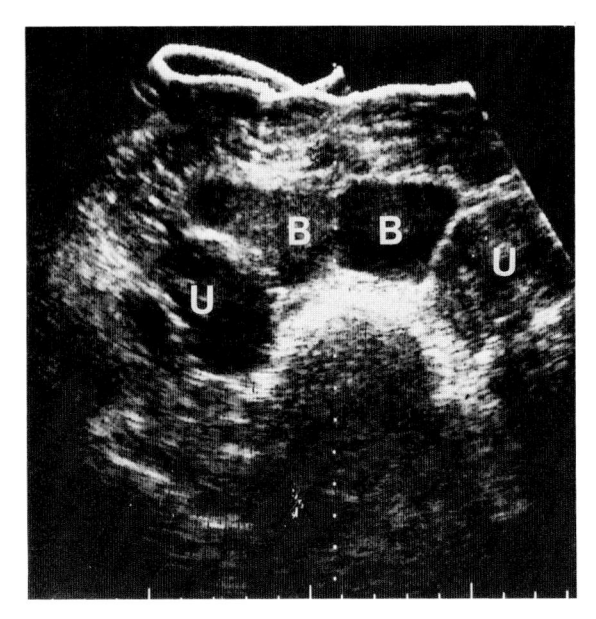

12.24 Calculi

A 5-year-old boy underwent repair of perineal hypospadia. A suprapubic cystostomy tube had been used for temporary urinary diversion; hematuria developed 2 months postoperatively. At that time, anteroposterior and lateral films of the pelvis (Figs. A and B, respectively) demonstrated two radiopaque densities believed to be bladder calculi. Ultrasonography was performed to verify the diagnosis since cystoscopy was impossible. Surgery was undesirable without determining the precise location of the stones. Figure C is a sonogram demonstrating a reflective area within the urinary bladder; these opacities shift in position and demonstrate acoustic shadowing, findings typical of bladder calculi.

(Figs. A & B and Scan C from Rosenfield AT, Taylor KJW, Weiss RM: Ultrasound evaluation of bladder calculi. J Urol 121:119–120, 1979. © 1979 The Williams & Wilkins Co., Baltimore.)

SUGGESTED READING

Rosenfield AT, Taylor KJW, Weiss RM: Ultrasound evaluation of bladder calculi. J Urol 121:119–120, 1979

A

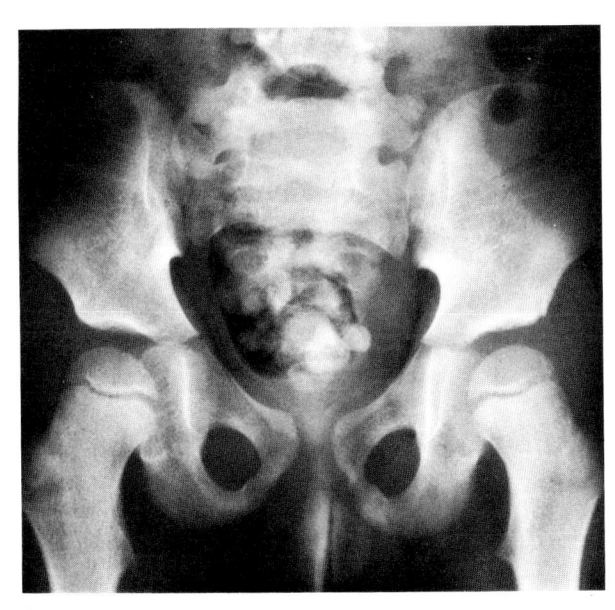

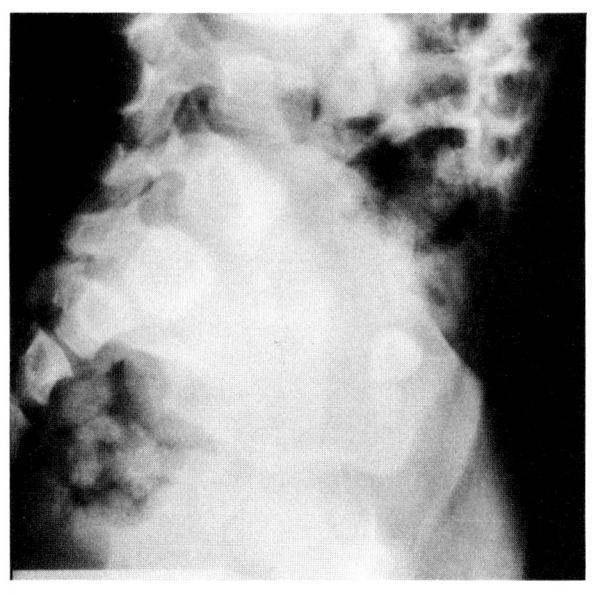

B

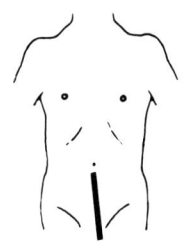

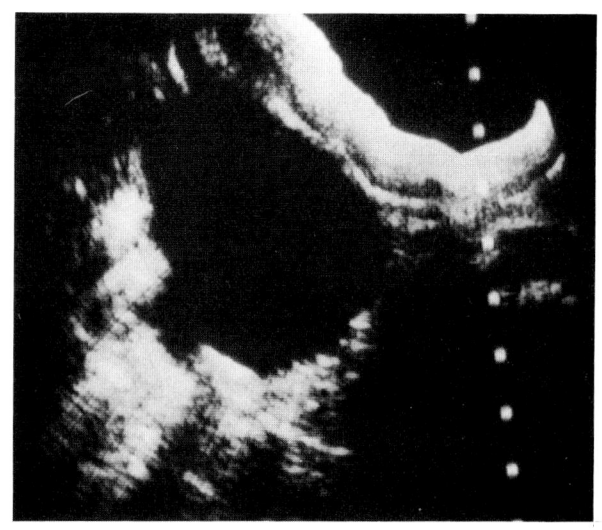

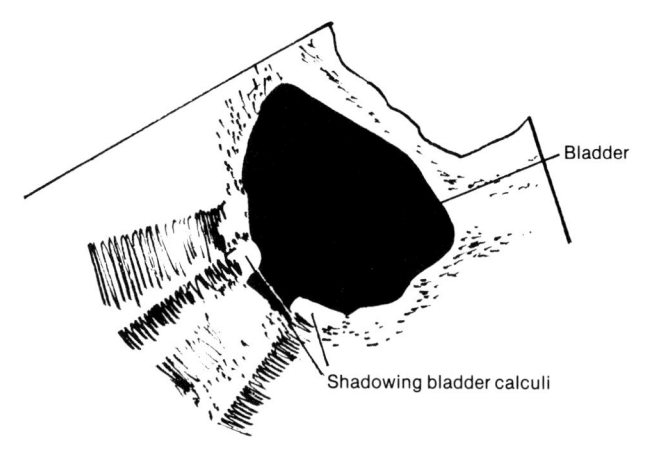

C

Bladder

Shadowing bladder calculi

896

12.25 Blood Clot

A patient who presented with hematuria underwent excretory urography which demonstrated a filling defect within the bladder (Fig. A). A transverse sonogram (Fig. B) showed a 2-cm echogenic mass on the left side of the bladder (open arrow) and a smaller echogenic mass just to the right of midline (closed arrow). A longitudinal scan through the left side of the bladder once again demonstrated the echogenic mass (Fig. C). Dynamic scanning of the bladder was then performed and, as the patient shifted position, the masses shifted in position as well, consistent with blood clot. The masses resolved spontaneously with time, presumably verifying the diagnosis.

(Figs. A–C from Zeman RK, Taylor KJW, Rosenfield AT: Kidney, adrenal, bladder. In Kossoff G, Fukuda M, (eds): Ultrasonic Differential Diagnosis of Tumors. Igaku-Shoin, Ltd., Japan, 1984.)

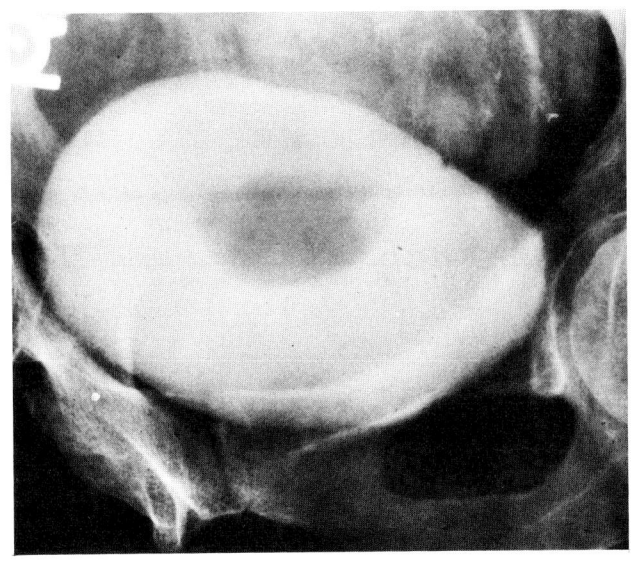

A

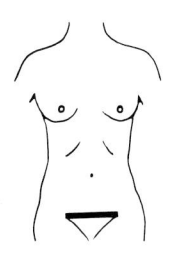

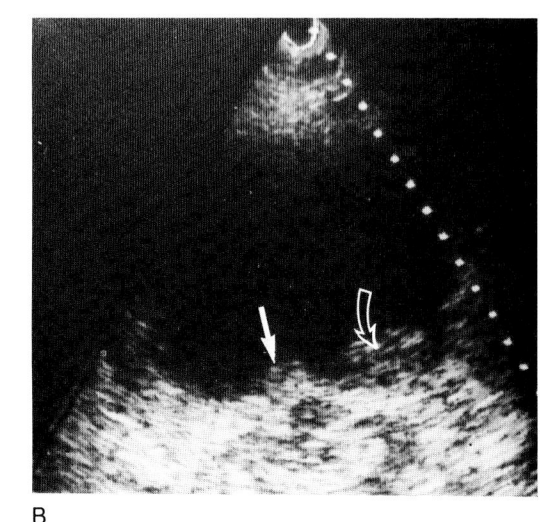

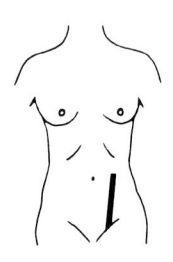

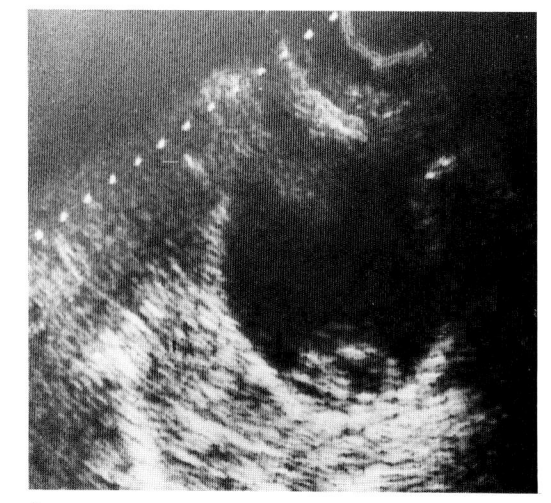

B

C

12.26 Diverticulum Containing Stone

An elderly man presented with signs and symptoms of prostatic enlargement. Excretory urography demonstrated a bladder diverticulum occupying much of the left hemipelvis (Fig. A). The patient subsequently underwent ultrasonography and computed tomography. On a transverse sonogram through the upper portion of the bladder, the bladder is seen as an echo-free mass in the right hemipelvis (Fig. B). Adjacent to the bladder is the diverticulum (D), seen as second echo-free mass.

Figures C and D demonstrate a sonogram and a CT scan, respectively, through the lower portion of the bladder. The bladder diverticulum is now less prominent. Note a focal zone of echogenicity (arrowed in Fig. C) without a well-defined acoustic shadow in the posterior portion of the diverticulum. Despite the lack of an acoustic shadow these findings are strongly suggestive of a stone within the diverticulum. Computed tomography at the same level demonstrates a stone within the calyceal diverticulum (arrowed in Fig. D). A portion of bowel containing gas is adjacent to the region of the stone on the CT scan; the shadowing caused by this gas probably precludes visualization of the acoustic shadow on the ultrasound study.

Figure E is a longitudinal scan through the true pelvis showing prostatic enlargement with a prominent median lobe, as well as the adjacent seminal vesicle.

Diverticula of the bladder may be any size and single or multiple. The classic diverticulum has its orifice adjacent to the ureteral meatus and protrudes lateral to the ureter. At times the ureter may enter directly into the diverticulum. Multiple diverticula may be associated with outlet obstruction. Because these bladder diverticula do not contain muscle within their wall but are outpouchings of mucosa, they frequently do not empty well. As a result, they may be missed on excretory urography. In addition, stasis can lead to infection, stone formation, or tumor within the diverticulum. Sonography can be of great value in identifying and examining these lesions.

SUGGESTED READING

Bree RL, Silver TM: Pictoral essay: sonography of the bladder and pelvocalyceal abnormalities. AJR 136:1101–1104, 1981

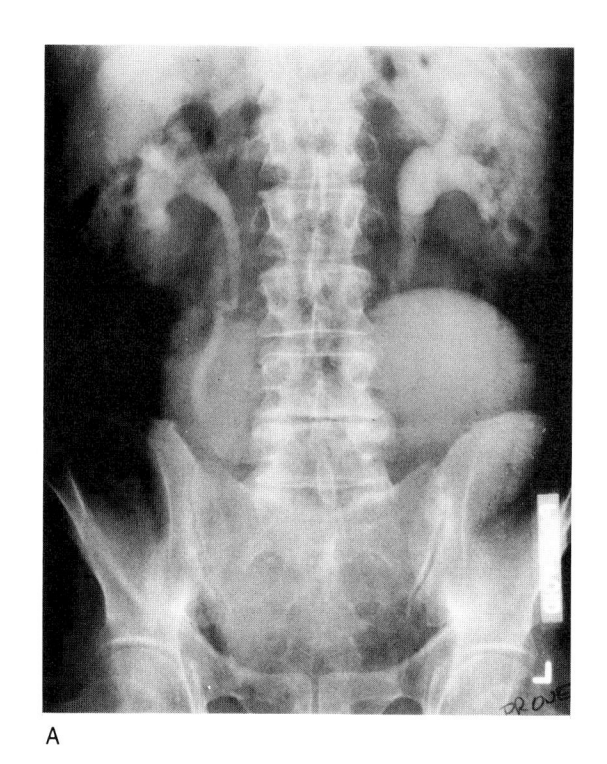

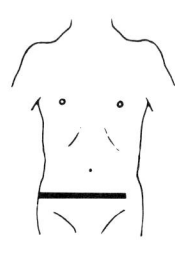

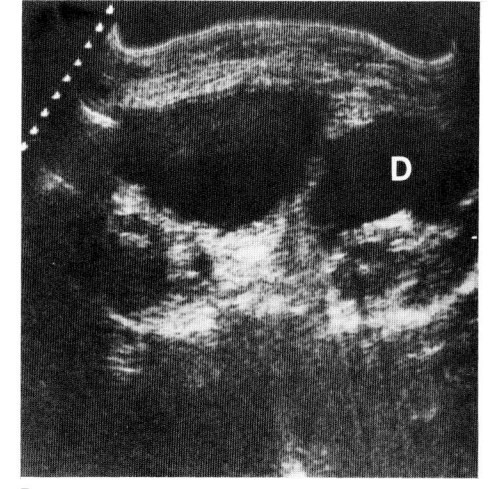

A

B

900

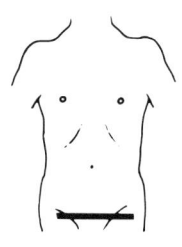

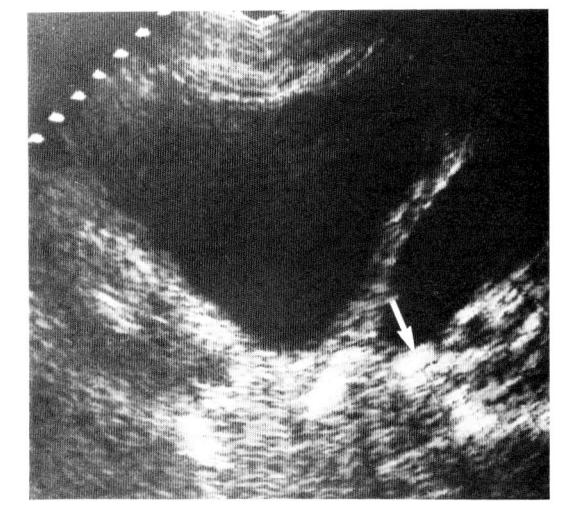

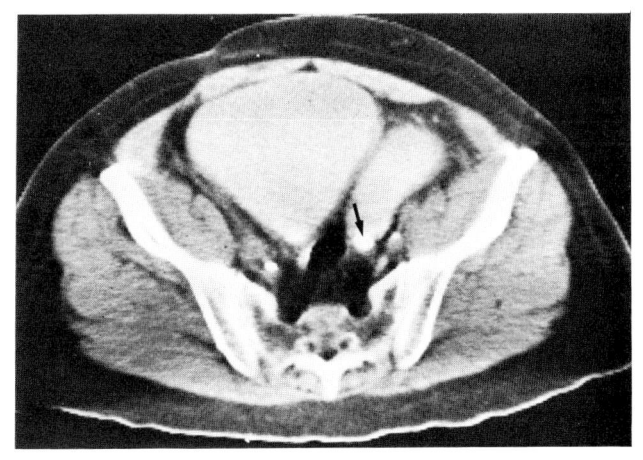

C

D

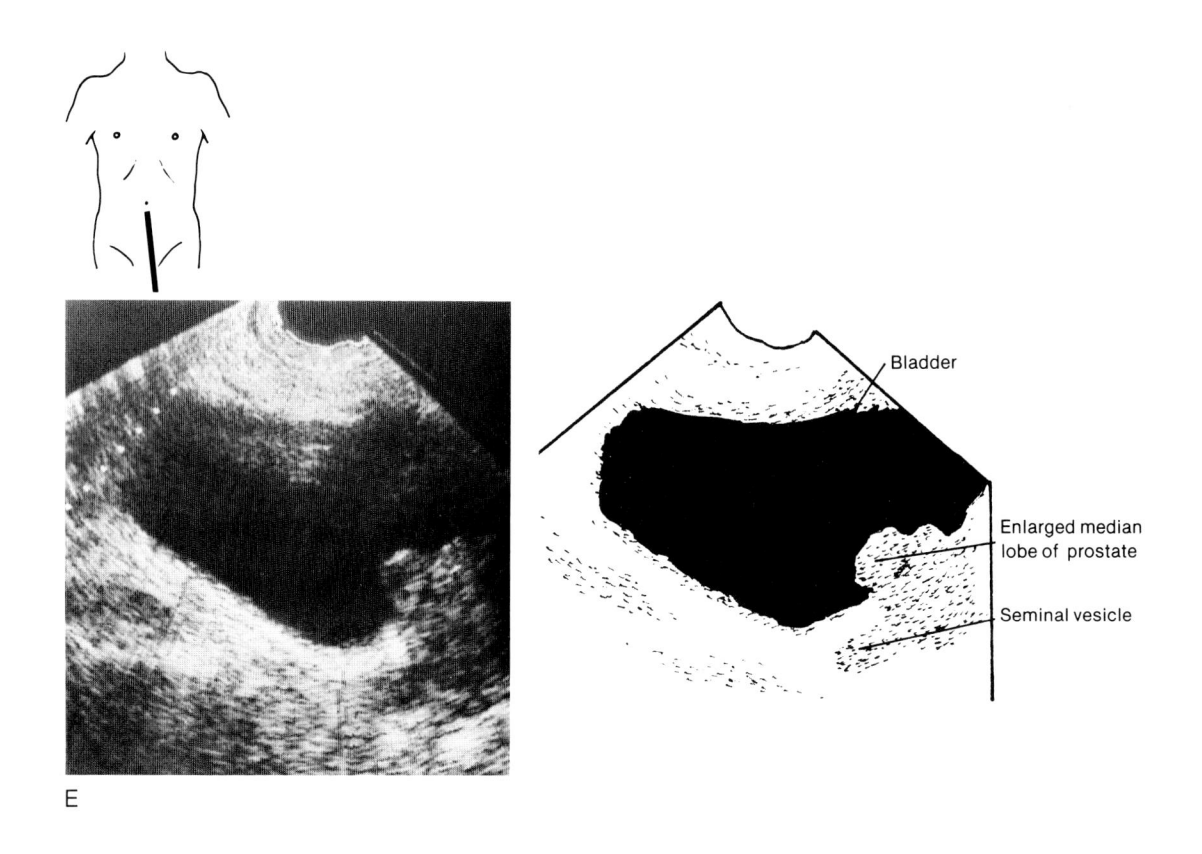

E

902

12.27 Transitional Cell Carcinoma

Ultrasonography has been used to screen for bladder tumors as well as stage them. Transabdominal (which we use at our institution), transrectal, and transurethral ultrasonography all have been used for this purpose. Ultrasonography can readily demonstrate a polypoid transitional cell carcinoma as shown in Figure A (arrowed). Widespread tumor can virtually fill the bladder, as shown in Figure B from another patient. Ultrasound cannot stage such tumors with respect to which layers of the bladder wall are involved, but may be able to show extension beyond the bladder.

A 66-year-old woman presented with hematuria. Clinical examination and cystoscopy showed an advanced bladder carcinoma. A transverse sonogram (Fig. C) shows a sessile tumor arising from the bladder wall, which is indurated and has lost its normal contour. Homogeneous strands of tumor material extending out toward the pelvic wall are also visible. These strands indicate invasion beyond the bladder wall.

The most common bladder tumor, transitional cell carcinoma, may occur in a benign superficial form or in a highly invasive and aggressive form. Other types of bladder tumors are much less common and include adenocarcinoma and squamous cell carcinoma. Adenocarcinoma is typically associated with cystitis glandularis, closure of exstrophy of the bladder, or a congenital diverticulum related to a urachal abnormality.

SUGGESTED READINGS

Bree RL, Silver TM: Pictorial essay: sonography of the bladder and pelvocalyceal abnormalities. AJR 136:1101–1104, 1981

Cronan JJ, Simeone JF, Pfister RC, et al: Cystosonography in the detection of bladder tumors: a prospective and retrospective study. J Ultrasound Med 1:237–241, 1981

Morley P: The bladder. p. 147. In Rosenfield AT (ed): Genitourinary Ultrasonography. Clinics in Diagnostic Ultrasound, vol 2. Churchill Livingstone, New York, 1979

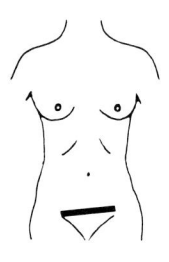

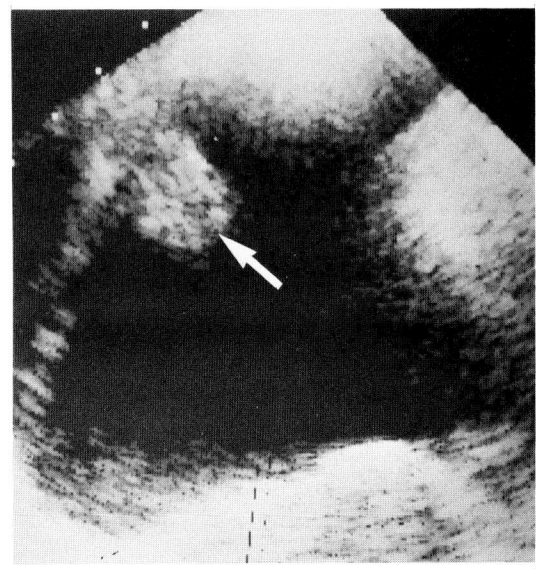

A

B

C

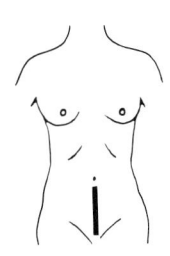

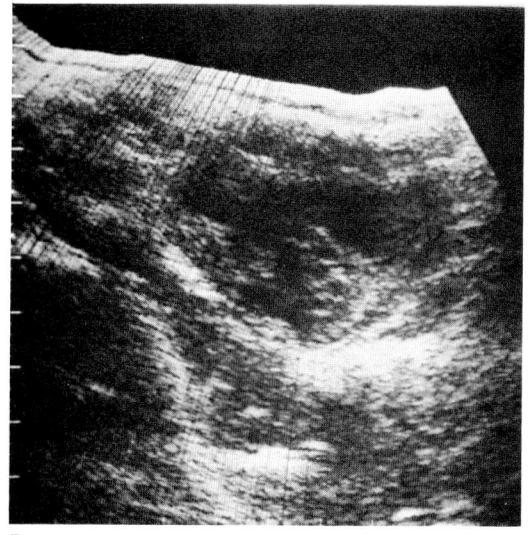

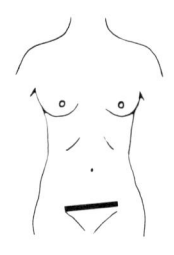

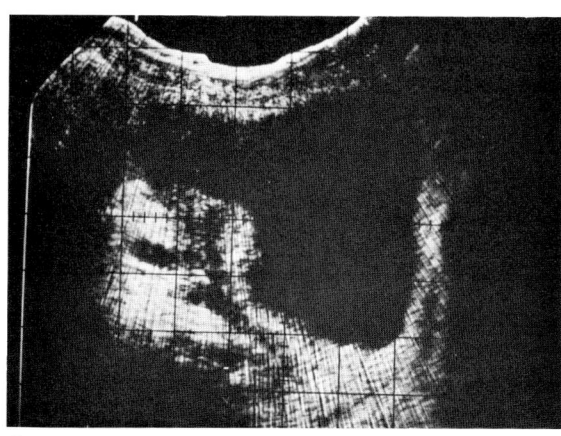

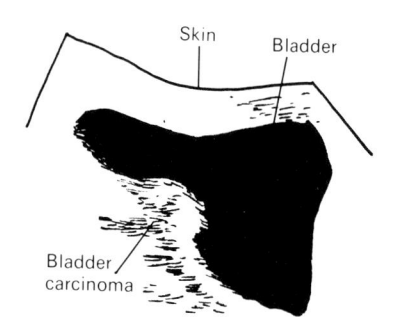

Transverse section
of bladder

905

Hematoma (12.28 to 12.30)

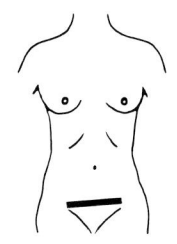

12.28 Anterior Deformity of the Bladder Secondary to Rectus Sheath Hematoma

A 25-year-old woman was hit by a bicycle and subsequently evaluated by ultrasonography. A transverse scan through the true pelvis (Fig. A) demonstrates an echo-free mass (H) displacing the bladder (B) posteriorly. The mass extends from the xiphoid to the true pelvis. To determine which fluid-filed mass was the bladder, the patient had a postvoid study (Fig. B). The bladder decreased in size while the mass remained constant.

Rectus sheath hematoma is one of the few cystic lesions that appear anterior to the bladder. Sonography is a useful technique to identify and follow these lesions.

(Figs. A & B from Gonzalez R, Rosenfield AT: Ultrasonography in the evaluation of abdominal trauma. pp. 33–54. In Taylor KJW, Viscomi GN (ed): Ultrasound in Emergency Medicine. Clinics in Diagnostic Ultrasound, vol 7. Churchill Livingstone, New York, 1981)

SUGGESTED READINGS

Conrad MR, Freedman M, Weiner C, et al: Sonography of the page kidney. J Urol 116:293–296, 1976

Gonzalez R, Rosenfield AT: Ultrasonography in the evaluation of abdominal trauma. pp. 33–54. In Taylor KJW, Viscomi GN (ed): Ultrasound in Emergency Medicine. Clinics in Diagnostic Ultrasound, vol. 7. Churchill Livingstone, New York, 1981

Kay CJ, Rosenfield AT, Armm M: Gray-scale ultrasonography in the evaluation of renal trauma. Radiology 134:461–466, 1980

Spitz HB, Weja HGM: Rectus sheath hematoma. J Clin Ultrasound 5:313–416, 1977

Wicks JD, Silver TM, Bree RL: Gray scale features of hematomas: an ultrasonic spectrum. AJR 131:977–980, 1978

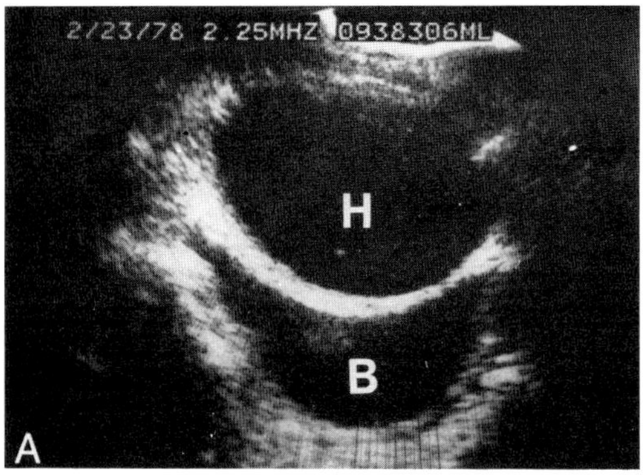
2/23/78 2.25MHZ 0938306ML
H
B
A

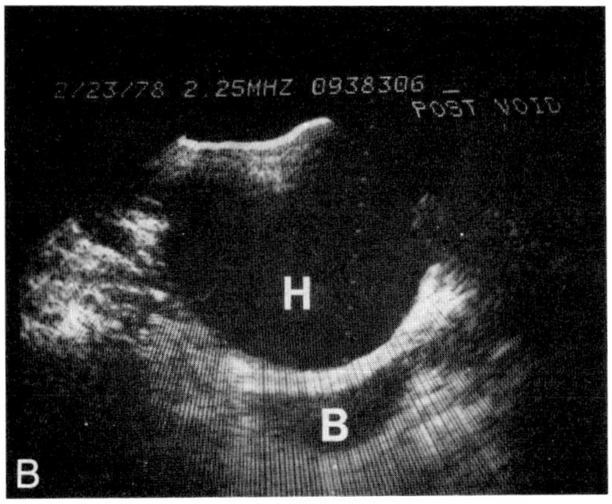
2/23/78 2.25MHZ 0938306
POST VOID
H
B
B

12.29 Old Rectus Sheath Hematoma

A 34-year-old hemophiliac man with an anterior abdominal wall mass, which had persisted for 4 years following mild abdominal trauma, underwent ultrasound and CT scans. Figure A shows transverse scans through the true pelvis, demonstrating an echo-poor mass (H) in the abdominal wall anterior to the bladder (B). Computed tomography of the same region shows a high density area (arrowed) anterior to the bladder (B) and within the rectus muscle (Fig. B). These findings are both consistent with an old hematoma located in the rectus sheath.

(Figs. A & B from Gonzalez-Gomez R, Rosenfield AT: Ultrasonography in the evaluation of abdominal trauma. pp. 33–54. In Taylor KJW, Viscomi GN (eds): Ultrasound in Emergency Medicine. Clinics in Diagnostic Ultrasound, vol. 7. Churchill Livingstone, New York, 1981.)

SUGGESTED READINGS

Conrad MR, Freedman M, Weiner C, et al: Sonography of the Page kidney. J Urol 116:293–296, 1976

Gonzalez-Gomez R, Rosenfield AT: Ultrasonography in the evaluation of abdominal trauma. pp. 33–54. In Taylor KJW, Viscomi GN (eds): Ultrasound in Emergency Medicine. Clinics in Diagnostic Ultrasound, vol. 7. Churchill Livingstone, New York, 1981

Spitz HB, Weja HGM: Rectus sheath hematoma. J Clin Ultrasound 5:313–416, 1977

Wicks JD, Silver TM, Bree RL: Gray scale features of hematomas: an ultrasonic spectrum. AJR 131:977–980, 1978

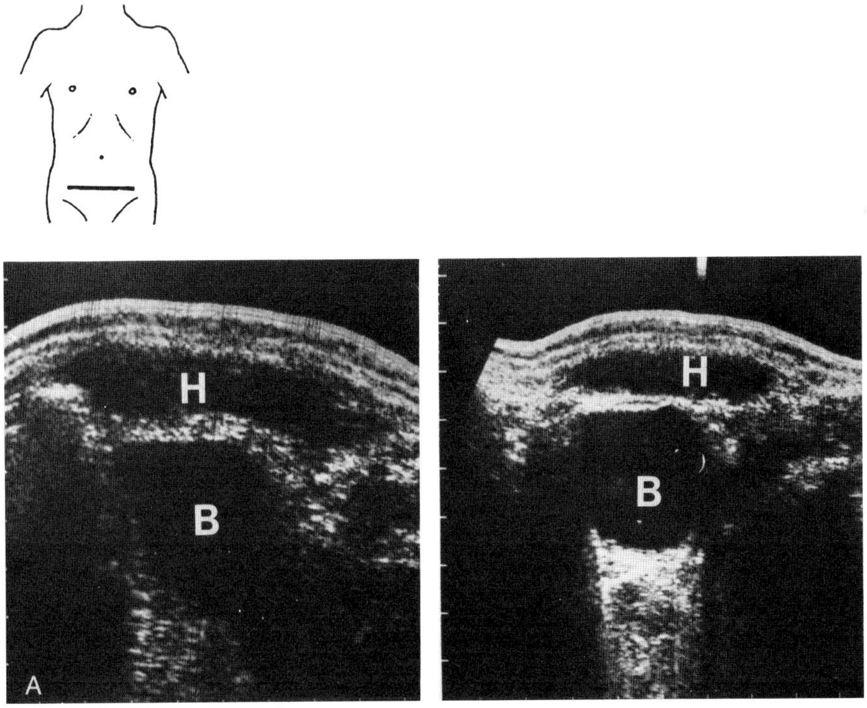
H
B
A
H
B

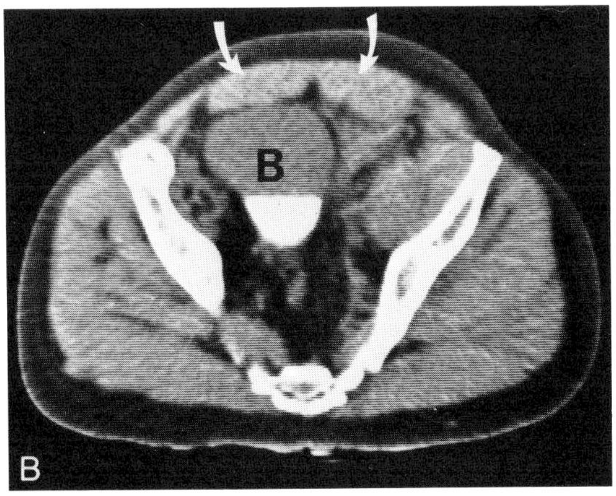
B
B

12.30 Perirenal Hematoma

A 60-year-old man had undergone left nephrectomy for a renal cell carcinoma. He also had a history of renal tuberculosis, diagnosed earlier in the year and was admitted with chief complaints of fever and watery diarrhea. At the time of admission, an intravenous urogram revealed acute obstruction of the right kidney and a percutaneous nephrostomy was performed. Ultrasound following percutaneous nephrostomy (shown in the figure) revealed a perirenal collection which compressed the kidney on its anterolateral aspect and contained low-level echoes. This was consistent with an acute perirenal hematoma.

Hematomas may be echogenic, echo-poor, or echo-free. Acutely, perirenal hematoma tends to be echo-free although as the clot organizes it may become echogenic. With time, hematomas become echo-poor and may then become echo-free. The findings of a complex perinephric fluid collection are nonspecific and may also be seen with abscess or urinoma.

SUGGESTED READINGS

Conrad MR, Freedman M, Weiner C, et al: Sonography of the Page kidney. J Urol 116:293–296, 1976

Gonzalez R, Rosenfield AT: Ultrasonography in the evaluation of abdominal trauma. pp. 33–54. In Taylor KJW, Viscomi GN (eds): Ultrasound in Emergency Medicine. Clinics in Diagnostic Ultrasound, vol. 7. Churchill Livingstone, New York, 1981

Kay CJ, Rosenfield AT, Armm M: Gray-scale ultrasonography in the evaluation of renal trauma. Radiology 134:461–466, 1980

Wicks JD, Silver TM, Bree RL: Gray scale features of hematomas: an ultrasonic spectrum. AJR 131:977–980, 1978

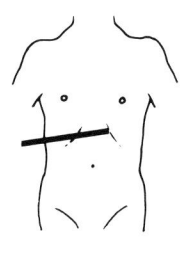

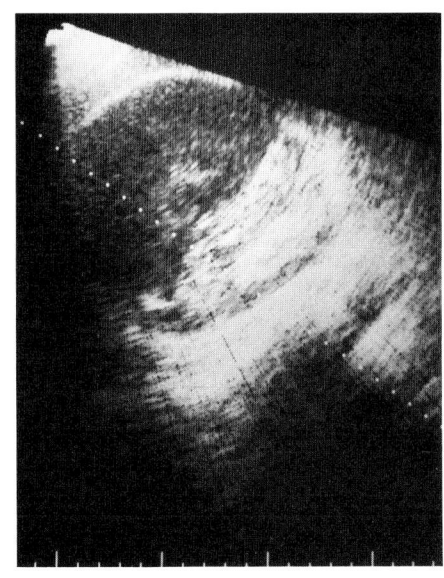

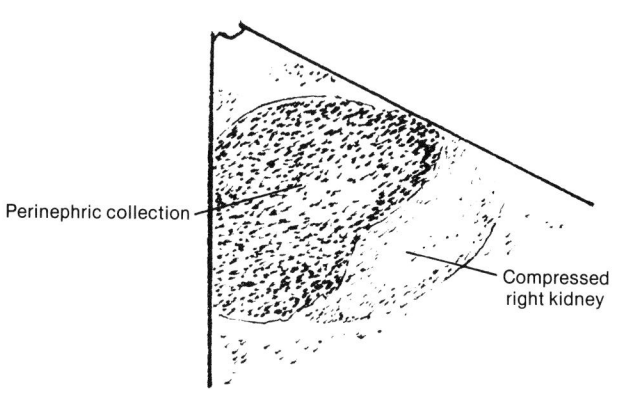

Perinephric collection

Compressed right kidney

12.31 Infected Urinoma

A 24-year-old man underwent abdominal surgery for perforated small bowel secondary to a gunshot wound. Two weeks later a large abdominal mass had developed. Plain film of the abdomen demonstrates a large mass (arrowed) occupying the midabdomen; a bullet is seen overlying the right sacrum (Fig. A).

Figure B is a transverse scan through the midabdomen demonstrating that the fluid-filled mass has a debris level (arrowed) within it. A longitudinal scan through the true pelvis (Fig. C) shows that the entire abdomen is filled by a large fluid-filled mass containing debris (arrowed) in its inferior aspect. The bladder (B) is seen inferiorly. Debris within a fluid-filled mass suggests a complicated mass such as one with infection or hemorrhage. At surgery, an infected urinoma was found, which was related to perforation of the right ureter.

(Figs. A–C from Gonzalez R, Rosenfield AT: Ultrasonography in the evaluation of abdominal trauma. pp. 33–54. In Taylor KJW, Viscomi GN (eds): Ultrasound in Emergency Medicine. Clinics in Diagnostic Ultrasound, vol. 7. Churchill Livingstone, New York, 1981.)

SUGGESTED READINGS

Gonzalez R, Rosenfield AT, Ultrasonography in the evaluation of abdominal trauma. pp. 33–54. In Taylor KJW, Viscomi GN (eds): Ultrasound in Emergency Medicine. Clinics in Diagnostic Ultrasound, vol. 7. Churchill Livingstone, New York, 1981

Kay CJ, Rosenfield AT, Armm M: Gray-scale ultrasonography in the evaluation of renal trauma. Radiology 134:461–466, 1980

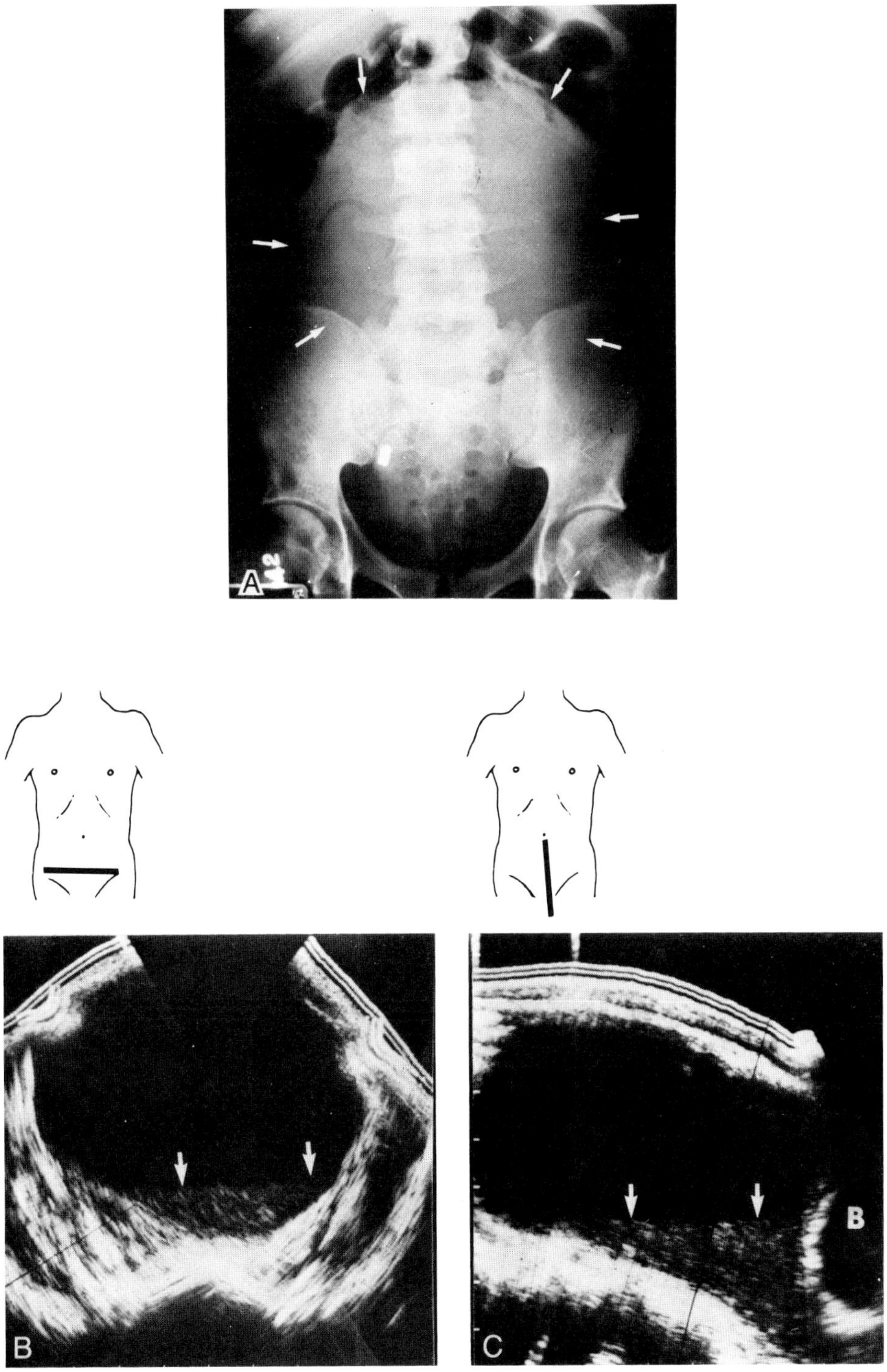
A
B
C
B

12.32 Normal Prostate and Seminal Vesicle

Figure A is a transverse sonogram through the prostate of a normal patient. The prostate is seen as a rounded structure behind the bladder. An echogenic focus at the center of the prostate represents the urethra and the periurethral glands. The proximal portions of the seminal vesicles, particularly the left seminal vesicle, can be identified. Figure B is an oblique scan through the left side of the true pelvis in the same patient. It demonstrates the prostate with a central linear echo focus representing the urethra and periurethral glands. The left seminal vesicle can be seen extending cranially. Figure C is a transverse scan at a more cephalad level than Figure A, demonstrating both seminal vesicles (arrowed) which are symmetrical. The seminal vesicles have echogenic fat around them. Loss of this echogenic fat in the presence of a prostatic or bladder mass indicates spread of a tumor beyond the bladder wall.

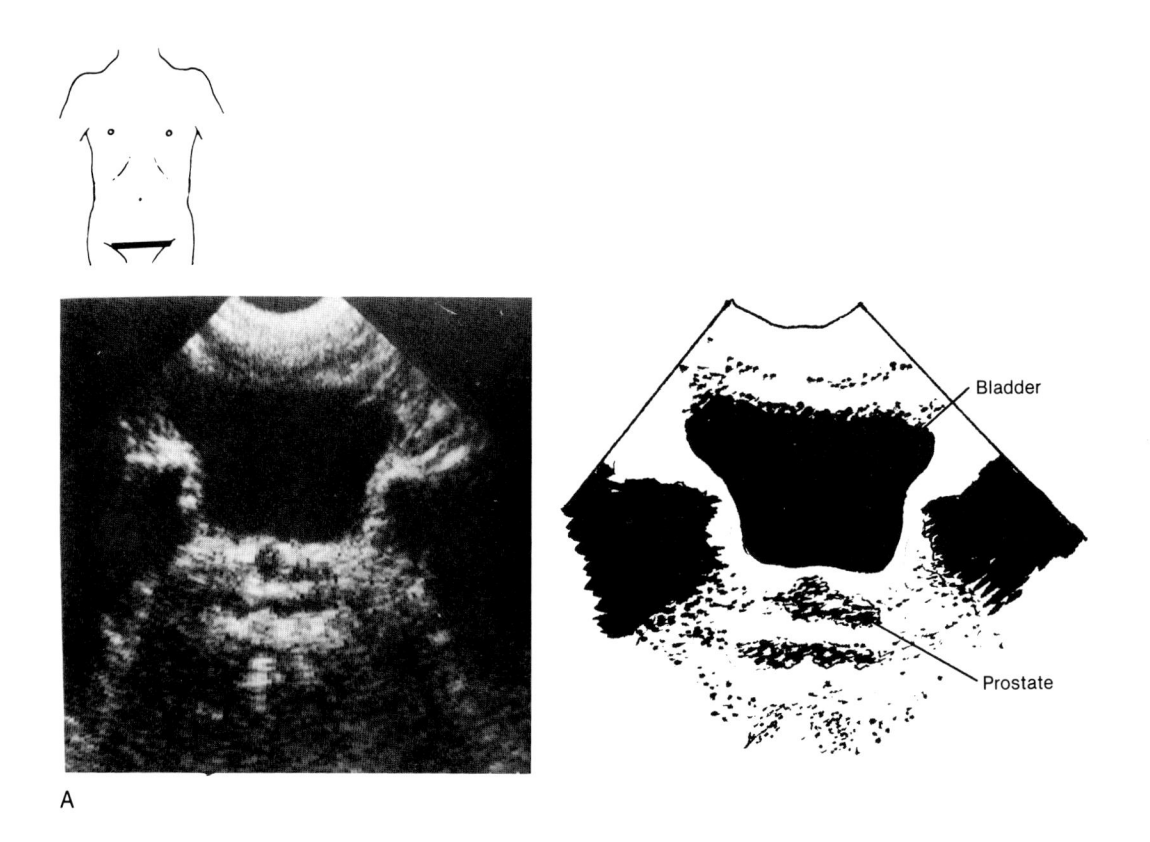

A

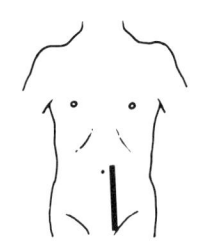

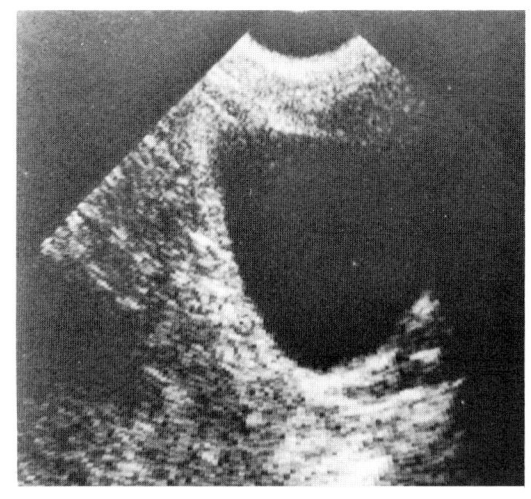

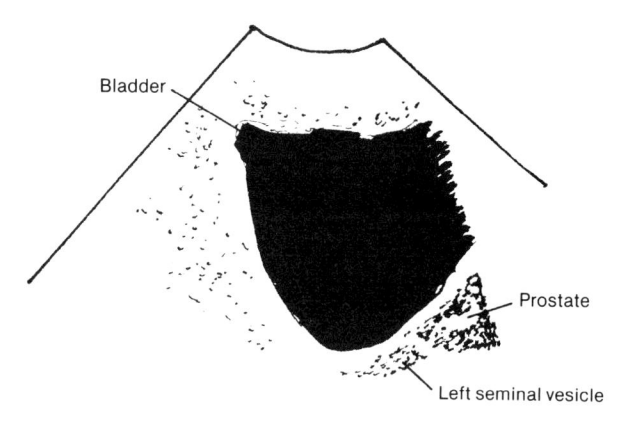

Bladder
Prostate
Left seminal vesicle

B

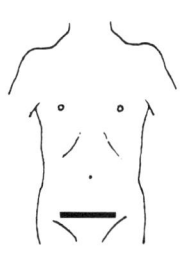

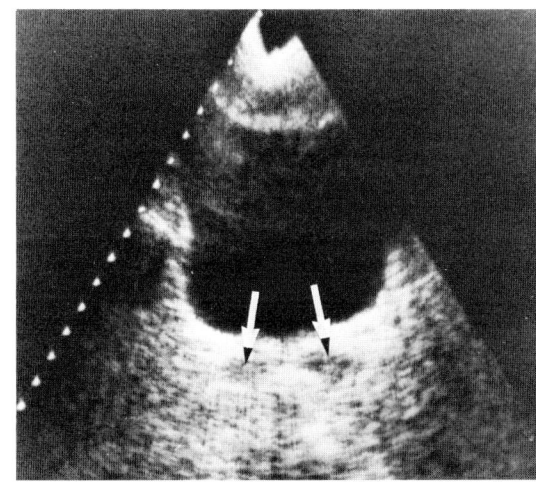

C

Benign Prostatic Hypertrophy (12.33 and 12.34)

12.33 Per Abdominal Scans

A 78-year-old man had a hard palpable prostate gland at clinical examination. Transabdominal suprapubic ultrasound was performed to evaluate the patient further. Figure A is a sonogram through the true pelvis at the level of the prostate showing bladder and prostate. Note the symmetrical enlargement of the prostate and the central echogenic focus from the region of the urethra. Figure B, the longitudinal scan through the true pelvis of the same patient, shows the prostatic enlargement and echogenic urethra. Note the normal seminal vesicles extending cephalad. Figure C is a transverse scan through both seminal vesicles showing that they are surrounded by normal echogenic fat. Symmetrical enlargement of the prostate with a homogeneous echo texture and the absence of any tumor spread beyond the prostate is typical of benign prostatic hypertrophy. As the gland enlarges; proliferation of glandular stroma elements in the periurethral tissues can lead to a pseudocapsule seen sonographically as a rind of increased echogenicity. The pseudocapsule is not present in this case.

SUGGESTED READING

Greenberg M, Neiman HL, Brandt BD, et al: Ultrasound of the prostate: analysis of tissue texture and abnormalities. Radiology 141:757–762, 1981

917

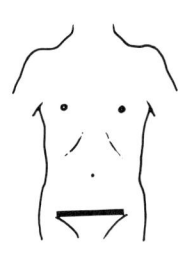

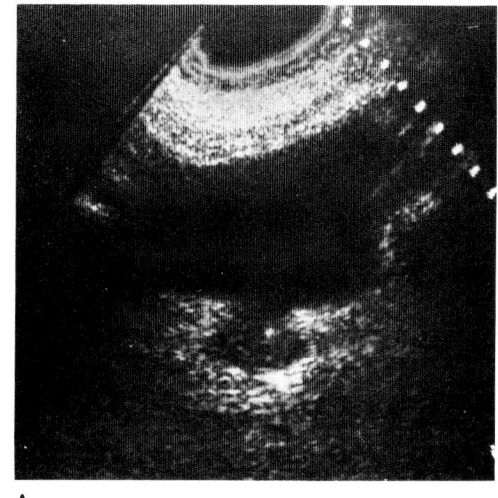

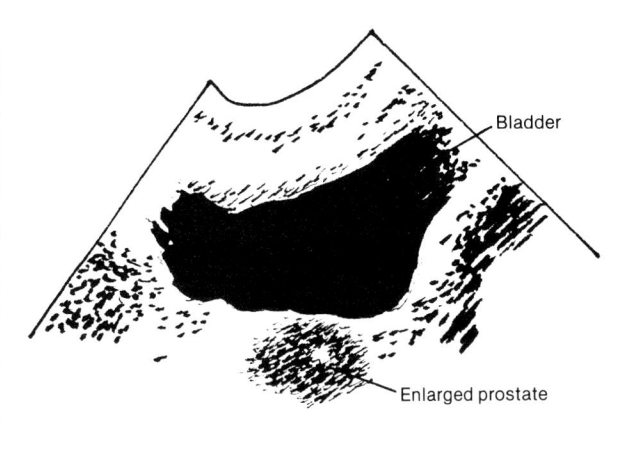

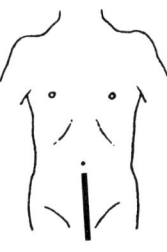

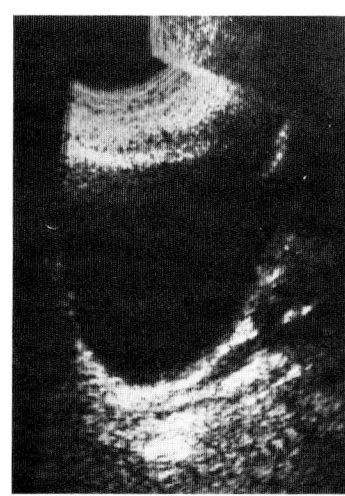

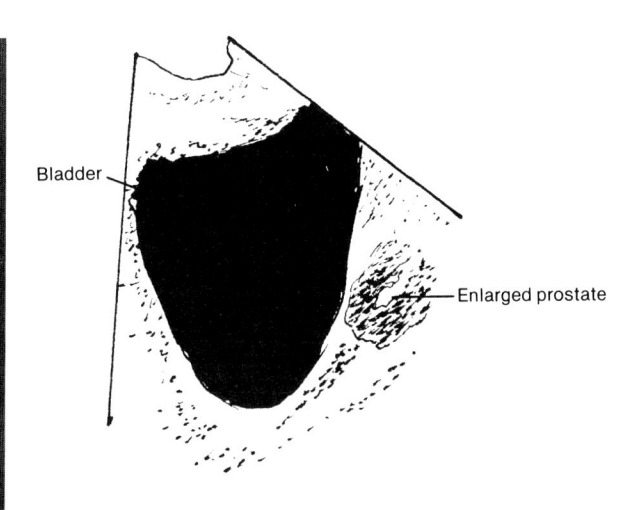

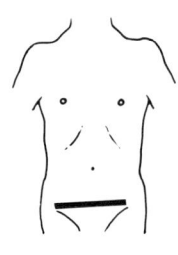

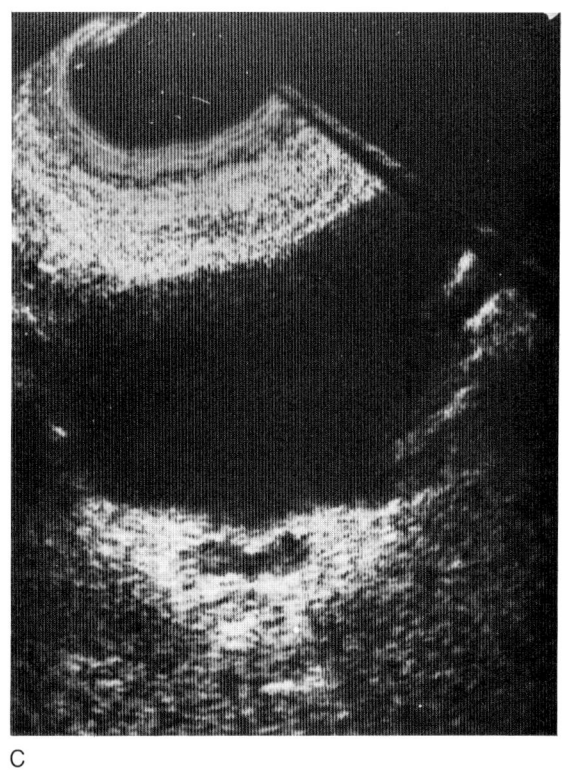

C

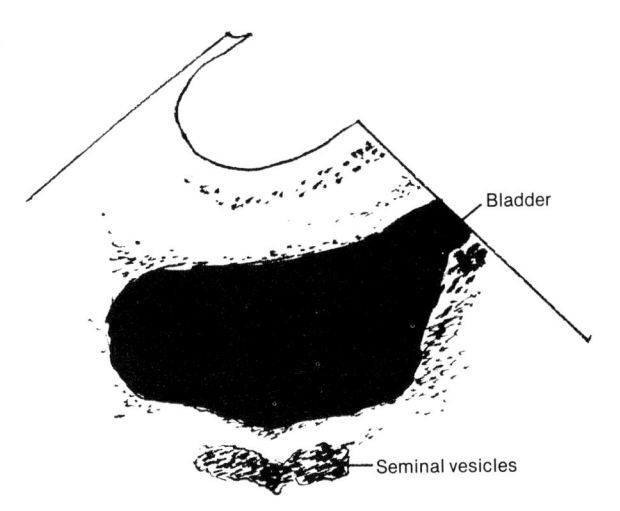

Bladder

Seminal vesicles

12.34 Hypertrophy with Bladder Wall Thickening

A 76-year-old man presented with a 10-year history of increasing difficulty voiding. Ultrasound clearly demonstrated a markedly trabeculated and thick-walled bladder on the transverse (Fig. A) and longitudinal scans (Fig. B). On the longitudinal scan the prostate itself is identified and is symmetrically enlarged. Note the echogenic line representing the thick capsule.

Ultrasonography also demonstrated bilateral hydronephrosis and incidental cysts (Fig. C shows the right kidney and Fig. D the left kidney).

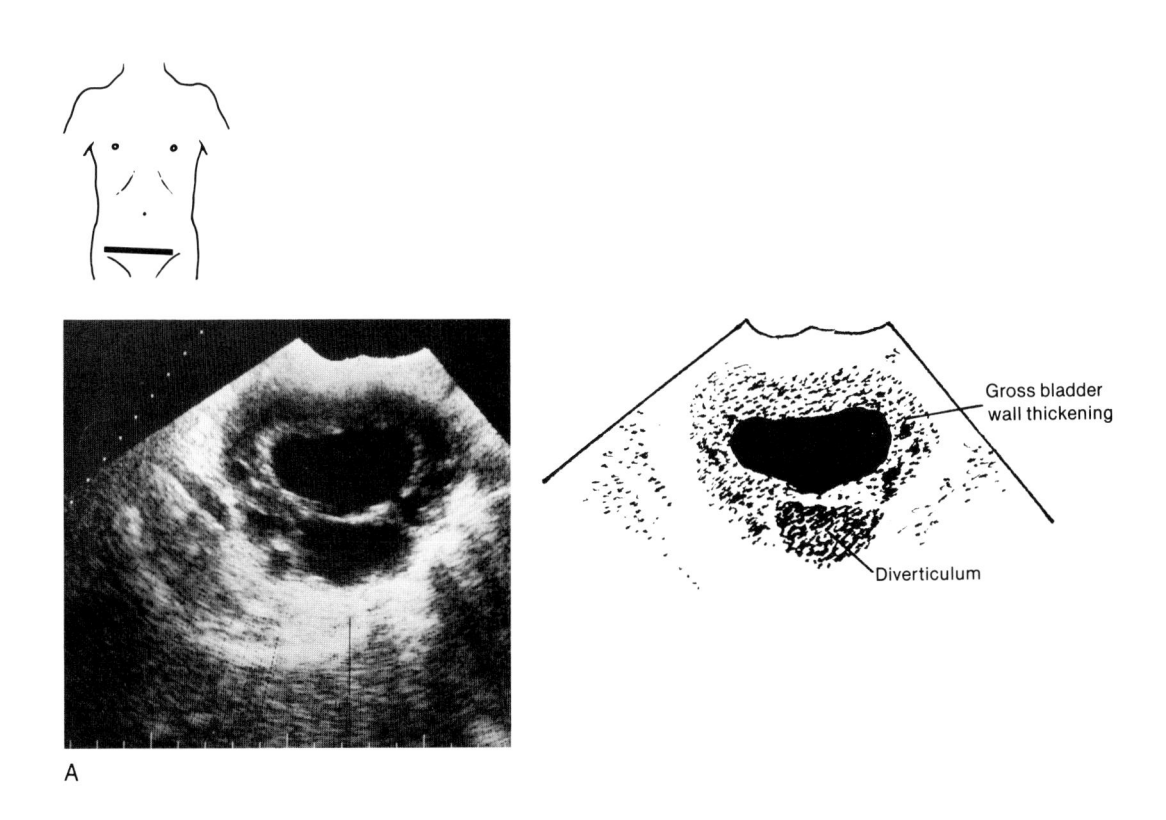

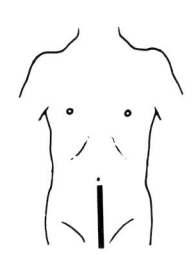

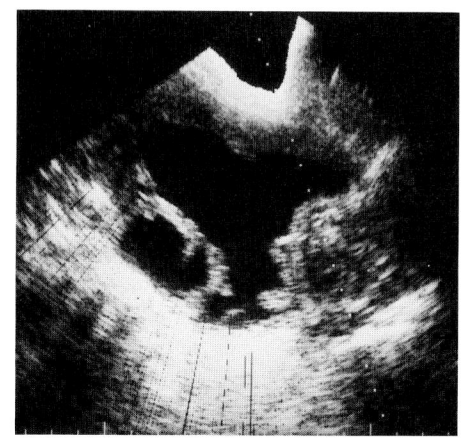

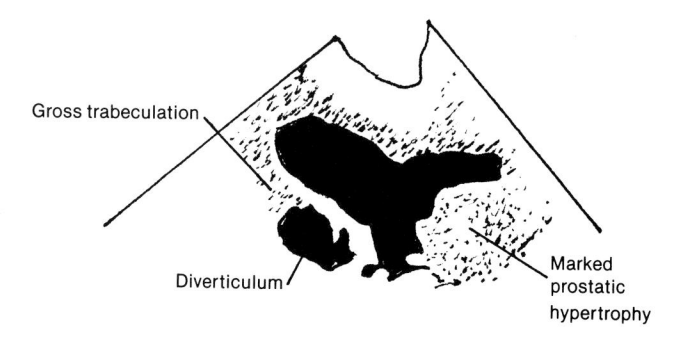

Gross trabeculation

Diverticulum

Marked prostatic hypertrophy

B

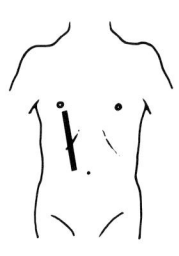

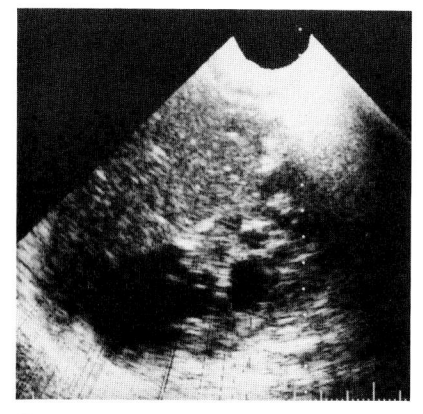

C

920

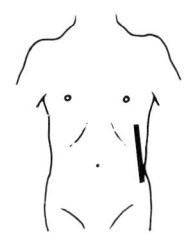

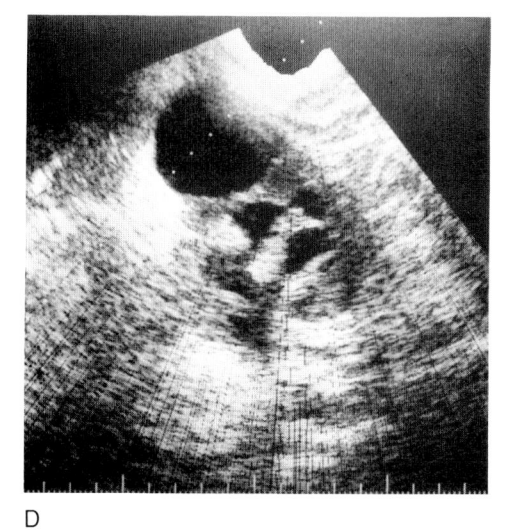

D

12.35 Prostatic Stones

Figure A is a longitudinal ultrasound study of the bladder and prostate in an elderly man. In addition to the enlarged prostate, note the zone of punctate echogenicities in the prostate with associated acoustic shadowing. These findings are typical of prostatic calculi. Figure B is from the excretory urogram and demonstrates both the prostatic enlargement and the calculi. Prostatic calculi can be identified routinely by ultrasound, but they are not of great clinical significance.

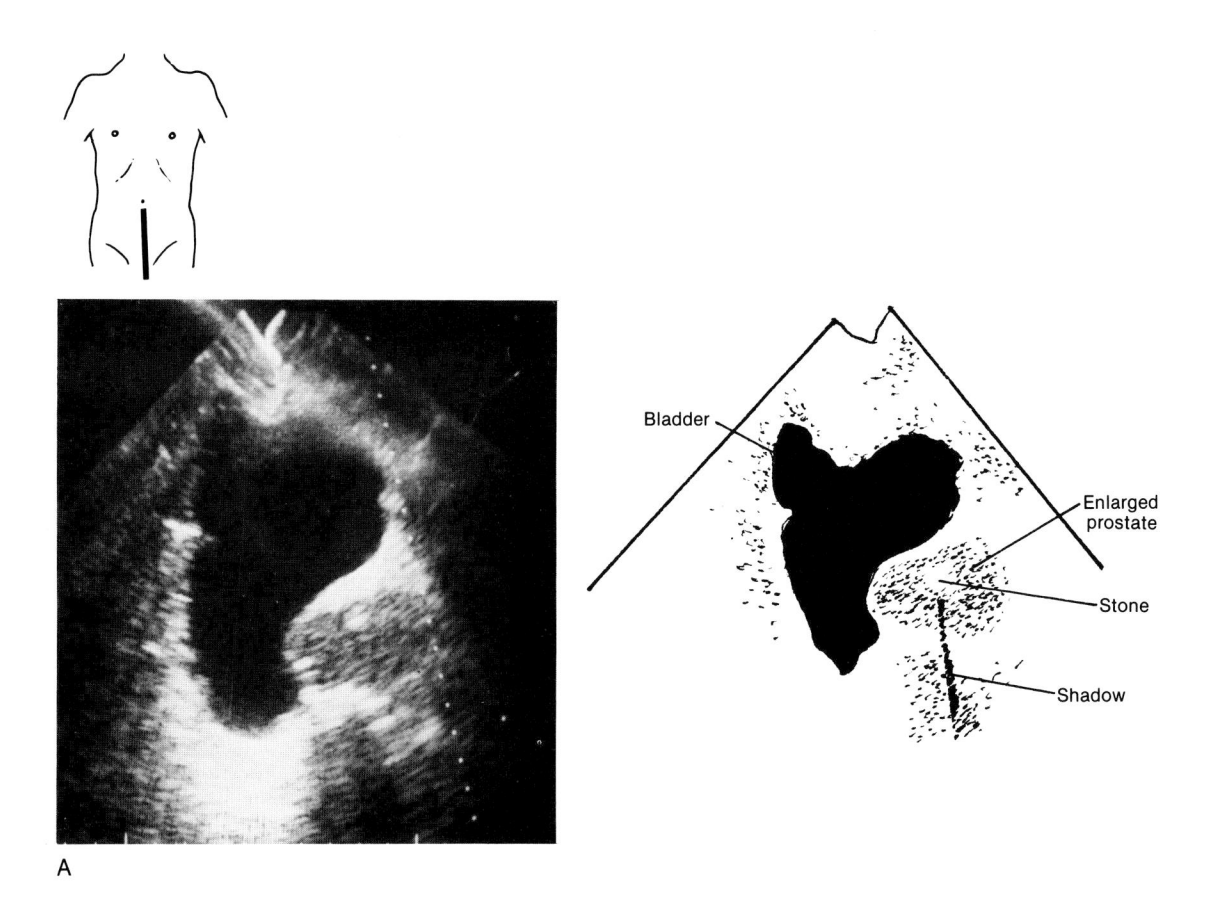

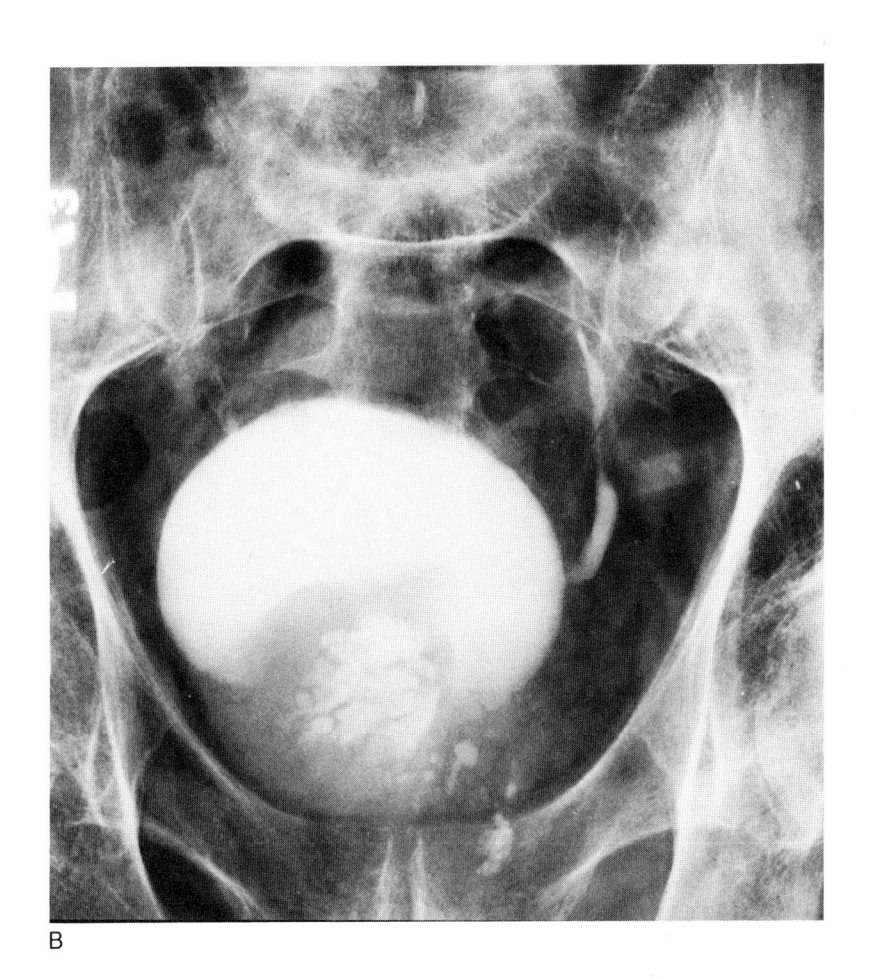

B

12.36 Prostatic Carcinoma

The figure shows a longitudinal midline sonogram through the bladder and prostate, demonstrating a distended bladder containing a Foley catheter balloon. Beneath the Foley balloon is the enlarged prostate which has an uneven echo texture with poor transmission. The entire visualized prostate was irregular in texture and contour on tomograms. These findings are more consistent with malignant than benign disease. Carcinoma of the prostate was found at surgery.

On a sonogram, prostatic carcinoma can present as increased or decreased echogenicity. However, asymmetrical enlargement of the prostate suggests malignancy.

SUGGESTED READING

Greenberg M, Neiman HL, Brandt BD, et al: Ultrasound of the prostate: analysis of tissue texture and abnormalities. Radiology 141:757–762, 1981

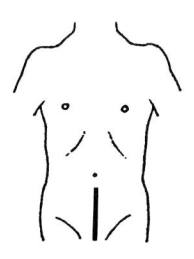

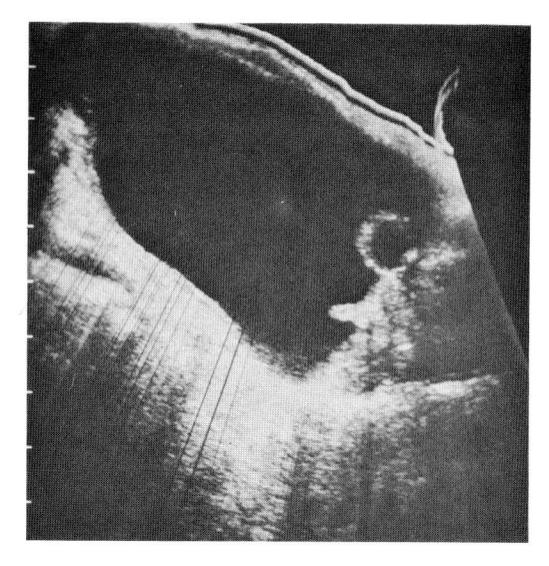

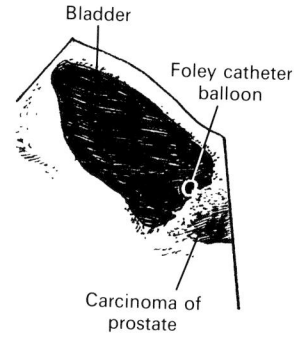

12.37 Posterior Urethral Valves with Secondary Bladder Outlet Obstruction

A 2-month-old boy had a recent urinary tract infection which was successfully treated with antibiotics. Excretory urography (Fig. A) was unremarkable except for minimal fullness to the left ureter. However, ultrasonography was performed and demonstrated a markedly thickened bladder wall as shown in transverse (Fig. B) and longitudinal scans (Fig. C). Voiding cystourethrography subsequently demonstrated both the trabeculated bladder and the dilated posterior urethra consistent with posterior urethral valves. There was also vesicoureteral reflux on the left.

This case demonstrates that posterior urethral valves can present with significant obstruction and bladder wall thickening without significant upper urinary tract dilatation. It also demonstrates the marked discrepancy between the bladder as it appeared on the IVP, at which time it was not definitely abnormal, and sonogram which demonstrated the markedly thickened wall. Sonography can demonstrate the abnormality in the posterior urethral valves even in utero and the dilated posterior urethra in utero may also be seen at times.

(Figs. A–C from Gonzalez-Gomez R, Richman AH, Taylor KJW. Urinary tract ultrasonography. pp. 29–52. In Finberg HJ ed: Case Studies in Diagnostic Ultrasound. Clinics in Diagnostic Ultrasound, vol. 9. Churchill Livingstone, New York, 1981.)

SUGGESTED READING

Gonzalez-Gomez R, Richman AH, Taylor KJW, et al: Urinary tract ultrasonography. pp. 29–52. In Finberg JH, (ed): Case Studies in Diagnostic Ultrasound. Clinics in Diagnostic Ultrasound, vol. 9. Churchill Livingstone, New York, 1981

A

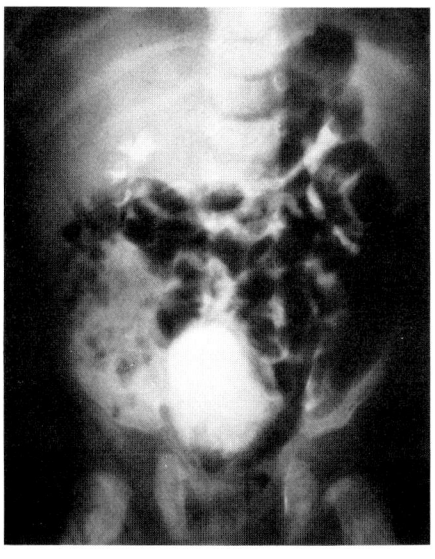

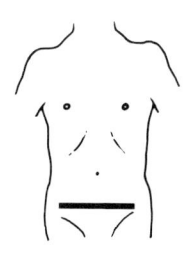

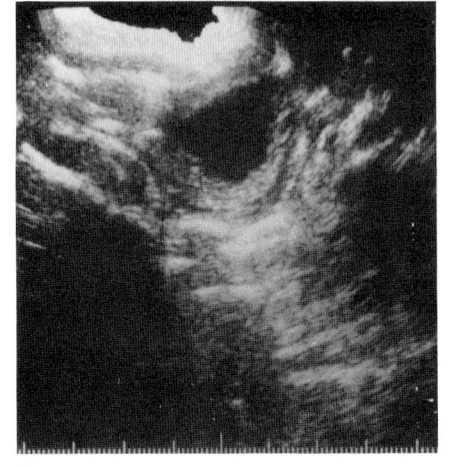

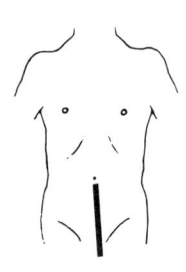

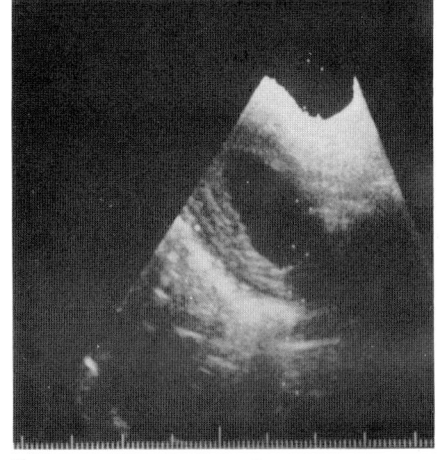

B

C

926

12.38 Pelvic Lipomatosis

An elderly man underwent excretory urography for hematuria. A preliminary urograph demonstrated no obvious pelvic mass, although significant fat was present in the pelvis. An excretory urograph (Fig. A) demonstrated the bladder to be elongated in a craniocaudad dimension and indented from the sides. A subsequent barium enema (Fig. B) also demonstrated the rectosigmoid to be vertically elongated by an apparent mass. The differential diagnosis for such an elongated bladder and rectosigmoid includes pelvic lipomatosis, collaterals associated with inferior vena caval thrombosis, psoas muscle hypertrophy, bilateral iliac artery aneurysms, lymphadenopathy, bilateral tumors, and bilateral lymphoceles.

Cross-sectional imaging can be a great aid in differentiating among these possibilities. Figure C is a transverse scan through the base of the bladder, demonstrating highly echogenic material around the bladder, consistent with fat. A longitudinal scan (Fig. D) demonstrated the elongated fluid-filled bladder compressed by highly echogenic fat posteriorly. The finding of echogenic fat about the bladder is consistent with pelvic lipomatosis. This was confirmed by a CT scan (Fig. E) which demonstrated the bladder to be surrounded by low-attenuating fat, a finding typical of pelvic lipomatosis.

Pelvic lipomatosis is the deposition of significant amounts of fat within the bony pelvis which typically affects middle-aged men. Although the entity is usually benign, causing impingement on the bladder or displacement of bowel, in its more aggressive form it can cause significant problems by obstructing the urinary tract.

(Case and figures courtesy of Louis Bader, M.D., Park City Hospital, Bridgeport, CT)

SUGGESTED READINGS

Crawford ED, Dumbadze I, Katz DL, Vester JW: Pelvic lipomatosis: diagnosis by computerized tomography scan. Am J Med 65:1021–1026, 1978

Susmano DE, Dolin EH: Computed tomography in diagnosis of pelvic lipomatosis. Urology 13:215–220, 1979

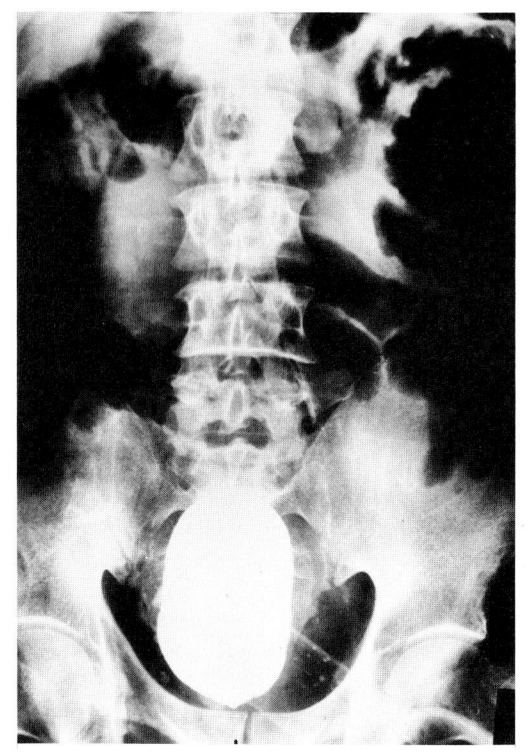

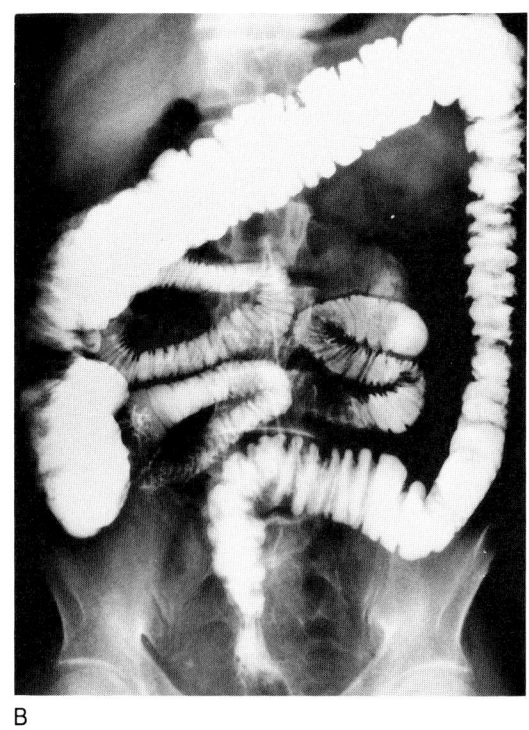

A

B

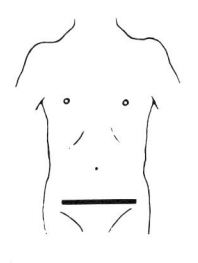

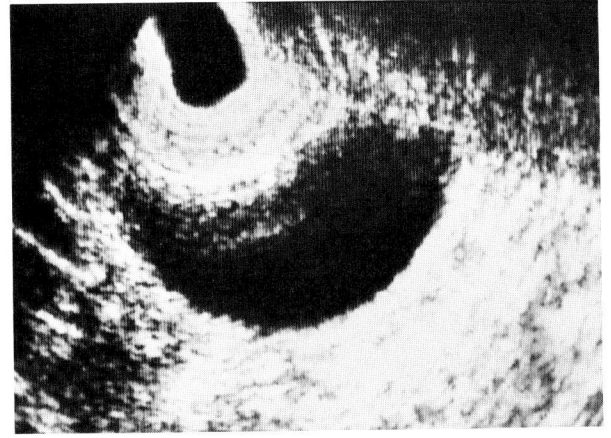

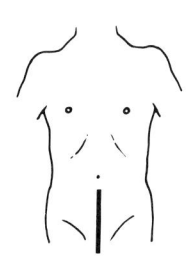

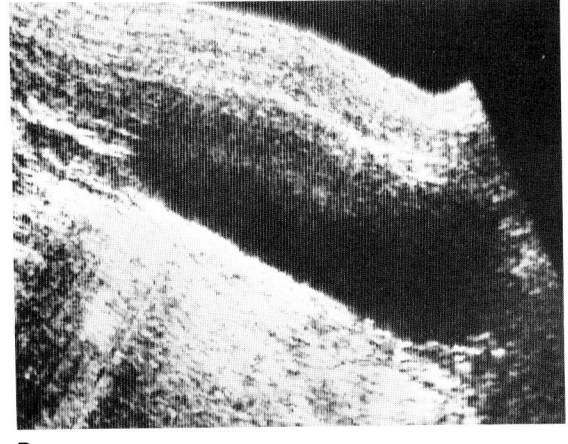

C

D

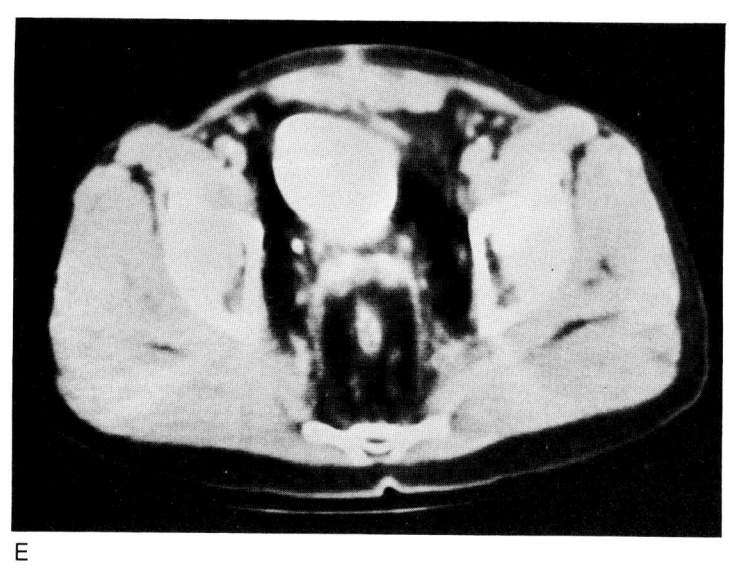

E

13 The Adrenal Gland

TINA RICHMAN and ARTHUR T. ROSENFIELD

The normal adrenal gland can be identified sonographically but generally is visualized more easily by CT. The right adrenal gland is above the kidney and is limited by the liver laterally, the inferior vena cava anteriorly, and right crus of the diaphragm medially. The left adrenal gland is both superior and medial to the left kidney and is bordered by the crus of the diaphragm medially, the tail of the pancreas anterolaterally, and the aorta anteromedially.

Ultrasonography and computed tomography can be employed to identify adrenal enlargement and to characterize adrenal masses; an advantage of CT is that it consistently permits identification of the normal adrenal gland when an extra-adrenal mass is present, while sonography does not. However, the longitudinal view of the upper abdomen obtained on sonography allows discrimination among adrenal, hepatic, and renal lesions with better accuracy than CT. Retroperitoneal fat is displaced away from the organ of origin. Ultrasound is particularly useful in children and thin adults.

Masses in the adrenal 2 cm or larger are usually identified. The adrenal gland is one of the most common sites of metastatic disease from the lung, breast, gastrointestinal (GI) or genitourinary (GU) tract, and the ovary. Adrenal carcinomas, most of which function, are usually poorly echogenic. Nonfunctioning tumors are commonly very large when first discovered. If hemorrhage occurs, the appearance may be echogenic or echo-poor. Central necrosis may appear echo-poor or totally anechoic, but the edges should be irregular. Tumors, benign or malignant, as well as hemorrhage, may calcify.

Adrenal adenomas, as well as hyperplasia, are also usually poorly echogenic. There is a 2 percent postmortem incidence of adenomas and these are found in 12–15 percent of patients with hypernephroma.

True adrenal cysts most commonly are lymphangiomatous epithelial cysts and are quite rare. Hemorrhagic pseudocysts also occur. Cyst puncture may be performed for cytologic study.

Pheochromocytomas arise from the adrenal medulla and should be considered in patients with hypertension. As with other adrenal masses, the ultrasound appearance is nonspecific.

Neuroblastomas differ from other adrenal masses because they are usually diffusely highly echogenic, unless hemorrhage or necrosis occurs. The cause of this echogenic appearance is unclear. Myelolipomas are also intensely echogenic, but this is due to the presence of fat within these benign tumors.

Other adrenal masses include connective tissue tumors, which are all quite rare, hemorrhage, and inflammatory disease. In the neonate, previous adrenal hemorrhage may become infected.

Since ultrasound is used routinely to examine the entire abdomen for disease, unsuspected adrenal disease may be identified and characterized.

SUGGESTED READINGS

Black HC, Mitty HA, Rose J, et al: Ultrasonography of adrenal masses: unusual features. Radiology 127:467–474, 1978

Crade M, Taylor KJW, Rosenfield AT: Discovery of an adrenal tumor by ultrasound: case report. J Clin Ultrasound 6:143–214, 1978

Gore RM, Callen PW, Filly RA: Displaced retroperitoneal fat: sonographic guide to right upper quadrant. Radiology 142:701–705, 1982

Mitty HA, Yeh HC: Radiology of the Adrenals with Sonography and CT. WB Saunders Co., Philadelphia, 1982

13.1 Normal Anatomy

Meticulous scanning technique, as described by Sample,[1,2] permits identification of both adrenal glands using coronal views. The left adrenal gland is defined by the spleen, left kidney, and aorta (Fig. A). The right adrenal can be identified on transverse sonograms through the liver in the region above the right kidney. Dynamic scanning permits rapid review of this region. Coronal scans through the right upper quadrant aligning the liver, inferior vena cava, and right kidney also may be used.

The neonatal and prenatal adrenal gland is large relative to the size of the kidney and indeed may be mistaken for it. Figure B is a coronal scan in a neonate. The large, right normal adrenal gland is easily seen lying above the right kidney.

REFERENCES

1. Sample WF: A new technique for the evaluation of the adrenal gland with gray scale ultrasonography. Radiology 124:463–469, 1977
2. Sample WF: Adrenal ultrasonography. Radiology 127:462–466, 1977

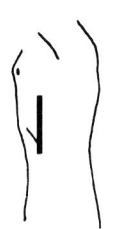

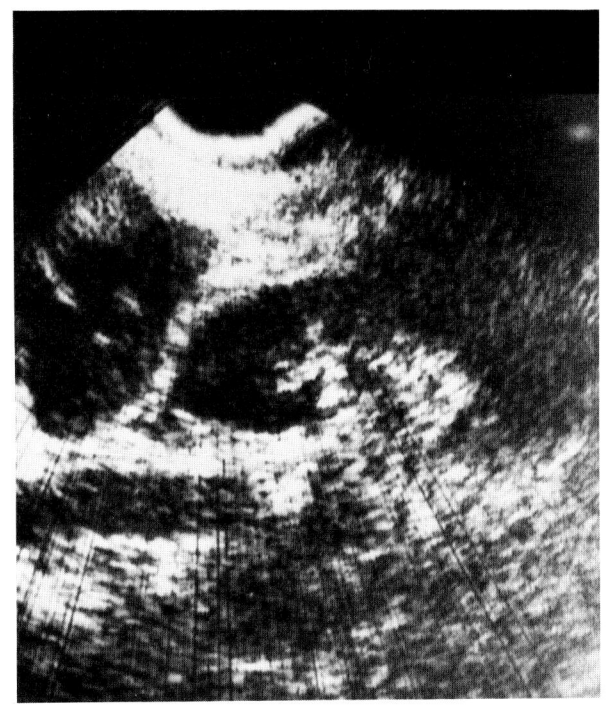

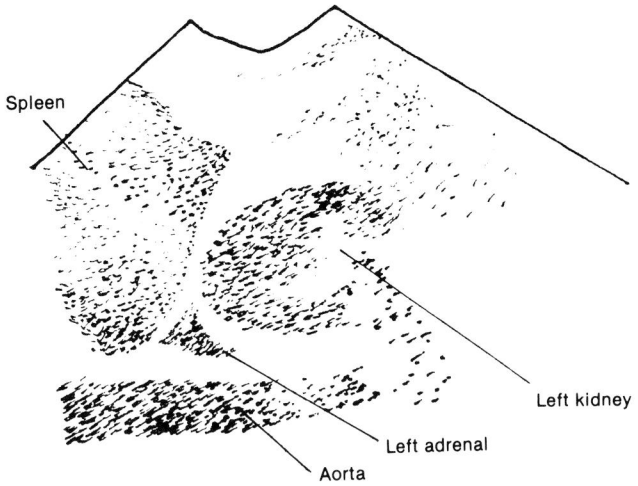

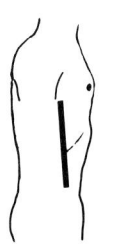

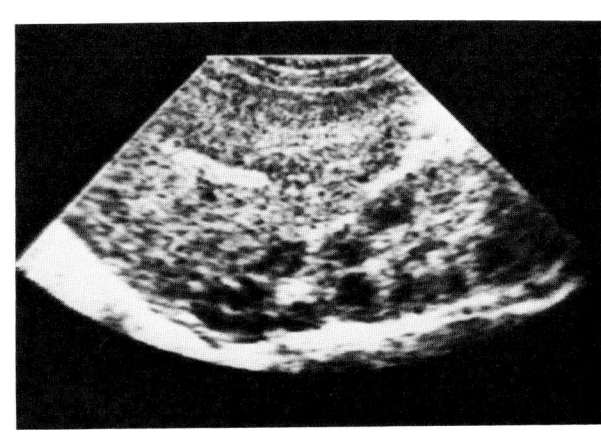

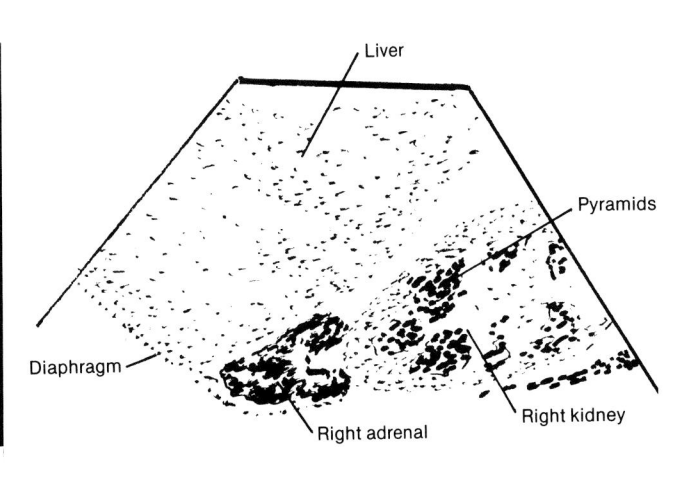

A

B

Hemorrhage (13.2 and 13.3)

13.2 Bilateral Hemorrhage

The hematocrit in a newborn infant dropped following a spontaneous vaginal delivery; ultrasonography was performed to exclude renal vein thrombosis. A longitudinal sonogram of the left flank (Fig. A) shows an echo-poor mass between the left kidney and the spleen. A longitudinal scan of the right flank shows a similar but smaller mass (Fig. B). The kidneys themselves are normal.

Adrenal hemorrhage in the newborn generally is attributed to blunt trauma. Clinical signs include a decrease in hematocrit and neonatal jaundice. Sonography is ideal for rapidly identifying this complication; although the kidneys may be displaced, they will be normal in texture. In the presence of a hematoma, the normally triangular adrenal, with echogenic central medulla and more echo-poor cortex, becomes enlarged and rounded and has a complex echo pattern within it. The mass begins to resolve within the first few days; calcification frequently occurs, and may be seen as early as 10 days after trauma.

SUGGESTED READINGS

Mineau DE, Koehler PR: Ultrasound diagnosis of neonatal adrenal hemorrhage. AJR 132:443–444, 1979

Lawson EE, Teele RL: Diagnosis of adrenal hemorrhage by ultrasound. J Pediatr 92:423–426, 1978

Pery M, Kaftori JK, Bar-Maor JA: Sonography for diagnosis and follow-up of neonatal adrenal hemorrhage. J Clin Ultrasound 9:397–401, 1981

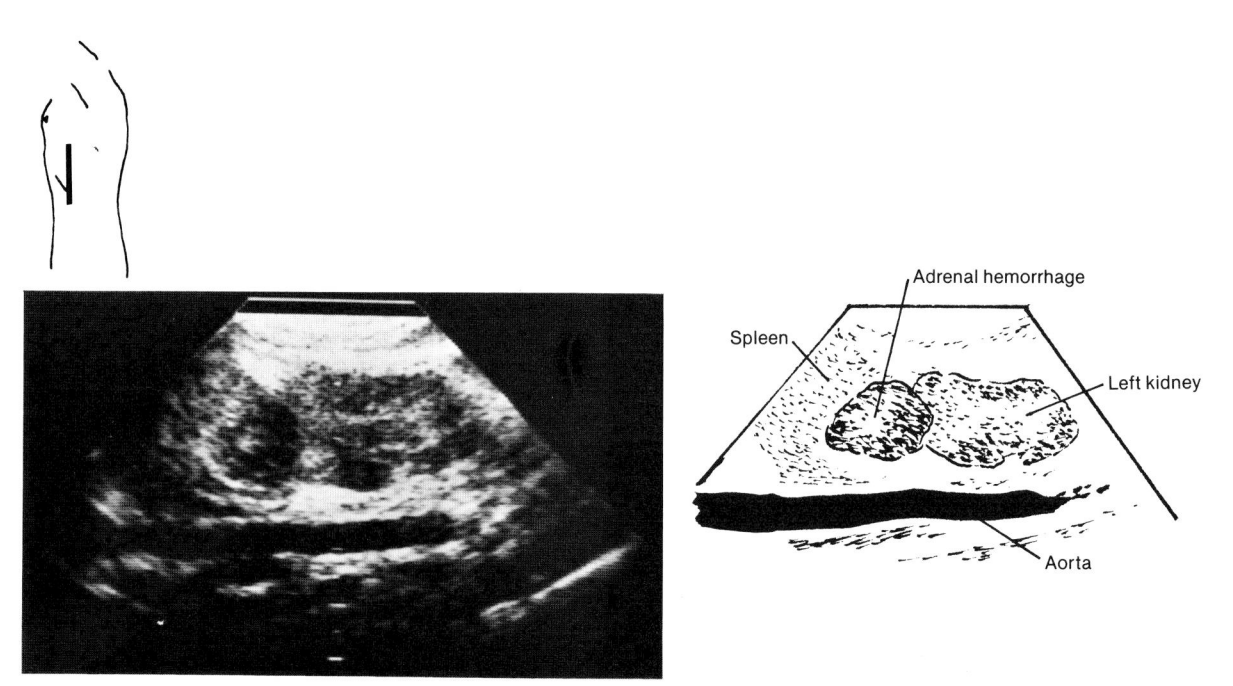

A

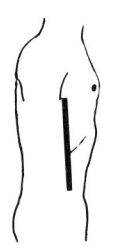

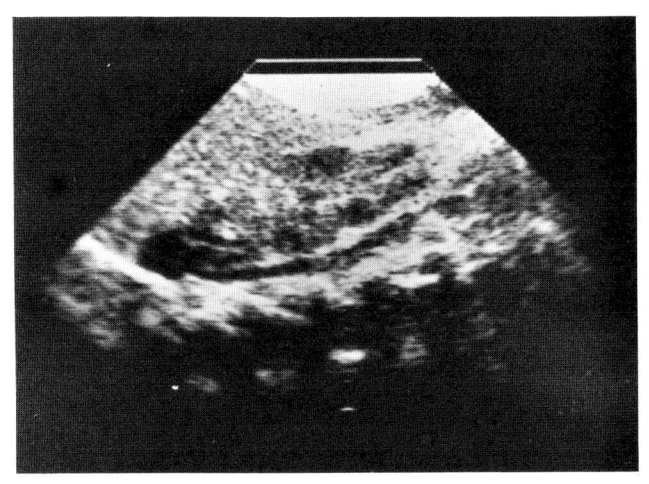

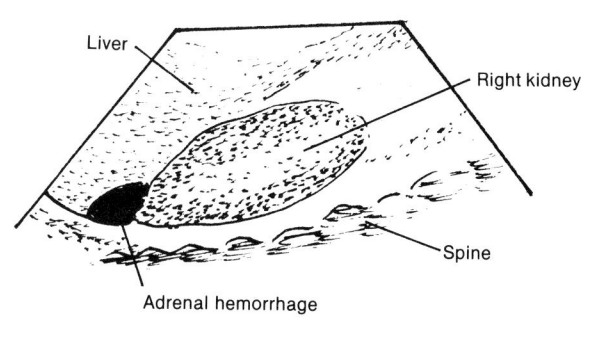

B

13.3 Infected Neonatal Hemorrhage

A 5-week-old infant presented with fever and bilateral palpable upper abdominal masses. An excretory urogram (Fig. A) demonstrates bilateral distortion of the collecting systems by masses above or in the upper portions of the kidneys. A longitudinal sonogram through the right upper quadrant (Fig. B), demonstrates a mass which is complex in nature impinging upon the liver (L) and inseparable from the upper portion of the right kidney (K). A coronal scan through the left upper quadrant (Fig. C) shows a mass in a similar position between the spleen (S) and left kidney (K). An acoustic shadow (R) is noted. Computed tomography demonstrates these masses to be fluid-filled (Fig. D).

The differential diagnosis of such masses includes bilateral duplicated collecting systems with obstruction to the upper pole moieties (and presumably pyonephrosis in light of the fever and debris), bilateral neuroblastomas, bilateral renal abscesses, and infected adrenal hematomas. Since the patient had pyuria and fever, the findings are not consistent with neuroblastomas. Infection of the upper pole moieties of duplicated collecting systems with the debris representing pyonephrosis is possible, but the absence of dilated ureters on the sonogram makes this diagnosis unlikely. Adrenal hemorrhage is a typical cause of bilateral abdominal masses in the newborn, but this type of lesion normally would be expected to have resolved by 5 weeks of age. However, infected hematomas would lead to persistent masses and this is the most likely diagnosis. At surgery, adrenal hemorrhage with bilateral secondary infection was identified.

(Figs. A–D from Gonzalez-Gomez R, Richman AH, Taylor KJW, et al: Urinary tract ultrasonography. pp. 29–52. In Finberg HJ, (ed): Case Studies in Diagnostic Ultrasound, Clinics in Diagnostic Ultrasound, Vol. 9. Churchill Livingstone, New York, 1981.)

SUGGESTED READINGS

Eklöf O, Grotte G, Jorulf H, et al: Perinatal hemorrhagic necrosis of the adrenal gland. Pediatr Radiol 4:31–36, 1975

Gonzalez Gomez R, Richman AH, Taylor KJW, and Rosenfield AT: Urinary tract ultrasonography. pp. 29–52. In Finberg JH (ed): Case Studies in Diagnostic Ultrasound, Clinics in Diagnostic Ultrasound, Vol 9. Churchill Livingstone, New York, 1981

Lawson EE, Teele RL: Diagnosis of adrenal hemorrhage by ultrasound. J Pediatr 92:423–426, 1978

Mineau DE, Kohler PR: Ultrasound diagnosis of neonatal adrenal hemorrhage. AJR 132:443–444, 1979

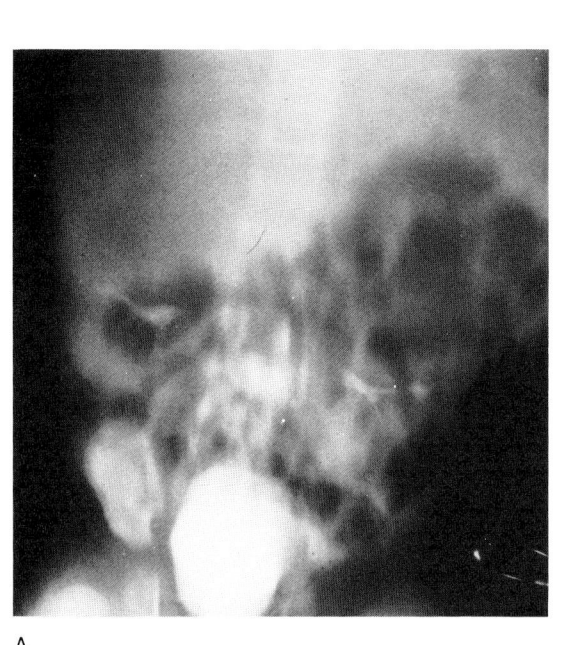

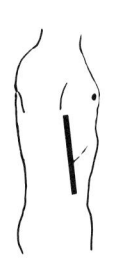

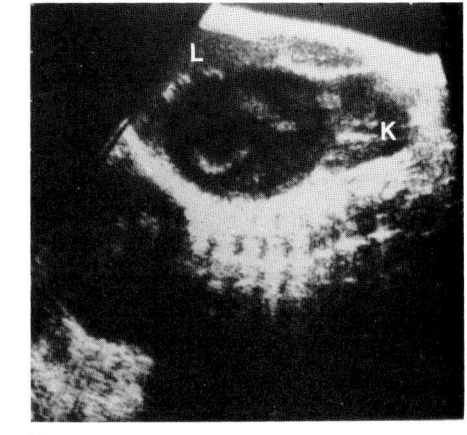

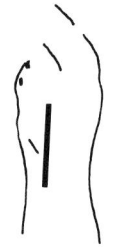

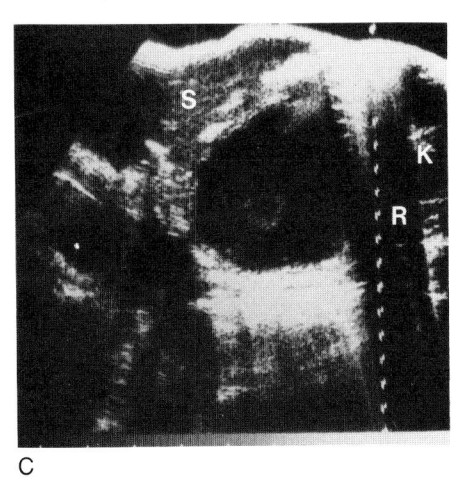

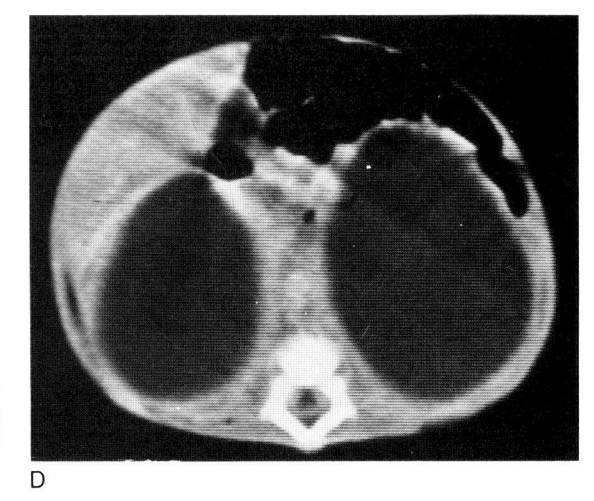

A

B

C

D

13.4 Myelolipoma

A 71-year-old woman with known cervical carcinoma was referred for staging. A large, echogenic mass was discovered in the right suprarenal position (Fig. A). The CT scan (Fig. B) revealed a mass of low attenuation (-25 to -83 Hounsfield Units) confirming the fatty nature of the tumor. The mass was asymptomatic and remained unchanged in size and appearance on a follow-up examination 7 months later.

The combination of a highly echogenic mass on ultrasound and low attenuation numbers in the range of fat on CT allows a presumptive diagnosis of myelolipoma of the adrenal gland. In addition, note the distal displacement of the diaphragm behind the mass due to the low propagation speed of sound through fat (Fig. A). This allows a diagnosis to be made by ultrasound alone.

Myelolipoma is a rare, nonfunctioning benign tumor of the adrenal gland. It is composed of varying proportions of fat and bone marrow elements. When lipomatous elements predominate, a presumptive diagnosis can be made by ultrasound. If the patient is asymptomatic, surgery can be avoided.

(This case and figures taken from Richman TS, Taylor KJW, Kremkau FW: Propagation speed artifact in a fatty tumor (myelolipoma): significance for tissue differential diagnosis. J Ultrasound Med 2:45–47, 1983.)

SUGGESTED READINGS

Behan M, Martin EC, Muecke EC, et al: Myelolipoma of the adrenal: two cases with ultrasound and CT findings. Am J Roentgenol 129:993–996, 1977

Fink DW, Wurtzeback LR: Symptomatic myelolipoma of the adrenal. Radiology 134:451–452, 1980

Plaut A: Myelolipoma in the adrenal cortex (myeloadipose structures). Am J Pathol 34:487, 1958

Richman TS, Taylor KJW, Kremkau FW: Propagation speed artifact in a fatty tumor (myelolipoma): significance for tissue differential diagnosis. J Ultrasound Med 2:45–47, 1983

Scheible W, Ellenbogen PH, Leopold GR, et al: Lipomatous tumors of the kidney and adrenal: apparent echographic specificity. Radiology 129:153–156, 1978

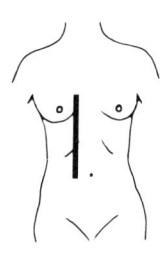

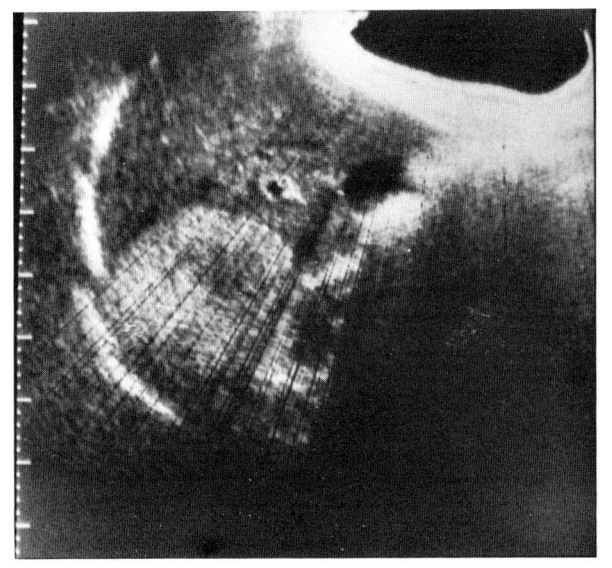

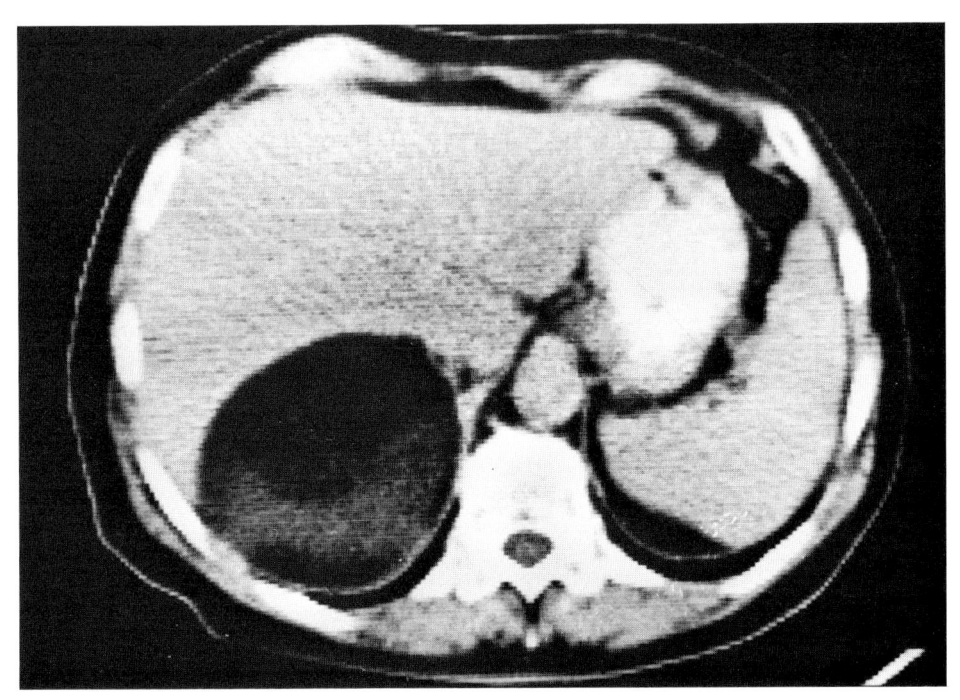

A

B

939

13.5 Pheochromocytoma

Coronal scans through the right upper quadrant in a patient with hypertension demonstrate a mass between the liver, kidney, and inferior vena cava as seen in the figure. The mass contains low-level echoes consistent with a solid tumor. A well-defined junction between the adrenal mass and the renal cortex without distortion of corticomedullary definition suggests that the origin of this lesion probably is extrarenal. Results of urine studies demonstrated abnormal vanillyl-mandelic acid (VMA) levels consistent with a pheochromocytoma.

Pheochromocytomas are solid and may be homogeneous or heterogeneous on sonography. Hemorrhage may lead to hyper- or hypoechoic areas, and necrosis may cause hypoechoic regions. Pheochromocytomas are tumors of the adrenal medulla although approximately 15 percent may be extra-adrenal, arising wherever chromaffin tissue is found. These tumors are catecholamine-producing lesions and may produce a distinctive clinical syndrome characterized by hypertension in young patients. An increased incidence of pheochromocytomas is associated with neurofibromatosis and with a familial syndrome characterized by a parathyroid hyperfunction and medullary carcinoma of the thyroid (Sipple's syndrome). In these two syndromes, the pheochromocytomas are almost always multiple.

Approximately 90 percent of extra-adrenal pheochromocytomas are below the diaphragm. Because of this, and the possibility of multiple tumors particularly in the familial syndromes, both adrenal areas, the retroperitoneum, and the true pelvis including the bladder should be examined when urinary catecholamine levels are elevated.

(Scan from Rosenfield AT, Taylor KJW, Crade M: Anatomy and pathology of the kidney by gray scale ultrasound. Radiology 128:737–744, 1978.)

SUGGESTED READINGS

Bernardino ME, Goldstein HM, Green B: Gray scale ultrasonography of adrenal neoplasms. AJR 130:741, 1978

Bowerman RA, Silver TM, Jaffe MH, et al: Sonography of adrenal pheochromocytomas. AJR 137:1227–1231, 1981

Rosenfield AT, Taylor JKW, Crade M: Anatomy and pathology of the kidney by gray scale ultrasound. Radiology 128:737–744, 1978

Yeh HC: Sonography of the adrenal glands: normal glands and small masses. AJR 135:1167–1177, 1980

Yeh HC, Mitty HA, Rose JS, et al: Ultrasonography of adrenal masses: usual features. Radiology 127:467–474, 1978

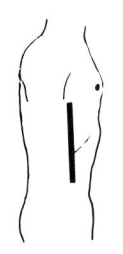

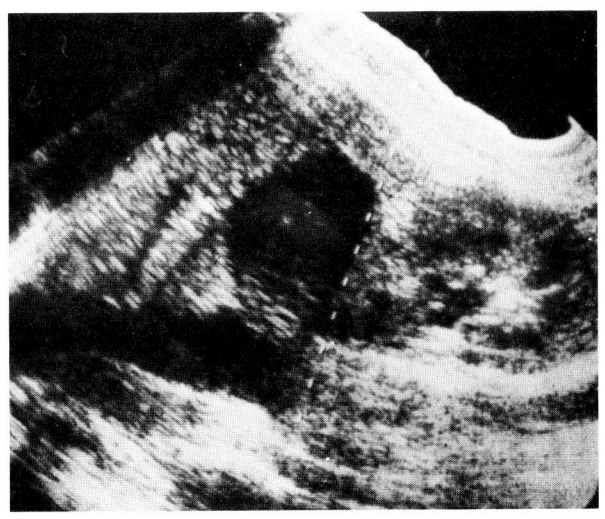

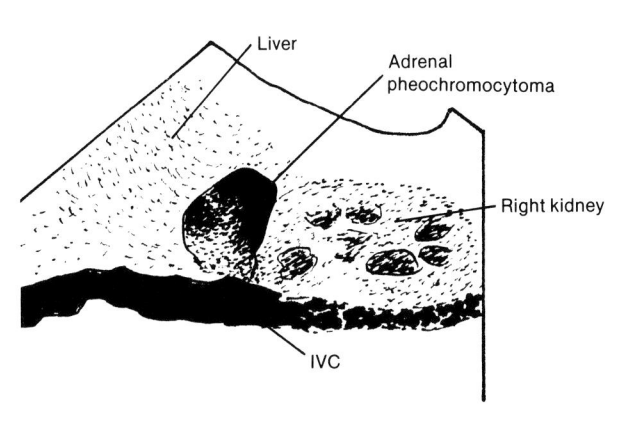

Liver

Adrenal pheochromocytoma

Right kidney

IVC

941

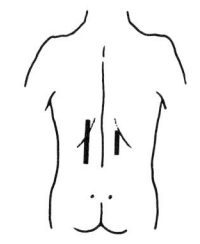

13.6 Neuroblastoma

A 4-month-old child presented with a palpable mass in the left upper quadrant. The coronal section through the left upper quadrant shown here demonstrated a 6-cm lesion above the left kidney. The mass contained irregular high-level echoes representing calcification, and was clearly solid with focal cystic areas. In a child, a solid lesion in the suprarenal area must be considered a neuroblastoma until proven otherwise. Subsequent surgery demonstrated neuroblastoma of the left adrenal.

Neuroblastoma is the most common solid abdominal mass in children. Approximately one-third of cases are seen within the first year of life and the frequency then decreases exponentially. The tumor is a malignancy that arises from embryonic sympathetic neuroblast. Approximately 37 percent of these lesions occur in the adrenal gland. Calcification of the tumor is common, and may be seen in metastases from the lesion as well. Sonographically, the lesion tends to be a mixture of high and low-level echoes, in contrast to Wilms' tumor, which tends to be more homogeneous except for areas of necrosis. Calcification within the neuroblastoma appears as a punctate zone of echogenicity with acoustic shadowing, as seen in the figure. This is an important diagnostic point since calcification is much more common in neuroblastoma than in Wilms' tumor, which is the other common solid abdominal tumor in infants and children.

SUGGESTED READINGS

Berger PE, Kuhn JP, Munshauer RW: Computed tomography in the diagnosis and management of neuroblastoma. Radiology 128:663–667, 1978

Gilchrist GS, Tank ES: Tumors of the adrenal medulla and sympathetic chain. pp. 975–989. In Kelais PP, King LR (eds): Clinical Pediatric Urology. WB Saunders Co., Philadelphia, 1976

White SJ, Stuck KJ, Blane CE, et al: Sonography of neuroblastoma. AJR 141:465–468, 1983

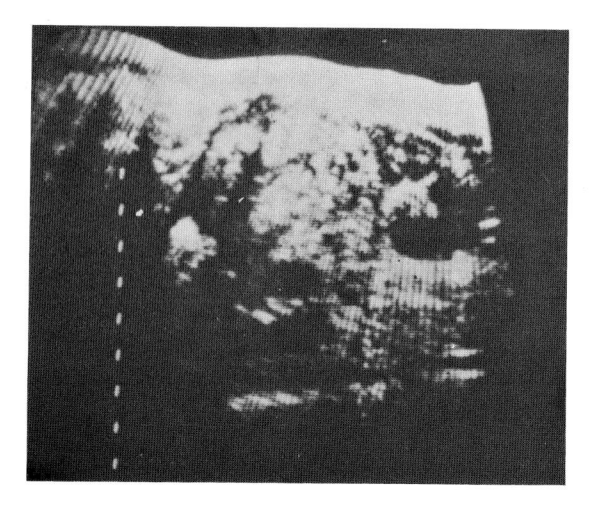

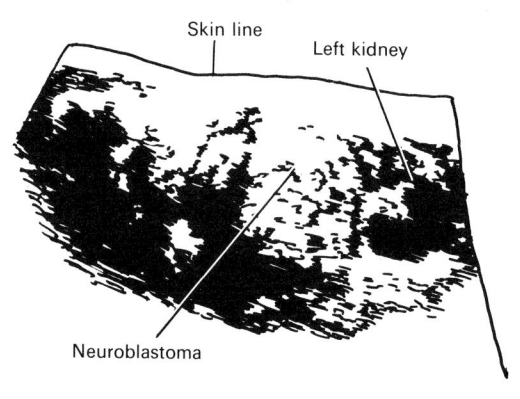

13.7 Metastases

Metastases to the adrenal gland are common in disseminated malignancy of many types. Bronchogenic carcinoma frequently metastasizes to the adrenal. Figure A is a chest radiograph in an elderly man demonstrating a perihilar mass due to bronchogenic carcinoma with associated right upper lobe collapse. In Figure B, a transverse scan through the liver, a solid mass extends behind the cava and the adjacent liver. Figure C is a sonogram at a lower level showing extension of the mass anterior to the right kidney. A coronal scan through the left upper quadrant (Fig. D) demonstrates an adrenal mass between the spleen and kidney which is defined as separate from both organs by the echogenic fat between the structures. The masses in the abdomen are consistent with solid adrenal masses and typical of adrenal metastases from the patient's known bronchogenic carcinoma.

Figure E is a longitudinal sonogram through the right upper quadrant in a 58-year-old woman who presented with a 3-month history of vaginal bleeding. Urinary tract work-up demonstrated a tumor of the urethra. A sonogram of the abdomen revealed a solid adrenal mass on the right side which proved to be a metastasis.

SUGGESTED READING

Forsythe JR, Gosink BB, Leopold GR: Ultrasound in the evaluation of adrenal metastases. J Clin Ultrasound 5:31–34, 1977

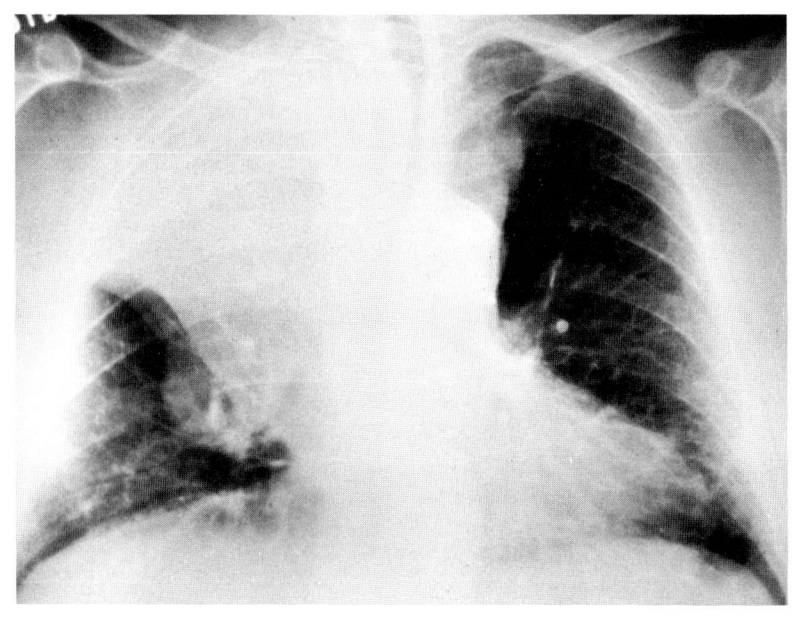

A

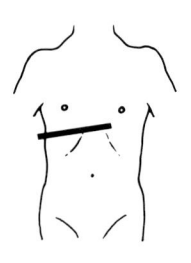

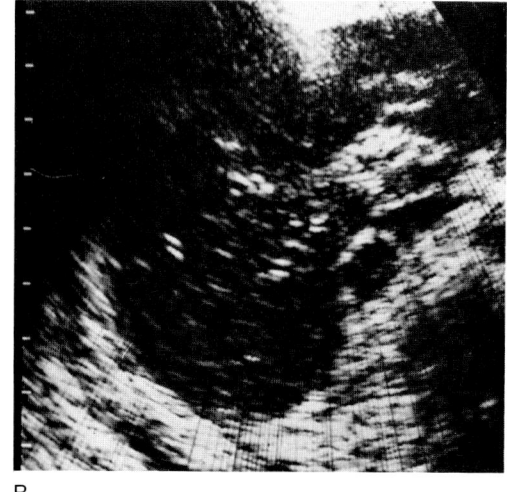

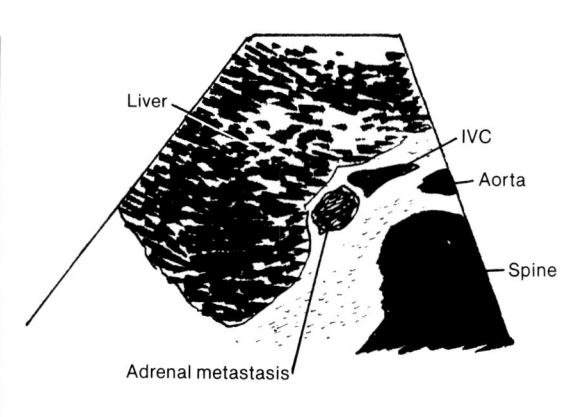

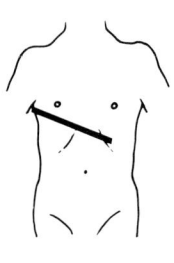

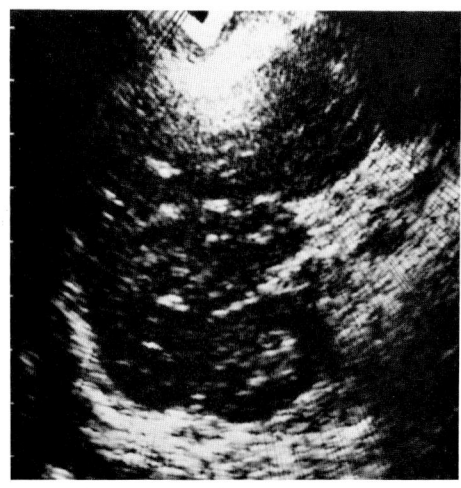

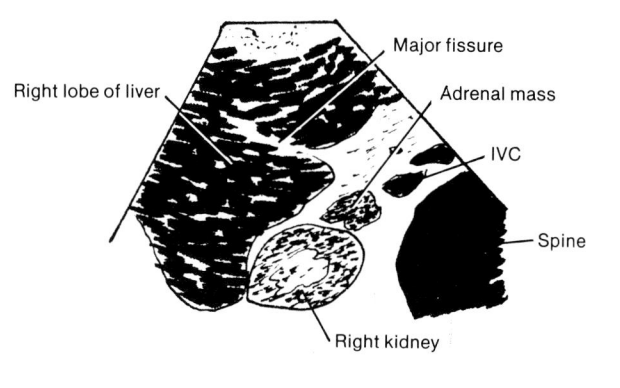

B

C

944

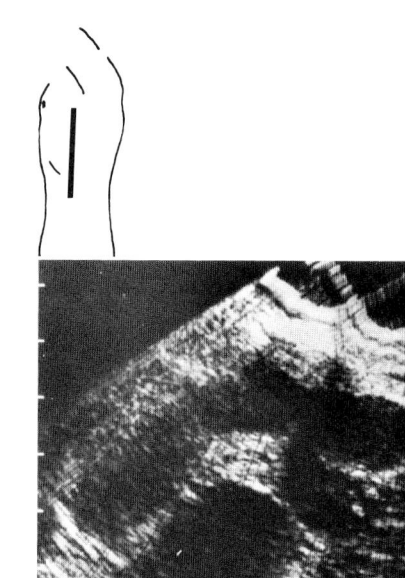

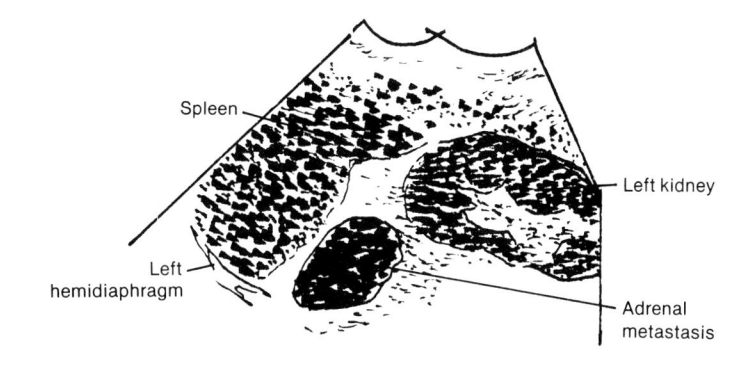

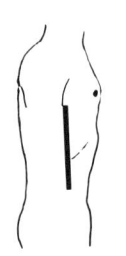

D

Spleen
Left hemidiaphragm
Left kidney
Adrenal metastasis

E

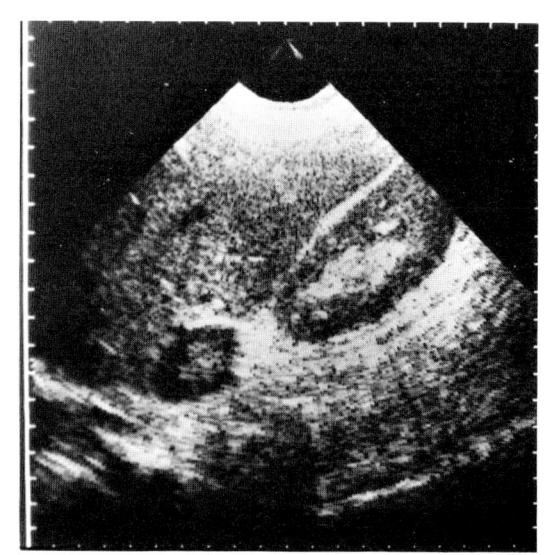

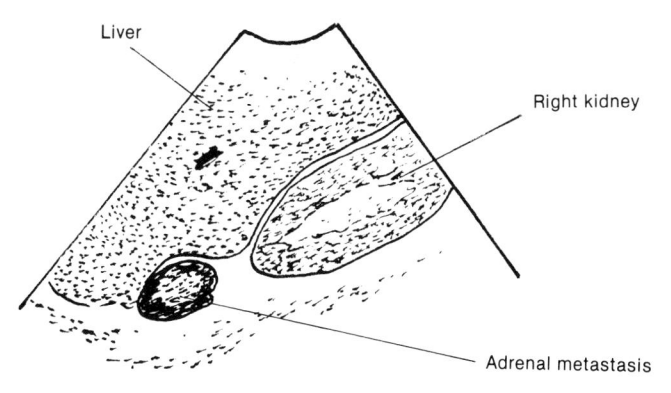

Liver
Right kidney
Adrenal metastasis

14 The Prostate

G. J. GRIFFITHS, W. B. PEELING, K. T. EVANS,
and E. E. ROBERTS

14.1 Indications for Scanning

ADVANTAGES OVER DIGITAL PALPATION

Digital palpation of the prostate has some well-known limitations, particularly for detecting prostatic cancers considered on clinical grounds to be confined within the prostatic capsule (stage B; stages T1/2). Clinical experience has shown that digital assessment is particularly unreliable for accurate diagnosis and localization of stage B cancers because they simulate prostatic calculi and areas of chronic prostatitis; and accurate staging of stage B cancers: 25 percent of those tumors assessed clinically as stage B have already broken through the capsule.[1] Stage B prostatic cancers are much less commonly encountered in clinical practice than invasive or metastatic tumors. However, since they are potentially curable either by excision with total prostatectomy or by eradication with an external beam or interstitially placed irradiation, any inaccuracy in diagnosis or staging would be particularly detrimental to the management of men with this type of disease. Incidentally diagnosed prostatic cancer (stage A; stage TO), detected microscopically from resected or enucleated adenomatous tissue, may be more common than previously believed.[2] By definition, this type of prostatic cancer is not diagnosed preoperatively by digital palpation.

Estimations of prostatic size by digital palpation can be unreliable particularly if the patient is obese or uncooperative. As clinical evaluation is a subjective method of measuring the prostate, attempts to monitor changes in size in response to treatment of prostatic cancer render comparisons difficult especially when assessed by different clinicians at different times.

Urologists have, therefore, been extremely interested in the development of methods of imaging the prostate which can overcome the limitations inherent in digital evaluation of the prostate. They welcome an objective means to:

1. Detect subclinical prostatic cancer which cannot be palpated (stage A; stage TO)
2. Differentiate cancer from benign conditions in nodules or areas of induration that simulate malignancy on digital palpation (stage B; stages T1/2)
3. Distinguish cancers confined to the prostatic capsule (stage A/B; stages TO/1/2) from those exhibiting local invasion (stage C; stages T 3/4)
4. Measure prostatic volume in initial and sequential examinations to monitor response to treatment, particularly of cancer

In cases where a prostatic cancer can be felt to be infiltrating the prostatic capsule or seminal vesicles, per rectal digital examination gives as much information as ultrasonic scanning.[3]

ANATOMY

Anatomically, the prostate has three main features:

1. Its capsule, which separates it from adjacent pelvic tissue and defines its margins
2. The urethra and periurethral glandular and

stromal tissue, which are anteriorly and superiorly placed
3. The glandular and stromal tissue of the bulk of the prostate, which is the functional part of the gland and lies outside the periurethral structures

The relation of the prostate to the surrounding organs is shown schematically in Figure A from the posterior aspect. The dotted B–B1 line shows the plane of section for Figure B. This scan shows a normal prostate which has a crescent shape in cross-section. The capsule appears intact at all levels and the internal echoes are, in general, homogeneous. Complete homogeneity of the parenchyma is rare. The urethra is rarely identified. The bull's eye posteriorly is the transducer in the rectum. Figure C shows the urethra and periurethral glandular and stromal tissue as a low-amplitude halo around an echogenic central area on the anterior aspect of the gland. The remainder of the glandular and stromal tissue has a homogeneous echo pattern.

Behind the upper part of the prostate (P) and the bladder neck are the seminal vesicles (S) in Figure A. These communicate with the vasa deferentia (V) to form the ejaculatory ducts which travel through the prostate to enter the urethra at the level of the veru montanum. These ducts are not generally visualized on per rectal scanning. The seminal vesicles (S) are demonstrated as curvilinear echo-free areas posterior to the bladder (B) in Figure D which is taken in the plane D–D1 in Figure A. However, at altered gain settings, it can be seen that the seminal vesicles (s) contain multiple low-amplitude echoes (Figure E).

Prostatic cancer, inflammatory disease, and calcification develop in peripheral zone tissue. These entities are shown schematically in Figure F. Therefore, all these conditions can be expected to lie outside the external margins of the periurethral zone elements or benign hyperplasia when present. In contrast, extensive benign nodular hyperplasia, shown schematically in Figure G, leads to compression of peripheral zone tissue in which an unsuspected carcinoma can develop. Similarly, prostatitis and calcification may occur here.

Any imaging technique will only arouse real interest among urologists if it is capable of representing the capsule of the prostate clearly as well as the seminal vesicles. It must also be able to demonstrate the internal architecture of the prostate in terms of periurethral structures as distinct from abnormalities in peripheral zone tissue. These are the criteria against which any imaging technique (or individual study) should be judged. Experience has shown that rectal ultrasound scanning gives the best results when compared with computed tomography, transabdominal ultrasound scanning,[4,5] or even the periurethral route.[6] The latter has been noted to cause some deformation of the periurethral part of the image due to the endoscope.[7]

(Fig. B from Brooman PJC, Griffiths GJ, Roberts EE, et al: Transrectal ultrasonography in the evaluation of cancer of the prostate. In Schulman CC (ed): Advances in Diagnostic Urology. Springer-Verlag, Berlin–Heidelberg–New York, 1981. Fig. D (scan) from Brooman PJC, Griffiths GJ, Roberts EE, et al: Per rectal ultrasound in investigation of prostatic disease. Clin Radiol, 32:669–676, 1981.)

REFERENCES

1. Byar DP, Mostofi FK, et al: Carcinoma of the prostate: prognostic evaluation of certain pathological features in 208 radical prostatectomies. Cancer 30:5–13, 1972
2. Chisholm GD, Beynon LL. The response of malignant prostate to endocrine treatment. p. 243 In Ghanadian R (ed): The Endrocrinology of Prostate Tumors. Lancaster, M.T.P. Press Limited, 1982
3. Brooman PJC, Griffiths GJ, Roberts EE, et al: Per rectal ultrasound in the investigation of prostatic disease. Clin Radiol 32:669–676, 1981
4. Sukov RJ, Scardino PT, Sample WF, et al: Computer tomography and transabdominal ultrasound in the evaluation of the prostate. J Comput Assist Tomogr 1:281–289, 1977
5. Richards D, Gowland M, Brooman PJC, et al: Computed tomography and transrectal ultrasound in the diagnosis of prostatic disease—a comparative study. Br J Urol 55:726–732, 1983
6. Gaamelgaard J, Holm HH; Transuretheral and transrectal ultrasonic scanning in urology. J Urol 124:863–868, 1980
7. Braeckman J, Denis L; The practice and pitfalls of ultrasonography of the lower urinary tract. Eur Urol 9:193–201 1983

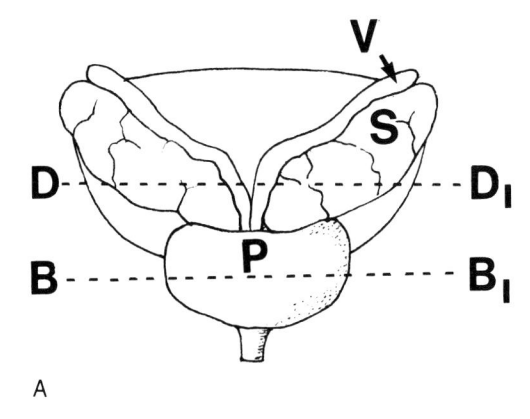

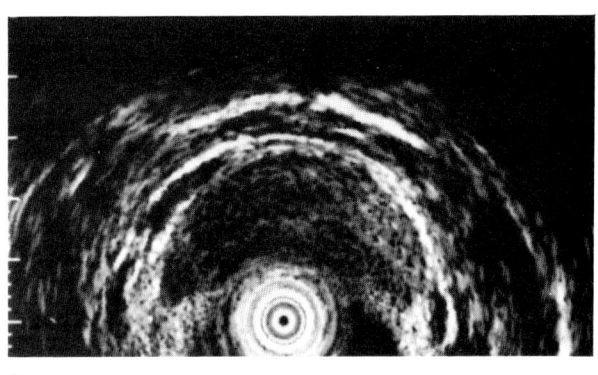

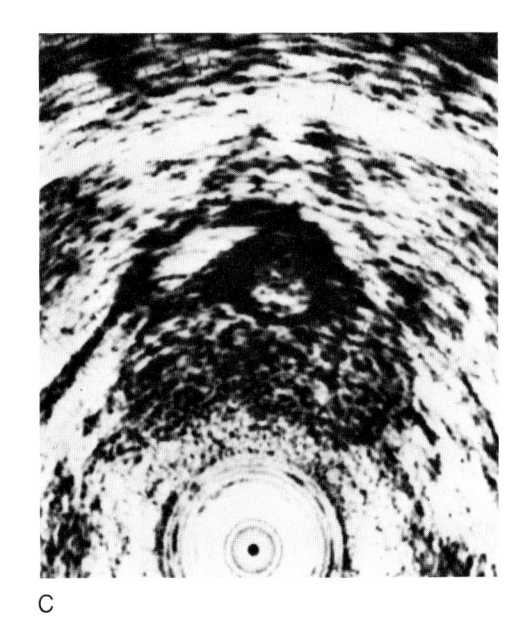

A

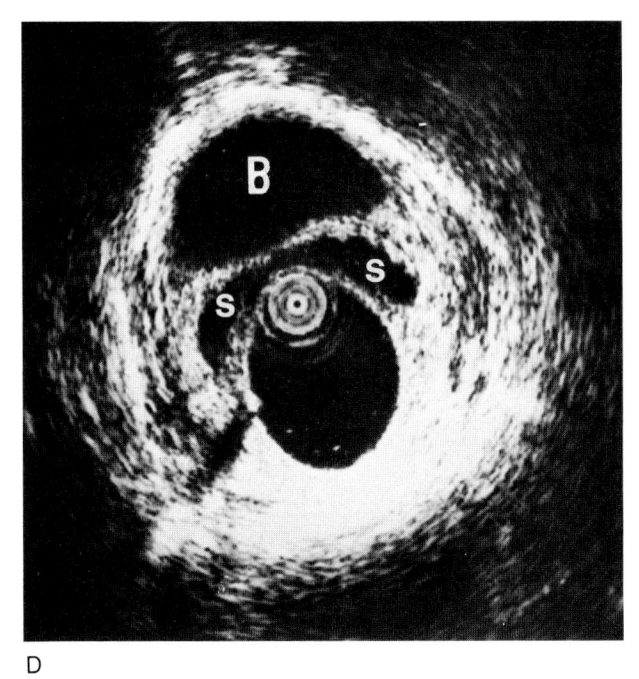

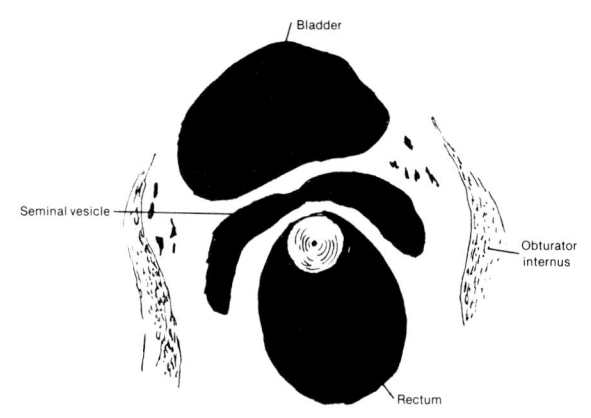

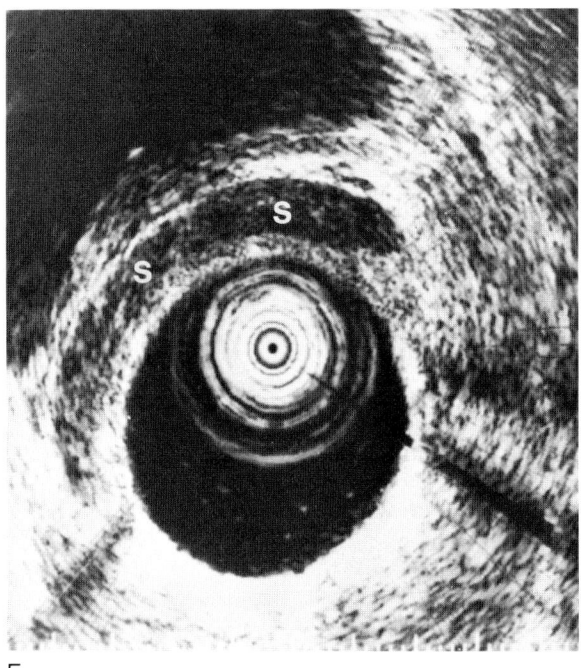

D

E

950

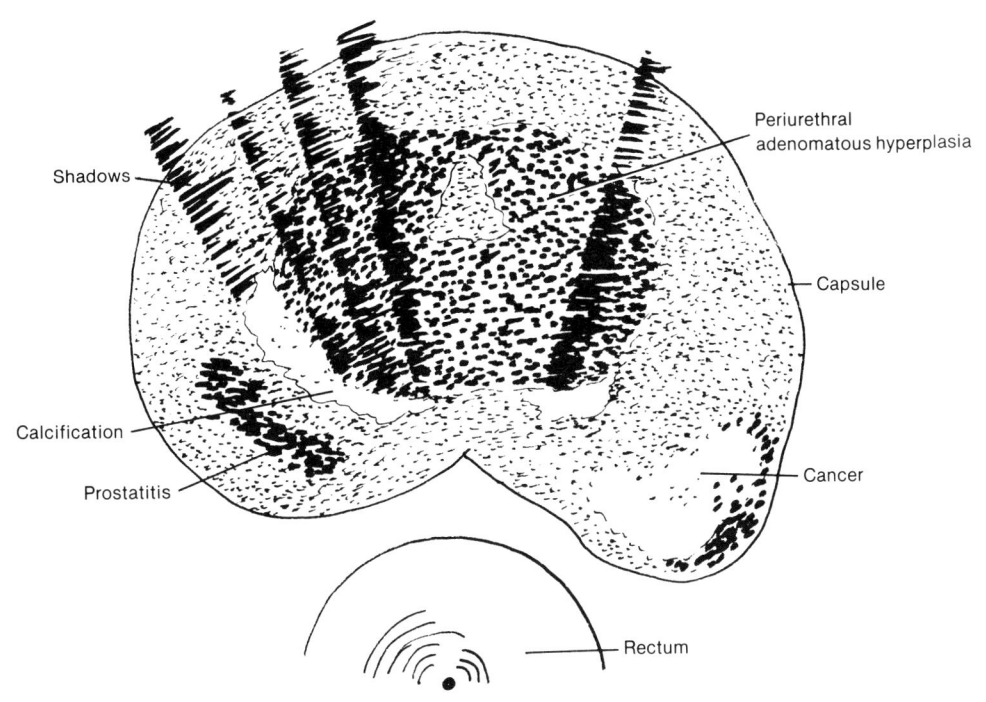

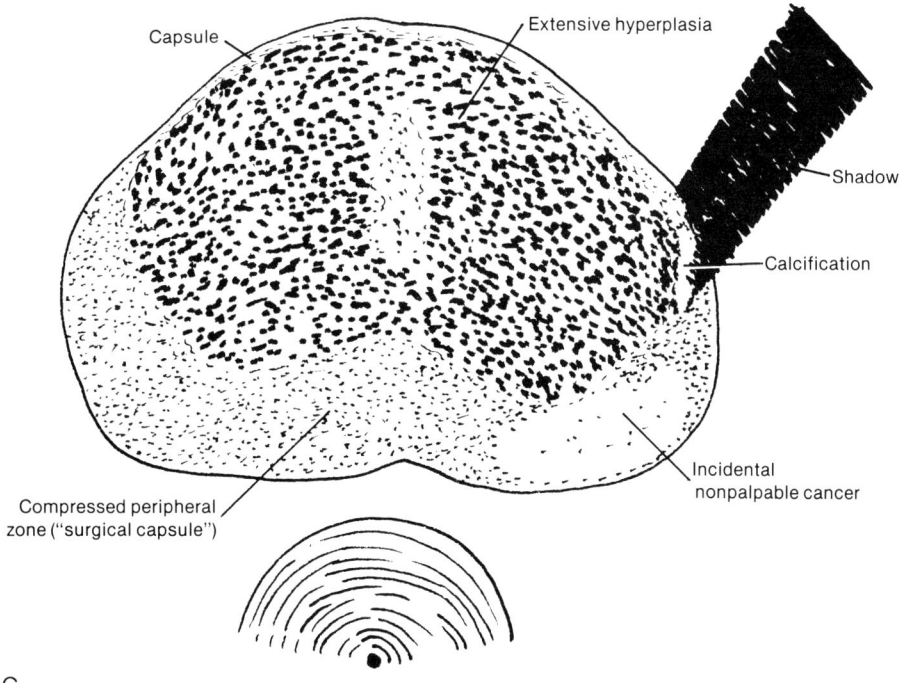

F

G

951

Benign Hyperplasia (14.2 and 14.3)

14.2 Nodular Hyperplasia

Benign nodular hyperplasia of the prostate develops in periurethral tissue and, as it enlarges, peripheral tissue becomes partially compressed around smaller adenomas. In Figure A the periurethral adenoma is seen anteriorly as an area of lower amplitude echoes (arrowed). The peripheral tissue is compressed posteriorly and laterally and appears as a more echogenic area. In large adenomas, the peripheral zone may be completely flattened (Fig. B). The prostate is now circular and the capsule intact. The gland is fairly homogeneous but the flattened periphery is just visible posteriorly as a slightly more echogenic rim of tissue (arrowed). Adenomatous tissue may be multinodular in texture but it essentially involves stromal fibromuscular tissue mixed with glandular elements. Small concretions called corpora amylacea may be present in adenomatous tissue.

(Fig. B from Brooman PJC, Griffiths GJ, Roberts EE, et al: Transrectal ultrasonography in the evaluation of cancer of the prostate. In Schulman CC (ed): Advances in Diagnostic Urology. Springer-Verlag, Berlin—Heidelberg—New York, 1981.)

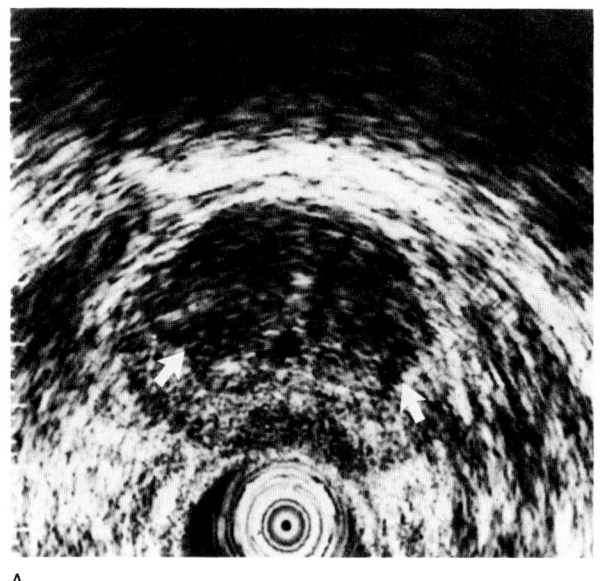

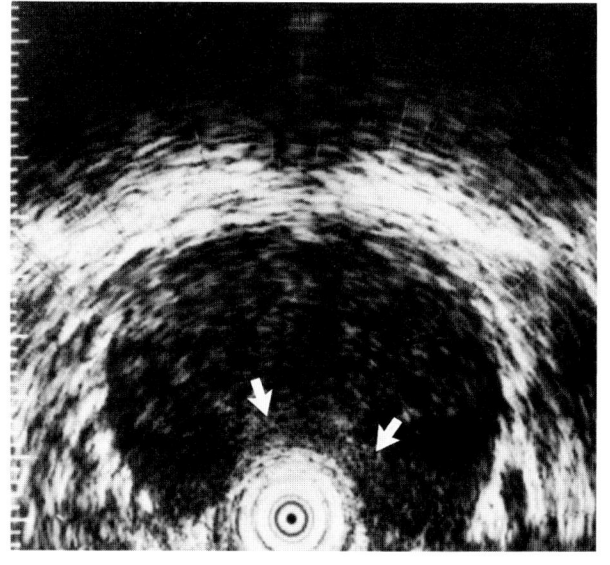

14.3 Benign Hyperplasia

A 65-year-old man presented with progressive hesitancy of micturition; a poor intermittent flow of urine that dribbled for several minutes at the end of voiding. There were no other urologic symptoms. Physical examination showed no general abnormalities and the prostate gland was judged, on digital palpation, to be enlarged due to benign prostatic hyperplasia.

This was confirmed by the sonogram (Fig. A) which shows the peripheral zone markedly compressed by large adenomas. The gland is rounded in shape and the capsule is intact. The large adenoma in the right lobe is clearly demarcated by an echo-free halo (arrowed).

Transurethral prostatectomy was carried out and the patient made an uneventful recovery. Histologically, the resected tissue showed the presence of benign nodular hyperplasia.

Figure B is another example of benign prostatic hypertrophy and demonstrates highly reflective calcifications (arrowed) appearing as a curvilinear area at the junction of the adenomatous tissue and the peripheral zone. This area is often referred to as the "surgical capsule." It provides a line of cleavage for enucleation of adenomas of the prostate. Calcification is rare in an adenoma but is most common in the peripheral zone near the junction with adenomas.

Calcification can occur anteriorly as shown in Figure C which also demonstrates distal acoustic shadowing (S). This should not be misinterpreted as an invasive carcinoma with an anterior breach of the capsule.

Figure D demonstrates the appearances of a gland with benign prostatic hyperplasia following transurethral resection. An echo-free area is seen in the center of the gland (arrowed) indicating the site of the transurethral resection.

(Fig. A from Brooman PJC, Griffiths GJ, Roberts EE, et al: Transrectal ultrasonography in the evaluation of cancer of the prostate. In Schulman CC (ed): Advances in Diagnostic Urology. Springer-Verlag, Berlin–Heidelberg–New York, 1981.)

954

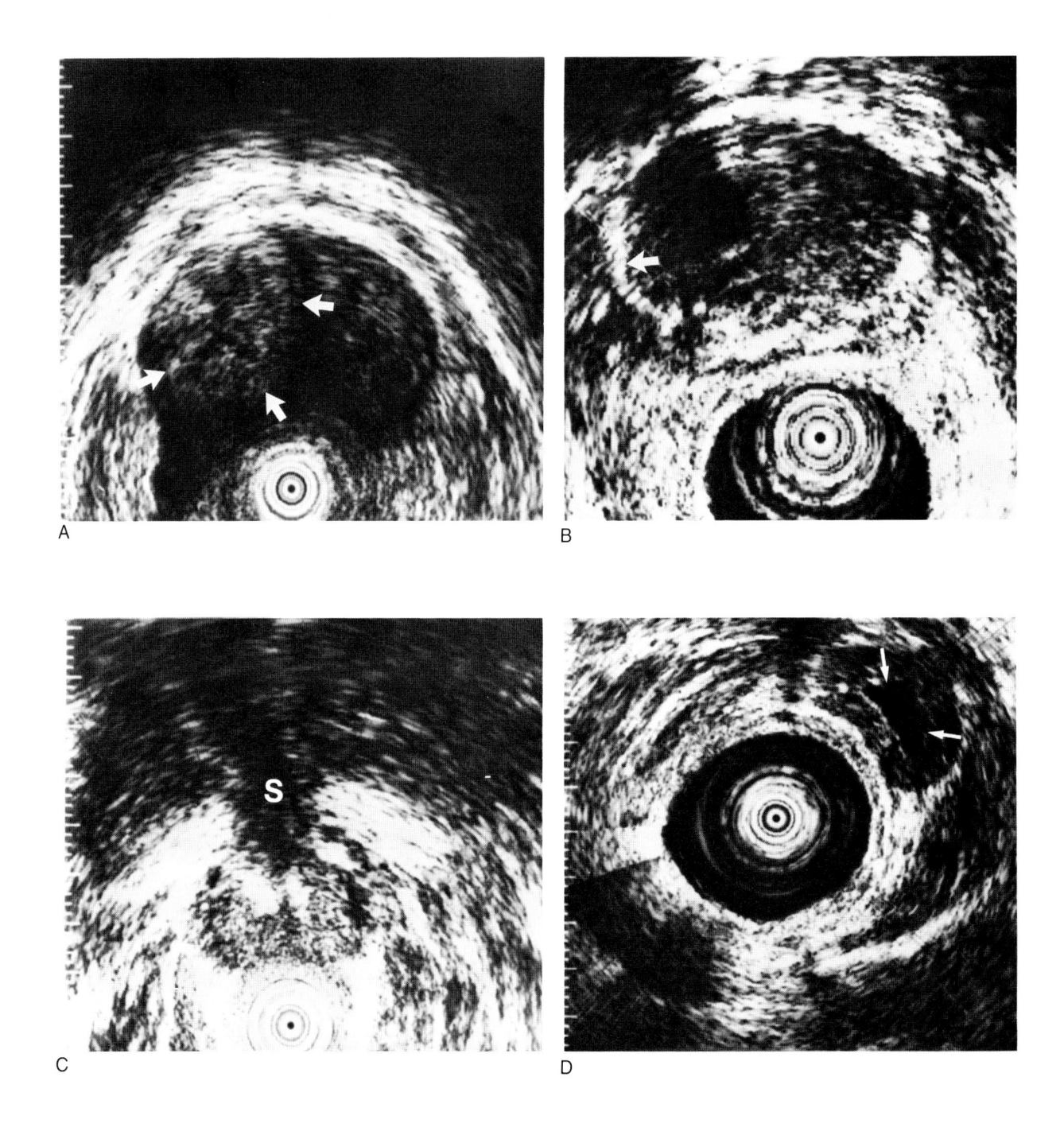

14.4 Bacterial and Nonbacterial Prostatitis

A 32-year-old man presented with terminal dysuria, frequency and urgency of micturition, with perineal aching; he also experienced penile and perineal pain on ejaculation. There was no history of urethral discharge. Palpation of the prostate indicated that it was mildly enlarged, rather boggy in consistency but had a number of tender indurated areas in its parenchyma. Expressed prostatic fluid had a pH of 8.0, and showed 15 white cells/high-power field. A diagnosis of nonbacterial prostatitis was made and the patient was treated with antibiotics with symptomatic relief.

Per rectal ultrasonography in bacterial and nonbacterial prostatitis shows three main features. The first is a heterogeneous echo pattern with multiple areas of low amplitude echoes in the gland parenchyma (Fig A). The appearances suggest multiple focal areas of prostatic infection. The prostatic capsule is ill-defined.

Tubular echo-free areas (arrowed in Figure B) are also seen adjacent to the prostate and extending from the anterior region of the gland around its lateral margins. These appearances are thought to be due to engorged and prominent veins in the prostatic venous plexus secondary to prostatic inflammation. Although the prostatic venous plexus is often demonstrated during per rectal ultrasonography, we have only seen the prostatic veins with this degree of prominence in prostatitis. Also demonstrated in this figure are areas with low-amplitude echoes, indicating inflammation, in the posterior parenchyma of the gland and as a halo in the periurethral area.

The third sign of prostatitis is shown in Figure 14.1C: the periurethral glandular and stromal tissue as a low-amplitude halo around a central echogenic area. We have seen this appearance in all proven cases of bacterial and nonbacterial prostatitis and we believe this to be a valid sign of prostatitis. However, others[1] only noted this appearance in 50 percent of their cases of prostatitis and also commented that it was visualized in 69 percent of normals. The specificity of this sign should, therefore, remain under review for the present.

REFERENCE

1. Harada K, Tanahashi Y, Igari D, et al: Clinical evaluation of inside echo patterns in gray scale prostatic echography. J Urol 124:216–220, 1980

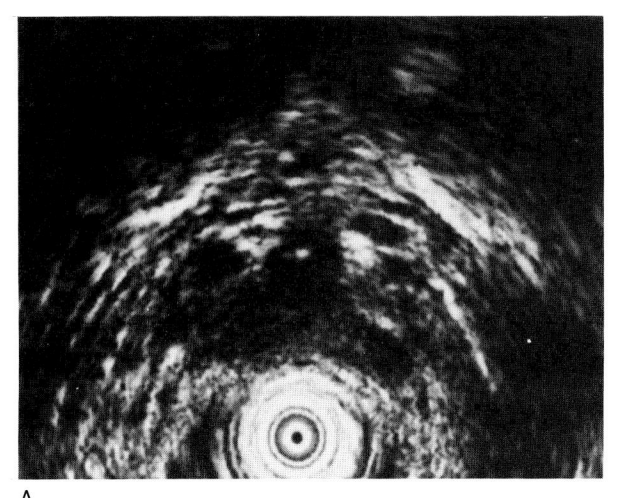

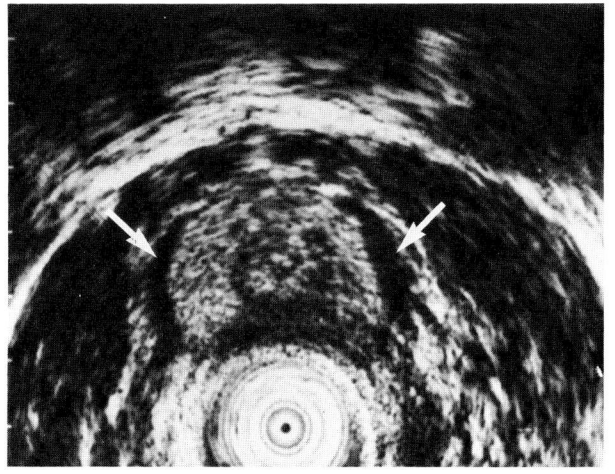

A

B

14.5 Cyst

A 45-year-old man injured his perineum and suffered subsequent pain and difficulty on micturition. Examination showed perineal bruising with prostatic tenderness on palpation. These features subsided but he experienced some residual difficulty in urination. Per rectal sonogram revealed a rounded echo-free area (arrowed in the figure) in the posterior part of the gland. Acoustic enhancement is seen anteriorly. The appearance is of a prostatic cyst thought to be due to the previous perineal trauma. We have seen two similar cysts in patients with a history of previous severe trauma to the perineum.

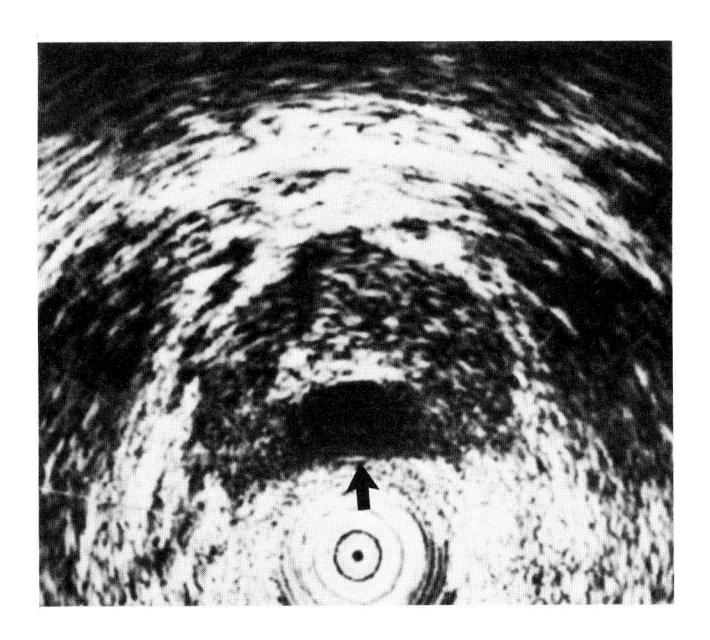

Cancer (14.6 to 14.10)

14.6 Incidental Cancer (Stage A)

A 70-year-old man presented with acute retention of urine after 3 years of varying but progressively difficult micturition. On admission to hospital, his bladder was grossly enlarged and painful, and after catheterization the prostate was felt on digital examination to be enlarged (50 g) due to benign prostatic hyperplasia. Per rectal ultrasonography was carried out to check the volume of the prostate so that a decision between transurethral or open prostatectomy could be made preoperatively. The figure shows a periurethral adenoma of benign prostatic hyperplasia which appears as the low-amplitude area (white arrows). However, an area showing increased echogenicity (black arrow) is in the left lobe of the prostate peripheral and lateral to the adenoma. At operation this area was biopsied with a Trucut needle and the adenoma was resected transurethrally. Histologically, a moderately differentiated adenocarcinoma of the prostate was confirmed from the needle biopsy specimen. Some of the transurethral chippings from the left posterior part of the prostatic capsule indicated an infiltrating tumor. Further investigations showed no metastatic disease; the patient was treated by external beam radical radiotherapy to the prostate.

This patient's cancer was not detected preoperatively by digital palpation but its presence was suggested by ultrasonography. It is likely that only the more developed incidental cancers (stage A2) are detectable ultrasonically since focal incidental cancer (stage A1) is a microscopic process which does not appear to produce detectable acoustic abnormalities.[1]

REFERENCE

1. Harada K, Tanahashi Y, Igari D, et al; Clinical evaluation of inside echo patterns in gray scale prostatic echography. J Urol 124:216–220, 1980

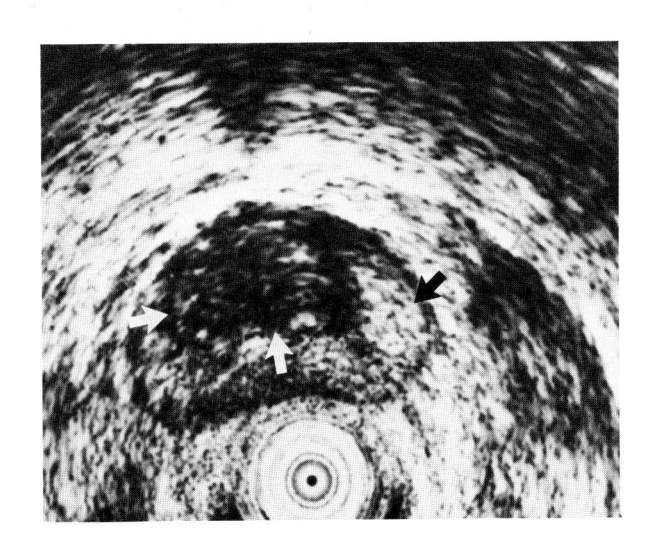

14.7 Clinically Confined Disease (Stage B: Stages T1/2)

A 55-year-old man presented having had two episodes of hemospermia; he had no difficulty urinating or other symptoms. On physical examination, the only abnormality was a hard nodule in the left lobe of the prostate which was considered on digital palpation to be a confined carcinoma (stage B). The diagnosis was proved by perineal Trucut needle biopsy and the clinical staging of the tumor was confirmed by rectal ultrasonography. Figure A demonstrates asymmetry of the gland: the left lobe is larger than the right due to the nodule. The gland has a heterogeneous echo pattern but the capsule, although distorted, is intact at all levels. These appearances confirm the presence of a confined carcinoma (stage B). The patient was treated by radical external beam irradiation to the prostate and has survived 4 years without further problems.

Despite this patient's presenting symptoms, hemospermia is an uncommon presentation of prostatic cancer.

A 61-year-old man presented with acute retention of urine after a 3-month period of increasing hesitancy, poor flow, urgency, and some suprapubic pain. On physical examination, the relevant abnormality was a tense painful bladder and, after catheterization, the prostate was felt to be hard, enlarged, and somewhat irregular in contour. A clinical diagnosis of carcinoma of the prostate was made but the tumor was considered on clinical grounds to be confined within the prostatic capsule (stage B). The diagnosis was confirmed by Trucut needle biopsy via the perineum. Per rectal sonogram (Fig. B) showed an unexpected capsular discontinuity anterolaterally (arrowed). The site of this defect was not accessible to digital palpation and it was inferred that this tumor, although apparently confined within the prostate on digital palpation, was actually infiltrating the capsule at a digital "blind spot." The patient was treated with radial external beam radiotherapy to the prostate but 18 months later developed overt metastatic disease.

Unexpected ultrasound evidence of capsular discontinuity is a bad prognostic sign particularly when extensive, as in this patient. Capsular discontinuity probably means that a prostatic cancer is locally invasive. Preliminary studies on cadaveric prostates show close correlation between interpretation of per rectal ultrasound features with histologic diagnosis and staging of prostatic cancer.[1]

(Fig. B from Brooman PJC, Griffiths GJ, Roberts EE, et al: Transrectal ultrasonography in the evaluation of cancer of the prostate. In Schulman CC (ed): Advances in Diagnostic Urology. Springer-Verlag, Berlin–Heidelberg–New York, 1981.)

REFERENCE

1. Brooman PJC, Griffiths GJ, Roberts EE, et al: Per rectal ultrasound in the investigation of prostatic disease. Clin Radiol 32:669–676, 1981

960

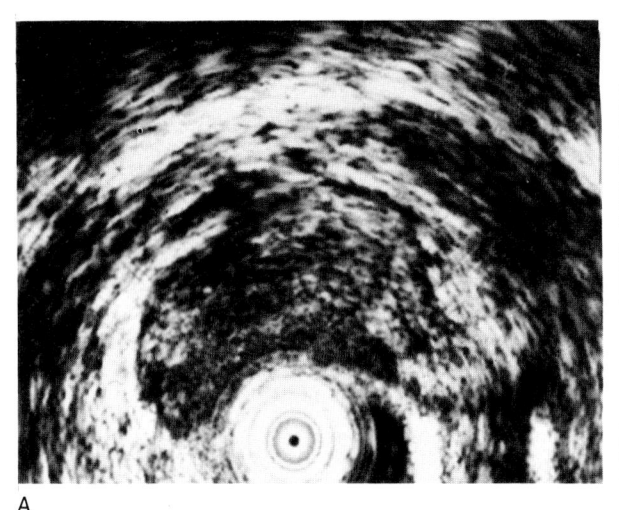

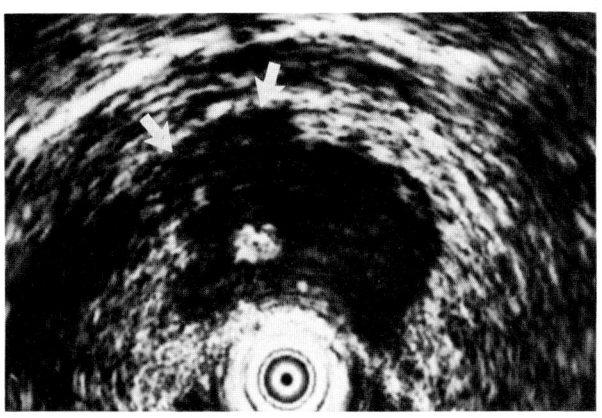

14.8 Invasive Cancer (Stage C; Stages T3/4)

A 72-year-old man had experienced mild bladder outflow symptoms for many years, but he presented with a rapidly worsening urinary flow associated with pain in the perineum, some blood-stained mucoid rectal discharge, and general malaise with weight loss. On examination, he looked ill, pale, and cachectic. On rectal examination, the prostate and anterior rectal wall were indurated, hard, and irregular and it was difficult to decide whether rectal or prostatic cancer was present. Prostatic cancer was confirmed by perineal Trucut needle biopsy and clinically the tumor was considered to be stage C (stage T4). Per rectal sonogram confirmed the presence of prostatic cancer with extensive extracapsular spread of the tumor, as shown in the figure. The gland has a heterogeneous echo pattern, particularly in its posterior part. The capsule is grossly distorted both anteriorly and on the left posterolateral aspect (arrowed), indicating a widespread breach of the capsule. Other investigations indicated the presence of metastatic disease. The patient was treated by transurethral prostatectomy to relieve bladder outflow problems, and bilateral subcapsular orchidectomy to treat the prostatic cancer. This was followed by regression of the primary tumor and the rectal symptoms.

(Figure from Brooman PJC, Griffiths GJ, Roberts EE, et al: Per rectal ultrasound in the investigation of prostatic disease. Clin Radiol 32:669–676, 1981.)

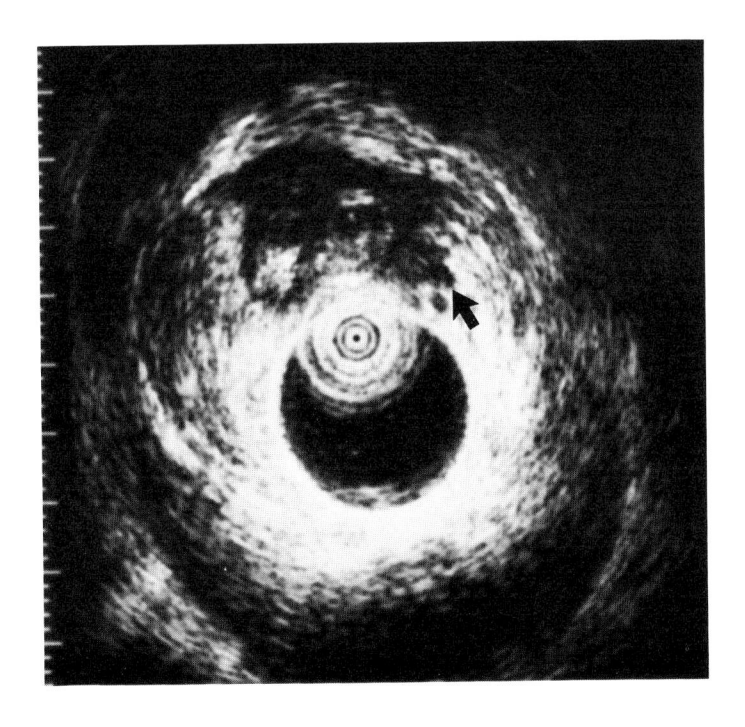

14.9 Monitoring Disease

A 68-year-old man presented with symptoms related to a large clinically confined stage B prostatic cancer. These features agreed with the findings from rectal ultrasonography. In Figure A, a large rounded gland (arrowed) is seen with a heterogeneous internal echo pattern. The capsule is intact and the estimated weight of the gland was 82.5 g. The diagnosis was confirmed histologically by perineal Trucut needle biopsy. The patient also had demonstrable metastatic disease and was treated by bilateral subcapsular orchidectomy. Clinically, the disease regressed and regression of the primary tumor was measurable ultrasonically. The sonogram shown in Figure B was taken 8 months after treatment and shows a marked decrease in size and change in shape of the prostate gland (arrowed; estimated weight 27 g). The internal echo pattern was still heterogeneous with an echogenic area in the right lobe. Calcification was seen posteriorly as an area of highly reflective echoes.

A 73-year-old man presented with symptoms related to a carcinoma of the right lobe of the prostate which, on digital assessment, was considered to be confined to the capsule of the prostate (stage B1). The diagnosis was confirmed histologically by Trucut needle biopsy and the tumor was shown to be well-differentiated. Per rectal sonogram (Fig. C) shows increased echogenicity (arrowed) suggesting a carcinoma in the right lobe of the prostate. On some of the sonograms there was possible discontinuity of the capsule anterolaterally on that side. A policy of "deferred" treatment was adopted and the patient's condition was reviewed regularly in the outpatient clinic. Clinically, there was no change in the size or consistency of the primary tumor but a follow-up sonogram (Fig. D) 9 months after the initial visit showed undoubted capsular discontinuity at the previously suspicious site. It was inferred that these features indicated the presence of progressive disease that was not detectable digitally, and the patient was treated with radical radiotherapy to the prostate.

Monitoring prostatic cancer either to measure a response to active treatment or to supervise the progress of the patients undergoing "deferred" nonactive treatment has been shown to be of great potential value.[1,2] Similarly, clinical responses to treatment of some patients with bacterial and nonbacterial prostatitis have also been accompanied by reductions in volume of the prostate as measured ultrasonically (Griffiths GJ, Buck AC, Crooks AJR, et al: unpublished data, 1983).

REFERENCES

1. Peeling WB: Castration for prostatic carcinoma still an alternative form of treatment? pp. 127–128. In Schroder FH (ed): Androgens and Anti-Androgens. Weesp, Schering, Nederland. 1983
2. Carpentier PJ, Schroder FH, Blom JHM: Transrectal ultrasonography in the follow-up of prostatic carcinoma patients. J Urol 128:742–746, 1982

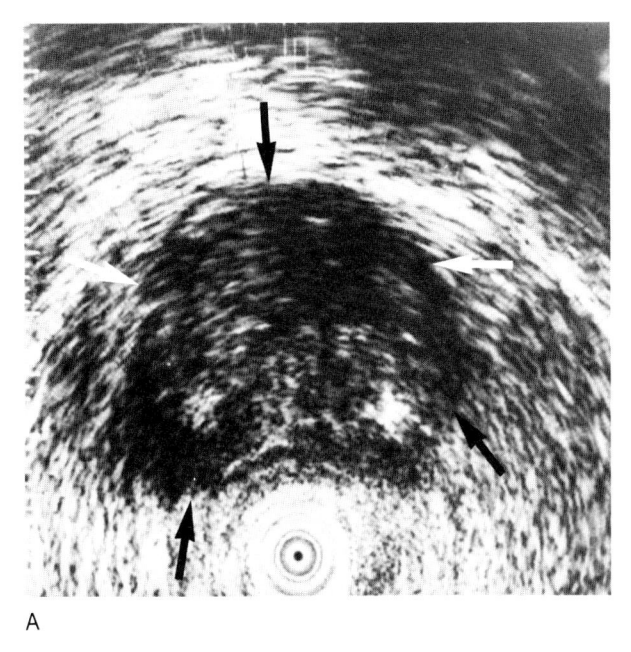

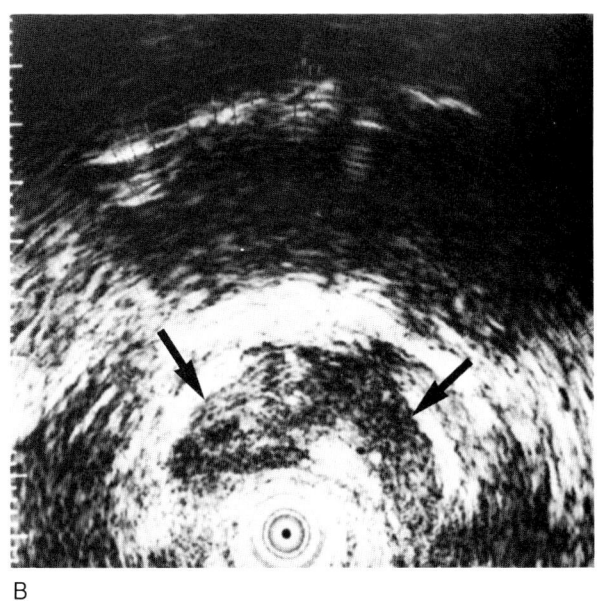

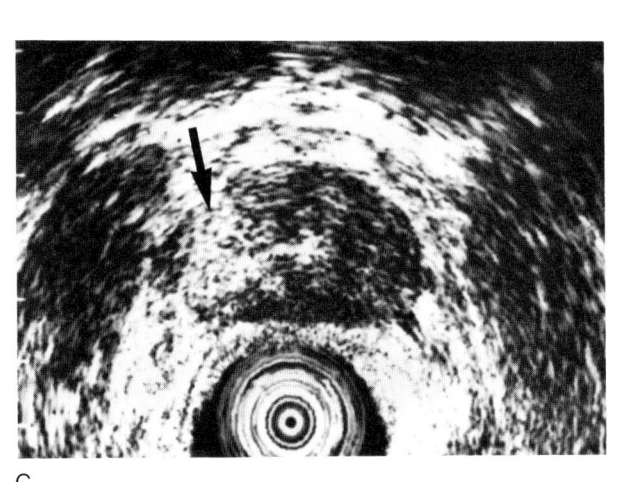

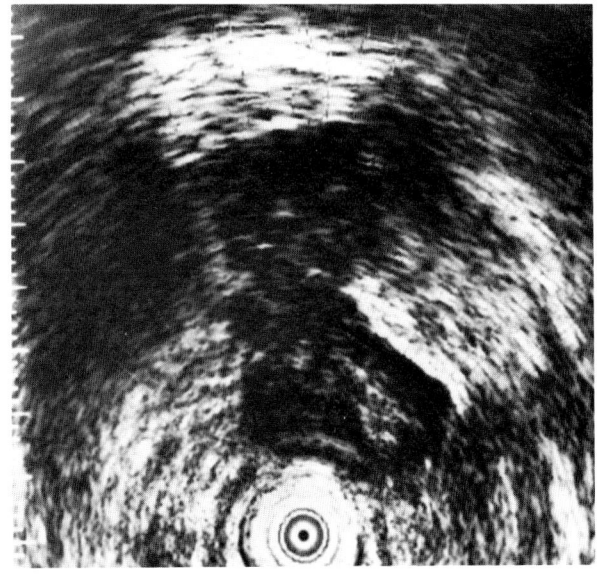

A

B

C

D

14.10 Incidental Bladder Cancer

Occasionally, an unsuspected bladder cancer is seen in the bladder base at the time of per rectal ultrasonography for suspected prostatic disease.

A 72-year-old man presented with difficulty micturating. There was no history of previous hematuria. On digital examination of the prostate, he was thought to have an irregular right lobe and ultrasound examination was requested.

Routine scanning of the bladder base, shown in the figure, revealed an unsuspected papillary carcinoma of the bladder (m) at the mouth of a bladder diverticulum. There is some irregularity of the bladder wall, suggesting local invasion.

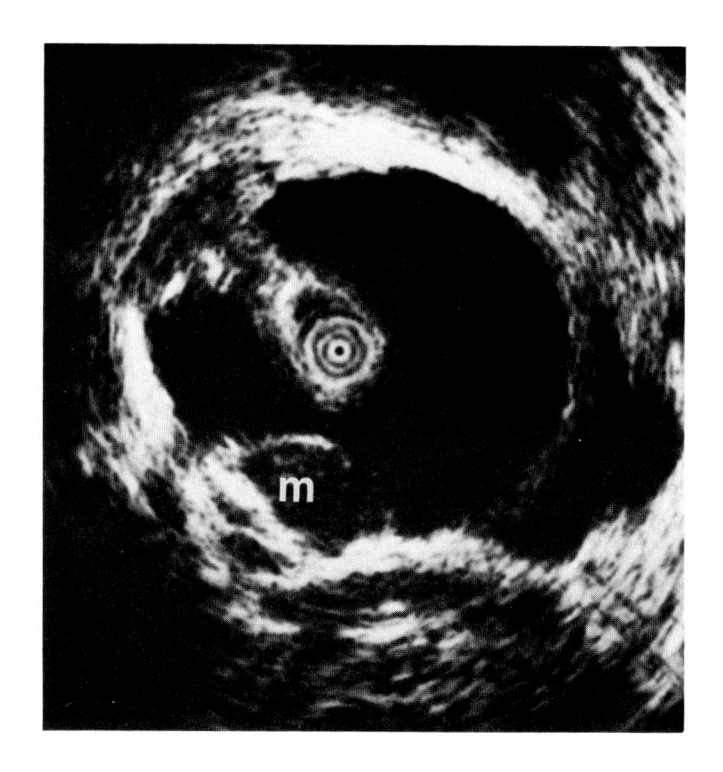

15 The Testes

C. WHITLEY VICK

High-resolution ultrasound study of the scrotal contents has proved to be a clinically efficacious method of evaluating suspected scrotal pathology. The technique entails negligible risk or discomfort, and it often complements other noninvasive diagnostic methods, including the physical examination and radionuclide scanning. Prognostic and management decisions can often be made on the basis of information provided by scrotal ultrasound.

INDICATIONS

Evaluation of a scrotal mass represents the most important and useful application of scrotal ultrasound. Even when the physical examination is limited by scrotal pain or swelling, ultrasound usually permits the presence of a mass to be confirmed and often provides precise anatomic localization of a scrotal lesion. Ultrasound may also be useful in evaluating scrotal trauma, nonresolving epididymo-orchitis, and orchalgia. A nonpalpable testicular tumor may be detected by ultrasound in a patient presenting with metastatic retroperitoneal lymph nodes or lung nodules. Finally, valuable information may be provided in selected patients with suspected testicular torsion.

INSTRUMENTATION

The scrotal contents can be successfully imaged with either dynamic or static gray-scale equipment. In general, dynamic scanning is less operator-dependent and requires slightly less time to complete a study than static scanning. However, static scanners have the advantage of being able to display a larger field of view than most dynamic scanners, allowing inclusion of the entire scrotal contents on one image.

For acceptable resolution, a high-frequency transducer (7.5-MHz or greater) should be used. Occasionally, it may be necessary to use a 5-MHz transducer to image a markedly swollen scrotum. High-frequency transducers appropriate for scrotal imaging may be purchased for use with most commercially available static and dynamic scanners.

To place the scrotal contents within the transducer's focal zone for optimum resolution, one may use either a short focal length contact transducer or a longer focal length transducer coupled to a water bath. Imaging of very superficial lesions is best achieved using a water bath, since even "short"-focused transducers (focal length 1–2 cm) are suboptimal.

EXAMINATION TECHNIQUE

Palpation of the scrotum is important to insure that the area of clinical suspicion is scanned, and the patient should be encouraged to help in localizing a small lesion. Gel is preferred as the coupling agent as it is easier to remove from the perineal area than mineral oil. Maintaining a thick coat of gel allows a more uniform contact over the irregularly rounded scrotal surface.

The patient is scanned in the supine position with a folded towel placed behind the scrotum. It may be helpful to tape the penis out of the way with gauze and a strip of tape. Stabilization of the scrotum is important. In some patients, the scrotum can be scanned satisfactorily without any specific external stabilization. The scrotum may also be stabilized by having the patient hold the ends of two folded towels, one in front of and the other behind the scrotum, immobilizing the scrotum between the two towels.[1] The examiner or patient may also stabilize the testis manually.

Longitudinal and transverse images of each hemiscrotum are made at approximately 5-mm intervals. An attempt should be made to image the long axis of the epididymis, a view which may be obtained by angling the transducer or gently rotating the testis to place its posterolateral surface in the field of view. If possible, a transverse view including both testes on one image should be made to compare the two sides for symmetry and echogenicity.

DIFFERENTIAL DIAGNOSIS OF A SCROTAL MASS

The ability to localize and characterize a scrotal mass by ultrasound is used to construct a differential diagnosis and, in some cases, provide a specific etiology for a scrotal mass. Sample et al.[2] classified scrotal lesions into three categories based on sonographic localization: testicular, extratesticular, or combined testicular and extratesticular (Table 15-1). This classification is useful because, in general, *extratesticular* lesions are likely to be benign and may often be managed medically.[2-4] (Exceptions to this generalization are discussed below.) On the other hand, *testicular* lesions may be benign or malignant, and most reports on scrotal ultrasound have indicated that it alone cannot reliably distinguish benign from malignant testicular disease.[2-4]

Acoustic characterization of a scrotal mass may also be prognostically useful. A totally cystic scrotal mass is almost always benign, often representing a hydrocele, spermatocele, or epididymal cyst. In addition, it has been our experience that a scrotal mass lesion which is homogeneously hyperechoic (relative to the testis) is likely to be benign, often representing scar.

Table 15-1. Differential Diagnosis of Scrotal Lesions Based on Ultrasound Localization

Extratesticular
  Epididymitis
  Spermatocele
  Epididymal cyst
  Hydrocele
  Varicocele
  Hematocele
  Paratesticular abscess
  Tumor: Adenomatoid
  Others: Mesothelioma, rhabdomyosarcoma, other sarcomas
Testicular
  Neoplasm
  Orchitis/abscess
  Torsion
  Granuloma
  Fracture/hematoma
Combined Extratesticular and Testicular
  Epididymitis and orchitis
  Epididymitis and neoplasm
  Hydrocele and orchitis or tumor
  Fractured testis and hematocele
  Hernia
  Torsion and epididymal swelling and/or hydrocele

REFERENCES

1. DiGiacinto TM, Pattne D, Willscher M, et al: Sonography of the scrotum. Med Ultrasound 6:95–101, 1982
2. Sample WF, Gottesman JE, Skinner DG, et al: Gray scale ultrasound of the scrotum. Radiology 127:225–228, 1978
3. Sample WF: Renal, adrenal, retroperitoneal and scrotal ultrasonography. pp. 276–279. In Sarti DA, Sample WF (eds): Diagnostic Ultrasound Text and Cases. G.K. Hall, Boston; 1980
4. Leopold GR, Woo VL, Scheible FW, et al: High resolution ultrasonography of scrotal pathology. Radiology 131:719–722, 1979

15.1 Normal Anatomy

The normal testis has a homogeneous, fine, granular echo texture, as illustrated in longitudinal (Fig. A) and transverse (Fig. B) sonograms made manually with a 7.5-MHz transducer. A longitudinal scan taken with the Picker Microview is shown in Figure C. The epididymis, extending longitudinally along the posterolateral surface of the testis, normally returns echoes equal to or greater in amplitude and coarser in texture than the testis. The head of the epididymis (globus major) can usually be seen capping the upper pole of the testis, and often a portion of the more narrow epididymal body can be visualized. The thin epididymal tail (globus minor) is infrequently visualized. The epididymis drains into the ductus deferens (vas) which is occasionally visualized as an echo-poor, tubular structure running longitudinally along the posteromedial aspect of the testis.

The scrotum, consisting of skin and dartos, and the various other tissue layers surrounding the testis are not individually imaged on ultrasound but instead are seen as an echogenic stripe several millimeters in thickness. The median raphe of the scrotum attenuates sound, causing an acoustic shadow between the testes on transverse images (arrowed, Fig. B).

A small amount of fluid is occasionally seen around the normal testis (Fig. C). The diagnosis of a hydrocele is usually not made unless there is enough fluid to cause palpable scrotal swelling.

The tunica albuginea, a fibrous membrane covering the testis, reflects into the testis as an incomplete longitudinal septum called the mediastinum testis which courses parallel to and identifies the location of the epididymis. The mediastinum serves as a support structure for vessels and ducts of the testis. Although the tunica albuginea is not seen separately on ultrasound, the mediastinum can sometimes be seen as a longitudinally oriented echogenic stripe in the testis near its posterolateral edge[1] (Fig. D). The mediastinum gives off numerous imperfect septa which divide the interior of the testis into a number of cone-shaped, incomplete lobules containing the sperm-producing seminiferous tubules and the hormonally active interstitial cells. The lobules are not separately identified on ultrasound, nor is the rete testis, an anastomosing network of sperm-conducting tubules within the mediastinum. At the upper pole of the testis, the vessels of the rete testis empty into multiple efferent ductules which conduct sperm from the testis to the epididymis.

Occasionally, small (1–2 mm), hyperechoic foci are seen within the normal testis[2] (arrowed, Fig. E). These are thought to be of no clinical significance, although their cause is unknown. The appendix testis (a mullerian duct remnant), the appendix epididymis (a detached efferent duct), and other less common small appendages are not usually seen, although occasionally one or more of these may be visualized when there is fluid around the testis.

REFERENCES

1. Wilson PC, Day DL, Valvo JR, Gramiak R: Scrotal scanning with an Octason™. RadioGraphics 1:24–39, 1982
2. Leopold GR, Wood VL, Scheible FW, et al: High-resolution ultrasonography of scrotal pathology. Radiology 131:719–722, 1979

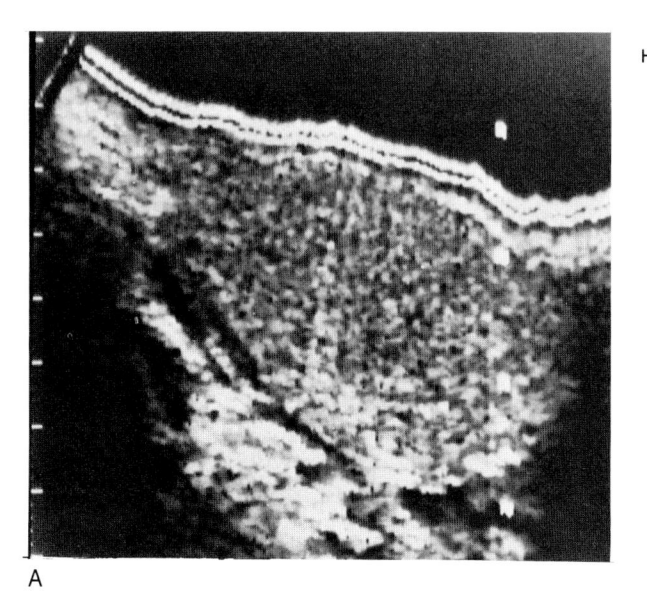

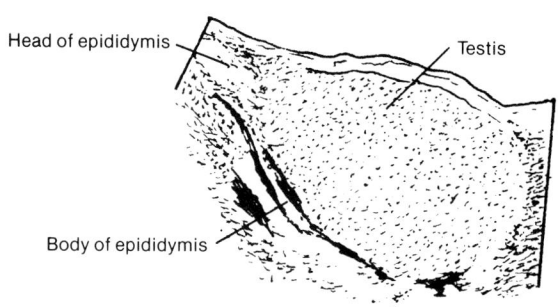

A

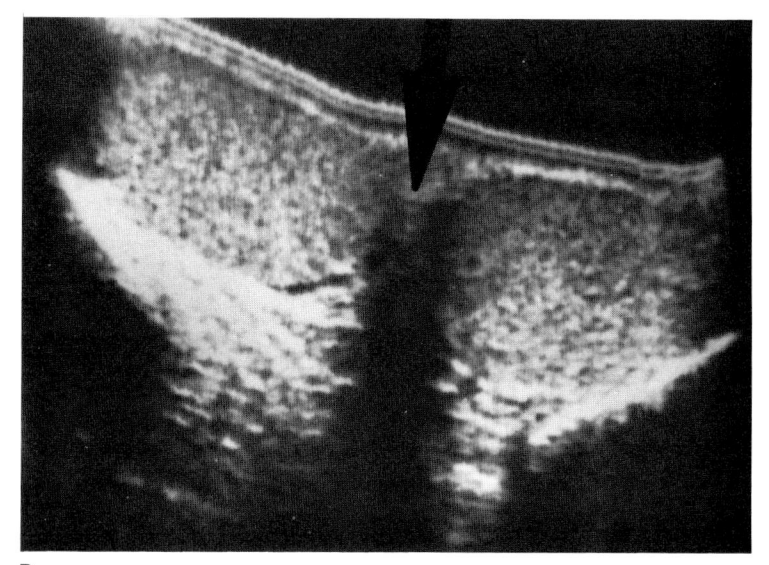

Head of epididymis — Testis
Body of epididymis

B

968

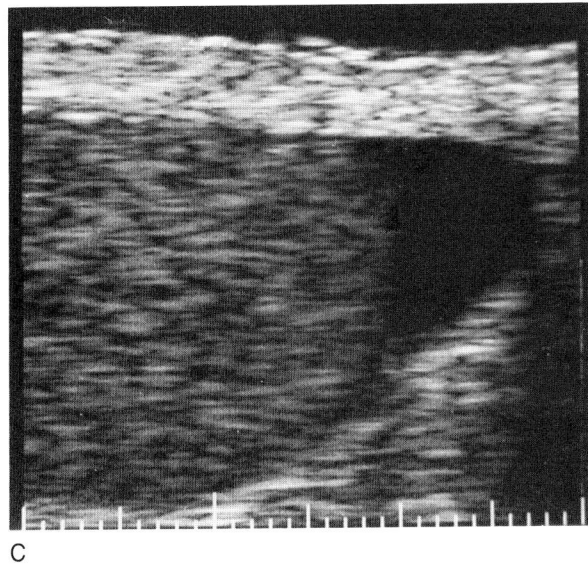

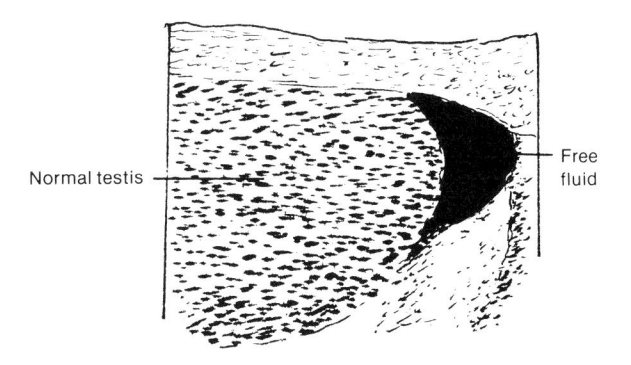

C

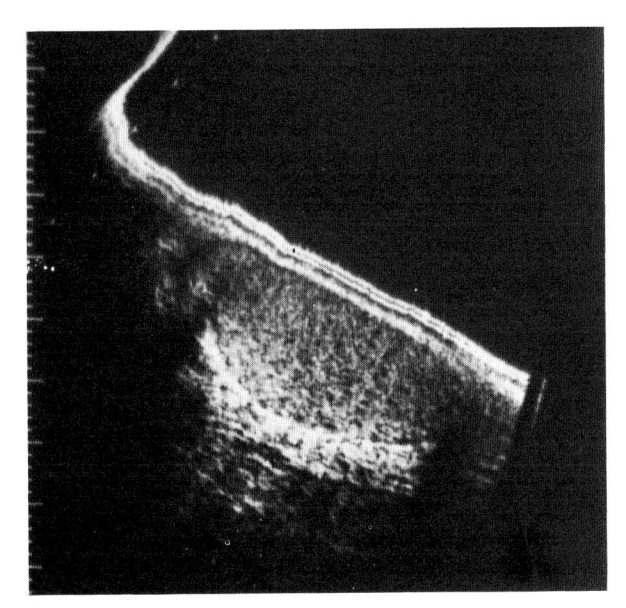

Normal testis — Free fluid

D

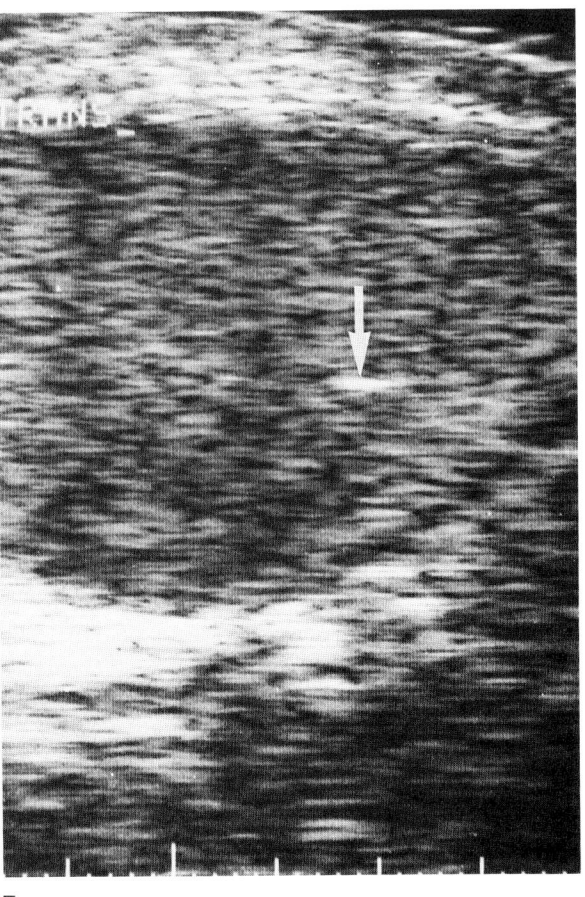

E

969

Extratesticular Pathology (15.2 to 15.6)

15.2 Epididymitis

Acute epididymitis is typically seen on ultrasound as diffuse or focal epididymal swelling, and the epididymis is often, but not always, abnormally sonolucent[1-3] (arrowed in the figure). The figure is a longitudinal sonogram of a 29-year-old man with a 6-day history of scrotal pain and fever. Symptoms in this patient resolved with antibiotic treatment.

Epididymitis is a frequent cause of scrotal pain and swelling. Characteristically, palpation reveals epididymal enlargement and tenderness. Epididymitis often results from retrograde extension along the vas deferens of a focus of infection in the bladder or prostate. Hence, the patient commonly has dysuria, pyuria, and fever. Causes include gonococcal, nonspecific pyogenic, or tuberculous infection and trauma.[1] Occasionally, epididymitis occurs secondary to mumps or syphilitic orchitis.

Ultrasound is usually not necessary to diagnose acute epididymitis, which has a typical clinical presentation and a rapid response to antibiotics. Ultrasound may be used to document or confirm epididymitis with an atypical presentation or a poor response to antibiotics. Ultrasound can also be used to identify associated abnormalities such as orchitis, testicular tumor (which occasionally occurs in conjunction with epididymitis), abscess, or hydrocele.[3] Since either orchitis or testicular tumor associated with epididymitis may be seen on ultrasound examination as a focal, echo-poor area in the testis, the two cannot be differentiated by ultrasound except with follow-up scans after treatment. These scans should show resolution of orchitis (or persistence of tumor).[3]

Chronic epididymitis may result from incompletely resolved acute epididymitis. The patient usually presents with a chronic, tender scrotal mass. With increasing duration of symptoms in epididymitis, there is a greater tendency for the epididymis to appear more echogenic, and epididymal thickening with normal or increased echogenicity may be seen. Chronic tuberculous epididymitis can produce a stony hard, nontender scrotal mass. Ultrasound may show foci of high-amplitude echoes with associated acoustic shadowing due to calcium.

(Fig. from Vick CW, Bird KI, Rosenfield AT, et al: Ultrasound of the scrotal contents. Urol Radiol 4:147–153, 1982.)

REFERENCES

1. Leopold GR, Woo VL, Scheible FW, et al: High-resolution ultrasonography of scrotal pathology. Radiology 131:719–722, 1979
2. Bird KI: Emergency testicular scanning. pp. 55–70 In Taylor KJW, Viscomi GN (eds): Clinics in Diagnostic Ultrasound, Volume 7, Ultrasound in Emergency Medicine. Churchill Livingstone, New York, 1981
3. Sample WF, Gottesman JE, Skinner DG, Erlich RM: Gray scale ultrasound of the scrotum. Radiology 127:225–228, 1978

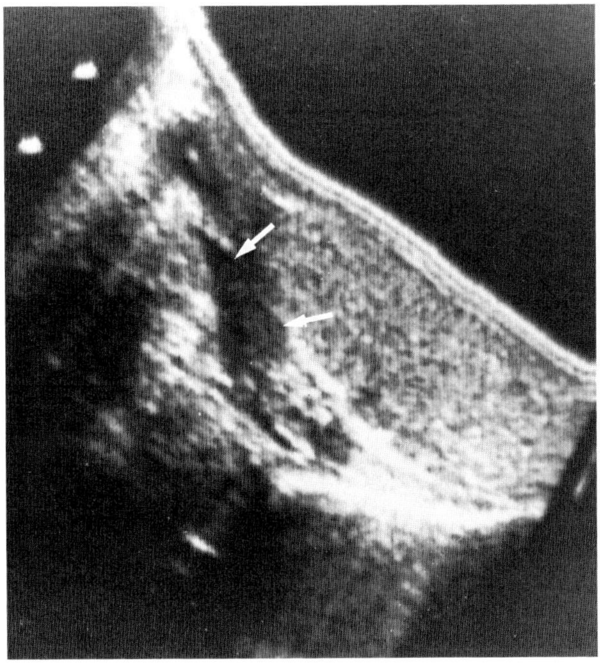

15.3 Cyst

A firm, nontender scrotal nodule was palpated in an 18-year-old patient. Ultrasound showed that the nodule represented an extratesticular simple cyst with no internal echoes and a smooth wall (arrowed in the figure). Differential diagnosis included epididymal cyst, spermatocele, and hydrocele of the cord. Surgical proof is often not obtained for such purely cystic lesions because they are considered benign. To our knowledge, a malignant scrotal tumor appearing as a simple cyst on ultrasound has not yet been reported. If aspirated, an epididymal cyst of a hydrocele yields serous fluid, while a spermatocele contains milky, sperm-laden fluid (which may cause dependently layering debris to be seen on ultrasound). Occasionally, an epididymal cyst may indent the testis and appear intratesticular, in which case differential diagnosis includes a benign mesothelial cyst of the tunica albuginea.

(Fig. from Vick CW, Bird KI, Rosenfield AT, et al: Ultrasound of the scrotal contents. Urol Radiol 4:147–153, 1982.)

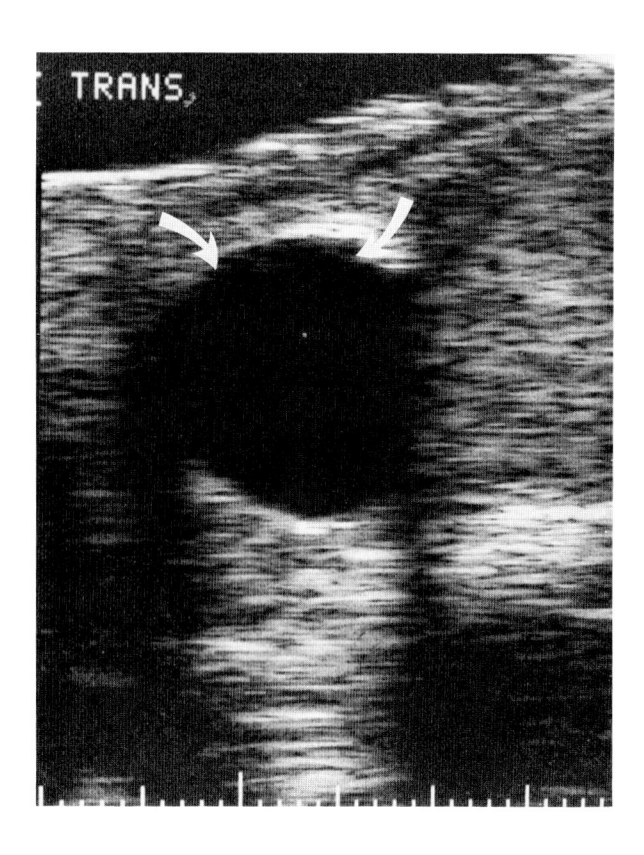

15.4 Hydrocele

An 81-year-old man complained of painless scrotal enlargement. Ultrasound showed the typical appearance of a large hydrocele as an anechoic fluid collection surrounding the testis except posterolaterally at the point where the epididymis attaches to the scrotum and the testis (arrowed, Fig. A).

A hydrocele consists of a collection of serous fluid in the scrotum, usually located within the tunica vaginalis. It represents one of the most common causes of scrotal swelling. Hydroceles may be idiopathic (primary) or secondary to almost any disease process in the scrotum, including tumor, epididymo-orchitis, trauma, or torsion. Transillumination of a hydrocele is characteristic, making the clinical diagnosis straightforward in most cases. Ultrasound may be used to look for possible underlying testicular pathology which may not be clinically evident. Ultrasound can also correctly diagnose a chronic hydrocele which has developed a thickened tunica vaginalis, preventing transillumination.

If a hydrocele is chronic, or follows infection or hemorrhage, septae may form. A noninfected hydrocele with septae is shown in Figure B. Based on the ultrasound appearance alone, one cannot differentiate this from an infected hydrocele, a paratesticular abscess, or a hematocele. However, often the clinical and sonographic findings considered together allow one to make the correct diagnosis.

(Fig. A from Vick CW, Bird KI, Rosenfield AT, et al: Ultrasound of the scrotal contents. Urol Radiol 4:147–153, 1982.)

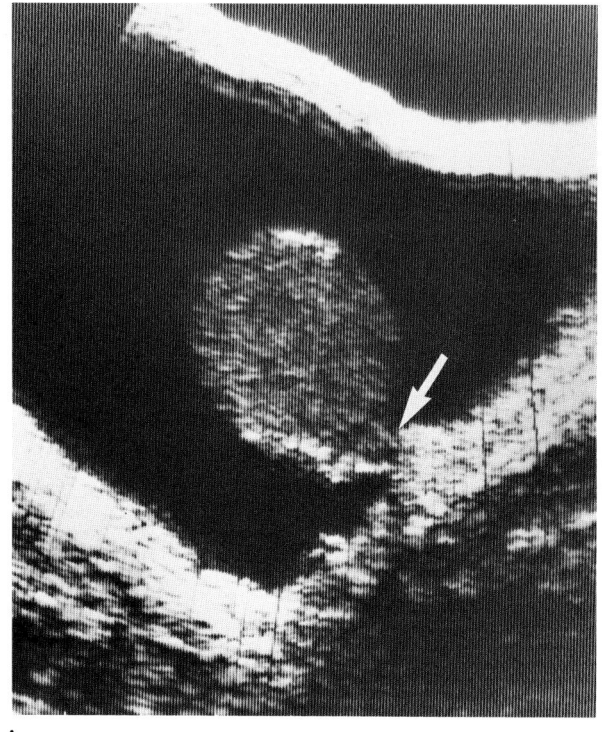

A

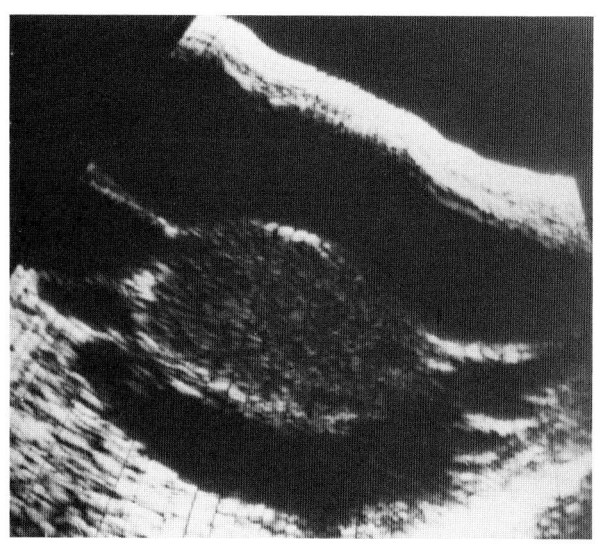

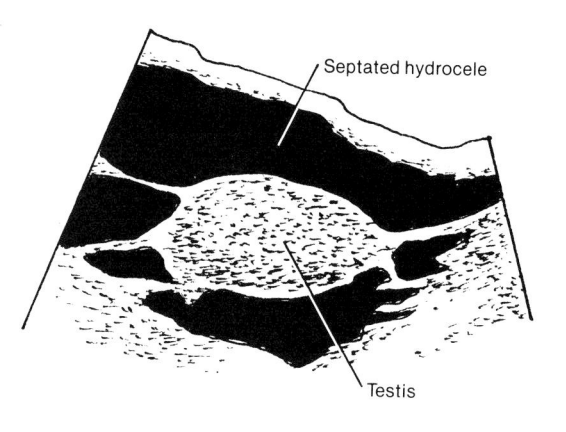

B

Septated hydrocele

Testis

974

15.5 Varicocele

An image taken superior to the testis in a 26-year-old man shows the typical sonographic appearance of a varicocele as an extratesticular lesion with multiple interconnected cystic areas representing the dilated veins of the pampiniform plexus. Although sonography is usually not necessary to diagnose a varicocele, because of the characteristic findings on palpation, one should be familiar with the sonographic appearance of this common lesion. It is likely that many varicoceles are not demonstrated by ultrasound because patients are scanned supine, causing most varicoceles to drain. Scanning a patient upright will distend a varicocele, enhancing its visibility. If a varicocele is right-sided, nonreducible, or first discovered in patients over age 40, one should consider evaluation of the abdomen for neoplastic obstruction of gonadal venous return.

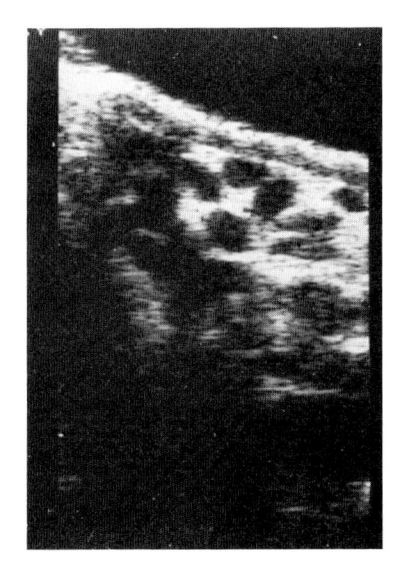

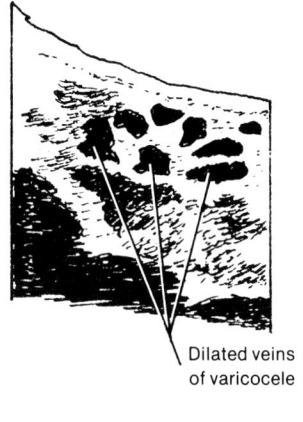

15.6 Tumor

A 23-year-old man had noted a painless scrotal mass for 2 months prior to seeking medical attention. The sonogram showed a solid extratesticular mass located inferior to the testis (Fig. A). The testis appeared normal on other images. At surgery this lesion proved to be a benign adenomatoid tumor arising from the epididymal tail.

A 6-year-old boy presented with an asymptomatic scrotal mass. Ultrasound demonstrated a large, complex extratesticular lesion displacing the normal-appearing testis (Fig. B). Surgery disclosed a rhabdomyosarcoma arising from the spermatic cord (and a normal testis).

Uncommonly, neoplasms may arise from the testicular adnexal structures. These can be identified by ultrasound as solid or complex extratesticular masses. The primary sonographic differential consideration is inflammatory swelling of the epididymis, a condition seen much more frequently than an extratesticular tumor. If there is no history typical of epididymitis (pain, fever, symptoms of urinary tract infection) and a noncystic extratesticular mass is found, the possibility of tumor should be considered. Extratesticular tumors may be benign, most commonly adenoma, adenomatoid tumor, or leiomyoma of the epididymis; or malignant, including sarcomas arising from the cord or epididymis (rhabdomyosarcoma, liposarcoma, and undifferentiated mesenchymal tumor) and mesothelioma arising from the tunica vaginalis.[1]

REFERENCE

1. Murphy GP, Gaeta JF: Tumors of the testicular adnexal structures and seminal vesicles. In: Harrison H, Gittes R, Perlmutter A, et al. (eds): Campbell's Urology, 4th edition. W.B. Saunders Co, Philadelphia: 1979

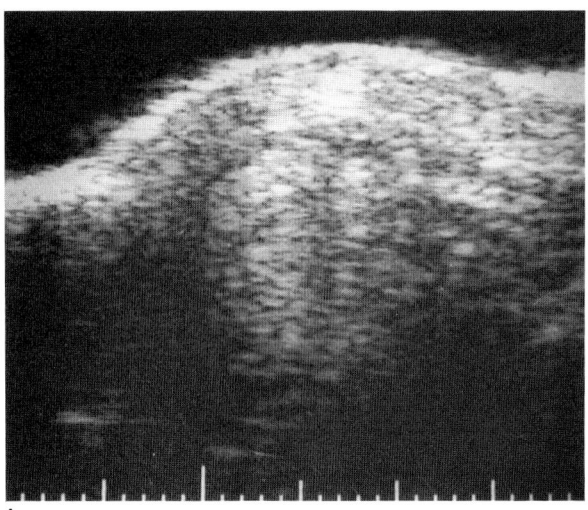

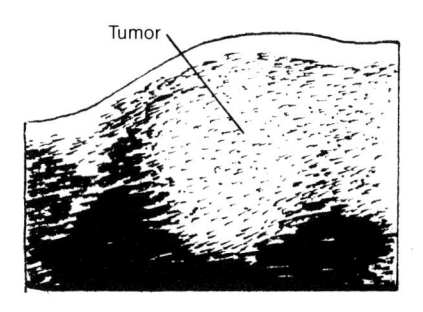

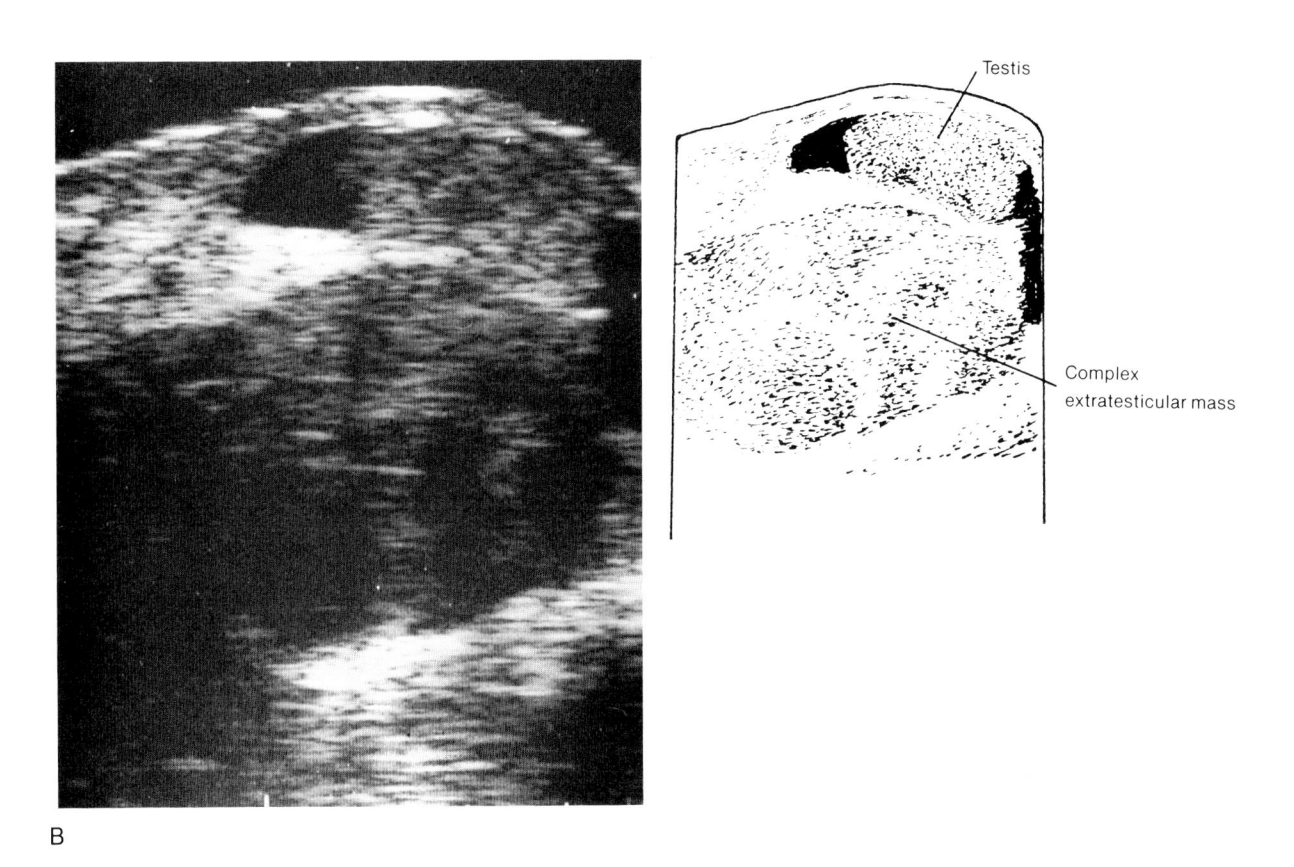

B

Testis

Complex extratesticular mass

Testicular Pathology (15.7 and 15.8)

15.7 Tumor

Testicular tumors are seen on ultrasound because they cause focal or diffuse distortion of the normally homogeneous echo texture of the testis. Echo amplitude and texture with testicular neoplasms vary depending on the presence of hemorrhage, necrosis, cystic change, fibrosis, calcium, etc. Most commonly, a tumor appears abnormally echo-poor compared to normal testicular parenchyma.[1] This is shown in the longitudinal scan of a 32-year-old man who presented with a painless testicular nodule. Ultrasound showed a focal, echo-poor testicular lesion (arrowed, Fig. A), which proved to be a seminoma at surgery. This case was also of interest because the abnormal testis had been undescended at birth and was placed in the scrotum by orchiopexy at age 13. The probability of developing tumor in an undescended testis has been estimated to be 5–100 times greater than in a normally descended testis.[2] In addition, orchiopexy after age 5 or 6 does not seem to reduce the risk of developing neoplasm in the undescended testis (data regarding the value of orchiopexy prior to this age are inconclusive).[2]

The peak incidence of testicular neoplasms is in early adulthood (20–40 years).[2] The most common presentation is as a painless scrotal mass, although pain may occur if there is associated hemorrhage or necrosis. In some patients (less than 25 percent), the presenting manifestations may be due to metastases, and, in a small percentage of these patients, the primary testicular neoplasm may be so small that it is clinically undetectable.[2] In this situation, ultrasound can be used to demonstrate the clinically occult testicular neoplasm.[1,3,4]

Ninety-five percent of testicular neoplasms are of germ cell origin, including seminoma, embryonal carcinoma, teratocarcinoma, choriocarcinoma, and mixed patterns.[2] The remainder consist of non-germ-cell primary tumors or metastases. In general, ultrasound cannot predict a tumor's histologic appearance, although teratocarcinoma has a propensity to contain cystic areas.[2,5] An example of a testicular teratocarcinoma is shown in Figures B and C.

(Fig. A from Vick CW, Bird KI, Rosenfield AT, et al: Ultrasound of the scrotal contents. Urol Radiol 4:147–153, 1982.)

REFERENCES

1. Leopold GR, Woo VL, Scheible FW, et al: High-resolution ultrasonography of scrotal pathology. Radiology 131:719–722, 1979
2. Barzell WEI, Whitmore WF: Neoplasms of the testis. pp. 1125–1169. In Harrison H, Gittes R, Perlmutter A, et al (eds): Campbell's Urology, 4th edition. W.B. Saunders Co., Philadelphia, 1979
3. Sample WF, Gottesman JE, Skinner DG, et al: Gray scale ultrasound of the scrotum. Radiology 127:225–228, 1978
4. Peterson LJ, Catalona WJ, Koehler RE: Ultrasound localization of a non-palpable testis tumor. J Urol 122:843–844, 1979
5. Leopold GR: Ultrasonography of superficially located structures. Radiol Clin North Am 18:161, 1980

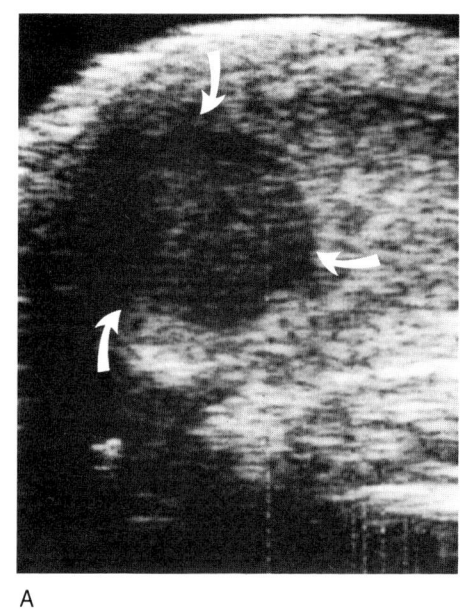

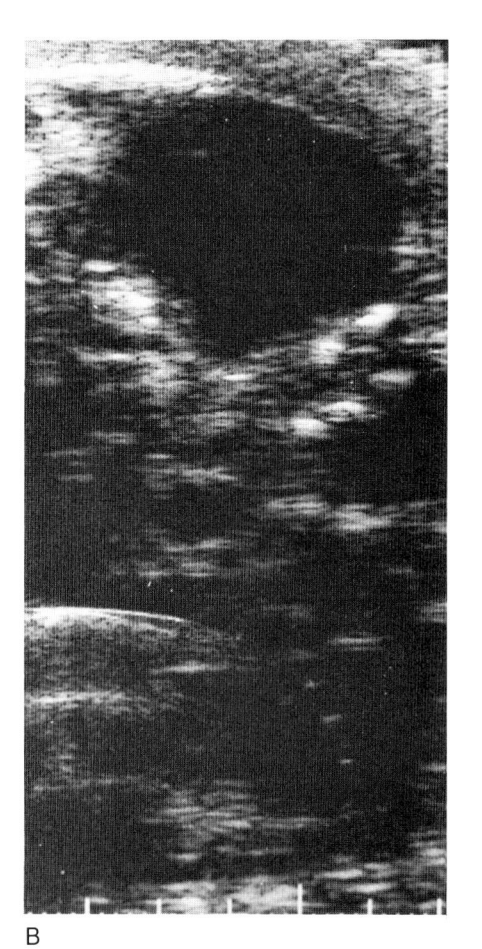

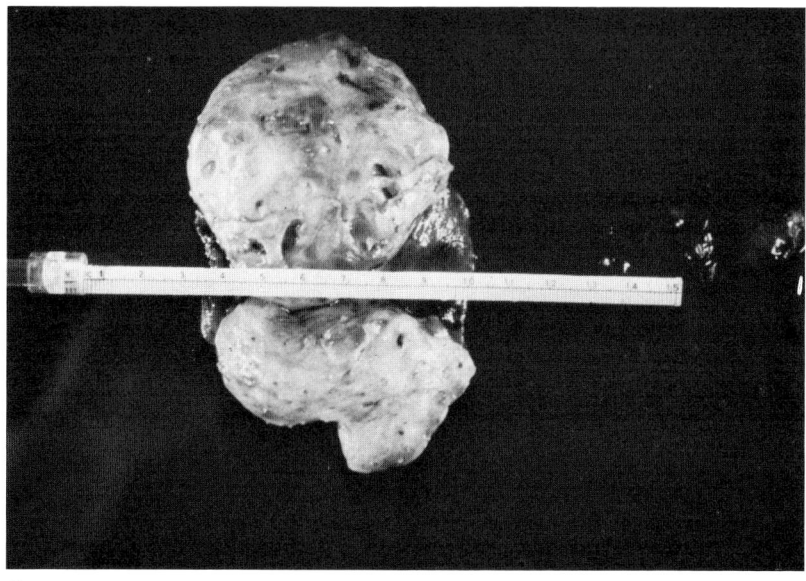

A

B

C

979

15.8 Tumor

Mild pain and swelling in the right testis occurred over the course of 2 months in a 24-year-old man. A sonogram showed that the symptomatic testis had a diffusely echo-poor and inhomogeneous appearance (Fig. A) compared to the normal side (Fig. B). Incidentally seen is a varicocele adjacent to the normal testis. There are no extratesticular abnormalities on the symptomatic side.

Differential diagnosis of an echo-poor or complex testicular abnormality found on ultrasound includes tumor, orchitis, torsion, and hemorrhage. In general, these various testicular lesions cannot be reliably differentiated based on their ultrasound appearances alone, although in some cases the clinical picture and/or ancillary ultrasound data may help to narrow the differential diagnosis.[1-3] For example, decreased testicular echogenicity without any associated peritesticular abnormalities (as in this case) suggests that tumor is more likely than a benign condition.[3] Radical orchiectomy in this patient revealed a mixed malignant tumor.

REFERENCES

1. Sample WF, Gottesman JE, Skinner DG, et al: Gray scale ultrasound of the scrotum. Radiology 127:225–228, 1978
2. Leopold GR, Woo VL, Scheible FW, et al: High-resolution ultrasonography of scrotal pathology. Radiology 131:719–722, 1979
3. Arger PH, Mulhem CF, Coleman BG, et al: Prospective analysis of the value of scrotal ultrasound. Radiology 141:763–766, 1981

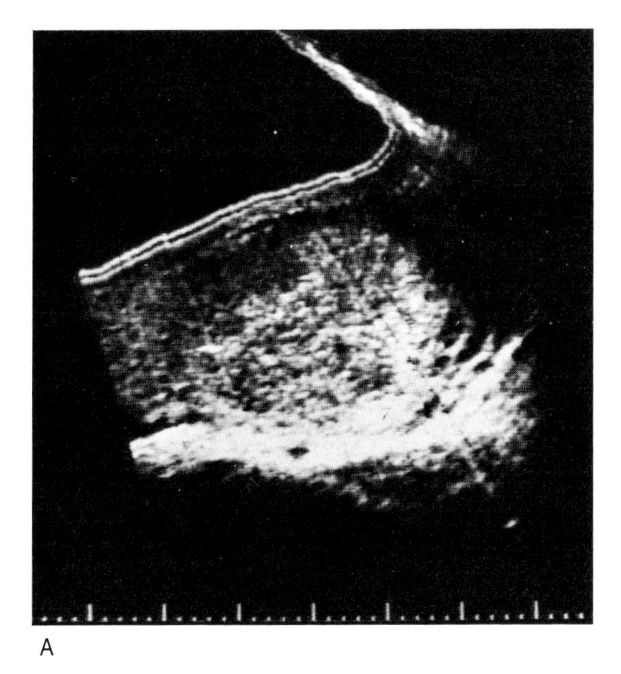

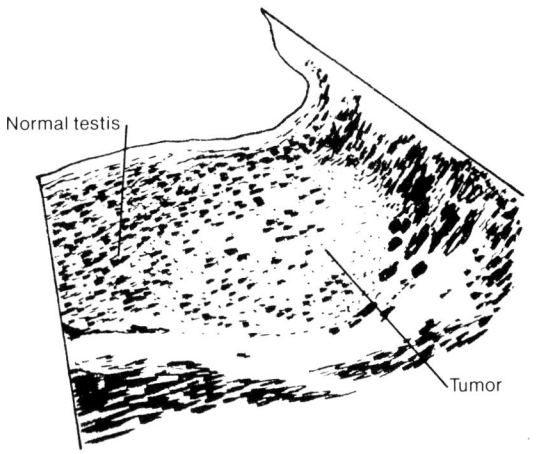

A

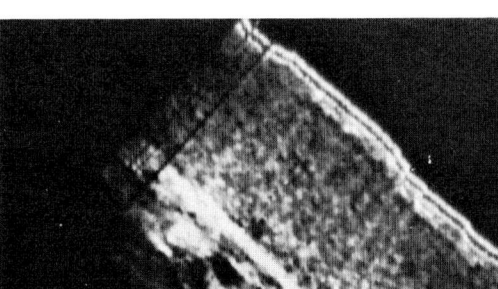

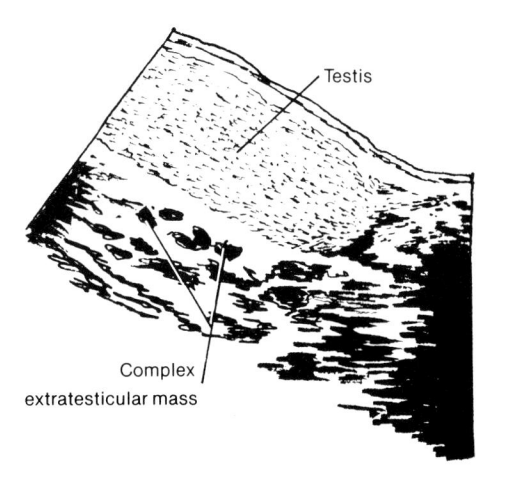

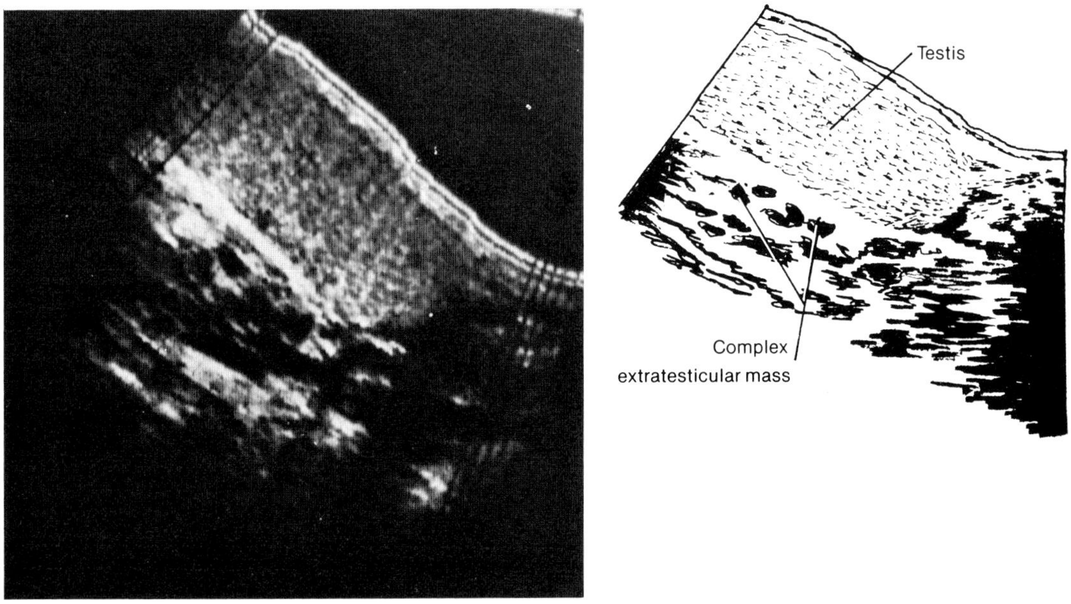

Normal testis

Tumor

B

Testis

Complex extratesticular mass

981

15.9 Combined Testicular and Extratesticular Pathology: Torsion

A 16-year-old boy was admitted with a 5-day history of right testicular pain and swelling. His temperature and white blood cell count were normal, and palpation revealed a tender, swollen right hemiscrotum. A transverse sonogram shows an abnormally sonolucent right testis with associated epididymal thickening and an echo-containing collection lateral to the testis (Fig. A). The left testis and epididymis are normal.

Combined testicular and extratesticular pathology on ultrasound generally has the same significance as testicular pathology alone: benign and malignant disease may be indistinguishable.[1,2] In some cases, the clinical presentation and/or ancillary ultrasound findings may suggest a particular diagnosis or direct further diagnostic work-up. For example, it has been reported that the sonographic findings of decreased testicular echogenicity associated with epididymal swelling, peritesticular fluid, and/or skin thickening suggest that a benign condition (i.e., orchitis or torsion) is more likely than tumor.[3]* Therefore, in the case illustrated here, initial work-up should be directed to exclude torsion or orchitis (based on the ultrasound findings of decreased testicular echogenicity, epididymal thickening, and a peritesticular collection). Since the patient's clinical picture made orchitis unlikely, torsion was believed to be the most likely diagnosis. A radionuclide scan (Fig. B) subsequently confirmed this diagnosis and surgery revealed an infarcted, gangrenous testicle twisted one-and-a-half times on its cord. Extratesticular hemorrhage accounted for the echo-containing collection seen lateral to the testis.

When torsion has a classic presentation with acute pain and swelling in a prepubertal boy, imaging is usually not considered appropriate or necessary, because prompt surgery is necessary to salvage the ischemic testis.[5]

Radionuclide testicular scanning traditionally has been the first imaging study ordered when torsion presents atypically and the clinical diagnosis is unclear. The potential role of ultrasound in the investigation of suspected torsion is evolving. A study from Yale demonstrates that the sonographic appearance of torsion is time-related following the onset of symptoms.[6] Very early, the involved testis may appear normal, but gradually it becomes swollen and its echo texture becomes disorganized. Echo amplitude within the torsed testis may be inhomogeneously decreased[6] or increased.[7] A chronically torsed testis may appear echo-poor and atrophic.[6] Other sonographic findings commonly associated with torsion include epididymal swelling (with variable echogenicity) and skin thickening.[6] All torsed testes in the Yale study appeared abnormally echo-poor by 6 hours following the onset of symptoms, so that the demonstration of a normal testis after at least 6 hours of symptoms appears to exclude torsion. In addition, since a torsed testis often appears normal prior to 6 hours of symptoms, there appears to be little indication for gray-scale ultrasound in this acute situation. Doppler ultrasound has been shown to be potentially useful in diagnosing torsion in the acute setting, because it can demonstrate absence of arterial flow in the spermatic cord.[8]

---

*It should be kept in mind that testicular tumors are occasionally associated with epididymitis, neoplastic invasion of the epididymis or cord, or hydrocele formation.[1,2,4] Therefore, whenever an echo-poor or complex testicular lesion is found on ultrasound, either alone or in combination with extratesticular pathology, tumor should be included in the differential diagnosis and appropriate follow-up is indicated to exclude this possibility.

REFERENCES

1. Sample WF, Gottesman JE, Skinner DG, et al: Gray scale ultrasound of the scrotum. Radiology 127:225–228, 1978
2. Sample WF: Renal, adrenal, retroperitoneal and scrotal ultrasonography. p 268. In Sarti D, Sample WF (eds): Diagnostic Ultrasound Text and Cases. C.G. Hall and Co., Boston, 1980
3. Arger PH, Mulhern CB, Coleman BG, et al: Prospective analysis of the value of scrotal ultrasound. Radiology 141:763–766, 1981
4. Barzell WEI, Whitmore WF: Neoplasms of the testis. pp. 1125–1169. In Harrison H, Gittes R, Perlmutter A, et al (eds): Campbell's Urology, 4th edition. W.B. Saunders, Philadelphia, 1979
5. Bird KI: Emergency testicular scanning. pp. 55–70. In Taylor KJW, Viscomi GN (eds): Clinics in Diagnostic Ultrasound, Volume 7, Ultrasound in Emergency Medicine. Churchill Livingstone, New York, 1981
6. Bird KI, Rosenfield AT, Taylor KJW: Ultrasound in testicular torsion. Radiology 147:527–534, 1983
7. Goodman JD, Haller JD: The scrotum in ultrasound in pediatrics. pp. 264–275. In Haller JD, Shkolnik A (eds): Clinics in Diagnostic Ultrasound, Volume 8, Diagnostic Ultrasound in Pediatrics. Churchill Livingstone, New York, 1981
8. Smith SP, King LR: Torsion of the testis: techniques of assessment. Urol Clin North Am 6:429–443. 1979

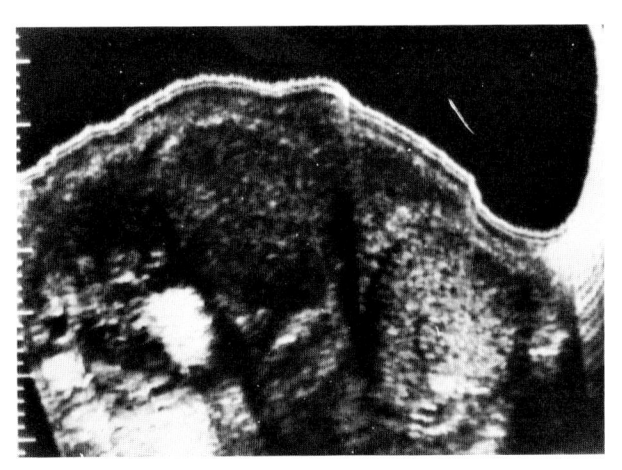

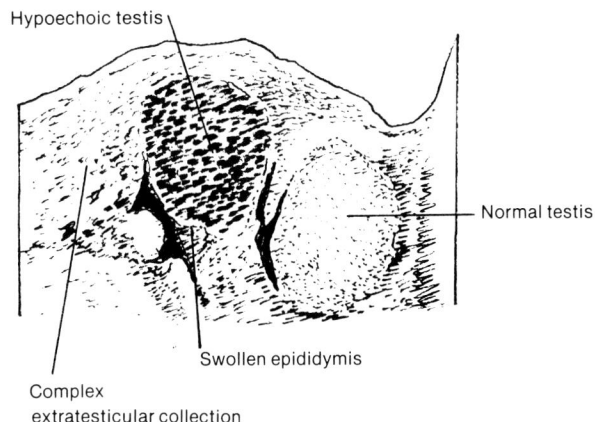

A

B

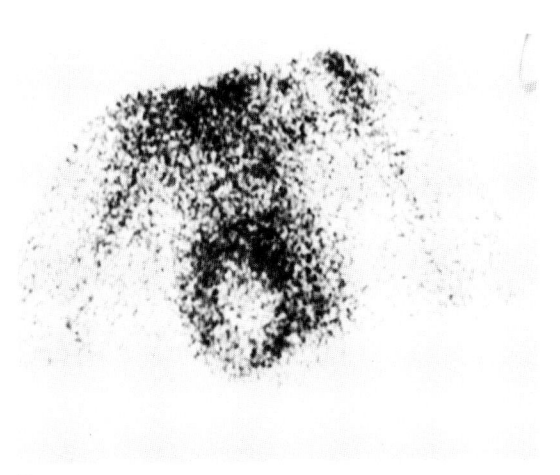

15.10 Trauma

A 30-year-old man was kicked in the scrotum 2 days before coming to the hospital. On physical examination, a large hematocele was evident, but the testis itself could not be palpated, and ultrasound was requested to evaluate the integrity of the testis. A longitudinal scan showed the testis to be intact, and the hematocele was seen as a complex extratesticular collection (Fig. A). The patient was successfully treated without surgery.

The sonographic appearance of blood varies depending on the amount of time which has elapsed since bleeding, the hematocrit of the blood, and the frequency of the transducer used to image it.[1] Consequently, a scrotal hematocele may range in appearance from a purely cystic extratesticular collection to a bizarre, complex scrotal mass. Since a scrotal abscess could look similar to a hematocele on ultrasound, clinical history is essential to make the correct diagnosis.

A patient who had been shot in the scrotum by a BB gun, underwent ultrasound prior to surgery to localize the BB shot. A longitudinal sonogram shows the BB (with a "comet-tail" artifact[2] arrowed) adjacent to the lower pole of the testis. The testis itself appears intact (Fig. B). These findings were confirmed at surgery.

(Fig. A scan from Vick CW, Bird KI, Rosenfield AT, et al: Ultrasound of the scrotal contents. Urol Radiol 4:147–153, 1982.)

REFERENCES

1. Coelho JCU, Siegel B, Ryva JC, et al: B-mode sonography of blood clots. J Clin Ultrasound 10:323–327, 1982
2. Ziskin MC, Thickman DI, Goldenberg NJ, et al: The comet tail artifact. J Ultrasound Med 1:1–7, 1982

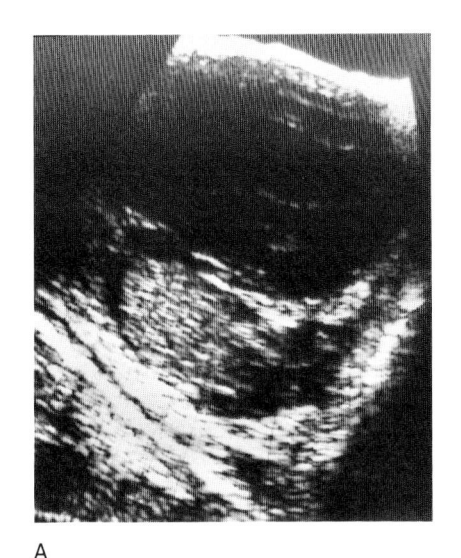

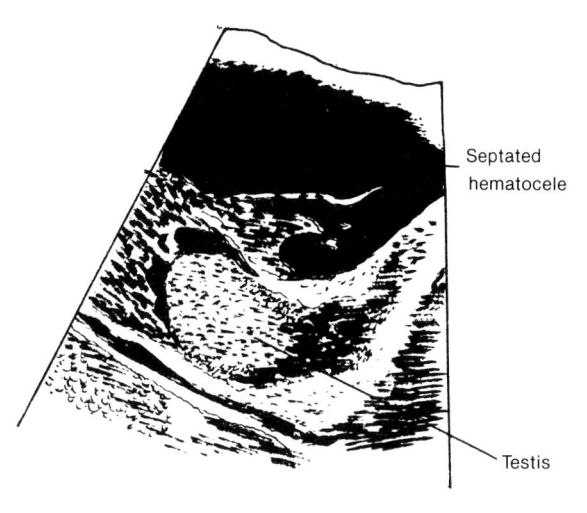

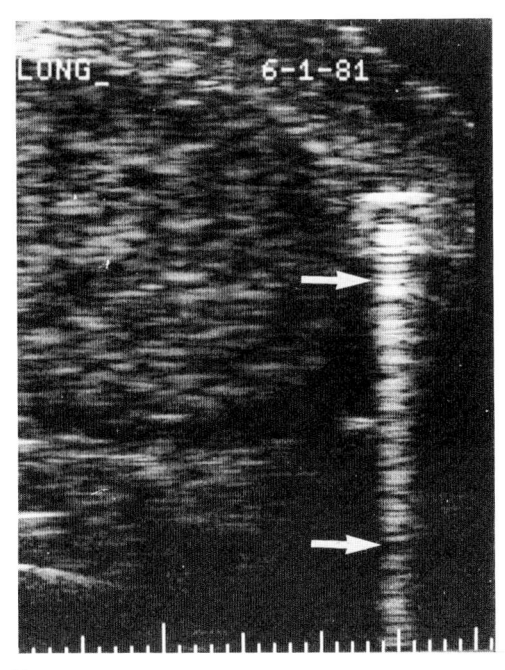

A

B

985

15.11 Benign Hyperechoic Scrotal Lesion

A 39-year-old man was referred for scrotal ultrasound study because of a palpable, nontender testicular nodule. Ultrasound scans showed a small, hyperechoic lesion along the testicular margin (arrowed, Fig. A). Surgery disclosed a benign adenomatoid tumor embedded in the tunica albuginea.

An adenomatoid tumor is a slowly growing benign tumor which usually arises from the epididymis or spermatic cord, but occasionally, as in this case, it may be found embedded in the tunica albuginea.[1] There is no known malignant potential.[1]

It has been our experience that scrotal lesions which are totally hyperechoic on ultrasound are likely to be benign, regardless of their intrascrotal location. Fibrosis or scar tissue usually corresponds to the hyperechoic area. Microscopic examination of the adenomatoid tumor illustrated here showed a dense fibrous stroma, which probably presumably accounted for the tumor's hyperechoic appearance on ultrasound.

A mass that is predominantly hyperechoic but also contains foci of lower-amplitude echoes may not necessarily prove to be benign. Figure B shows an example of an inhomogeneous, predominantly hyperechoic testicular lesion which proved to be a teratoma. It has also been observed that metastases to the testis (most commonly from lymphoma, or from renal or prostate primaries) may appear hyperechoic on ultrasound.[2] However, this should rarely cause a diagnostic problem, because metastases to the testis are usually discovered incidentally in patients with widespread metastatic disease.[3] Multiple lesions may be imaged by ultrasound.[2]

(Fig. A and Fig. B scan from Vick CW, Bird KI, Rosenfield AT, et al: Scrotal masses with a uniformly hyperechoic pattern. Radiology 148:209–211, 1983.)

REFERENCES

1. Murphy GP, Gaeta JE: Tumors of testicular adnexal structures and seminal vesicles. pp. 1200–1212. In Harrison H, Gittes R, Perlmutter A, et al (eds.): Campbell's Urology, 4th edition. W.B. Saunders, Philadelphia, 1979
2. Carroll BA: Real-time small parts scanning. pp. 167–170. In Winsberg F, Cooperberg PL (eds): Clinics in Diagnostic Ultrasound, Volume 10, Real-time Ultrasonography. Churchill Livingstone, New York, 1982
3. Barzell WEI, Whitmore WF: Neoplasms of the testis. p. 1162. In Harrison H, Gittes R, Perlmutter A, et al (eds): Campbell's Urology, 4th edition. W.B. Saunders, Philadelphia, 1979

Testis

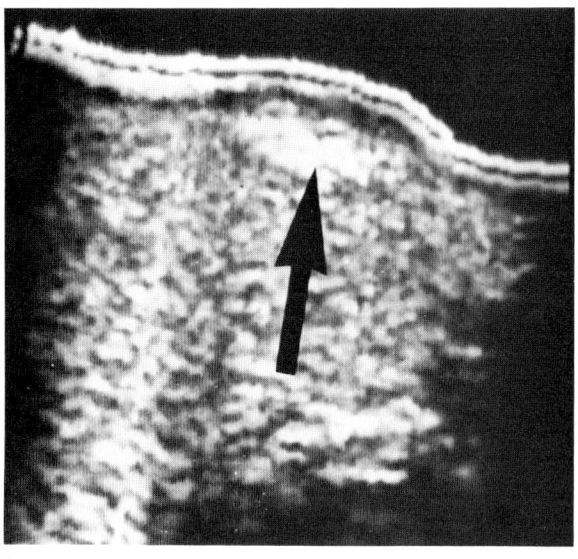

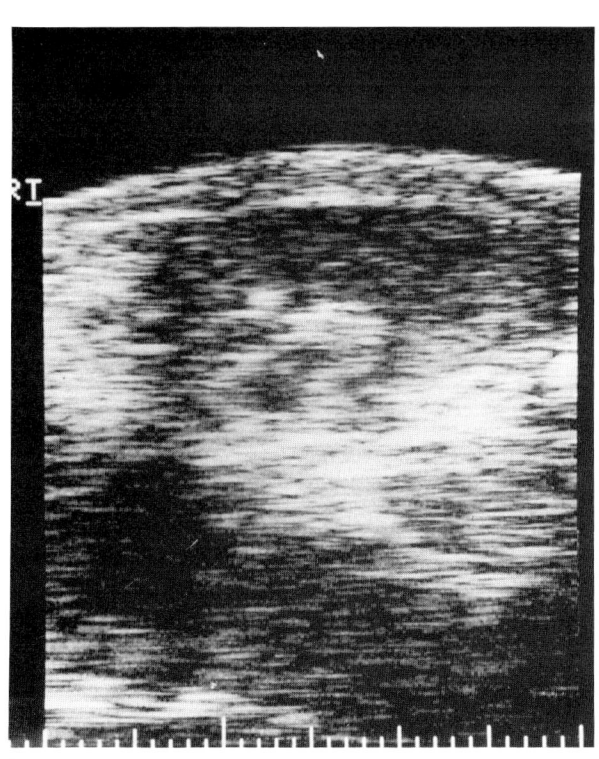

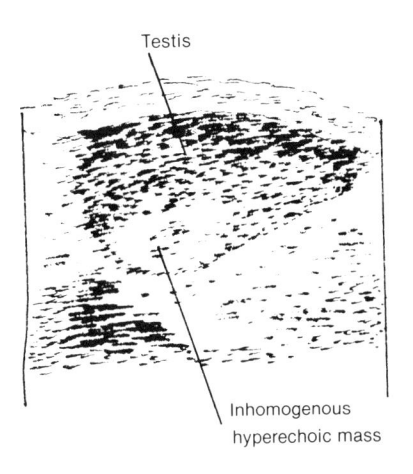

Inhomogenous hyperechoic mass

16 The Retroperitoneum

KENNETH J. W. TAYLOR

Retroperitoneal Fat (16.1 and 16.2)

16.1 Reflective Fat

In a patient referred for ultrasonography of the retroperitoneum, although the aorta was seen, the quality of the images of the retroperitoneum was suboptimal (Figs. A and B). Note that the patient had ample subcutaneous fat. Although "air in the bowel" is often blamed for such appearances, Bree and Schwab pointed out that excessive retroperitoneal or mesenteric fat rather than air interferes with ultrasonic visualization.[1] A CT scan of this patient demonstrated very extensive intraabdominal fat with comparatively little air contained in the bowel (Fig. C).

As is apparent from the echogenicity of a dermoid cyst or angiomyelolipoma, fat particles are extremely effective at scattering the ultrasound beam, presumably due to the quite large differences between the acoustic properties of fat and those of other biologic tissues. This case demonstrates the deterioration of the ultrasound images induced by such excessive fat.

REFERENCE

1. Bree RL, Schwab RE: Contribution of mesenteric fat to unsatisfactory abdominal and pelvic ultrasonography. Radiology 140:773–776, 1981

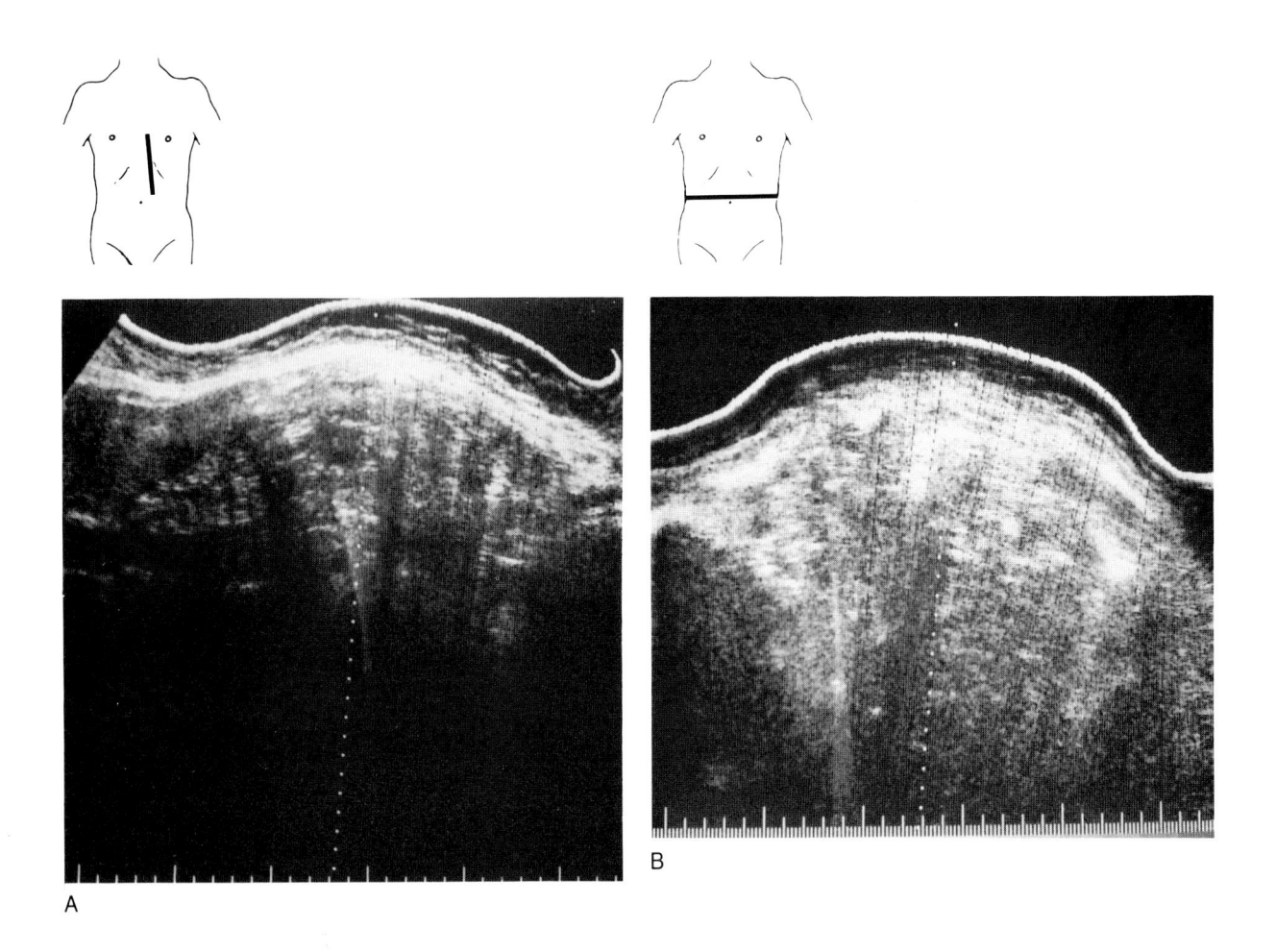

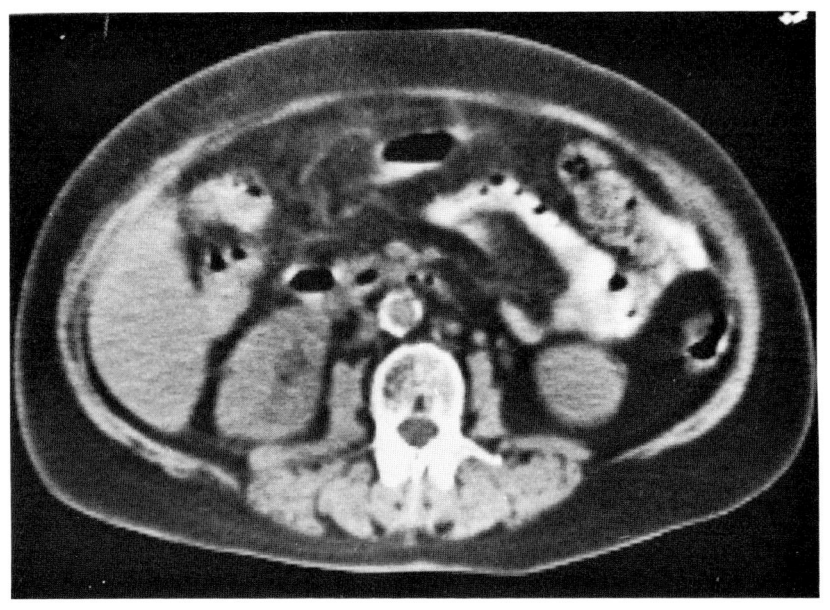

A

B

C

990

16.2 Fat Displacement

A 50-year-old woman with a long history of intermittent attacks of vertigo and palpitations was referred for ultrasound evaluation. Previous radiologic studies had been negative and the patient's symptoms were considered to be psychogenic.

A longitudinal scan of the right upper quadrant showed a large mass above the right kidney (arrowed, Fig. A). Note that a triangular tongue of retroperitoneal fat (arrowhead) was seen between the mass and the kidney, which was displaced inferiorly. This was useful in localizing the origin of the mass. A transverse sonogram (Fig. B) confirmed the presence of the mass (arrowed). The appearances were consistent with an adrenal mass such as pheochromocytoma. The patient's history of intermittent vertigo, blanching, and palpitations was consistent with this diagnosis.

Gore et al. noted the value of displaced retroperitoneal fat to localize the origin of a right upper quadrant mass. Hepatic and subhepatic masses displace this fat posteriorly, while renal and adrenal lesions displace it anteriorly, as in this patient. In particular, the formation of a wedge of this reflective material situated near the upper pole of the right kidney indicates an adrenal tumor, as in this patient.

REFERENCE

1. Gore RM, Callen PW, Filly RA: Displaced retroperitoneal fat: sonographic guide to right upper quadrant mass localization. Radiology 142:701–705, 1982

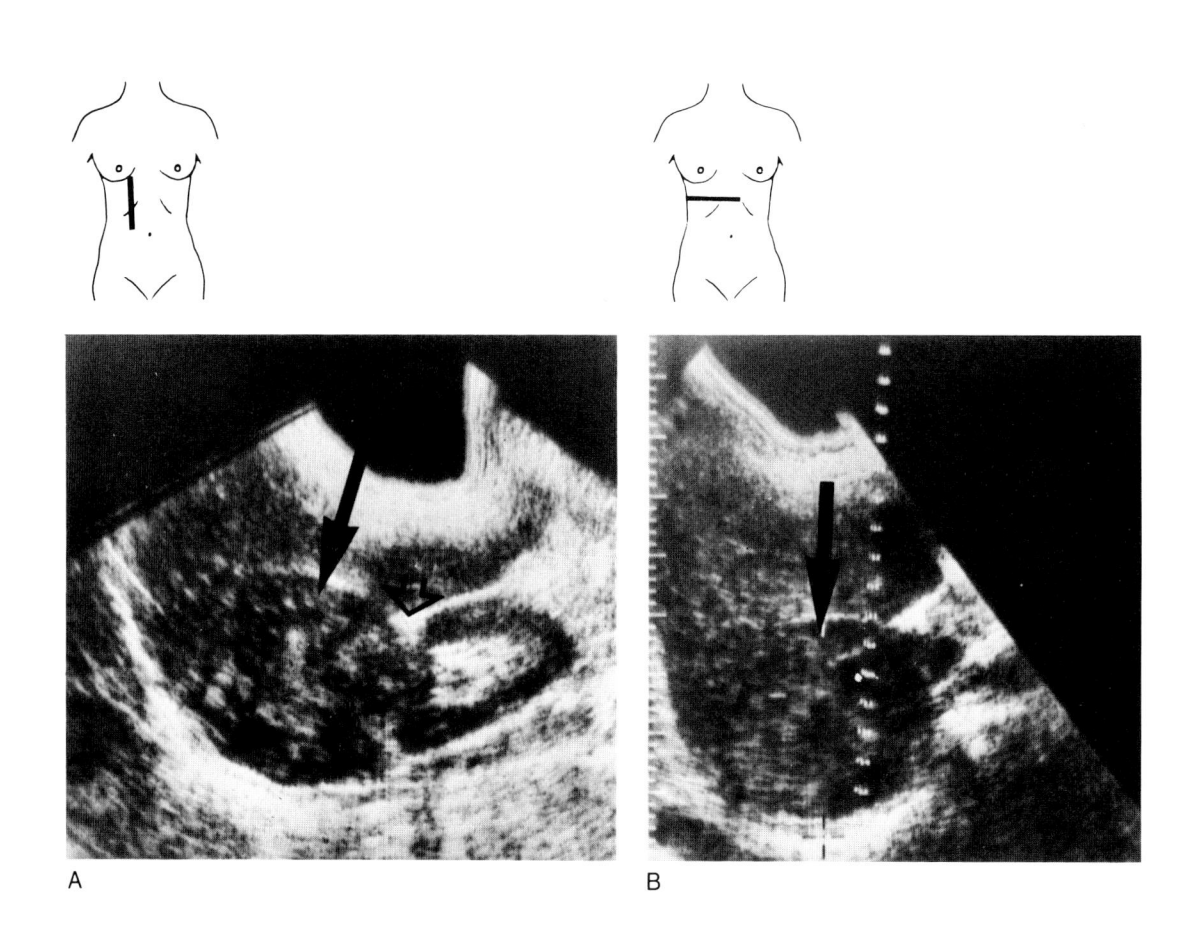

A

B

992

16.3 Paraaortic Lymphadenopathy

A 60-year-old woman was known to have had chronic lymphatic leukemia for 4 years, for which she had received extensive chemotherapy. She was referred for ultrasound evaluation of the upper abdomen.

A transverse sonogram immediately below the xiphisternum (Fig. A) showed the prevertebral vessels, including a large splenic vein joining the superior mesenteric vein to form the portal vein, the superior mesenteric artery, left renal vein, and aorta. Anterior to these vessels, lobulated homogeneous masses were seen.

A hemisection through the right side of the abdomen at this level (Fig. B) showed the right kidney again with a large lobulated mass anterior to it, consistent with paraaortic lymphadenopathy. These appearances were confirmed on the longitudinal scan 2 cm to the left of the midline (arrowed, Fig. C), which showed lobulated masses anterior to the aorta. A longitudinal sonogram through the plane of the inferior vena cava showed a lobulated mass mainly anterior to it (arrowed, Fig. D). A mainly retrocaval mass which compressed the caval lumen was seen in Figure E (arrows). The main differential diagnosis of such retrocaval masses is adrenal tumor.

Most radiologists prefer CT to ultrasound for the diagnosis of lymphadenopathy. However, Burney et al. compared ultrasound and CT in the staging and management of testicular carcinoma in 136 patients.[1] Although CT was more reproducible, the overall accuracy of the two techniques was similar, at around 75 percent. These authors used a second-generation CT scanner; a higher accuracy might be expected with a fourth-generation scanner.

REFERENCE

1. Burney BT, Klatte EC: Ultrasound and computed tomography of the abdomen in the staging and management of testicular carcinoma. Radiology 132:415–419, 1979

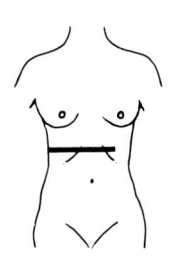

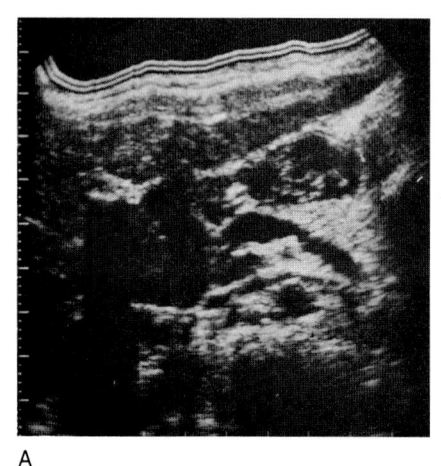

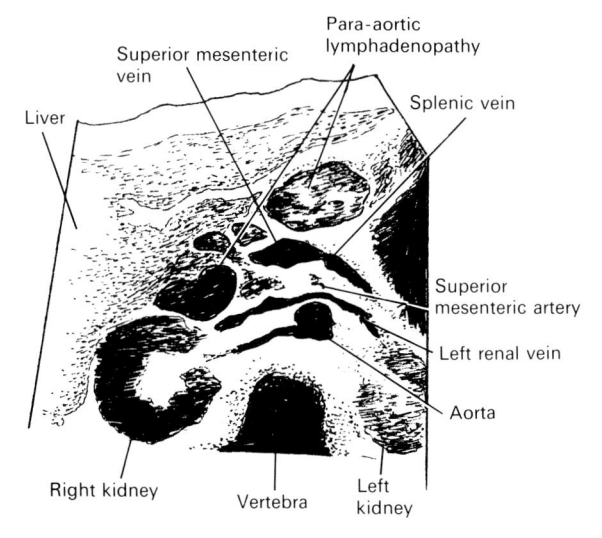

A

Liver	Superior mesenteric vein — Para-aortic lymphadenopathy — Splenic vein
	Superior mesenteric artery
	Left renal vein
	Aorta
Right kidney	Vertebra — Left kidney

B

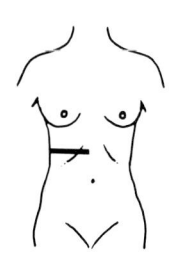

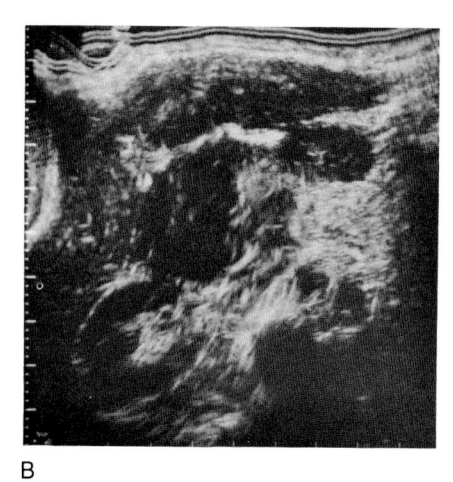

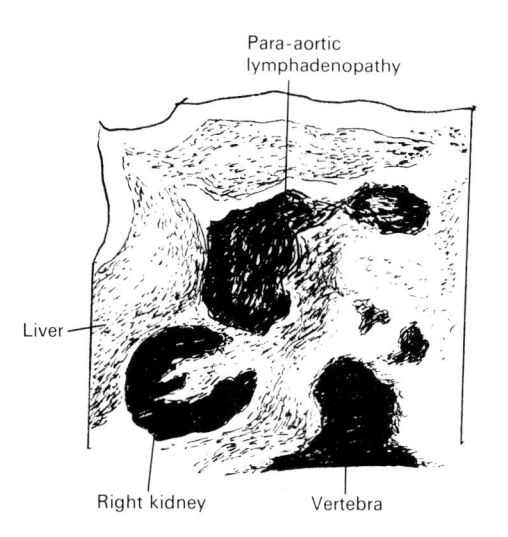

Para-aortic lymphadenopathy

Liver

Right kidney — Vertebra

994

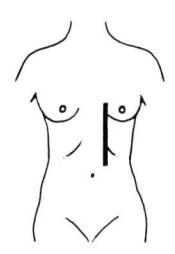

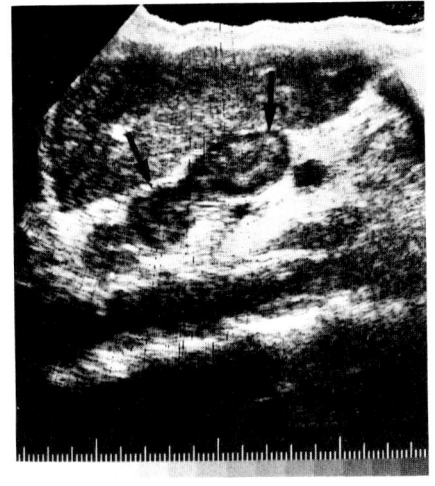

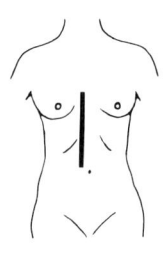

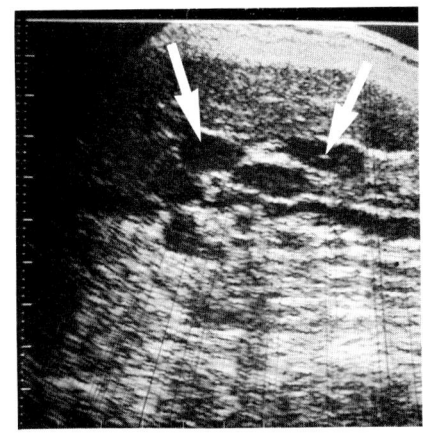

C

D

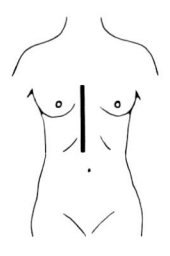

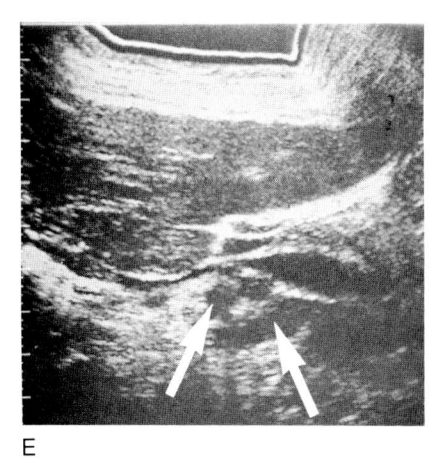

E

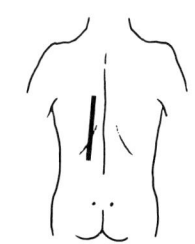

16.4 Left Upper Quadrant Abscess

A 20-year-old man presented with symptoms attributable to an islet cell tumor of the pancreas. A 2-cm lesion was defined on pancreatic examination and excised at surgery. Two weeks after surgery, the patient developed fever, left pleural opacity, and leukocytosis, and was referred for ultrasound investigation and localization of a possible abdominal abscess.

A paramedian sonogram through the left upper quadrant from the posterior aspect (Fig. A) showed the left kidney in longitudinal section and a triangular homogeneous mass between the anterior surface of the kidney and the diaphragm. The left hemidiaphragm appeared abnormally flat, suggesting possible hemiparesis. These appearances were considered to be consistent with a left subphrenic abscess, and surgery was undertaken at which the abscess was drained.

Repeat examination 3 days after surgery showed the left kidney in longitudinal section with a small homogeneous mass near the lower pole (Fig. B), which is the residual abscess cavity after drainage of the left subphrenic abscess.

Subphrenic abscesses are very accurately diagnosed and localized on the right side and with an accuracy of approximately 90 percent on the left side. Colonic contents, fluid in the stomach, and air in the bowel all make visualization of the left hemidiaphragm much more difficult than on the right side, in which the liver provides a good acoustic window toward the right hemidiaphragm.

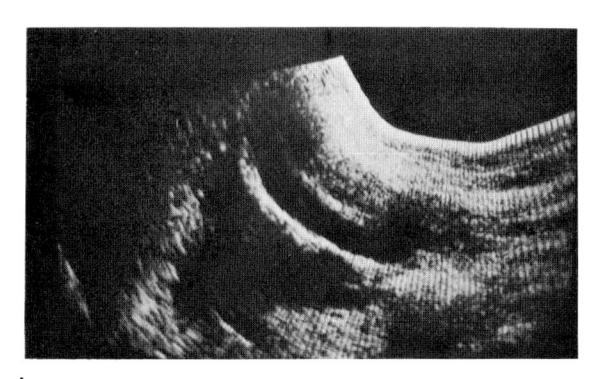

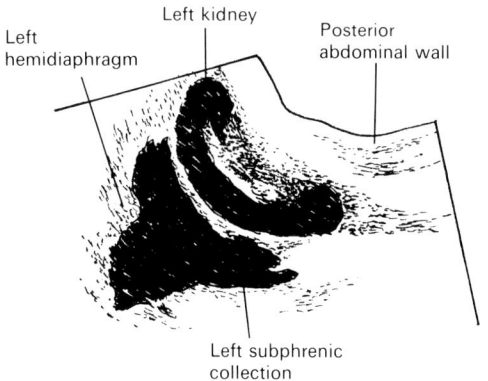

A

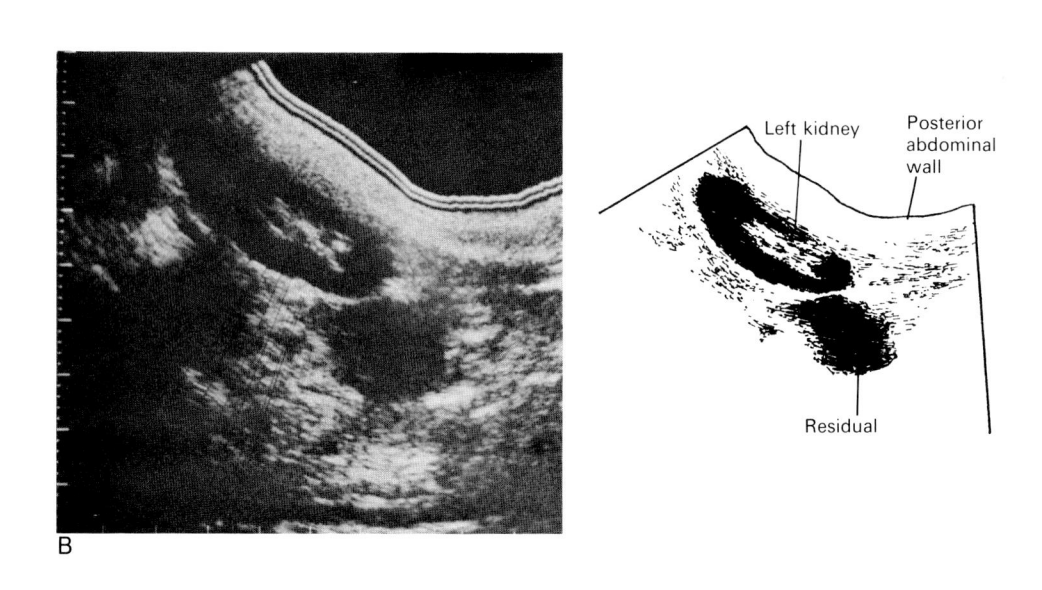

B

Left kidney
Posterior abdominal wall
Residual

16.5 Neurofibrosarcoma

A palpable mass was noted in the right upper quadrant on physical examination of an 11-year-old girl with known neurofibromatosis. She was referred for ultrasound to differentiate the nature of this mass.

A longitudinal sonogram through the right lobe of the liver and subcostal region (Fig. A) showed a large mass immediately below the liver. This mass was irregular in contour and echo amplitude and showed cystic components characteristic of central necrosis. There was evidence of an irregular junction between the liver and the mass, suggesting local invasion of the liver substance. These appearances were characteristic of a subhepatic malignant tumor.

The right kidney was displaced upwards by the mass and was immediately subdiaphragmatic in position. In this patient, who was known to have neurofibromatosis, the appearance of a malignant mass immediately below the right kidney, and displacing it upwards, strongly suggested malignant transformation in a neurofibroma arising in the lumbar ganglia. At surgery, a neurofibrosarcoma was found. This tumor was only partially excised. Repeat sonograms showed the residual tumor and were used to plan radiation therapy.

The response of the tumor to therapy was monitored by repeated ultrasound examinations. A sudden increase in the size of the mass necessitated a further examination. The transverse sonogram (Fig. B) showed a large cystic cavity within the tumor mass. This was aspirated under ultrasound visualization. Nine hundred ml of serosanguinous fluid was aspirated. Ultrasound examination after aspiration (Fig. C) showed evidence of a highly reflective recurrent tumor mass in the liver substance, but little fluid remained. Repeated hemorrhage into the tumor area necessitated several aspirations under ultrasound guidance.

This case demonstrates the practical use of ultrasound in the initial diagnosis and clinical management of a young patient with a malignant tumor. Twelve examinations were carried out over 6 months and the sonograms record her clinical course. In pediatric patients, the noninvasive and painless method of repeated examination is of particular value.

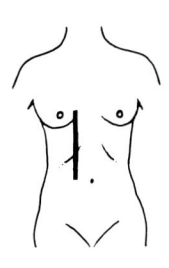

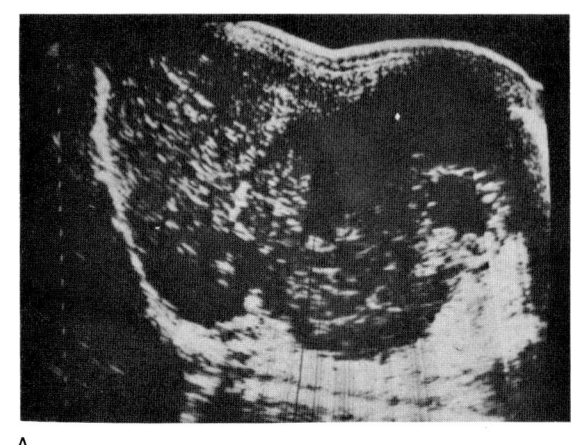

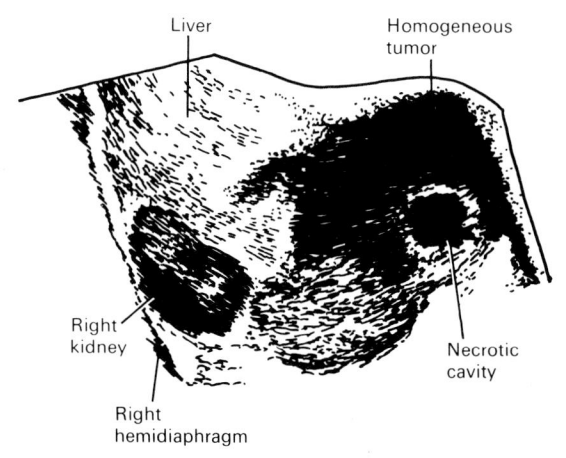

A

Liver · Homogeneous tumor

Right kidney

Necrotic cavity

Right hemidiaphragm

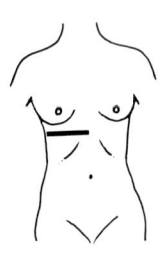

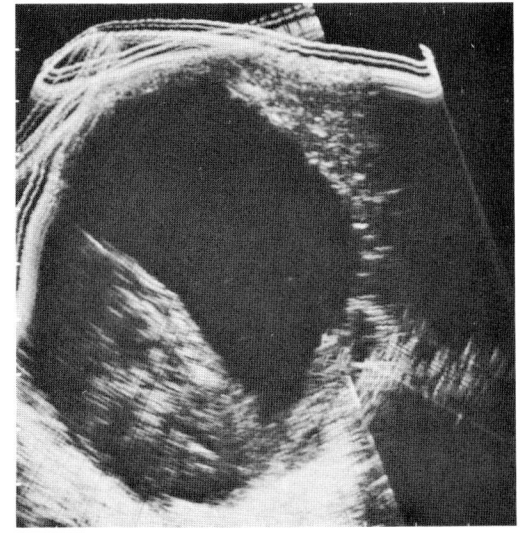

B

1000

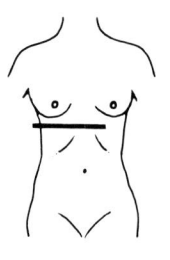

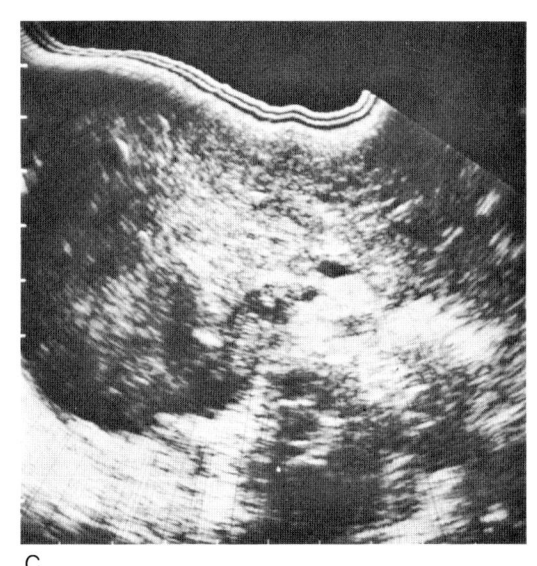

C

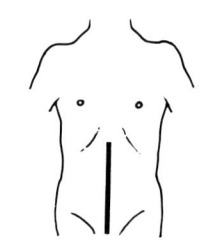

16.6 Leiomyoblastoma: Response to Therapy

An 18-year-old man presented with a large abdominal and pelvic tumor which biopsy revealed to be a leiomyoblastoma. On the longitudinal sonogram shown, the tumor was seen filling the abdomen and the rectovesical pouch. A large cystic mass was seen superior to the bladder; this was a central necrotic cavity. Despite treatment, the overall size of tumor increased and solid tumor encroached on the cystic necrotic area when the patient was rescanned 1 month later.

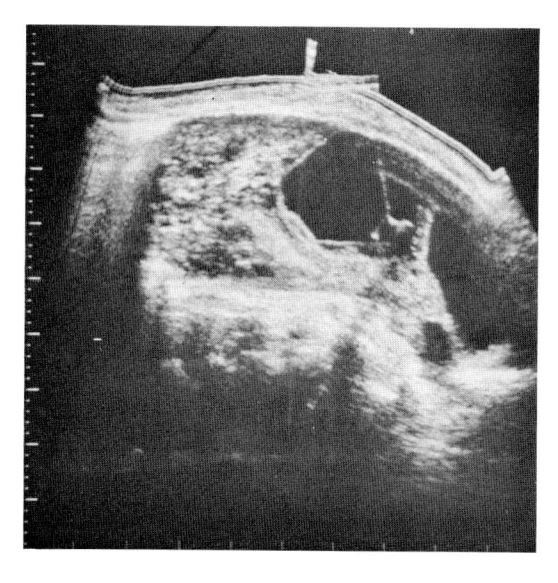

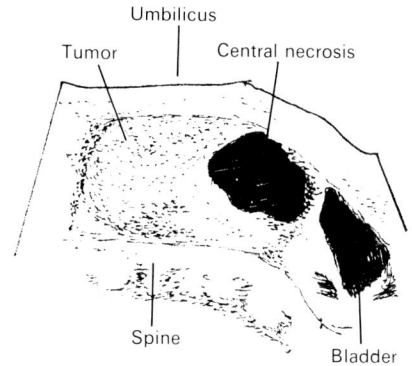

16.7 Urachal Histiocytoma

A 13-year-old girl presented with a 2-day history of fever and abdominal pain. On examination there appeared to be a midline abdominal mass just below the umbilicus. Intravenous pyelography and upper and lower GI series revealed no abnormality. Transverse (Fig. A) and midline longitudinal (Fig. B) sonograms showed a highly homogeneous tumor returning low-level echoes. The mass was well-encapsulated and situated immediately deep to the anterior abdominal wall. The appearances were those of a homogeneous mass, either an abscess or a tumor, lying deep to the rectus abdominus muscle.

Exploratory laparotomy revealed a pseudoencapsulated urachal tumor locally adherent to the omentum. This tumor had cystic elements in it which were ruptured during removal. Histologically, this proved to be a fibrous histiocytoma.

This patient was treated with radiotherapy and chemotherapy; ultrasound examination 6 months later revealed a definite 2 × 5 cm mass in the right pelvis, although results of lymphangiography were normal. Two months later, the patient presented again with fever and an obviously enlarging abdominal mass. Repeat ultrasound examination showed that on both transverse and longitudinal scans (Figs. C and D), the entire pelvis was filled with irregular tumor material, with obvious areas of necrosis. At surgery this extensive tumor infiltration was confirmed and numerous peritoneal seedings were noted.

This case illustrates the value of ultrasound not only as an initial diagnostic modality, but also for the follow-up of patients after treatment of primary tumor even when results of all other investigations are negative. Of more importance, ultrasound demonstrated recurrence of the tumor, but this finding was ignored in the presence of a normal lymphangiogram. A normal lymphangiogram may exclude disease in the lymph nodes, but extranodal tumor recurrence is best visualized by ultrasound or CT scanning. In this patient, who had already received the maximum radiotherapy and chemotherapy, the delay in any further therapy resulting from the false assurance of a normal lymphangiogram was clinically unimportant.

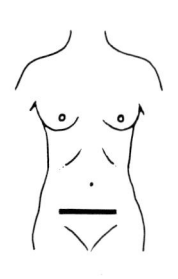

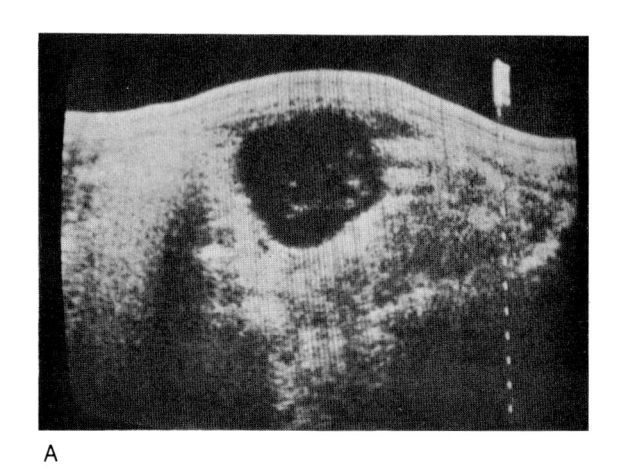

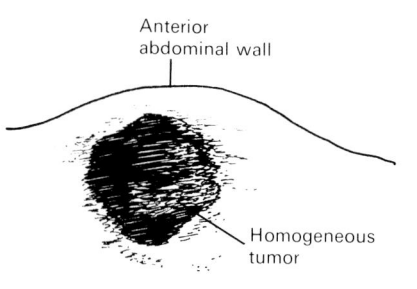

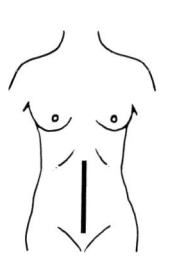

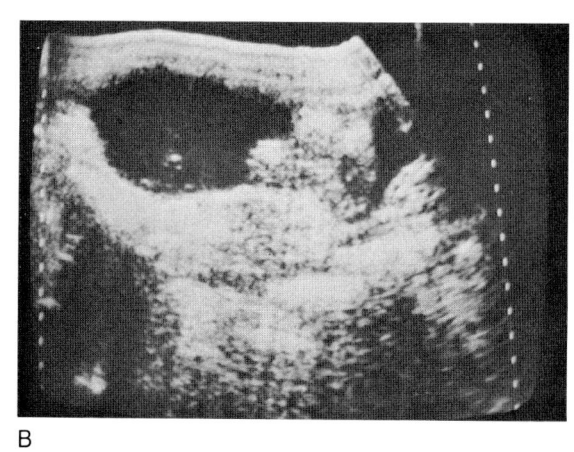

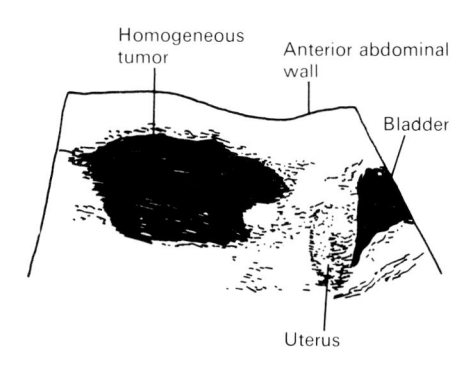

A

B

1004

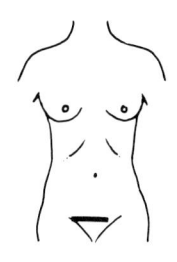

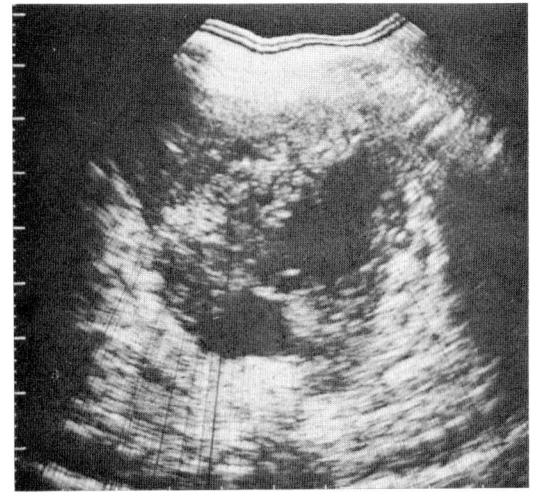

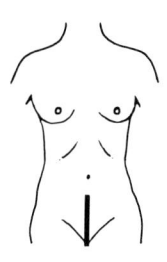

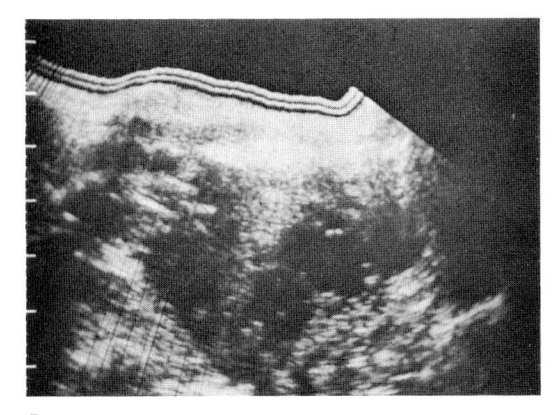

C

D

16.8 Abdominopelvic Mass

An 18-year-old man was admitted with gunshot wounds to the abdomen involving the bowel and necessitating immediate repair. He subsequently developed fever and a palpable suprapubic mass. A large cystic cavity was seen on transverse sonogram (Fig. A) 4 cm below the umbilicus, while the longitudinal sonogram (Fig. B) showed the same predominantly cystic cavity above the bladder. Posteriorly, debris was seen. Preoperatively, the differential diagnosis was between a pseudocyst of the pancreas and an abdominal abscess. A sterile abscess was drained.

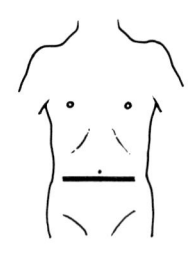

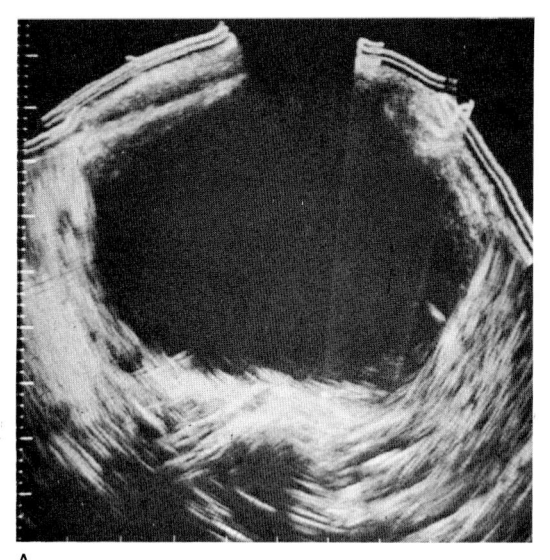

A

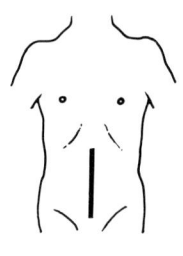

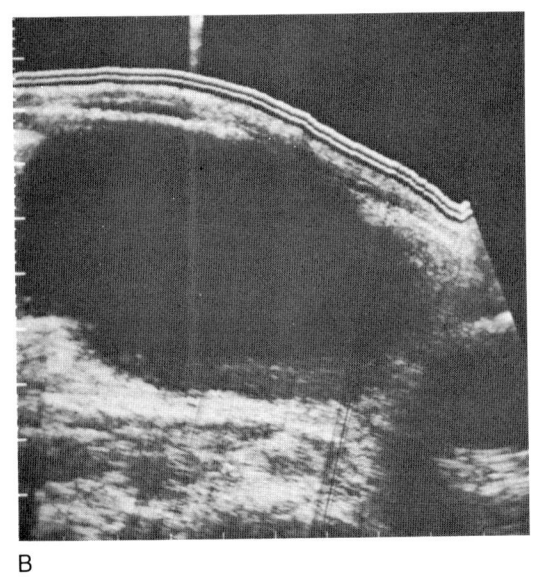

B

1007

16.9 Retroperitoneal Lymphangiomyomatosis

A 24-year-old woman presented with abdominal swelling, and ascites was noted. A lymphangiogram at another hospital had demonstrated obstruction to the iliac paraaortic nodes with saccular lymphatic dilatation.

A longitudinal sonogram 2 cm to the right of the midline (Fig. A) showed the liver lying anterior to the inferior vena cava. The prevertebral region showed multiple cystlike masses extending throughout the abdomen and pelvis. A pleural effusion was noted above the diaphragm.

A transverse sonogram at the level of the umbilicus (Fig. B) revealed similar cystic masses in the pre- and paraaortic positions, consistent with retroperitoneal lymphangiomyomatosis.

At laparotomy, chylous peritoneal fluid was found with multiple diffuse saccular masses extending from the retroperitoneum to the right common iliac area. Biopsy specimens of the sac wall and nodes at the root of the mesentery disclosed lymphangiomata. Treatment with medium-chain triglycerides and low-fat diet resulted in no recurrent ascites.

McQuown et al. reported the bistable ultrasound appearances of two cases of lymphangiomatosis arising in the root of the greater omentum.[1] They noted that the appearances varied with the size of the cystic spaces, which can range from capillary to cavernous. In addition, bleeding may occur into the lymph spaces and produce a more complex appearance.

(This case and scans taken from Walsh JW, Taylor KJW, Rosenfield AT: Gray scale ultrasonography in retroperitoneal lymphangiomyomatosis. Am J Roentgenol 129:1101–1102, 1977. © 1977 Am Roentgen Ray Soc.)

REFERENCE

1. McQuown DS, Fishbein MC, Moran ET, et al: Abdominal cystic lymphangiomatosis: report of a case involving the liver and spleen and illustration of two cases with origin in the greater omentum and root of the mesentery. J Clin Ultrasound 3:291–296, 1975

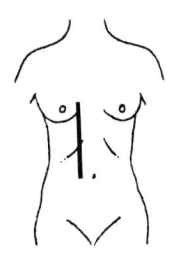

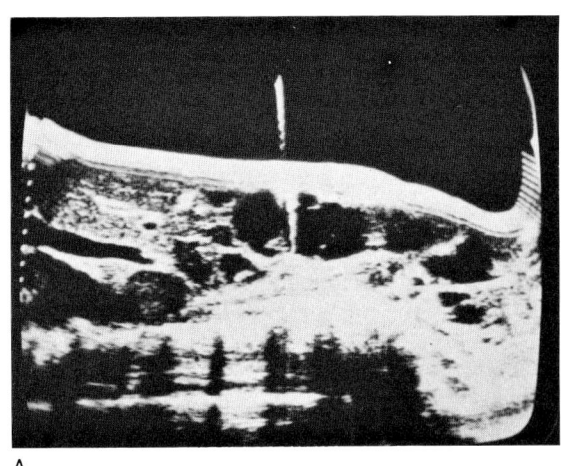

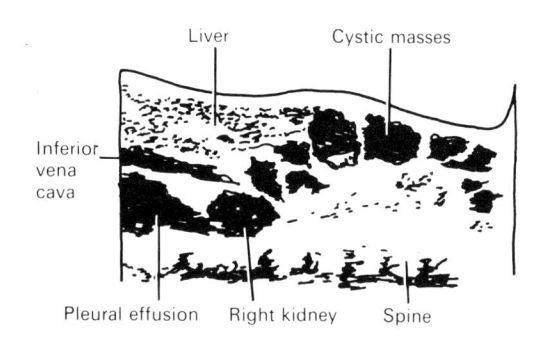

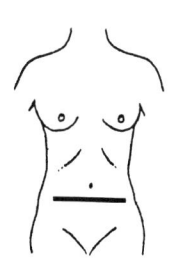

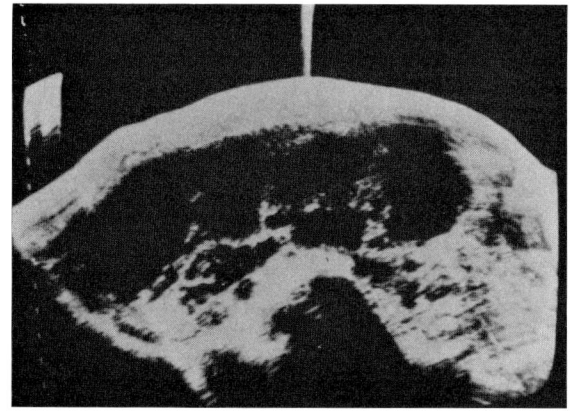

A

B

1009

Cysts (16.10 and 16.11)

16.10 Lymphangiectatic Cyst

An 18-year-old woman presented with increasing acute abdominal pain 3 days after minor trauma to the right lower quadrant. On direct questioning, her history included a recent disturbance and irregularity of menses for the previous 3 months, but she denied any increase in abdominal girth.

Examination revealed a dehydrated ill young woman with diffuse abdominal tenderness, but no definite palpable masses were appreciated. Her white cell count was 21,000/mm^3, her temperature was 101°F, and hematocrit was 41. Plain radiography of the abdomen was remarkable for demonstrating a gasless small bowel (Fig. A). The obvious diagnosis of hemoperitoneum seemed unlikely in view of her normal hematocrit. A liver/spleen scan showed normal findings and no evidence of splenic rupture.

Longitudinal and transverse sonograms disclosed multilocular cystic areas with contained debris filling the entire abdomen (Fig. B) and pelvis (Fig. C). The possibility was entertained that this was paralytic ileus with distended bowel loops. A more likely diagnosis was that of a preexisting mass, perhaps a teratoma, which had hemorrhaged in response to the moderate preceding trauma.

Surgery revealed a multicystic abdominopelvic mass attached only to the tail of the pancreas (Fig. D). When opened, the cystic areas contained considerable hemorrhage and thrombus. Histologic study revealed a lymphangiectatic cyst with recurrent hemorrhage and thrombus, consistent with a cystic lymphangioma of the mesentery.

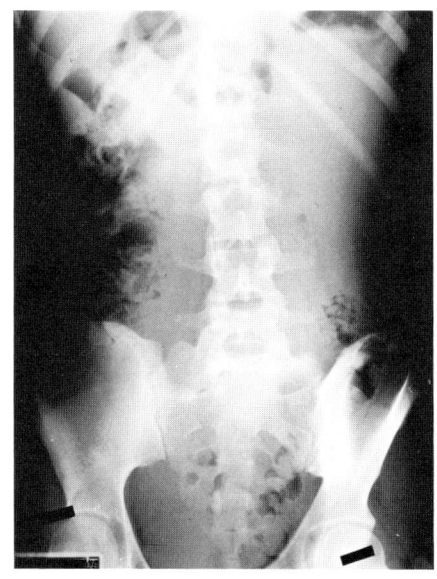

A

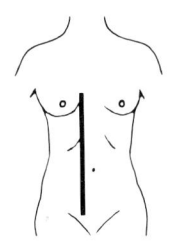

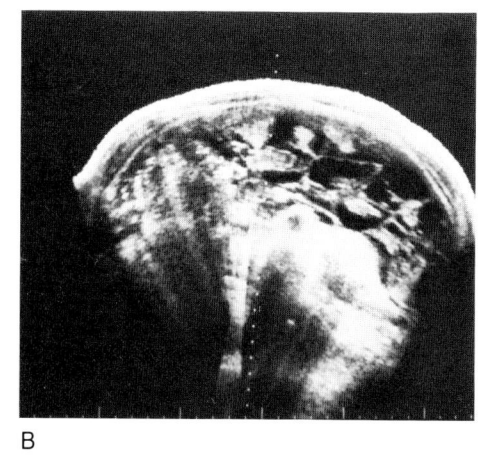

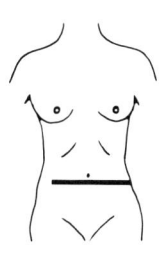

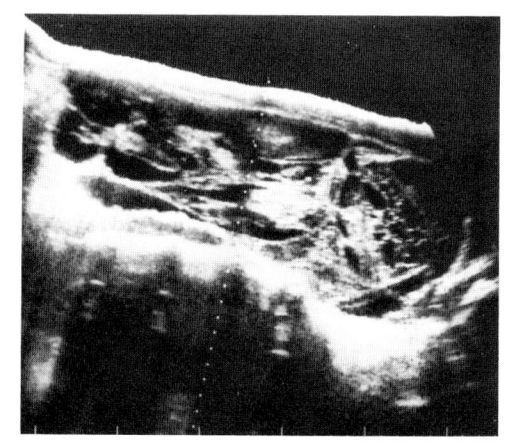

B

C

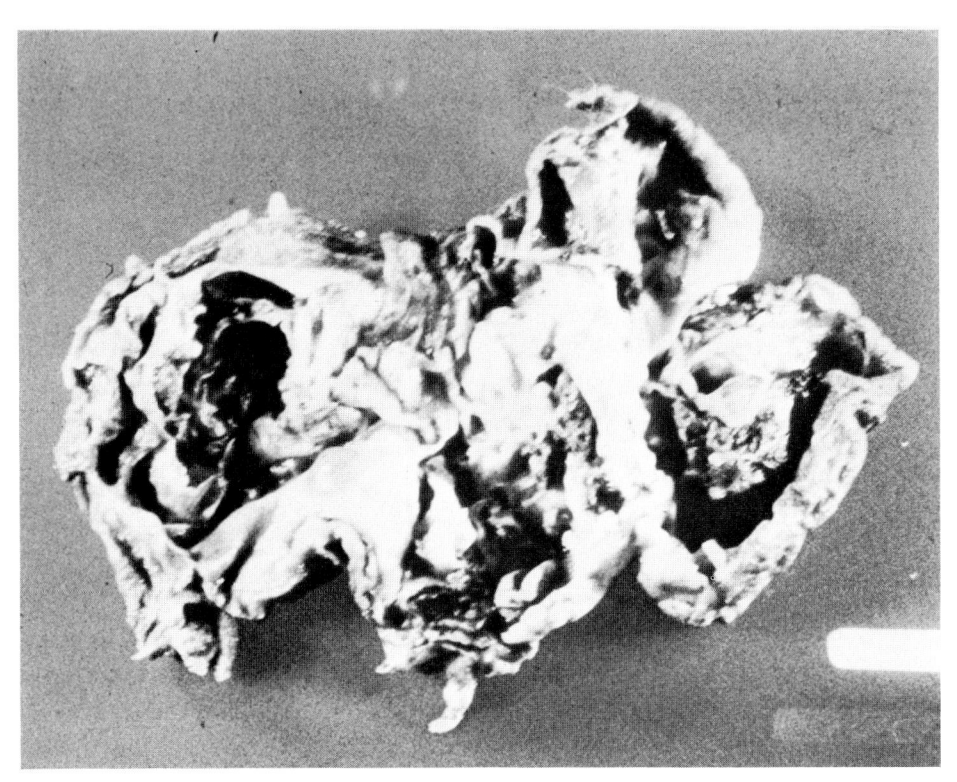

D

16.11 Retroperitoneal Cystic Mass in an Infant

A 2-month-old infant presented with a right flank mass noted by her pediatrician on routine examination. This mass was watched for 1 month, during which it appeared to increase in size. The patient was referred for an ultrasound examination to investigate this mass further. The longitudinal sonogram demonstrated a complex, partially cystic mass lying anterior to the right kidney and inferior to the right lobe of the liver (Fig. A). The transverse scan again demonstrated the septate, cystic nature of the mass (Fig. B). The mass appeared to be separate from both the kidney and the liver.

In view of our past experience of ovarian masses in neonates, the differential diagnosis included an ovarian cyst, a teratoma, or hematoma. Surgery revealed multiple benign ovarian cysts.

The primitive gonad arises from the genital ridge in the dorsal root of the mesentery during the 6th week of gestation. The cortex proliferates to form the primordial follicles until approximately 6 months' gestation. The ovary subsequently descends from its lumbar origin to its definitive pelvic site.

Ovarian cysts occur commonly in newborn girls. Small follicular cysts were found in 34 percent of 332 stillborns or neonatal deaths.[1] Most cysts are small and insignificant, but large cysts may produce respiratory distress, rupture and produce intraperitoneal bleeding, or present as abdominal masses, as in this patient.

The possibility of an ovarian cyst should be considered in any neonatal girl presenting with a lumbar mass. Because of the complex nature of the mass in this patient, excision was indicated to exclude the possibility of a teratoma.

REFERENCE

1. DeSa DJ: Follicular ovarian cysts in stillbirths and neonates. Arch Dis Child 50:45–50, 1975

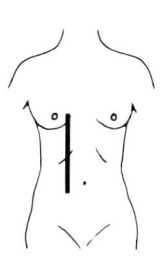

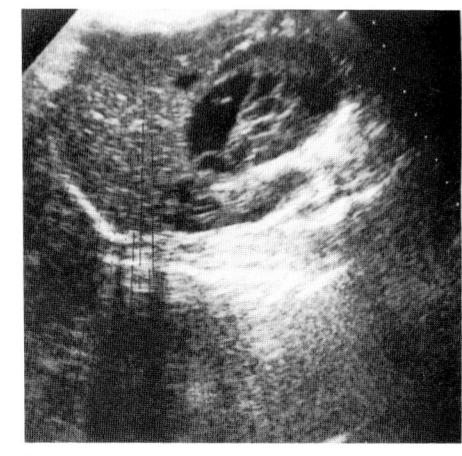

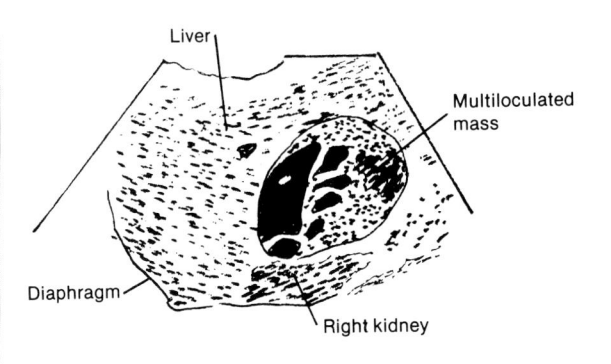

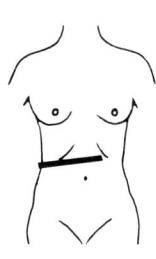

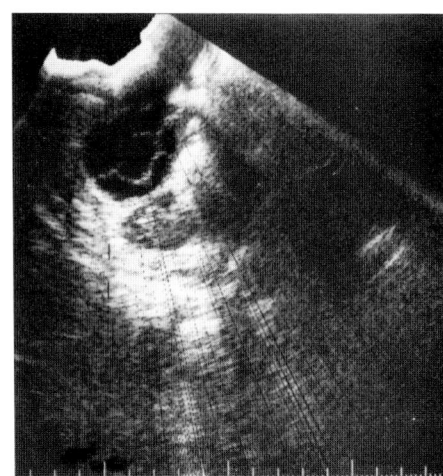

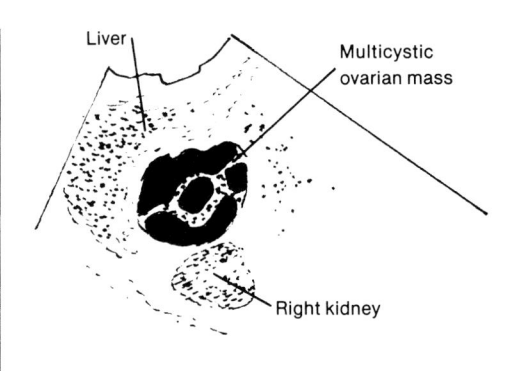

A

B

16.12 Left Upper Quadrant Mass: CSF Collection

An 8-year-old child with a malignant glioblastoma presented with vomiting and an enlarging head. A ventricular shunt had been inserted earlier, and symptoms were suggestive of an obstructed shunt. A plain film of the abdomen (Fig. A) demonstrated a fluid collection (arrowed) around the end of the catheter. Ultrasound examination of the left upper quadrant confirmed this (Fig. B), while a contact scan of the head demonstrated gross ventricular dilatation (Fig. C).

This case demonstrates well the value of ultrasound for surveying the entire body, including the brain in the very young. In this patient, both ends of the catheter could be examined, allowing the diagnosis of a loculated fluid collection around the lower end of the catheter and the resulting hydrocephalus.

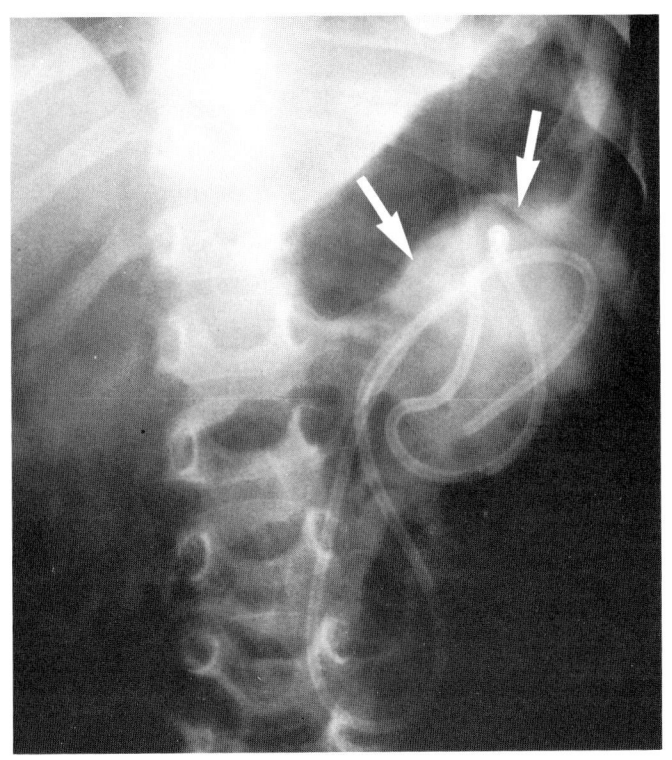

A

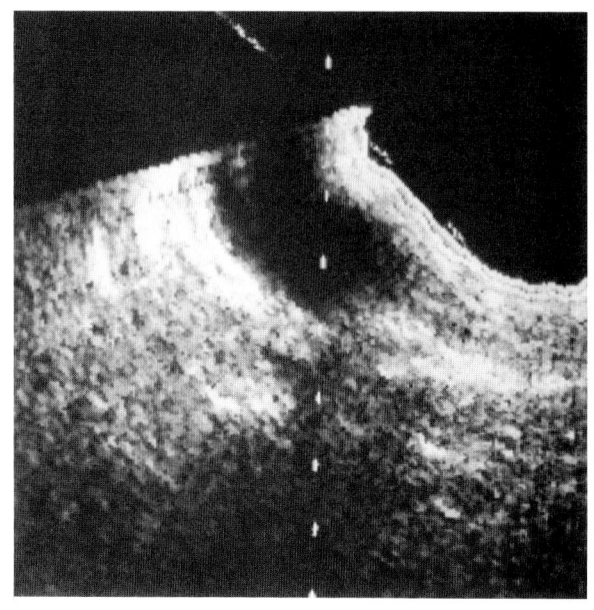

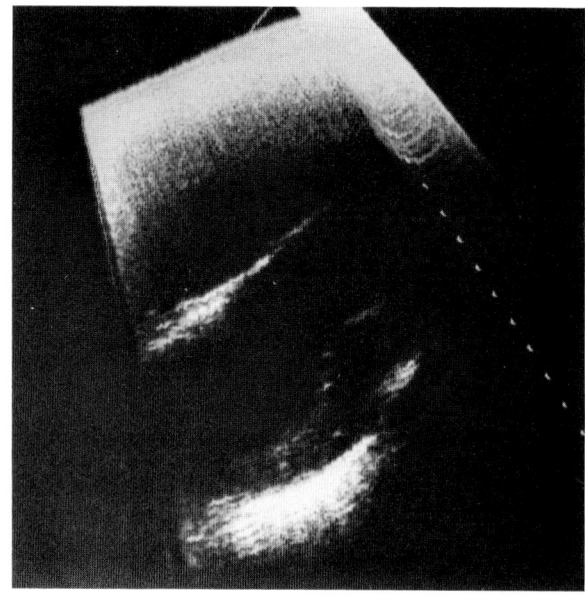

B

C

16.13 Psoas Abscess

A 20-year-old basketball player experienced pain in his right hip for a period of 9 months. He was treated with physical therapy with slight improvement. The pain subsequently worsened, requiring him to use crutches. There was a recent onset of chills and night sweats.

On physical examination the right leg was partially flexed. There was minimal tenderness in the right lower quadrant. The right leg was held in flexion and there was a suggestion of psoas muscle enlargement.

On admission he was referred for ultrasound examination. Two longitudinal sections (Figs. A and B) demonstrated gross enlargement of the right psoas muscle, with a huge cystic cavity consistent with an abscess or necrotic tumor. A CT scan (Fig. C) showed a biloculated right psoas collection (arrowed). Serial sections demonstrated pointing below the inguinal ligament. A [67]gallium study demonstrated uptake in the right paravertebral gutter (Fig. D). These appearances were consistent with a huge right psoas abscess.

At surgery, a thick-walled abscess was found containing more than 3 L of caseous material. Histologic study demonstrated a granulomatous reaction to acid-fast bacilli. The patient responded well to antituberculous therapy.

This case illustrates dramatically the huge abdominal abscesses that occasionally occur with little constitutional disturbance. A psoas abscess is the classic manifestation of tuberculosis. The abscess cavity is constrained by the thick lumbar fascia surrounding the psoas major muscle, so that the abscess contents point below the inguinal ligament.

(This case and Scans A & B and Figs. C & D taken from Andriole VT: The clinician's viewpoint. pp. 1. In Joseph AEA, Cosgrove D, (eds): Clinics in Diagnostic Ultrasound, Volume 11, Ultrasound in Inflammatory Disease. Churchill Livingstone, New York, 1983.)

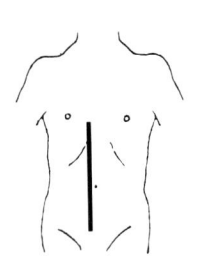

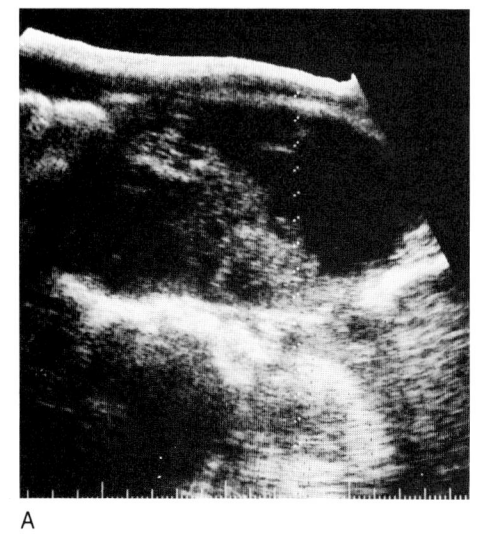

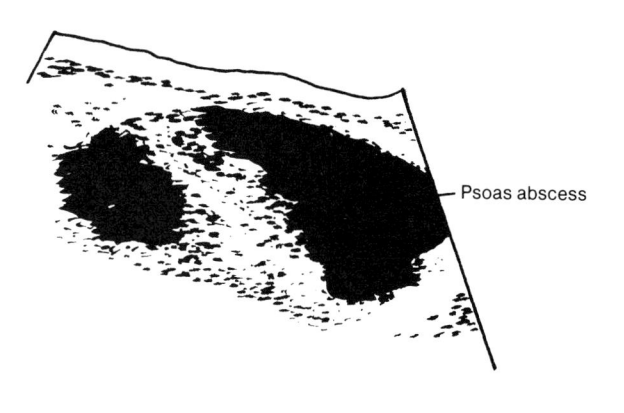

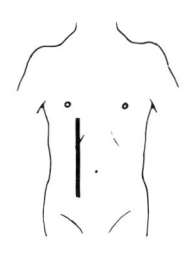

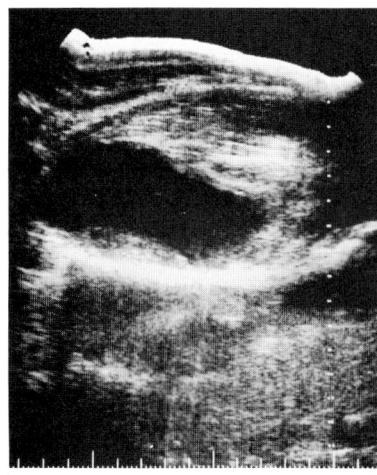

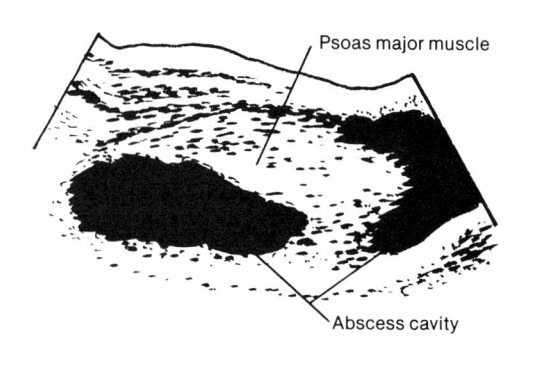

A

B

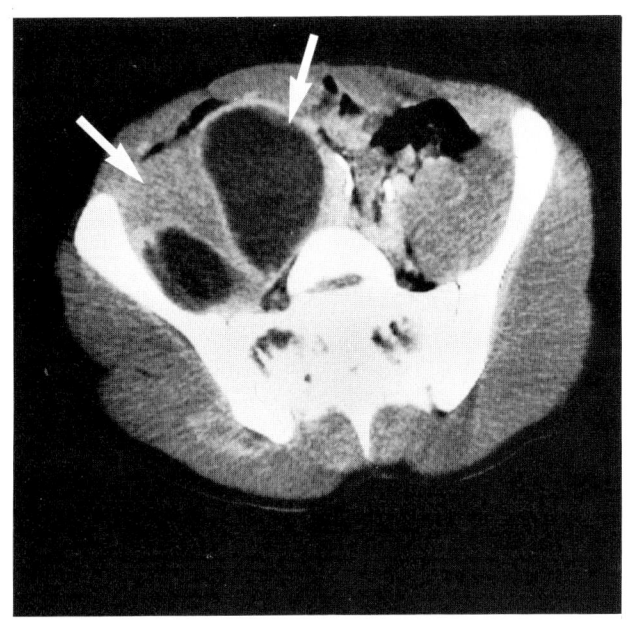

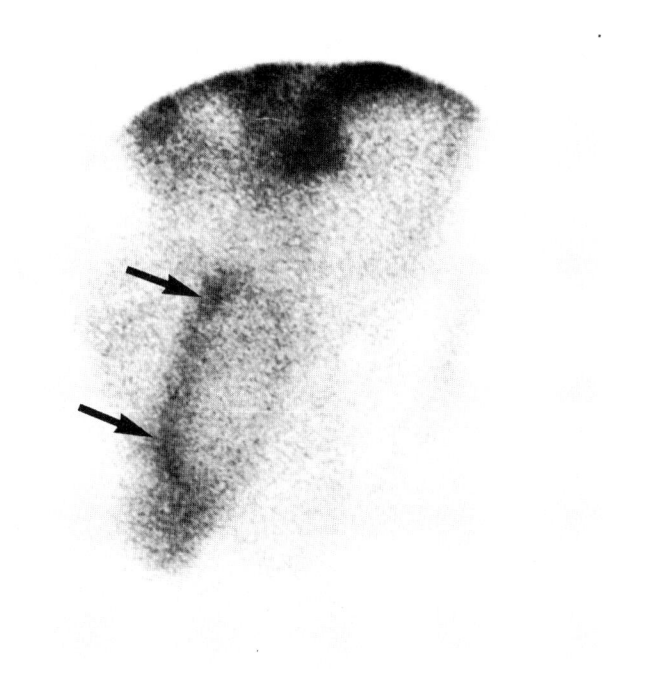

C

D

1019

16.14 Superficial Lumbar Mass

An 80-year-old diabetic woman developed a large, tender mass in the left loin over a period of 3 days. On examination, a tender but firm mass was appreciated apparently in the subcutaneous tissues of the posterior abdominal wall. Ultrasound demonstrated an irregular mass of homogeneous consistency with some contained debris (arrowed in the figure). The differential diagnosis was between a tumor and an abscess, with an abscess being more likely. Needle aspiration of the most homogeneous part of the mass yielded thin pus and gram stain demonstrated both gram-positive cocci and gram-negative rods. An incision performed in the ultrasound examination room demonstrated a small quantity of pus.

The patient was seen 2 days later after treatment with antibiotics. A large quantity of pus was present and easily expressed through the incision. The abscess resolved without further intervention.

The echogenicity of a mass gives little indication of the viscosity of contained material. Recently, clotted blood has been reported to appear as anechoic as a clear fluid collection. On the other hand, abscesses may be highly echogenic, especially where a small quantity of contained air has been produced by air-containing organisms. In this patient, differentiation between a phlegmon and liquid pus could not be made adequately either by ultrasound or other modalities. Such patients are most expeditiously treated by early aspiration and drainage, leading directly to bacteriologic diagnosis, appropriate therapy, and subsequent resolution of the abscess.

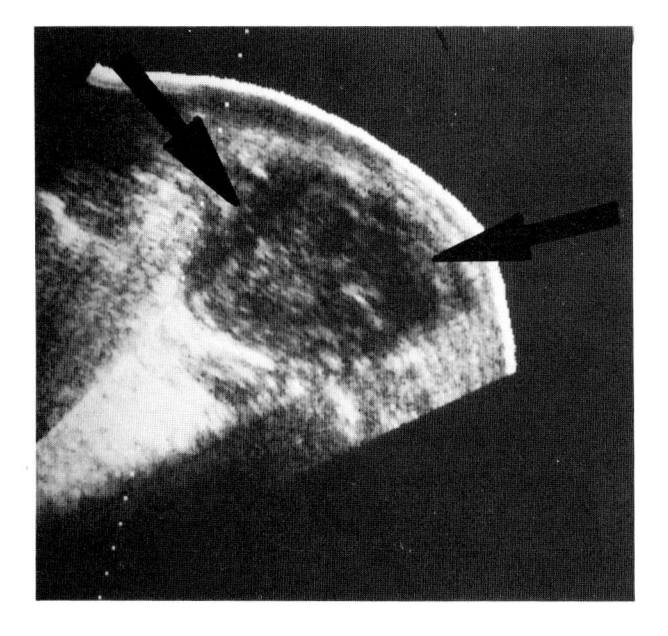

16.15 Recurrent Keloid Formation

A 21-year-old white woman presented with a mass in the anterior abdominal wall which was considered to be due to keloid formation. There was a long history of exuberant keloid formation in response to any surgical incision.

The transverse (Fig. A) and oblique (Fig. B) sonograms demonstrated a rather homogeneous mass (arrowed) probably arising from the rectus sheath. This was excised and proved to be a keloid.

The ultrasound characteristics of this mass appear to be surprising. Collagen has a high bulk modulus and therefore is considered to be an important source of echo formation. However, the change of acoustic impedance is responsible for the appearance of echogenicity. A mass of fairly pure collagen, therefore, would produce high-amplitude echoes at its junction with other tissues, but would not necessarily demonstrate high echogenicity within it.

A keloid is the abnormal accumulation of excessive amounts of collagen. Collagen accumulation in a healing wound reflects a balance between synthesis and lysis; keloid formation is due to an inadequate rate of lysis. Keloid formation appears to be an individual predisposition which is more common in blacks.

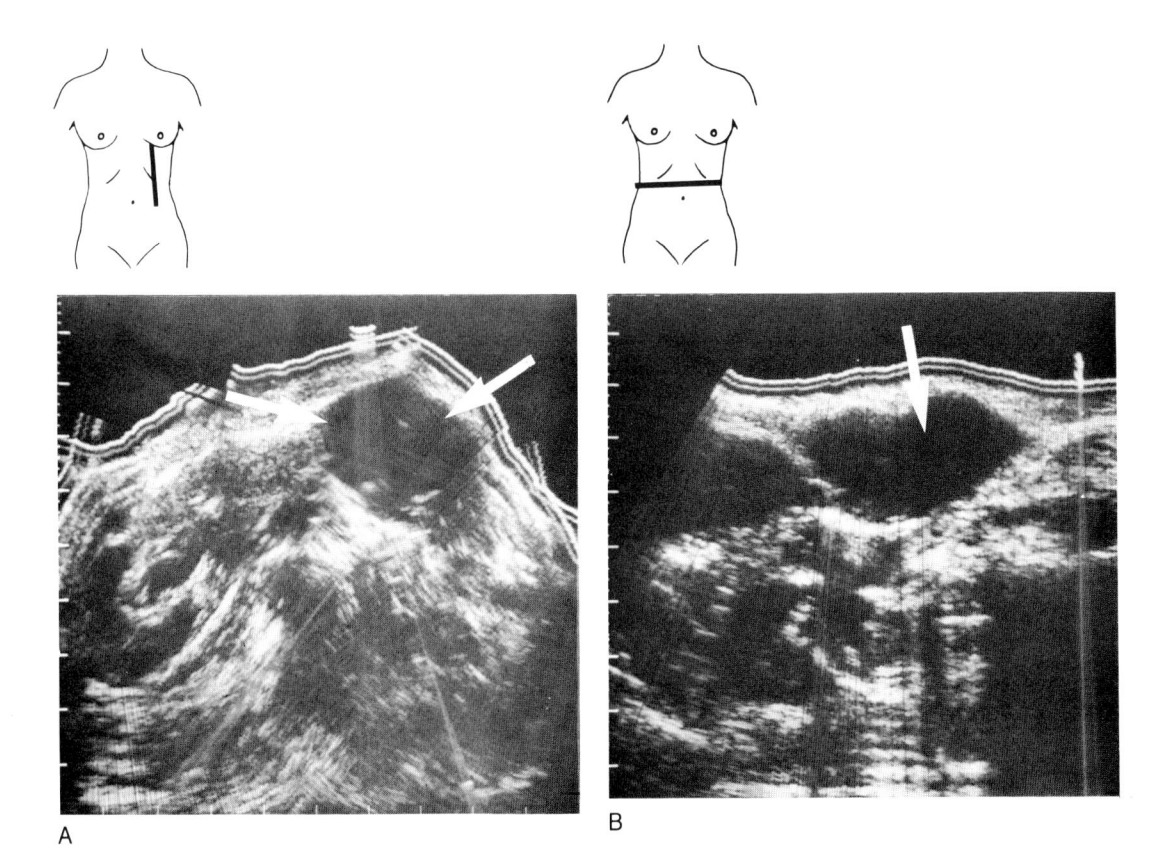

A

B

17 The Bowel

KENNETH J. W. TAYLOR

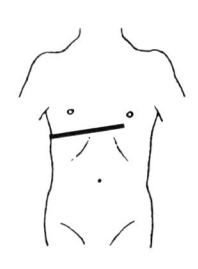

17.1 Normal Pylorus and Duodenum

The normal stomach (S) can be seen after ingestion of water, as in this figure. Fluid can be traced through the pylorus into the duodenum (D) thereby outlining the head, neck, and body of the pancreas which lie in the bed of the stomach. The common bile duct is arrowed, lying in the head of the pancreas. Gastric polyps and other tumors may be discovered serendipitously. In addition, thickening of the stomach wall due to linitis plastica or lymphoma can be assessed and any therapeutic response evaluated.

Kremer and Grobner described four patients with small focal gastric wall lesions observed by the fluid-filled-stomach method.[1] We and many other sonologists have used these methods routinely to view the pancreas.[2-4] During a real-time examination, the stomach wall should also be searched for polyps or other masses.

REFERENCES

1. Kremer H, Grobner W: Sonography of polypoid gastric lesions by the fluid-filled stomach method. J Clin Ultrasound 9:51–54, 1981
2. Crade M, Taylor KJW, Rosenfield AT: Water distention of the gut in the evaluation of the pancreas by ultrasound. AJR 131:348–349, 1978
3. Warren PS, Garrett WJ, Kossoff G: The liquid-filled stomach—an ultrasonic window to the upper abdomen. J Clin Ultrasound 6:315–320, 1978
4. Weighall SL, Wolfmann NT, Watson N: The fluid-filled stomach: a new sonic window. J Clin Ultrasound 7:353–356, 1979

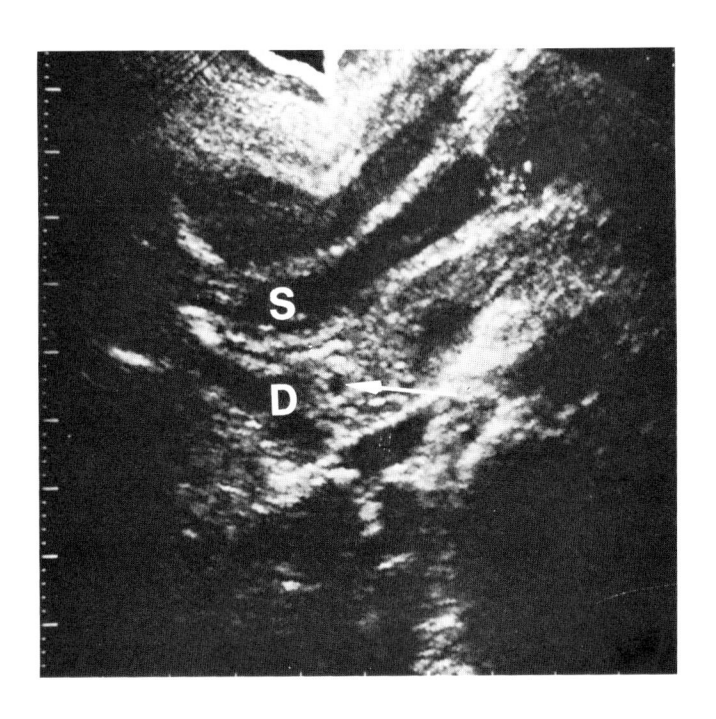

17.2 Hypertrophic Pyloric Stenosis

A newborn infant presented with vomiting and a palpable mass in the right side of the epigastrium. High-resolution real-time examination of this area after ingestion of water demonstrated the fluid-filled stomach converging onto the hypertrophied pylorus (Fig. A). The pylorus measured 2.4 cm in cross-section. An upper GI examination (Fig. B) demonstrated persistent antral indentation, which is characteristic of this condition (arrowed, Fig. B).

Strauss et al. reported the sonographic findings in 20 children with suspected hypertrophic pyloric stenosis. The pylorus was considered abnormal if it measured 15 mm or more in diameter. Of 16 infants with a mass of this size, 15 underwent surgery and the diagnosis was confirmed.

(Case and scans used courtesy of Dr. Yakcov Itzchak, Chaim Sheba Medical Center, Tel Aviv, Israel.)

REFERENCE

1. Strauss, S, Itzchak Y, Manor A, et al: Sonography of hypertrophic pyloric stenosis. AJR 136:1057–1058, 1981

Rectus abdominus muscle

Fluid filled stomach

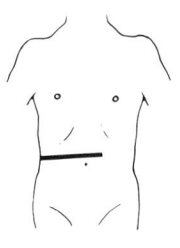

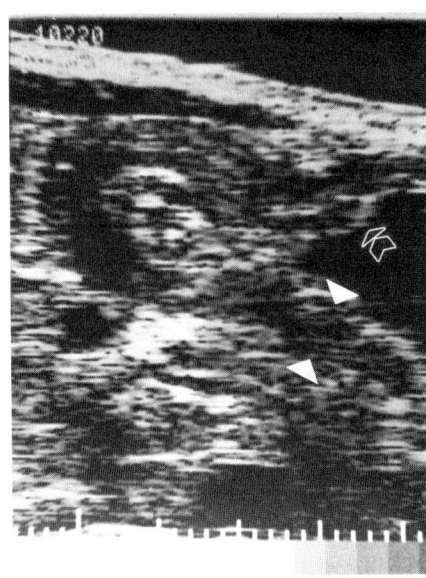

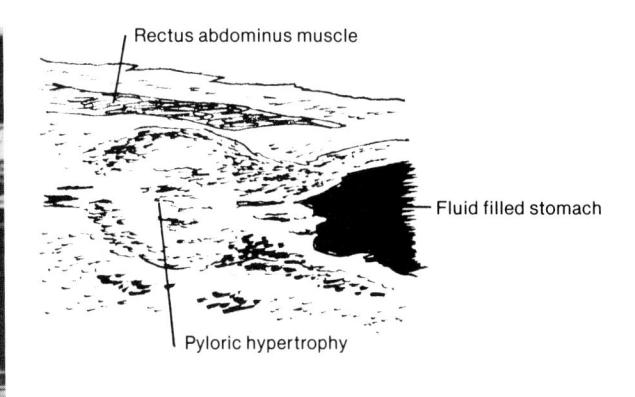

Pyloric hypertrophy

Bowel—pyloric stenosis

A

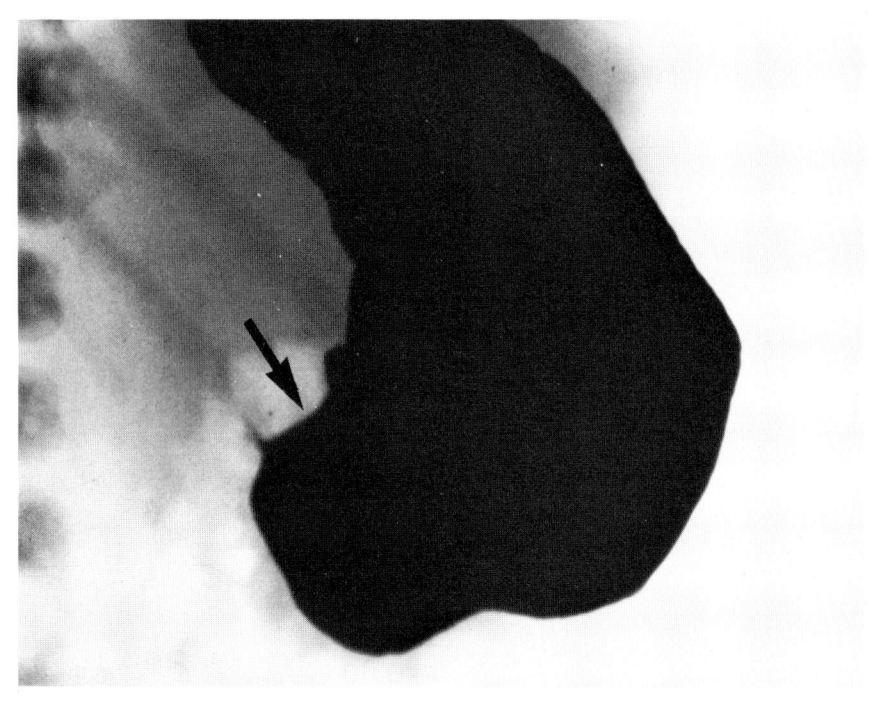

B

17.3 Left Upper Quadrant Mass: Stomach or Pseudocyst?

A 46-year-old woman was referred for a follow-up examination after a severe attack of alcohol-induced pancreatitis. No mass was appreciated on physical examination. An oblique sonogram (Fig. A) showed a large, cystic mass 6 cm in diameter in the left hypochondrium lying anterior to the left kidney and continuous with the tail of the pancreas. This was confirmed by a longitudinal sonogram (Fig. B), which showed the cystic mass anterior to, but separate from, the upper half of the kidney.

Occasionally such appearances are due to a distended stomach with gastric outlet obstruction. The patient can be given a drink of water or a carbonated beverage to see if bubbles appear in the cystic structure, or a nasogastric tube can be passed and the stomach contents aspirated. The appearances here are consistent with a pseudocyst in the tail of the pancreas.

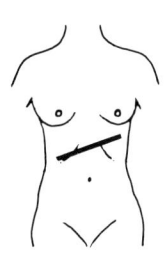

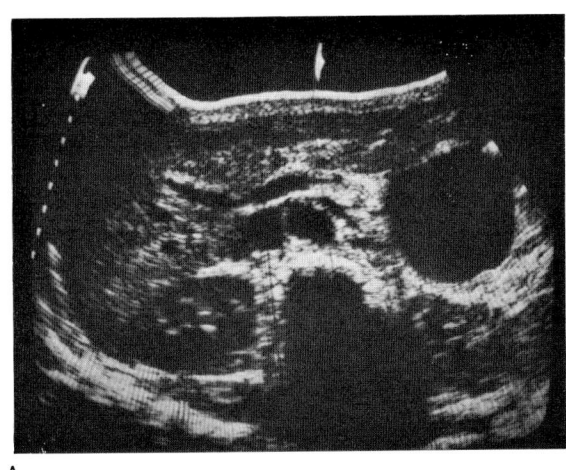

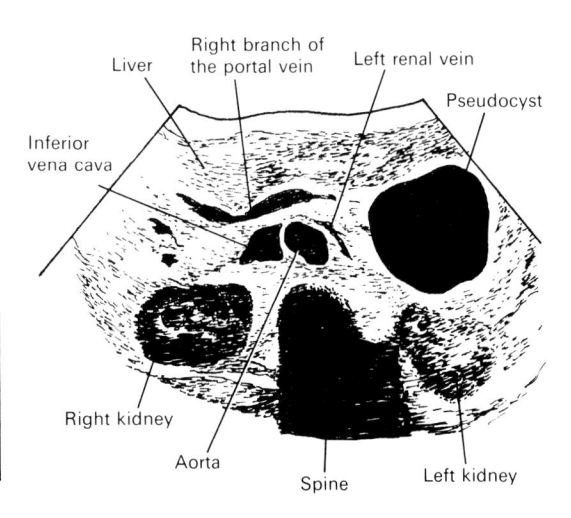

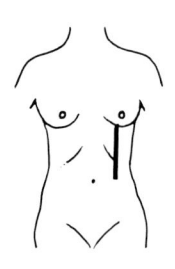

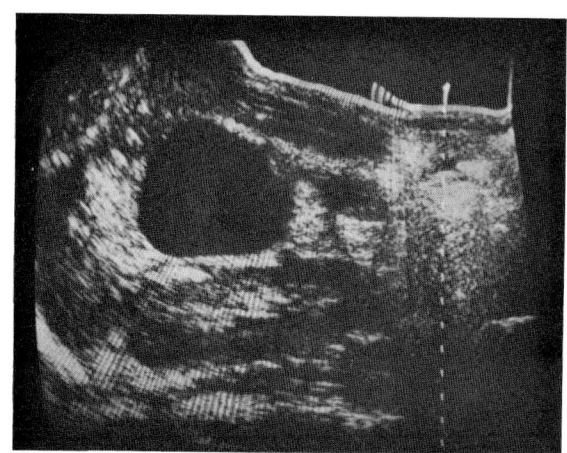

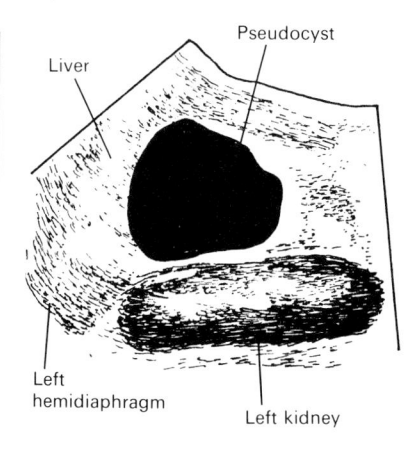

B

1028

17.4 Stomach Lymphoma

A 73-year-old man with a 28-year history of recurrent gastric polyps underwent endoscopic biopsy which produced profuse bleeding. He was transferred to a tertiary care hospital where investigation indicated that bleeding was due to idiopathic thrombocytopenia (ITP).

On physical examination, a palpable mass was appreciated in the left upper quadrant. A longitudinal sonogram (Fig. A) demonstrated marked thickening of the stomach wall, suggesting an infiltrating cancer or lymphoma. The transverse scan also documented gross thickening of the gastric wall (Fig. B).

An upper GI examination (Fig. C) showed tumor infiltration with thickening of the gastric folds, most marked on the greater and lesser curvatures (arrowed). The patient underwent a splenectomy for his ITP, which had proven resistant to steroid therapy. A needle biopsy specimen of the stomach at that time disclosed lymphocytic lymphoma.

A further case of lymphomatous infiltration of the bowel is shown in Figures D and E. Figure D demonstrates gross thickening of the gastric wall, which also showed poor compliance. Figure E demonstrates gross thickening of the wall of the small bowel.

The ultrasound appearances of gut tumors on bistable instrumentation were described by Walls[1] in 1976. Subsequently, named signs have been assigned to these appearances. Peterson et al. considered the "doughnut sign" to be specific for lesions of the GI tract.[2] Other authors[3] have used the term "pseudo-kidney sign" to describe the ultrasound appearances of a hypoechoic mass with a central echogenic lumen seen in this patient. Such appearances are characteristic of a diffuse infiltrating process which is usually, but not invariably, malignant.

REFERENCES

1. Walls WJ: The evaluation of malignant gastric neoplasms by ultrasonic B-scanning. Radiology 118:159–163, 1976
2. Peterson CR, Cooperberg PL: Ultrasonic demonstration of lesions of the gastrointestinal tract. Gastrointest Radiol 3:303–306, 1978
3. Bluth EI, Merritt CRB, Sullivan MA: Ultrasonic evaluation of the stomach, small bowel and colon. Radiology 133:677–680, 1979

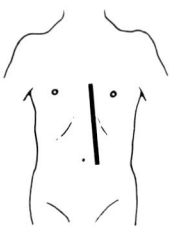

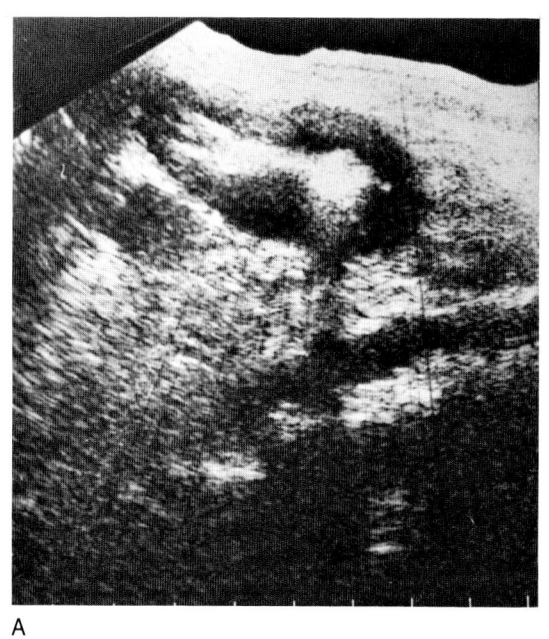

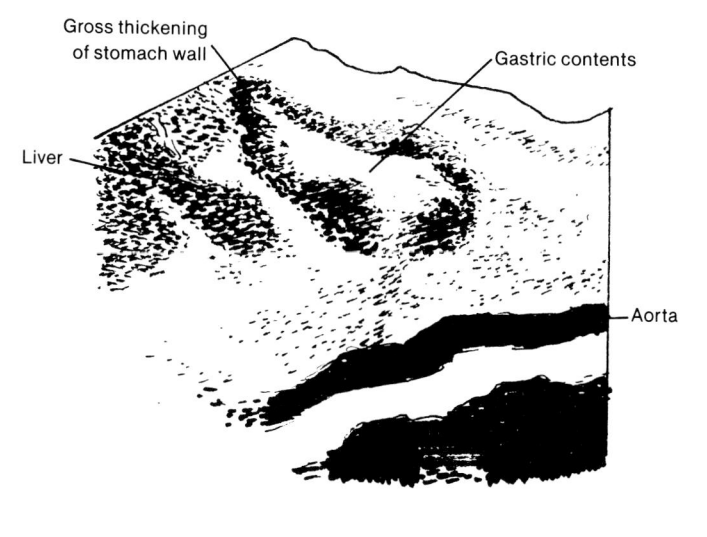

A

Gross thickening of stomach wall

Gastric contents

Liver

Aorta

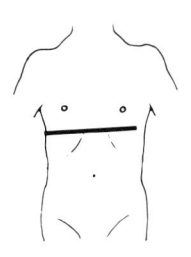

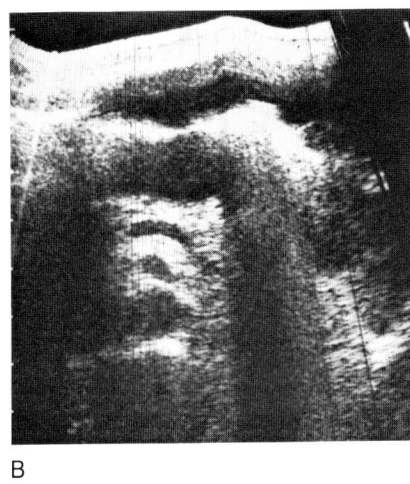

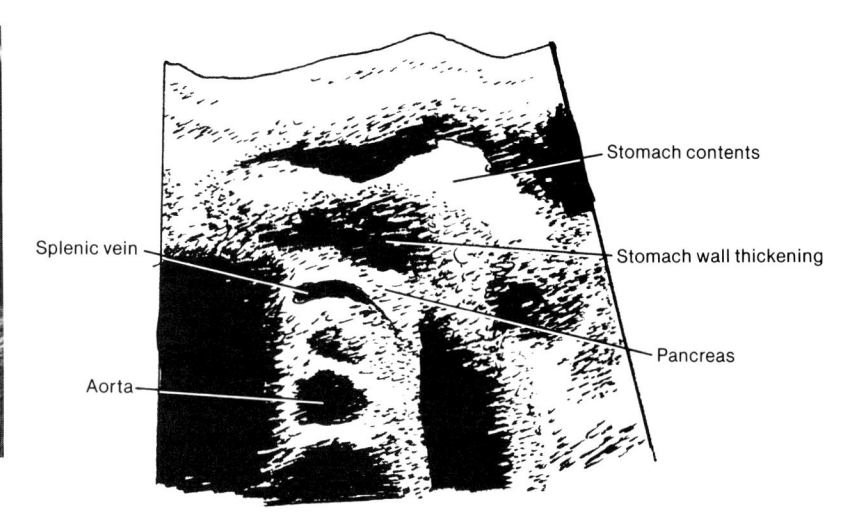

Stomach contents

Splenic vein

Stomach wall thickening

Pancreas

Aorta

B

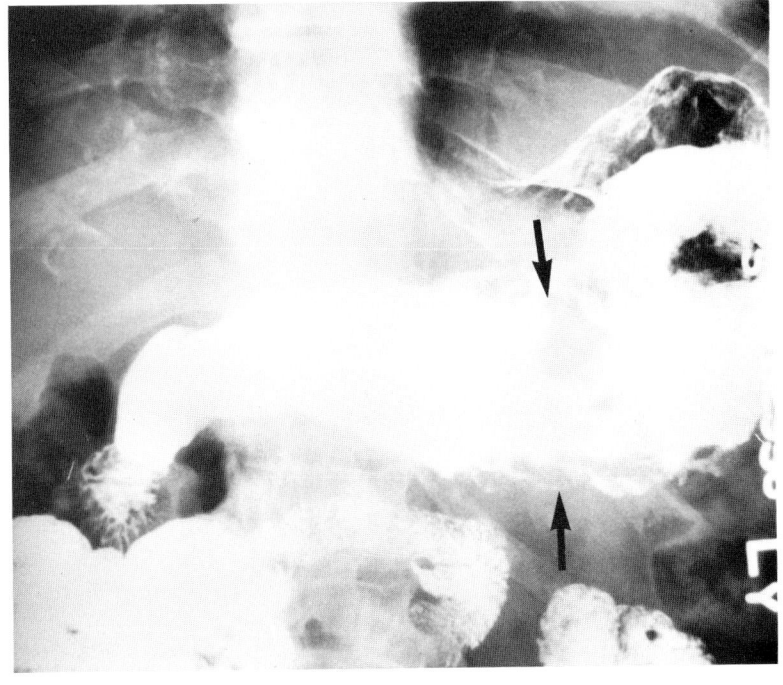

C

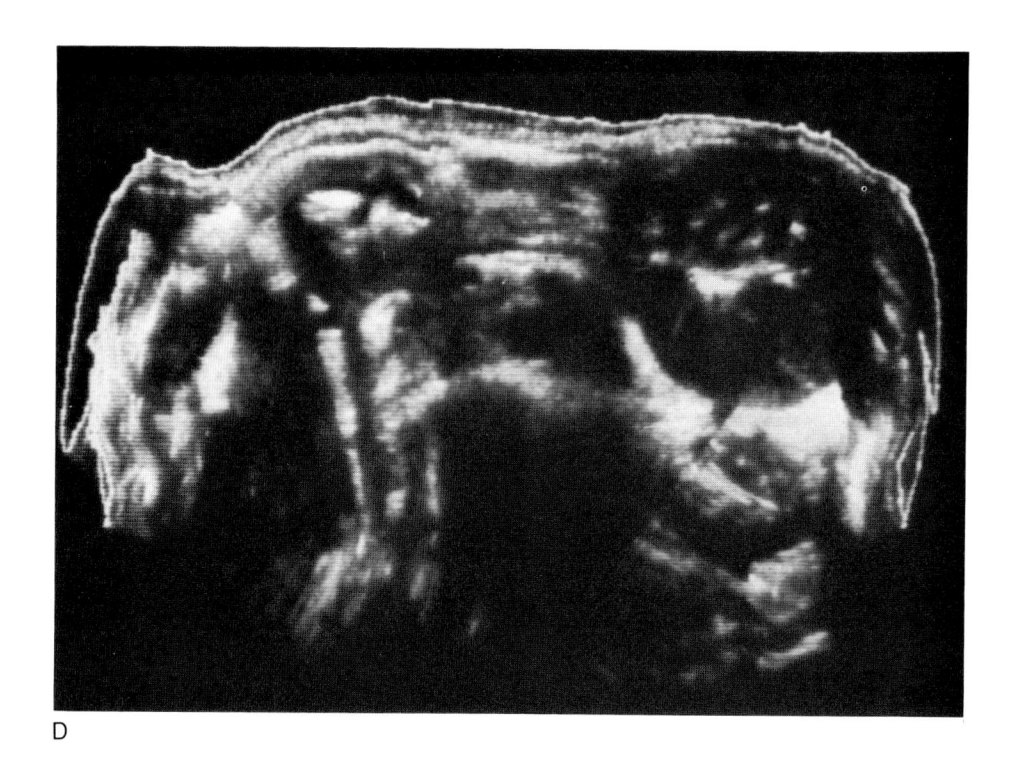

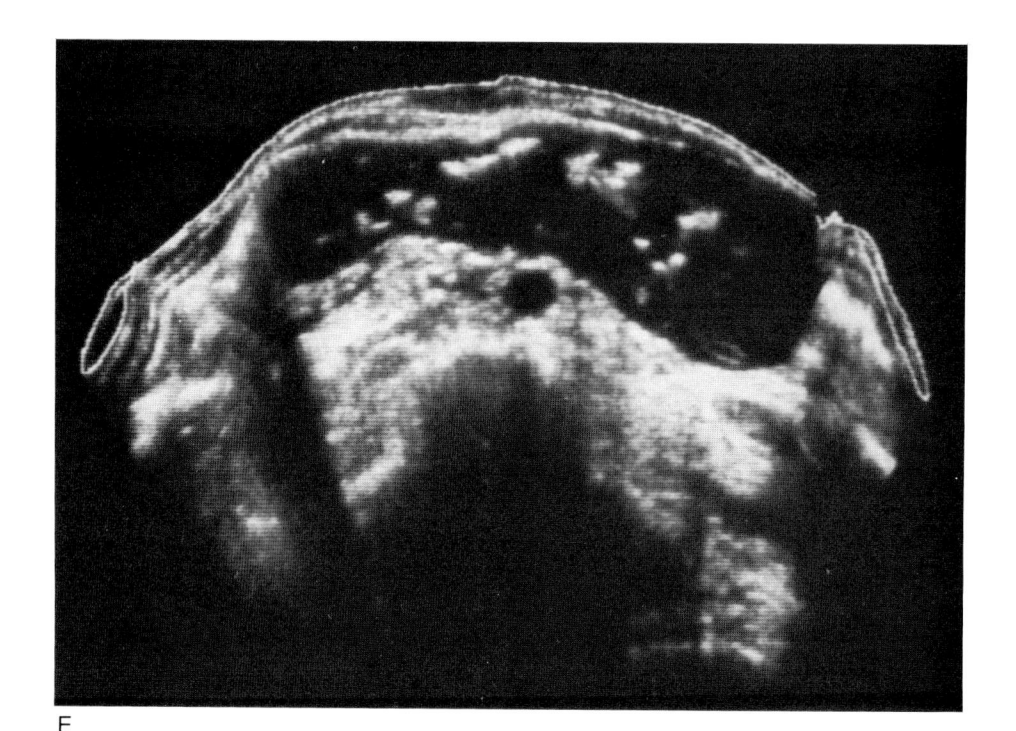

D

E

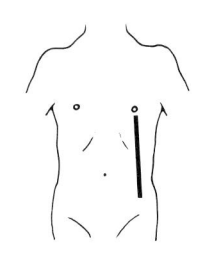

17.5 Trichobezoar

A mentally impaired patient developed upper abdominal pain and a palpable epigastric mass and was referred for ultrasound examination. The longitudinal scan shown in the figure demonstrated a highly reflective mass (arrowed) lying within the stomach deep to the liver. There was virtually no beam transmission through the mass. A trichobezoar was removed at surgery.

Ingestion of hair is comparatively rare, but does occur among the mentally handicapped. The sonographic appearances of a hairball have been described.[1] Although these appearances are similar to those of air in the stomach, the condition should be suspected when a mass is palpated.

(Case and figure courtesy of Dr. Lacoste, Bologna, Italy.)

REFERENCE

1. Ratcliffe JF: The ultrasonographic appearance of a trichobezoar. Br J Radiol: 55:166–167, 1982

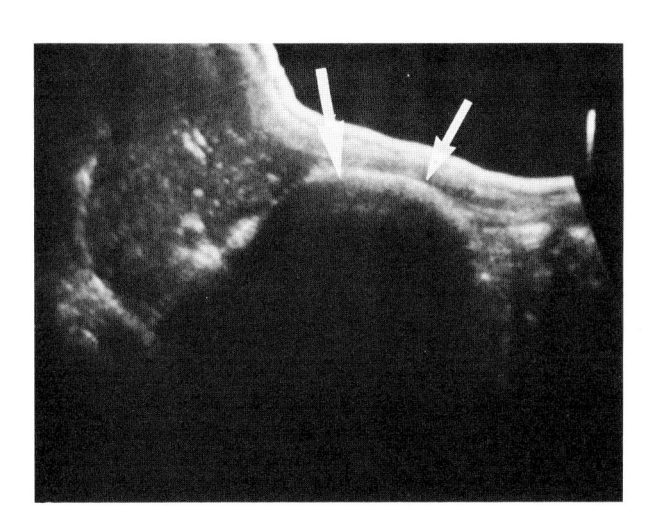

17.6 Perforated Duodenal Ulcer with Subphrenic Abscess

This is a highly unusual case of an 8-year-old with a perforated duodenal ulcer. The plain film showed mottled air in the right subphrenic space (Fig. A). Ultrasound examination with the patient in the decubitus position (Fig. B) showed a homogeneous collection under the right hemidiaphragm which returned high-level echoes. This was highly suggestive of an air-containing subphrenic abscess. The patient was treated with antibiotics.

This patient illustrates a number of important points about the ultrasonic detection of abscesses. Plain films of the chest and abdomen are worthwhile in the search for extraluminal gas collections. Allowance must be made for postoperative air. Evidence of air under the diaphragm, increasing with time, strongly suggests an abscess rather than postoperative air. Although air reputedly gives rise to difficulty in ultrasound diagnosis, its appearance can also be very helpful as indicated in this case. A relatively anechoic fluid collection containing high-amplitude echoes suggests air and is highly suspicious for abscess formation. The technique employed in ultrasound examination in such cases is critical for success.

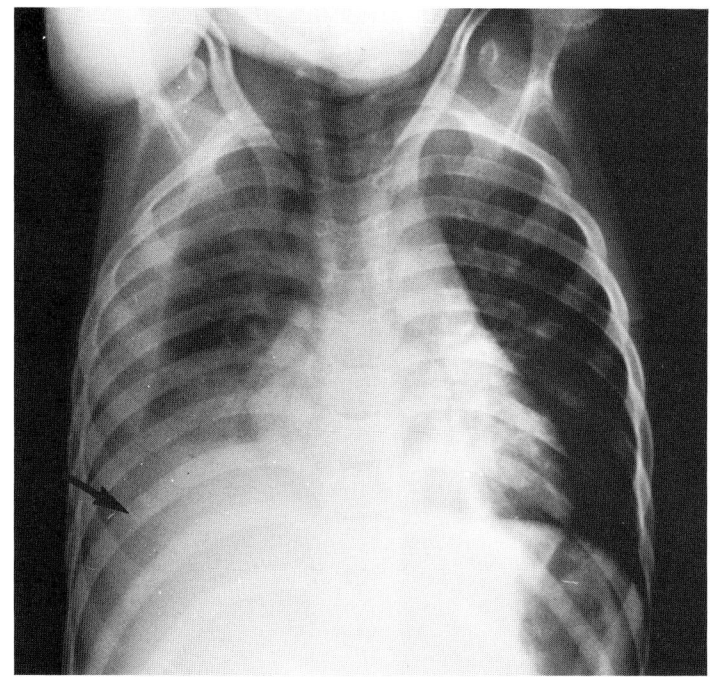

A

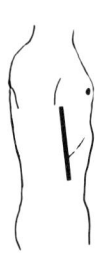

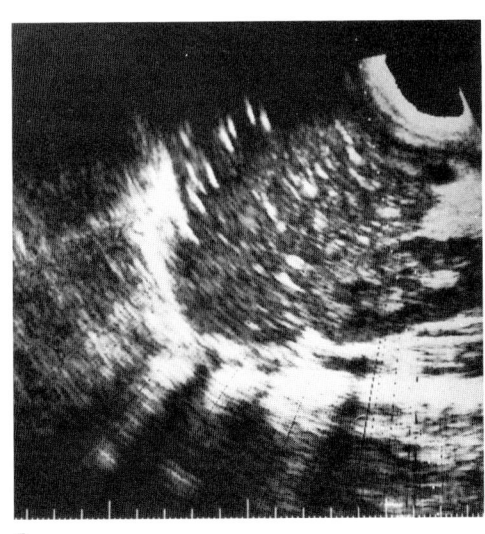

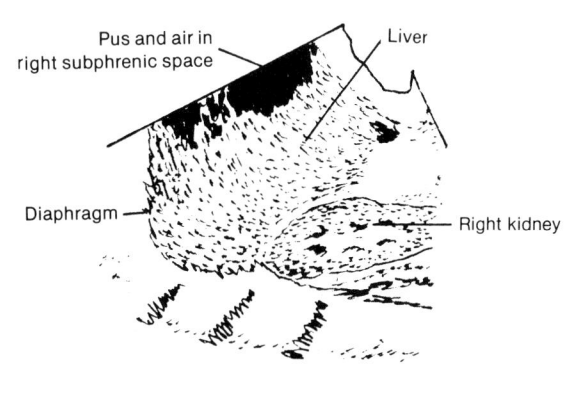

B

17.7 Epigastric Abscess Due to Perforation of Gut

A 72-year-old black woman presented to the emergency room with abdominal pain, fever, anorexia, nausea, and vomiting. These symptoms had been present for 3 months prior to admission. The patient had also undergone right mastectomy for carcinoma of the breast 13 months previously. She had received chemotherapy for her breast cancer since all axillary nodes were positive.

A kidney/ureter/bladder radiograph (Fig. A) demonstrated a needle (arrowed) in the right subxiphoid region in the middle of the soft-tissue density. A sonogram revealed a predominantly cystic mass lying anterior to the aorta with some contained debris (Fig. B). The differential diagnosis included an abscess or pseudocyst arising from the pancreas. Surgery revealed an abscess which was presumably secondary to perforation by the needle.

The patient was explored and 400 ml of foul-smelling pus was drained from a well-localized abdominal abscess. Subsequent ultrasonography was unable to locate the needle. Eventually the wound was reexplored under fluoroscopy and the needle was found and removed.

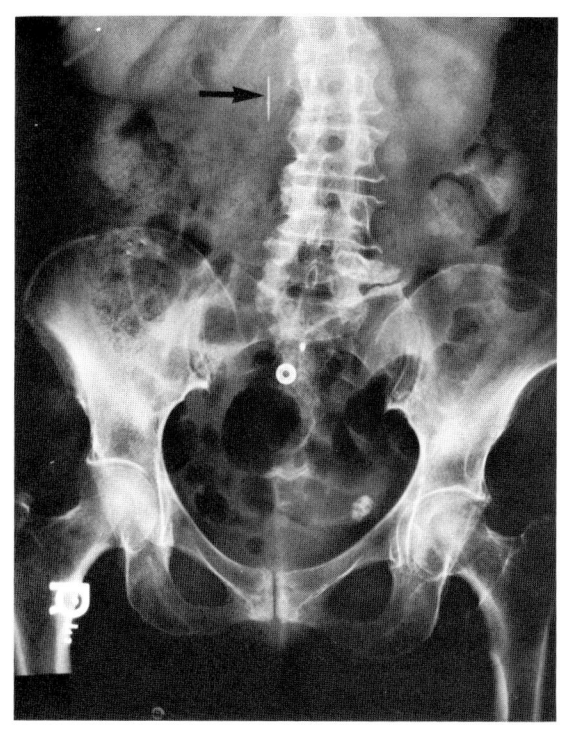

A

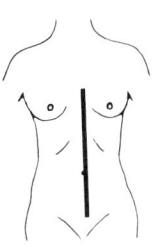

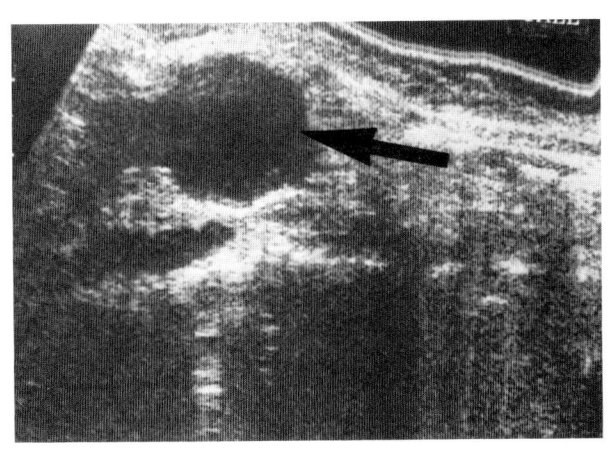

B

17.8 Mucocele of the Appendix

A 35-year-old woman was referred because of the incidental discovery of a right adnexal pelvic mass. A transverse sonogram (Fig. A) demonstrated an irregular cystic mass (arrowed) apparently separate from the right ovary. Part of this irregular mass (arrowed) was seen in the cul-de-sac lying posterior to the uterus (Fig. B). Debris was seen within the gut. Predominantly cystic pelvic masses are nearly always of ovarian origin and surgery was undertaken in this patient because of the irregular contour of this mass. Surgery disclosed a mucocele of the appendix which was benign on histologic examination.

A mucocele of the appendix is usually a benign condition; only 10 percent are malignant. It is a progressive, cystic dilatation of the distal part of the appendix by mucus.[1] Obstruction is usually by inflammatory stricture or fecolith. Sterile mucus accumulates, producing a cystic mass up to 15 cm in diameter. The wall is thin so that the cyst may appear translucent. Rarely, the cysts may rupture and because they are sterile, the resulting inflammatory reaction is mild. However, pseudomyxoma peritonei may result.[2]

A malignant mucocele arises from a mucinous cystadenocarcinoma of the appendix. Such tumors are more common in the ovary. Up to 25 percent of these tumors rupture and the peritoneum becomes seeded with tumor cells causing pseudomyxoma peritonei. This condition results more frequently from implanation of cystadenoma or cystadenocarcinoma cells of ovarian origin.

Li et al. reported the sonographic diagnosis of a mucocele of the appendix.[3] They noted that the appearances on ultrasound examination were nonspecific. However, they claimed that the combination of the ultrasound findings, a calcified rim on a plain film, and nonfilling of the appendix on a barium enema was virtually diagnostic.

REFERENCES

1. Hellsten S: Mucocele and carcinoma of the appendix. Acta Pathol Microbiol Scand 60:473–482, 1964
2. Elliott CE: Two cases of pseudomyxoma peritonei from mucocele of the appendix. Br J Surg 45:15–18, 1957
3. Li YP, Morin ME, Tan A: Ultrasound findings in mucocele of the appendix. J Clin Ultrasound 9:406–408, 1981

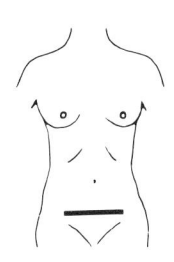

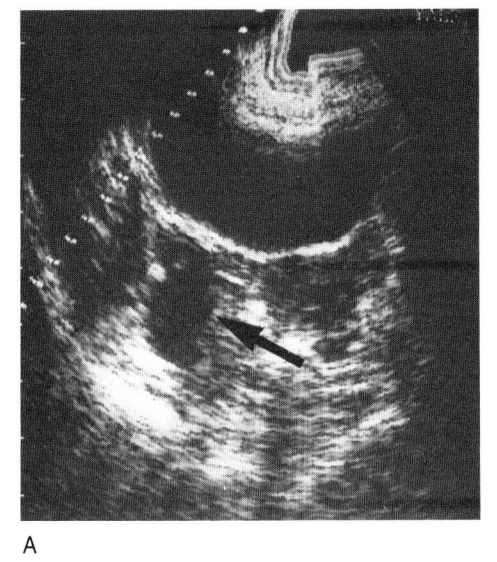

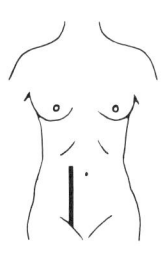

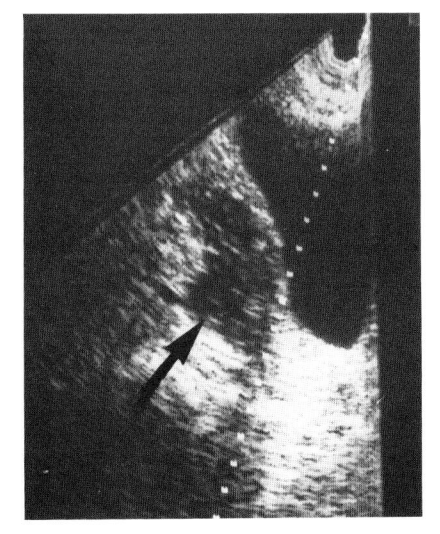

A

B

17.9 Abscess Due to Ruptured Appendix

A 13-year-old white girl presented with lower abdominal pain, vomiting, and diarrhea. She had had a low-grade fever for 10 days. Her maximum temperature had been 100°F. On examination she was febrile with an enlarged liver and a bulge above the pubis. Bowel sounds were active. Her white cell count was 23,800/mm^3 with 17 percent band cells. A kidney/ureter/bladder radiograph (Fig. A) demonstrated multiple air/fluid levels with a mass and some suprapubic air apparently displacing the bowel. A longitudinal sonogram (Fig. B) showed a huge fluid collection lying superior to the bladder. Anteriorly, within this mass the typical reverberating shadow of an air collection was seen. The appearances, therefore, were those of a large pelvic fluid collection which also contained air and were highly suggestive of a pelvic abscess.

Surgery disclosed a huge pelvic abscess secondary to a ruptured appendix.

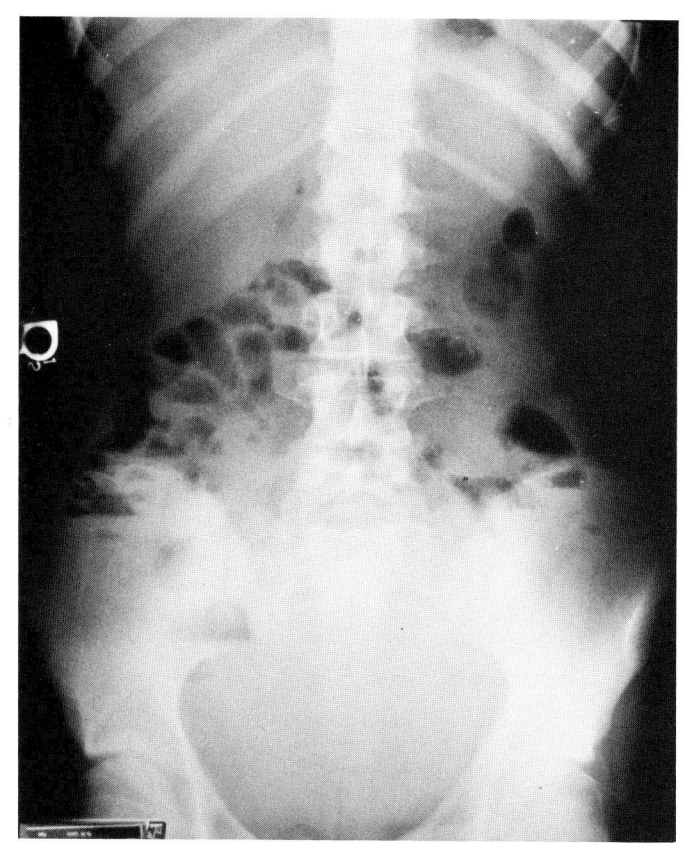

A

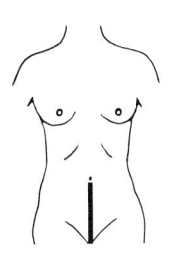

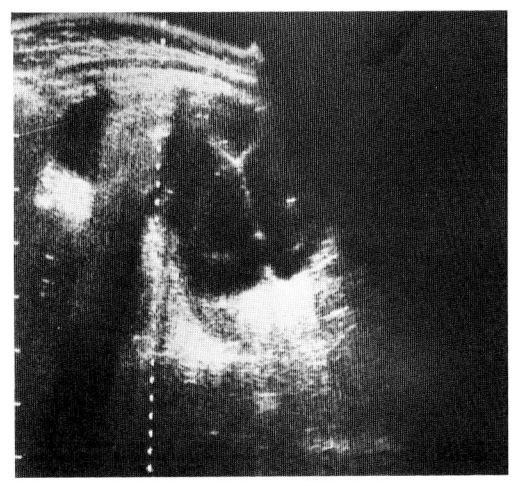

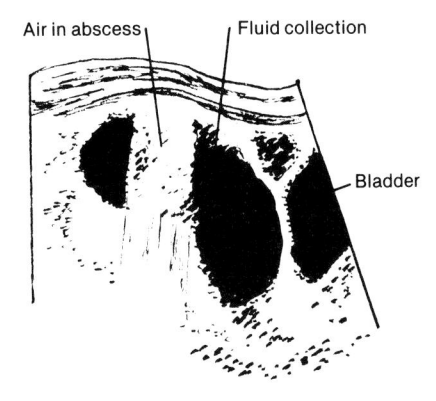

Air in abscess — Fluid collection — Bladder

B

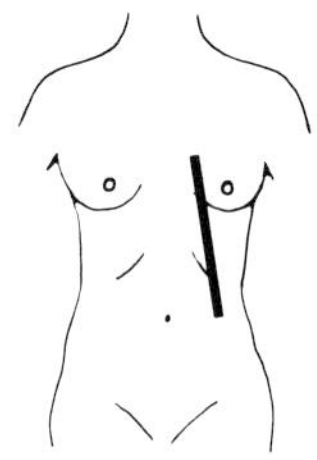

17.10 The Intestine

A 65-year-old woman who had undergone radical hysterectomy for stage 2 carcinoma of the cervix presented with abdominal pain of 3 years' duration. There was nausea and vomiting. An abdominal radiograph demonstrated dilated small bowel loops with multiple air/fluid levels consistent with early small-bowel obstruction. A small-bowel study performed via a Cantor tube demonstrated narrowed, nodular loops of distal ileum, probably due to metastatic disease to the mesentery and bowel wall. Longitudinal sonograms showed free ascites and dilated loops of intestine (Fig. A). Multiple nondistended intestinal loops are also seen in another patient with ascites (Fig. B).

In general, ultrasound is the worst modality for visualizing the bowel. However, the presence of ascites provides a contrast medium which facilitates visualization of gut. In addition, fluid distention of the gut because of obstruction may produce excellent visualization of the gut with its contained valvulae conniventes.[1] Real-time scans are particularly helpful, since they can demonstrate the presence or absence of peristalsis.

REFERENCE

1. Morgan CL, Trought WS, Oddson TA, et al: Ultrasound patterns of disorders affecting the gastrointestinal tract. Radiology 135:129–135, 1980

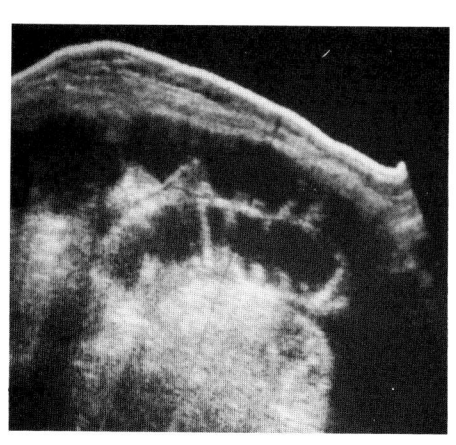

A

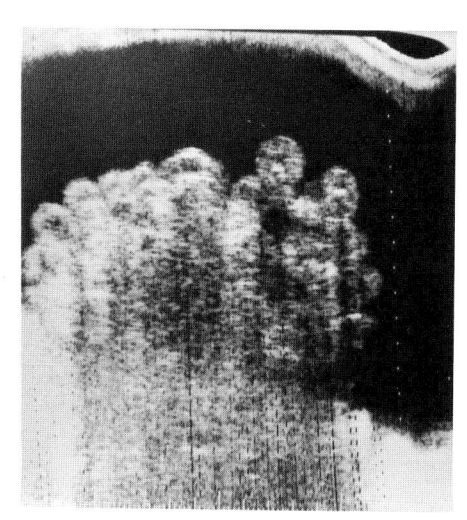

B

17.11 Colon Simulating Dermoid Cyst

A 23-year-old woman was referred for ultrasound investigation of a right adnexal mass. Clinically, this mass was believed to be cystic. A transverse sonogram (Fig. A) demonstrated an echogenic oval mass in the right adnexal position. The combination of the clinical impression of a cyst and an echogenic, complex mass on ultrasound, suggested the diagnosis of a dermoid cyst. Subsequently, this patient underwent exploratory laparotomy for excision of a dermoid cyst but no tumor was found on either ovary.

A sagittal section through the pelvis of another patient (Fig. B) demonstrated a large, echogenic mass (M) lying superior to a retroverted uterus (U). Again, the appearances of a large dermoid cyst are closely simulated. Repeat scanning of this patient on the following day showed disappearance of this mass, indicating that the mass was bowel contents and not due to true pathologic change.

The ultrasound appearances of dermoid cysts can be protean.[1] A mass that both feels cystic on clinical examination and is echogenic on ultrasound is highly suggestive of a dermoid cyst. However, in this case, the gynecologist had felt a 2 cm mass which was obviously a transient follicular cyst while a 5-cm pseudomass had been demonstrated by ultrasound. The importance of good communication between the sonographer and the clinician cannot be overstressed. In addition, the difficulties of diagnosing a dermoid cyst should be appreciated. Frequently these patients have to be examined on two occasions, occasionally with the use of a water enema.

REFERENCE

1. Sandler MA, Silver TM, Karo JJ: Gray-scale ultrasonic features of ovarian teratomas. Radiology 131:705–709, 1979

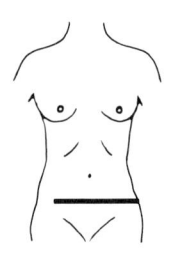

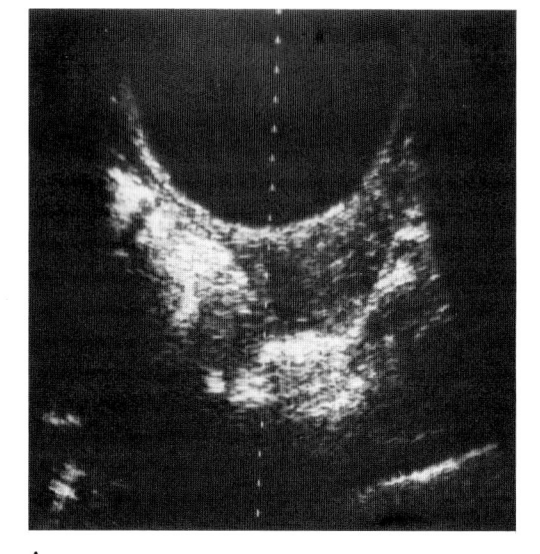

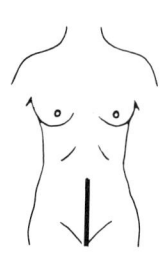

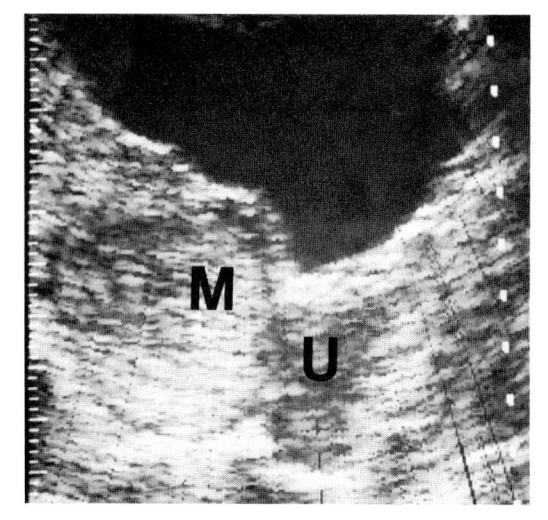

A

B

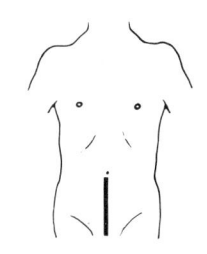

17.12 Carcinoma of the Colon

A 54-year-old man had a large palpable pelvic and abdominal mass which was known to be carcinoma of the colon. He was referred for ultrasound examination to obtain a baseline value for tumor size and to mark ports of entry for subsequent radiotherapy.

A midline section through the abdomen and pelvis revealed a large, solid tumor surrounded by free ascites, as shown in the figure. This solid mass contained many irregular, echo-free areas which were consistent with central necrosis. This evidence of irregularity in contour and level of echoes was strongly suggestive of malignancy.

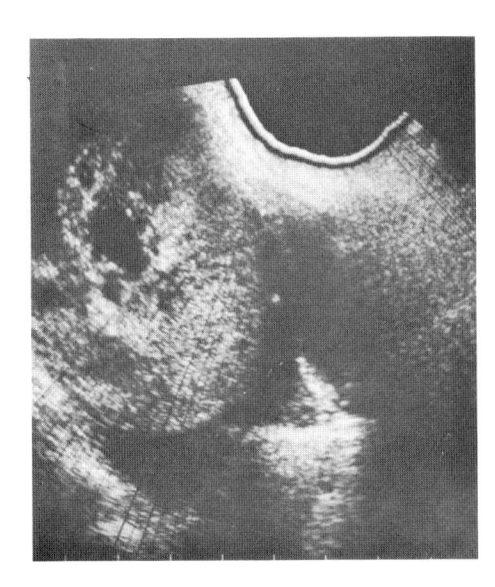

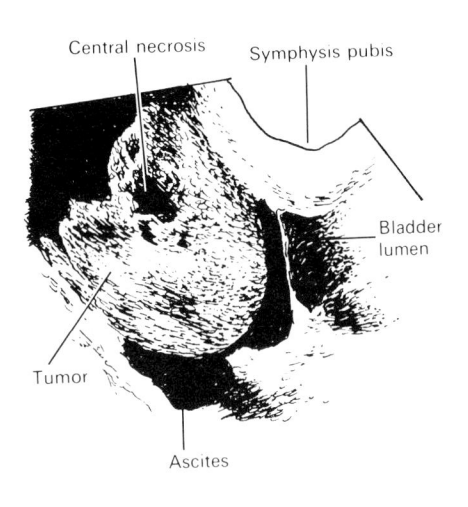

Rectum (17.13 and 17.14)

17.13 Normal Rectum

The lower gut is not usually visualized due to its contained air, but the longitudinal scan of a normal female pelvis shown here was carried out soon after an enema. The bladder was almost empty, but the normal uterus and vagina were seen. The rectum was seen lying within the concavity of the sacrum. The rectal walls were visible due to a small amount of fluid retained in the rectal lumen.

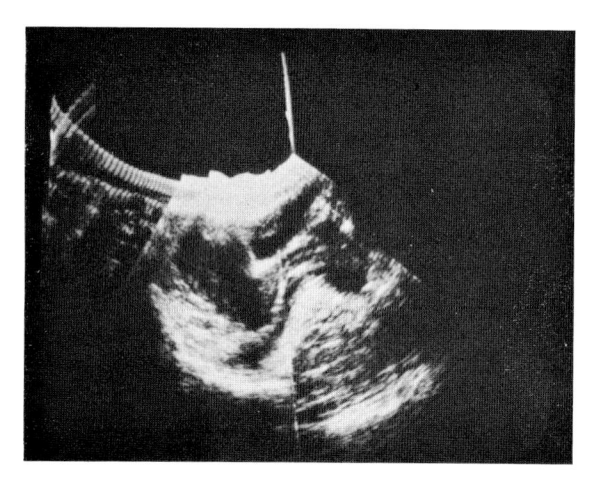

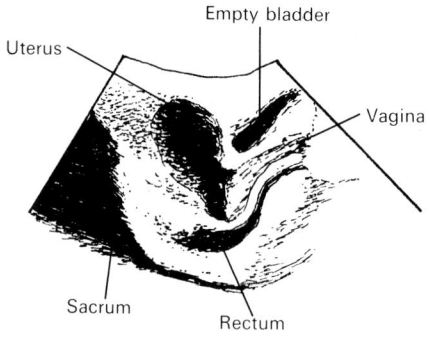

17.14 Rectal Bladder

A 32-year-old man was born with a defect of the bladder wall, and both ureters had been transplanted into the rectum. His bowel ended in a colostomy, and the sigmoid colon and rectum were functioning as a bladder. A longitudinal sonogram (Fig. A) demonstrated marked distention of the rectum with urine, while scans towards the right of the midline demonstrated sections through loops of bowel distended with fluid (Fig. B).

Transplantation of the ureters into the bowel was once in vogue as a treatment for carcinoma of the bladder. This practice was abandoned due to the resulting severe electrolyte imbalance caused by resorption of chloride. However, these scans demonstrate the excellent visualization of gut that can be obtained when it is distended with fluid and free of gas and feces. Iatrogenic distention of the bowel has been used to clarify the nature of pelvic masses.[1] In the presence of equivocal pelvic masses, dramatic improvement in the technical quality of the image can be obtained by the use of a water enema. However, the technique has failed to become popular with either patients or sonographers. In practice, most of these problems can be solved by real-time scanning and repeat scanning, since bowel masses are transient whereas true pathologic masses are permanent.

REFERENCE

1. Kurtz AB, Rubin CS, Kramer FL, et al: Ultrasound evaluation of the posterior pelvic compartment. Radiology 132: 677–682, 1979

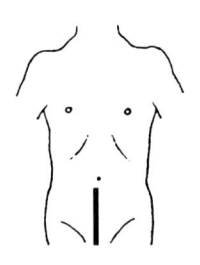

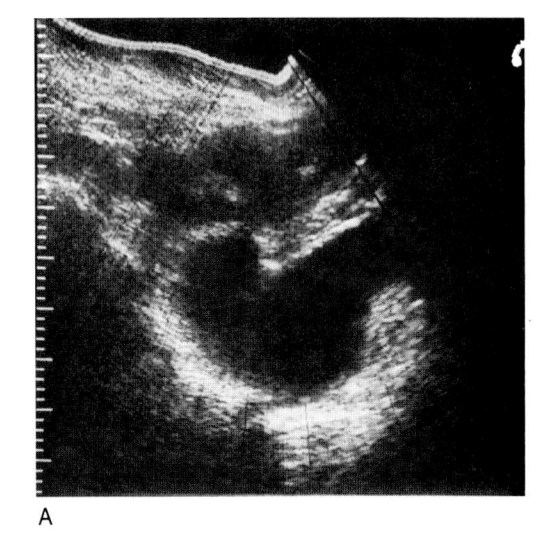

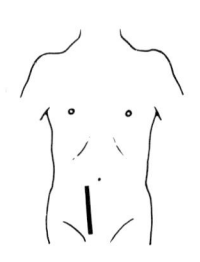

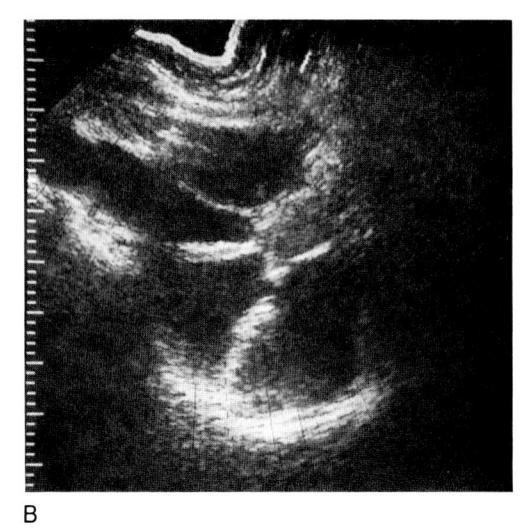

A

B

1048

17.15 Subphrenic and Pelvic Abscess Following Appendicitis

An 11-year-old white boy presented with a 5-day history of spiking fevers, low abdominal pain, and anorexia. The diagnosis of appendicitis was made on clinical grounds. He was taken to the operating room where a large pelvic abscess was drained and an appendectomy performed. Two days later a chest x-ray demonstrated a large left pleural effusion and ultrasound examination was requested to rule out a subphrenic abscess.

Ultrasound in the left decubitus position demonstrated a huge fluid-filled mass containing debris lying lateral to the spleen and a large left pleural effusion (Fig. A). A transverse sonogram (Fig. B) also demonstrated a large fluid collection lateral to the spleen. This was reported as consistent with a huge left subphrenic abscess.

The patient was returned to the operating room where 250 ml of foul-smelling pus was drained. The abscess was situated in the infrahepatic area of the left lobe, anterior to the spleen.

Seven days later he was again feverish and was referred for ultrasound. A transverse sonogram (Fig. C) demonstrated a homogeneous mass posterior to the bladder, while a longitudinal sonogram (Fig. D) demonstrated free fluid posterior and superior to the bladder with minimal thickening of the bladder wall. The patient was again referred to the operating room where a foul, purulent collection was drained. The patient progressed to an uneventful recovery.

This case demonstrates well the value of ultrasound for screening the entire abdomen and pelvis for pus collections. The status of such patients after surgery may change rapidly and several imaging procedures may be required during their hospitalization. Because of anatomic considerations, the subphrenic and perihepatic spaces and pelvis are the most common sites of postoperative abdominal and pelvic abscesses.[1] These can be easily and well-visualized by ultrasound.

REFERENCE

1. Meyers M: Intraperitoneal spread of infections. pp. 20–54. In Meyers M (ed): Dynamic Radiology of the Abdomen. Normal and Pathologic Anatomy, 2nd edition. Springer-Verlag, New York, 1982

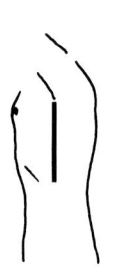

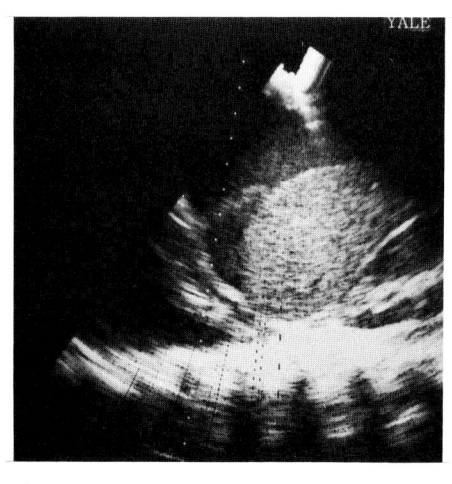

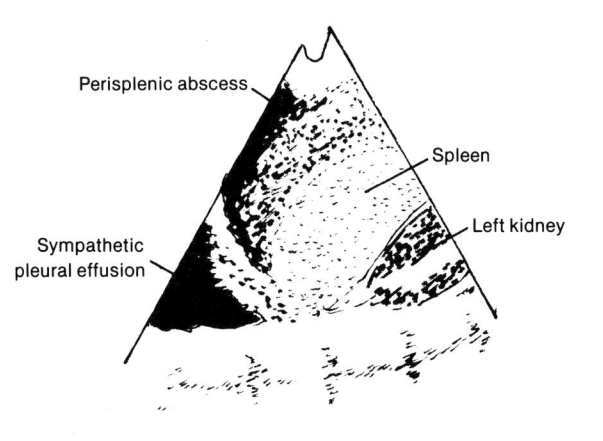

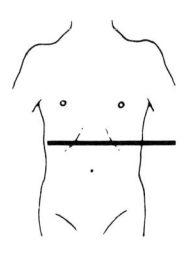

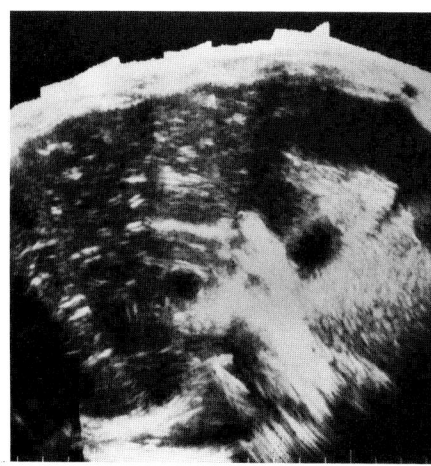

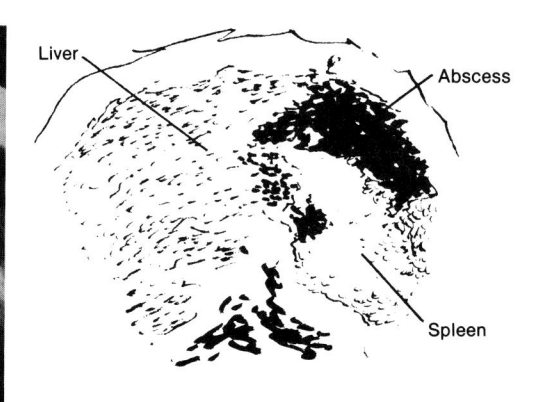

A

B

1050

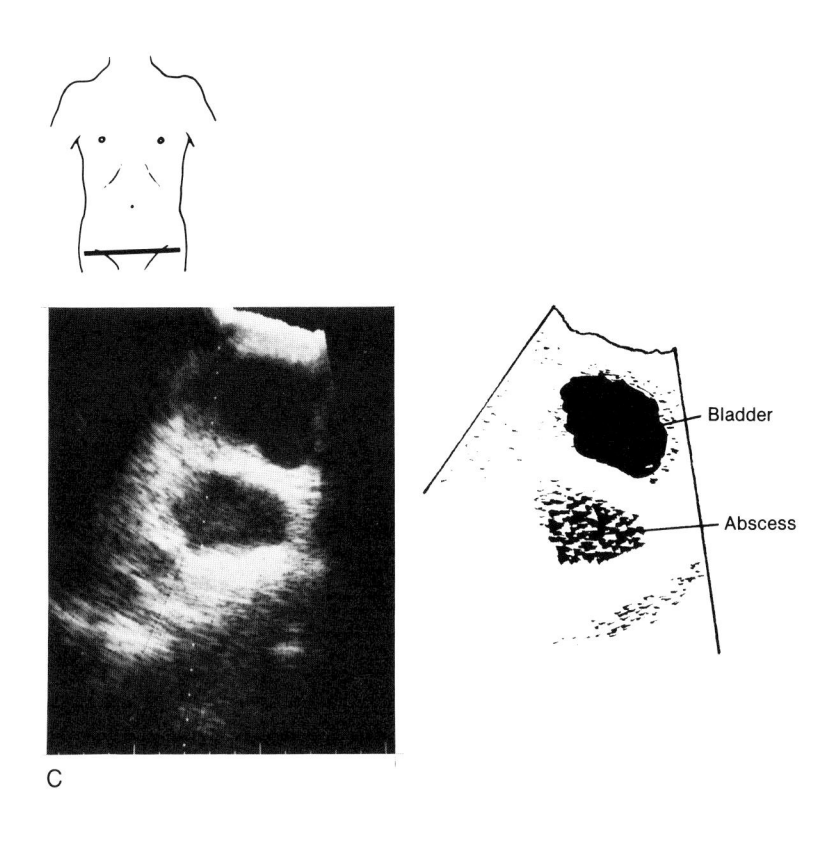

C

Bladder

Abscess

D

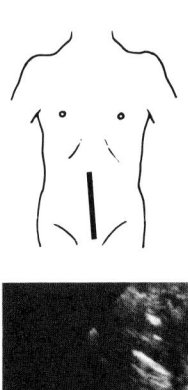

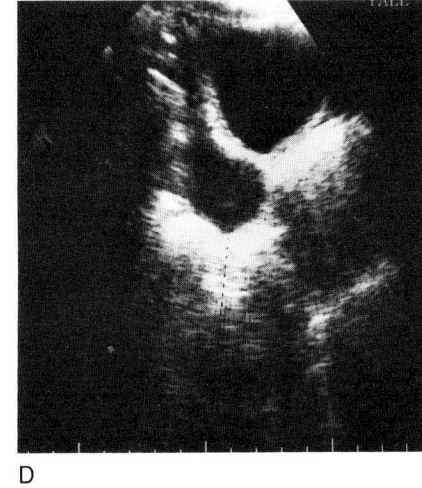

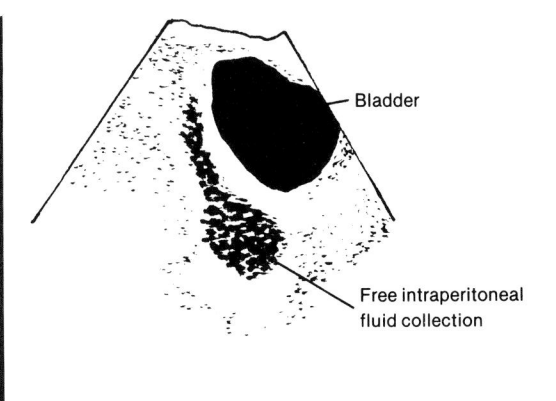

Bladder

Free intraperitoneal fluid collection

1051

18 The Thyroid and Parathyroid Glands

JOSEPH F. SIMEONE and PETER R. MUELLER

The Thyroid Gland (18.1 to 18.10)

APPLICATIONS OF ULTRASOUND

After examining approximately 750 patients with high-resolution real-time ultrasound equipment, we find that the benefits and disadvantages of this technique have become more obvious. While it had been hoped that high-resolution imaging of the thyroid gland would enable the radiologist to distinguish benign from malignant disease, that has proven impossible.

However, a few advantages and primary uses of the technique have become obvious. High-resolution real-time sonography of the thyroid has proved most useful for:

1. Detecting multinodularity of the thyroid gland
2. Finding occult carcinomas of the thyroid gland when metastatic disease from that primary carcinoma is present elsewhere
3. Finding recurrent thyroid carcinoma of the neck in postoperative patients; these nodules are often not palpable and are discovered by laboratory evidence or clinical suspicion of recurrent tumor.

Secondary uses of thyroid ultrasound include determination of the size and volume of the gland, determination of the size and volume of a nodule, determination of the cystic or solid nature of a nodule, and follow-up of patients with a history of neck irradiation to look for change in nodule size. These secondary uses, however, are less important and infrequently employed compared with the primary uses.

EQUIPMENT

Two commercially produced high-resolution 10-MHz real-time ultrasound scanners are currently available: The Picker Microview and the Diasonics-Wide View small-parts scanner. The Picker Microview is out of production but is still available for purchase. While adequate examinations of the thyroid and parathyroid can probably be done with a 7.5-MHz transducer, to achieve the highest quality of scanning, 10-MHz equipment should be used. Since one of the major advantages of the technique is in finding small lesions of both the thyroid and parathyroid, the highest-resolution equipment will provide the most information. All of the sonograms reproduced in this chapter have been performed with 10-MHz transducers using the equipment mentioned above.

18.1 Anatomy

Figure A is a transverse sonogram of the left half of the neck. The normal thyroid gland generally measures a maximum of 5–6 cm in length and 2 cm in height and width. It is easily distinguished on routine neck sonography from the normal surrounding structures. The lateral borders include the carotid artery (1) and jugular vein. The medial border is the trachea (2). Posterior to the thyroid gland the longus colli muscle is often seen, which generally appears as a triangular hypoechoic mass (4). Anterior to the longus colli muscle is the minor neurovascular bundle which contains the recurrent laryngeal nerve and inferior and superior thyroid arteries. Often the longus colli muscle and minor neurovascular bundle blend into one structure and cannot be separated. Posterior to the thyroid gland on the left side, just beside the trachea, the esophagus is seen in almost 50 percent of patients. Under real-time examination the esophagus is easily differentiated from a posterior thyroid mass by asking the patient to swallow and observing the resultant peristalsis. Anterior to the thyroid gland numerous muscle bundles are seen. The most frequently encountered muscles include the sternocleidomastoid (5), the sternohyoid, and sternothyroid muscles (3), the latter being applied to the most anterior portion of the thyroid gland.

Figure B is a sagittal section showing thyroid gland tissue between the strap muscles (3) and the longus colli muscle (4). The four normal parathyroid glands are found at each pole of the thyroid lobes. They are separated from the thyroid gland by an aponeurotic sheath which is not visible sonographically in normal parathyroid glands. However, this sheath may occasionally be seen in enlarged parathyroid glands as a linear echogenic line separating the thyroid from the parathyroid.

Numerous vascular structures may be seen posterior and inferior to the thyroid gland which, because of their hypoechoic nature, may mimic parathyroid enlargement. However, the branching nature of these structures can often be ascertained by real-time sonography and easily differentiated from parathyroid neoplasms.

(Figures from Simeone JF, Daniels GH, Mueller PR, et al: High-resolution real time sonography of the thyroid. Radiology 145:431–435, 1982.)

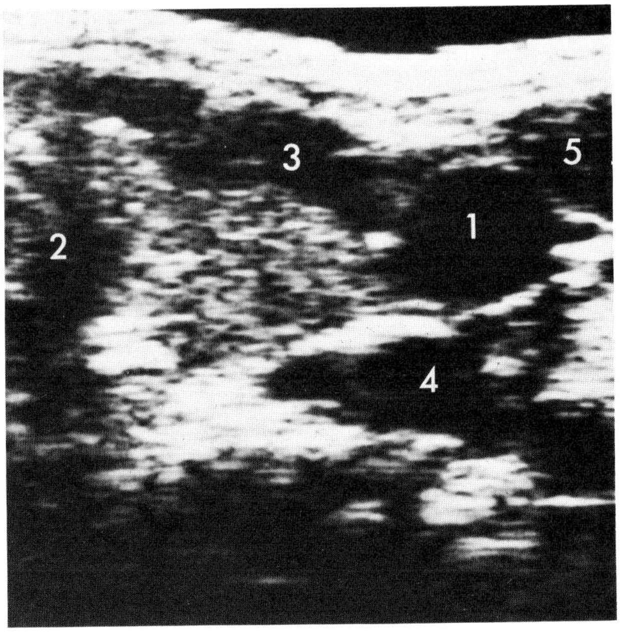

A

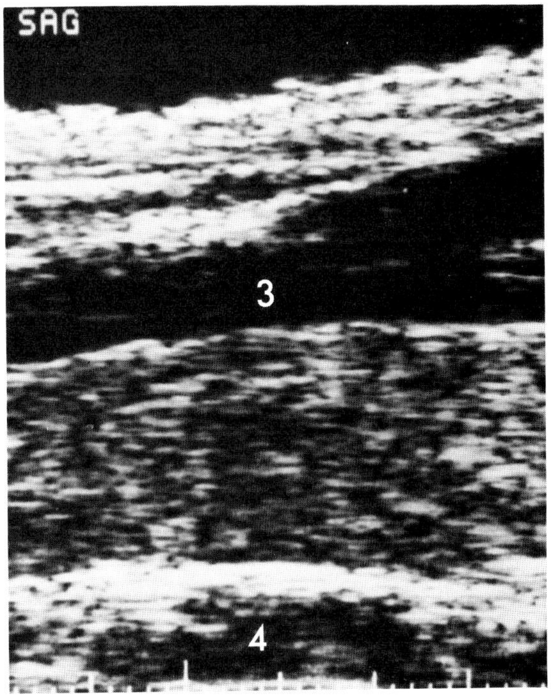

B

18.2 Follicular Adenoma

A 50-year-old woman presented with an asymptomatic thyroid mass. Scintigraphy demonstrated this to be a cold area. A transverse sonogram demonstrated a slightly enlarged thyroid gland with an echogenic nodule surrounded by a well-defined halo (arrowed in the figure). Findings on biopsy specimens were consistent with follicular adenoma.

Follicular adenomas are often seen on thyroid sonograms since these single solitary nodules, generally cold on nuclear medicine scan, are biopsied percutaneously. Numerous histologic subtypes of follicular adenomas exist but there is no distinguishing feature on ultrasound which permits differentiation between these histologic variations. Often the histologic diagnosis is made by observing the lining of cells within the wall of the adenoma. Such observation is impossible by ultrasound. Follicular adenoma, like adenomatous nodules, may be hypoechoic, isoechoic, or echogenic relative to the normal thyroid gland.

After discovery of a thyroid nodule by physical examination, the first examination is usually an isotopic study. If this study demonstrates a single, solitary hot nodule, no further work-up is generally done since the vast majority of hot nodules are benign. If the scintigraphic study indicates multinodularity of the gland, further diagnostic work-up with ultrasound is again not indicated because this is a rather accurate diagnosis by nuclear medicine. Ultrasound becomes important in the diagnosis when patients have a thyroid nodule which is cold on the nuclear medicine scan. A single solitary cold nodule carries a rate of malignancy of between 15 and 25 percent. In most cases, biopsy of this nodule will be indicated to exclude malignancy. However, since the resolution of the nuclear medicine scan is approximately 1–2 cm, nodules smaller than this will not be detected. The resolution of 10-MHz ultrasound transducers approaches 1 mm. Therefore, nodules measuring 2–10 mm will be easily detected by ultrasound and can be diagnosed as multinodular goiter rather than single cold nodules.

(Figure from Simeone JF, Daniels GH, Mueller PR, et al: High-resolution real time sonography of the thyroid. Radiology 145:431–435, 1982.)

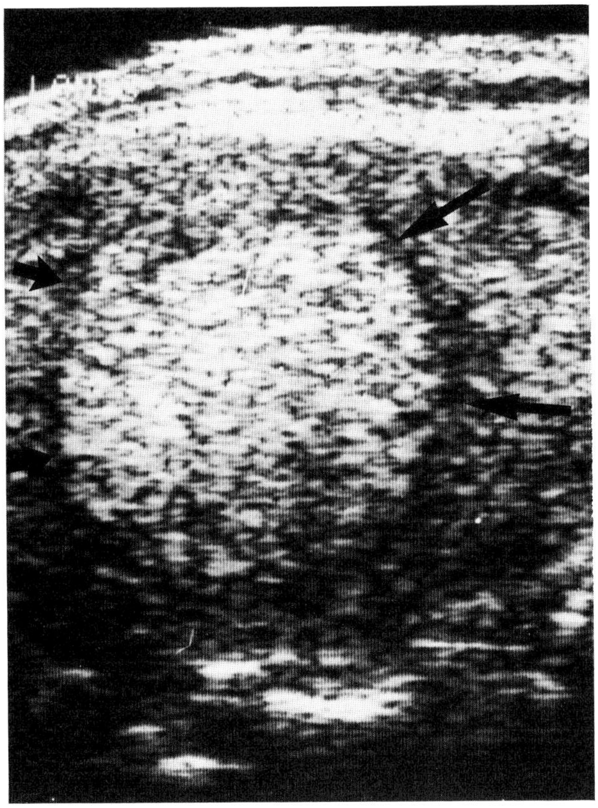

18.3 Adenomatous Nodules

A 45-year-old woman presented with a gradually enlarging but otherwise asymptomatic neck mass. A transverse sonogram demonstrated a gland three to four times normal size (Fig. A). Multiple small nodules, as well as calcification with shadowing (S) were noted. A larger nodule was present on the opposite side which proved to be echogenic but nonhomogeneous in texture (Fig. B). Appearances were consistent with a multinodular goiter.

Multinodular goiter is the most common cause of nodules found on a thyroid sonogram. Although there are histologic differences between an adenomatous nodule in a multinodular gland and a follicular adenoma, microscopic differentiation cannot always be made and there are no differences in their ultrasound appearances. Adenomatous nodules of a multinodular gland can appear hypoechoic, isoechoic, or echogenic relative to the normal thyroid gland. In our experience, approximately 50 percent of the nodules of a multinodular gland contain some fluid. This reflects their hemorrhagic or cystic degeneration. In clinical practice, the discovery of two nodules within a thyroid gland is enough to make the diagnosis of multinodularity. Nodules 2–3 mm in size are routinely discovered in the thyroid glands of normal patients and patients undergoing examination for other neck conditions.

(Figures from Simeone JF, Daniels GH, Mueller PR, et al: High-resolution real time sonography of the thyroid. Radiology 145:431–435, 1982.)

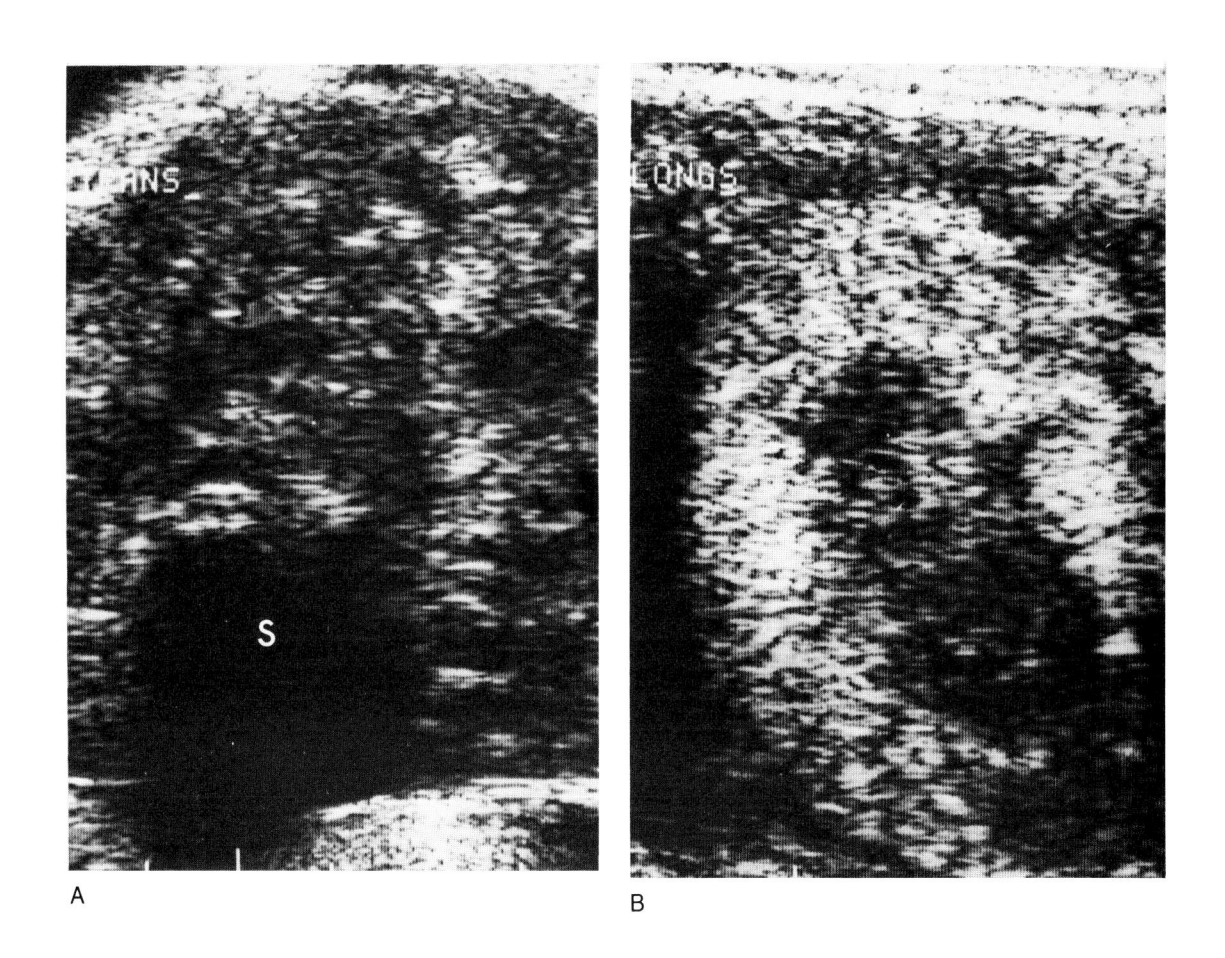

A

B

18.4 Multinodular Goiter

A 27-year-old woman presented with an asymptomatic neck mass which was cold on scintigraphy. Multiple nodules were seen on one side. Transverse sonograms of the right lobe (Fig. A) showed cystic components within one of these nodules (arrowed). This cystic component caused it to appear cold on scintigraphy. A transverse sonogram of the left lobe demonstrated multiple nodules (arrowed) within a normal-sized gland (Fig. B). These nodules were all under 5 mm and were undetected by the nuclear scan.

Autopsy studies have shown that a multinodular gland is three times more prevalent than a gland with a single nodule.[1] These multinodular areas are frequently undetectable by either physical examination or nuclear scintigraphy because of the small size of the nodules. High-resolution, 10-MHz ultrasound equipment, however, permits the diagnosis of multinodular goiter even when nodules are only 1–2 mm in size.

The importance of this diagnosis lies in the fact that the multinodular gland carries, at maximum, a risk of malignancy of no greater than 6 percent.[2] In our institution, a multinodular gland is considered benign and invasive techniques, such as biopsy, are generally not performed. Patients with a multinodular gland are usually followed clinically without treatment. They may, however, be treated with thyroid suppression if a nodule is large. Only if the nodule does not respond to suppression therapy need a biopsy be taken.

The importance of ultrasound lies in its ability to image small lesions within the thyroid gland. Ten-MHz transducers make such high resolution possible. This capability often converts the diagnosis of a single solitary cold nodule into that of a multinodular gland and the risk of malignancy is diminished from a maximum of 25 percent to a maximum of 6 percent. When a multinodular gland is considered to be benign, the patient may be assured that the rate of malignancy is close to zero.

(Figures from Simeone JF, Daniels GH, Mueller PR, et al: High-resolution real time sonography of the thyroid. Radiology 145:431–435, 1982.)

REFERENCES

1. Mortensen JD, Woolner LB, Bennett WA: Gross and microscopic findings in clinically normal thyroid glands. J Clin Endocrinol Metab 15:1270–1280, 1955
2. Brown CL: Pathology of the cold nodule. Clin Endocrinol Metab 10:235, 1981

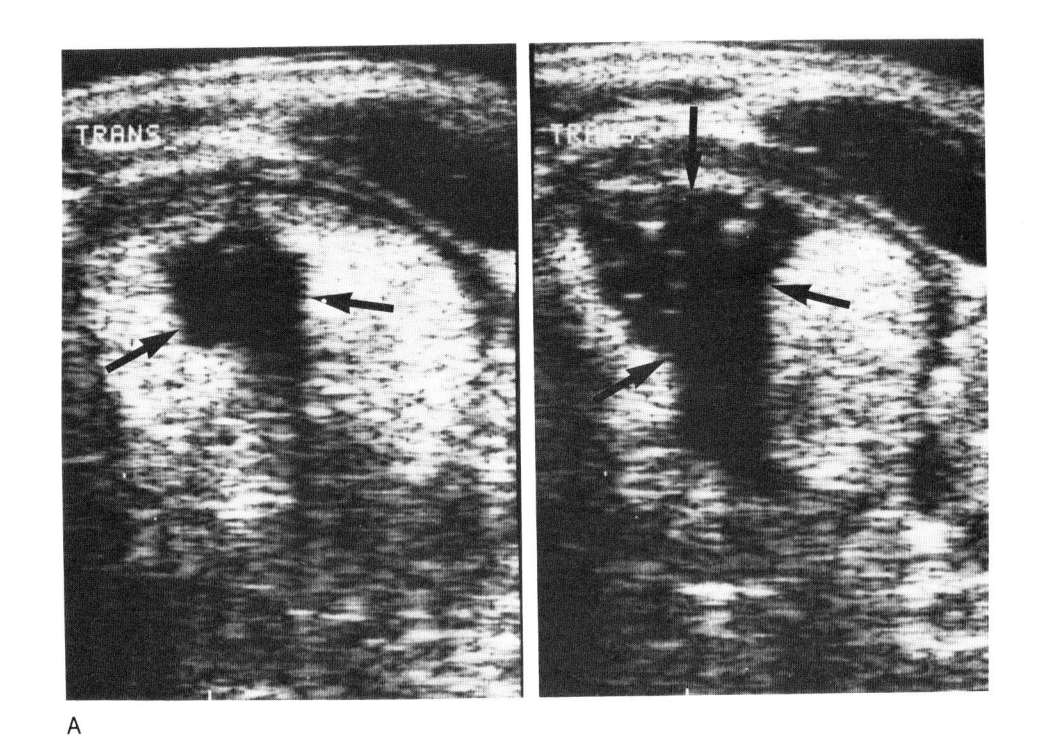

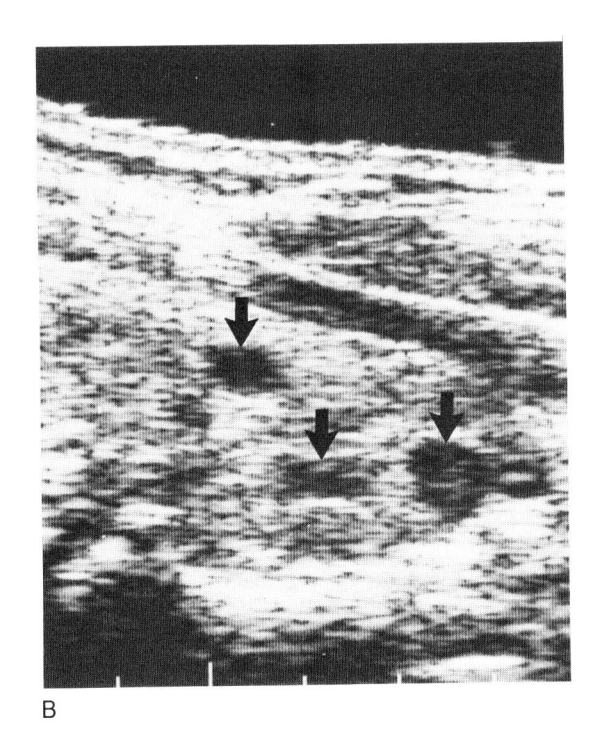

A

B

18.5 Hashimoto's Thyroiditis

A 38-year-old woman had a long history of thyroid disease. Results of previous blood tests demonstrated antithyroid antibodies. A transverse sonogram (Fig. A) showed the right side of the gland to be slightly enlarged, with disorganized texture and decreased echogenicity. The gland also contained calcification, with obvious posterior acoustic shadowing (arrowed). The opposite (left) side of the thyroid was also mildly enlarged, but a well-defined anterior nodule was demonstrated (arrowed, Fig. B). This proved to be Hashimoto's thyroiditis.

Hashimoto's thyroiditis is a clinical diagnosis, confirmed by the presence of serum thyroid antibodies. Ultrasound is of no value in making this diagnosis. However, it is of some value in detecting or excluding the presence of nodularity within Hashimoto's thyroiditis. This nodularity is indistinguishable from that of multinodular goiter or a follicular adenoma. In most cases of Hashimoto's thyroiditis, the thyroid gland is enlarged, hypoechoic, and contains numerous low-level echoes which are smaller than usual.

(Figures from Simeone JF, Daniels GH, Mueller PR, et al: High-resolution real time sonography of the thyroid. Radiology 145:431–435, 1982.)

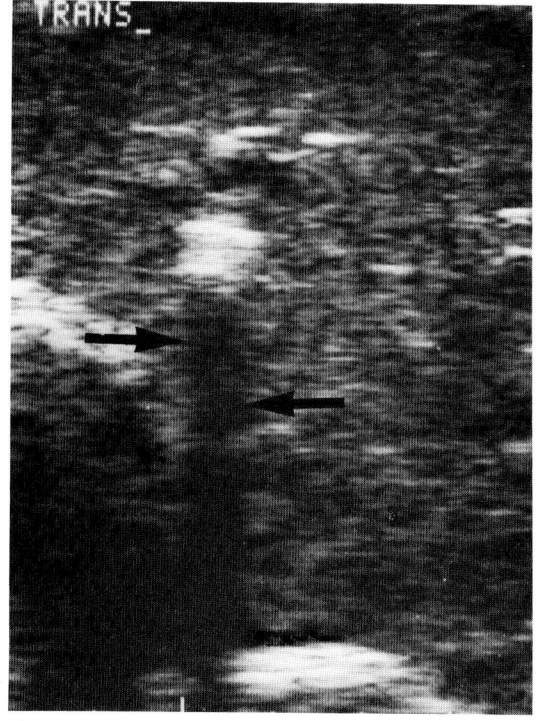

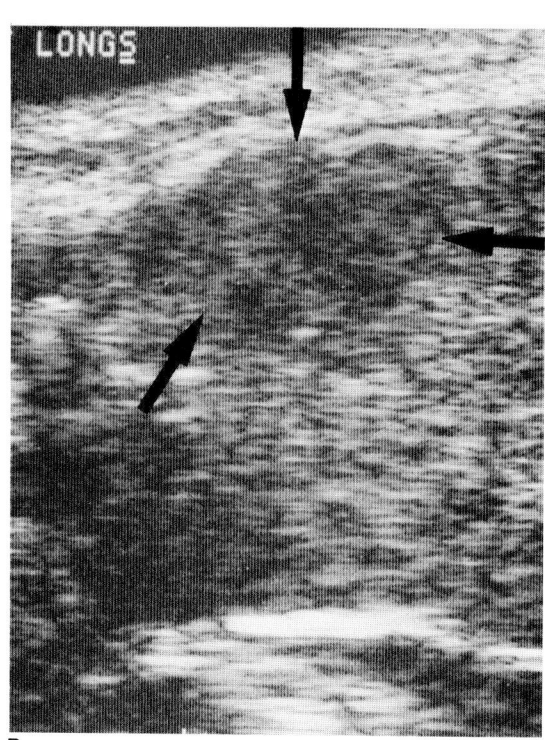

A

B

18.6 Hemorrhagic Cyst

A 16-year-old girl was hit in the neck with a rubber baseball bat. The following morning she awoke with a swelling in her neck which she had never previously noticed. A longitudinal sonogram showed the typical appearance of a hemorrhagic cyst. The enlarged gland deformed the skin. Normal thyroid tissue was seen surrounding a cystic area which contained multiple septa and had irregular borders.

A hemorrhagic cyst has the constant and classic appearance of a multiseptate fluid-containing mass, with irregular borders. Often, one can elicit from the patient a history of recent enlargement of a mass or trauma to the neck. If a sonogram is taken soon after the enlargement is detected, these septa will be seen. While there is no known cause of these septa, blood is assumed to dissect through the interstices of the thyroid gland, with septa representing residual thyroid tissue. The septa could also represent blood undergoing lysis or clot formation. The thyroid tissue or blood clot eventually breaks down and a more cystic lesion appears.

Hemorrhagic cysts also result from acute hemorrhage into a previously existing adenomatous nodule or follicular adenoma.

(Figure from Simeone JF, Daniels GH, Mueller PR, et al: High-resolution real time sonography of the thyroid. Radiology 145:431–435, 1982.)

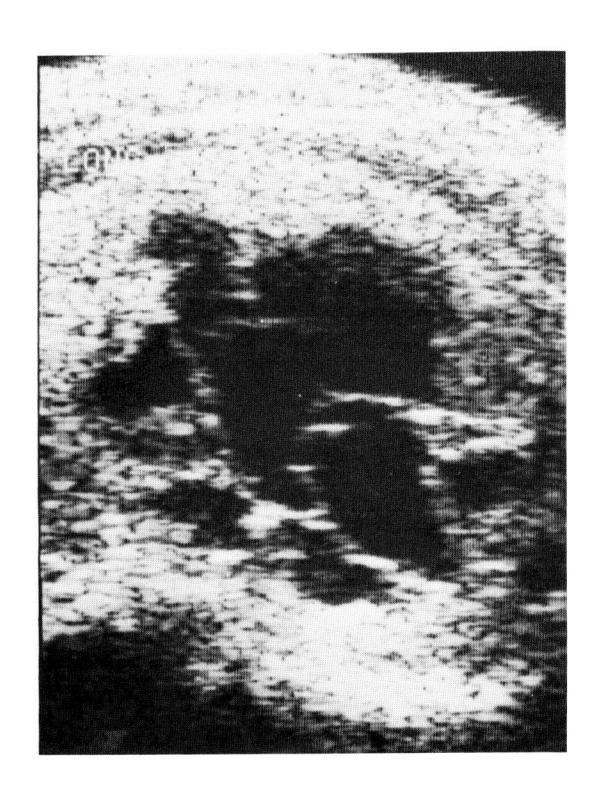

18.7 Cyst

A 48-year-old man was noted to have a neck mass on routine physical examination. He was asymptomatic and had never noticed its presence previously. A sonogram demonstrated a simple cyst (Fig. A), an unusual finding in a thyroid gland. Another classic appearance of a cyst is shown in Figure B. This could represent a thyroid cyst, however, percutaneous aspiration disclosed markedly elevated parathormone levels within the fluid suggesting a parathyroid cyst rather than a thyroid cyst. Note the low-level artifact through the center of the cyst (arrowed).

A simple cyst is an obviously benign lesion of the thyroid gland. We have only seen one proven simple cyst of the thyroid in more than 750 patients examined. If a purely cystic lesion of the thyroid gland is encountered which meets all of the classic criteria of a cyst including good through-transmission, a well-defined back wall, and absence of internal echoes, we are now highly suspicious that this represents a parathyroid cyst rather than a thyroid cyst. Most cystic lesions of the thyroid gland are follicular adenomas or adenomatous nodules which have undergone cystic or hemorrhagic degeneration.

(Figures from Simeone JF, Daniels GH, Mueller PR, et al: High-resolution real time sonography of the thyroid. Radiology 145:431–435, 1982.)

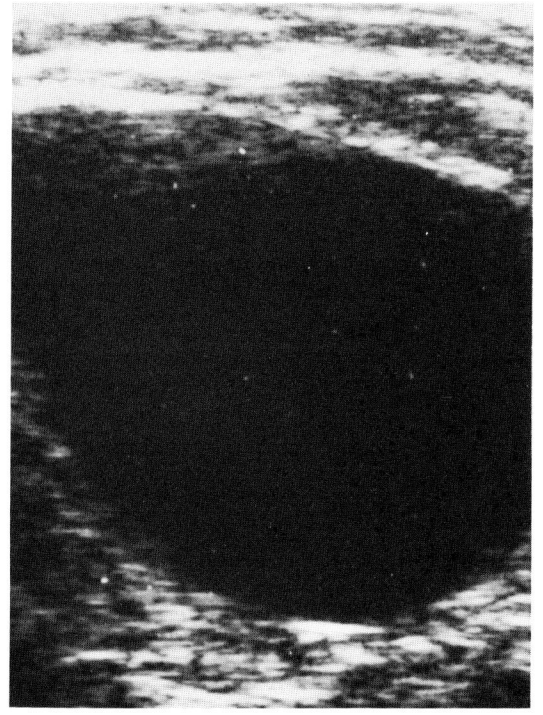

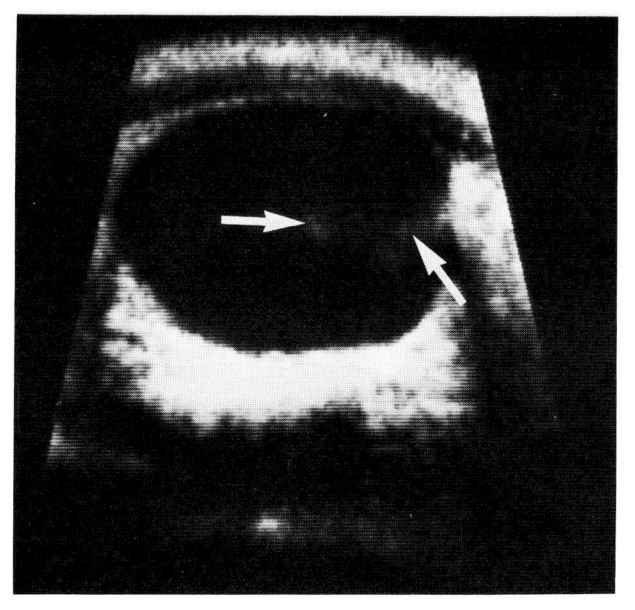

A

B

18.8 Papillary Carcinoma

A 37-year-old man presented with a right-sided neck mass. The biopsy specimen revealed histology compatible with a metastatic papillary carcinoma of the thyroid. The sonogram showed a small mass of diminished echogenicity (arrowed in the figure) within the otherwise normal thyroid gland. This appearance was consistent with a papillary carcinoma.

In our experience nearly all malignant lesions of the thyroid gland have been hypoechoic. One papillary carcinoma exhibited a halo and was isoechoic. Another papillary carcinoma was of mixed echogenicity with the majority of the nodule being echogenic, but with areas of decreased echogenicity. Papillary carcinoma of the thyroid generally presents as a small (2–6 mm) hypoechoic mass within the parenchyma of the thyroid and does not deform the gland. These small papillary carcinomas usually cannot be palpated and are not visible by scintigraphy. If they grow to a larger size before metastasizing, they can occasionally be palpated or visualized on an isotope scan. Papillary carcinomas may also be cystic and can mimic the exact appearance of cystic follicular adenomas. They appear as round, well-defined masses with a small area of echogenicity projecting into a cystic nodule. Only direct biopsy or excision can make the diagnosis.

Our experience with other forms of malignant disease of the thyroid is limited. Medullary carcinoma of the thyroid also presents as a hypoechoic mass. Only three lesions of the thyroid gland have proven to be metastatic disease. These were metastatic deposits from adenocarcinoma of the colon and breast. These appeared as large hypoechoic nodules within the thyroid gland and were indistinguishable from other thyroid nodules.

(Figure from Simeone JF, Daniels GH, Mueller PR, et al: High-resolution real time sonography of the thyroid. Radiology 145:431–435, 1982.)

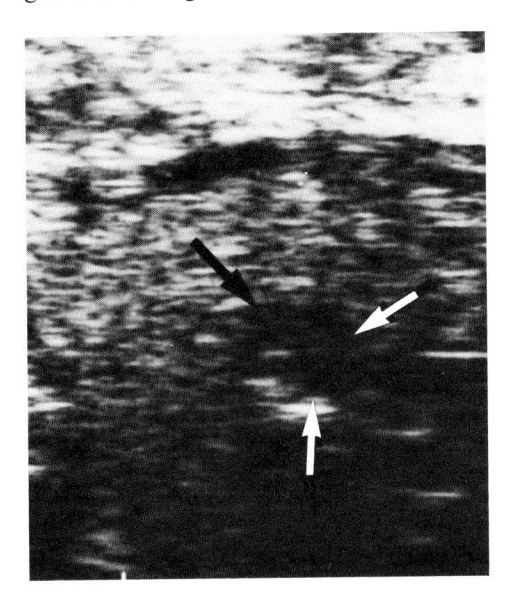

18.9 Papillary Carcinoma

A 25-year-old pregnant woman noted the presence of a small thyroid nodule. The nodule was cold on scintigraphy. A transverse sonogram demonstrated an irregular, oblong, fluid-containing mass with a small nodule projecting into the mass (arrowed in Fig. A). A transverse sonogram through a separate portion of the mass demonstrated the totally cystic nature of this area of the mass (Fig. B). This proved to be a papillary carcinoma.

Many articles have appeared in the radiologic literature in the past several years noting the virtues of ultrasound in differentiating cystic from solid lesions of the thyroid gland. This is not a productive use of the technique. In our experience, almost all cystic lesions of the neck are follicular adenomas which have undergone cystic or hemorrhagic degeneration. Papillary carcinomas of the thyroid gland can also be cystic. We have seen only one proven purely cystic lesion of the thyroid gland in more than 750 patients examined. When an apparent pure cyst of the thyroid gland is detected, we now assume it to be a parathyroid cyst since, to date, all but one such lesion have been subsequently proven to be parathyroid cysts.

(Figures from Simeone JF, Daniels GH, Mueller PR, et al: High-resolution real time sonography of the thyroid. Radiology 145:431–435, 1982.)

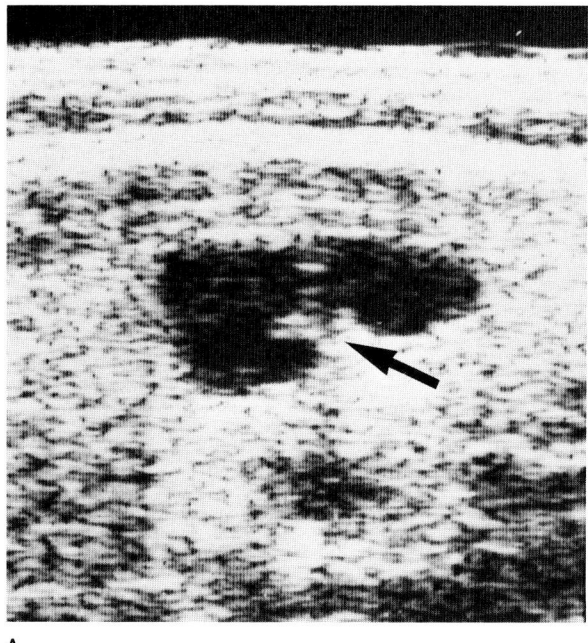

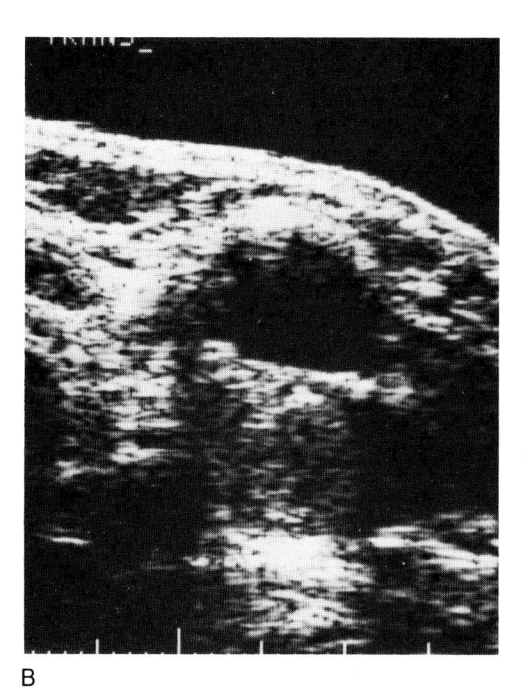

A

B

18.10 Papillary Carcinoma

A 45-year-old pregnant woman presented with a neck mass which, on biopsy, proved to be papillary carcinoma. Ultrasound of the thyroid gland revealed an isoechoic mass with a halo (arrowed in the figure).

It was initially thought that the presence of a "halo sign"—a sonolucent curvilinear line of demarcation—indicated that a nodule was benign. Numerous articles, however, have now shown that the "halo" may be present in follicular adenomas as well as papillary carcinomas.[1] The thickness and uniformity of the halo appear to have no diagnostic significance.

In our experience, no completely echogenic lesion has been malignant. A minority of follicular adenomas are totally echogenic. However, in approximately 20 solitary echogenic lesions, not one has proved malignant. Almost every malignant lesion detected has been hypoechoic compared with normal thyroid tissue. We have occasionally encountered lesions of mixed echogenicity which were primarily echogenic with some hypoechoic areas. These lesions have proven to be malignant.

An important application of thyroid ultrasound is the detection of occult carcinomas of the thyroid. Studies have shown that a high percentage of occult papillary carcinomas of the thyroid exist at autopsy and have never metastasized. In one study, papillary carcinomas were found incidentally at surgery in 82 of 140 cases (59 percent) without evidence of metastatic disease.[2] These lesions all were under 1.5 cm and were nonpalpable. Such studies indicate that papillary carcinoma is generally a subclinical entity which becomes clincially apparent only when it metastasizes to lymph nodes or elsewhere in the body.

When a patient presents with metastatic papillary carcinoma of the thyroid, ultrasound can be used to locate the primary lesion in the thyroid gland. This diagnosis permits a hemithyroidectomy rather than bilateral thyroidectomy to be performed. Patients undergoing hemithyroidectomy do not require subsequent thyroid replacement therapy. In every case we have seen at ultrasound, when metastatic disease has been present in neck nodes, the primary lesion has been in the ipsilateral thyroid lobe. All of the primary lesions in these patients have been 2–6 mm in size. None of the primary lesions were clinically palpable. A blind surgical exploration would have led to total thyroidectomy in all of these patients. Because of the findings on ultrasound, only a hemithyroidectomy was performed.

A last primary use of thyroid ultrasound is in the discovery of recurrent thyroid carcinoma in the neck in patients who have undergone previous total thyroidectomy and/or neck exploration. Often these patients present with clinical or laboratory evidence of recurrent tumor which is not palpable in the neck. Ultrasound examination of the thyroid bed is easy to perform since recurrent thyroid carcinoma presents as a hypoechoic mass in the midst of echogenic scar material. A marker may be placed on the skin to direct the surgeon to the exact spot for exploration if surgery is to be performed.

(Figure from Simeone JF, Daniels GH, Mueller PR, et al: High-resolution real time sonography of the thyroid. Radiology 145:431–435, 1982.)

REFERENCES

1. Simeone JF, Daniels GH, Mueller PR, et al: High-resolution real-time sonography of the thyroid. Radiology 145:431–435, 1982
2. Wollner LB, Lemmon ML, Beahrs OH: Occult papillary carcinoma of the thyroid gland: a study of 140 cases observed in a 30 year period. J Clin Endocrinol Metab 20:89–105, 1960

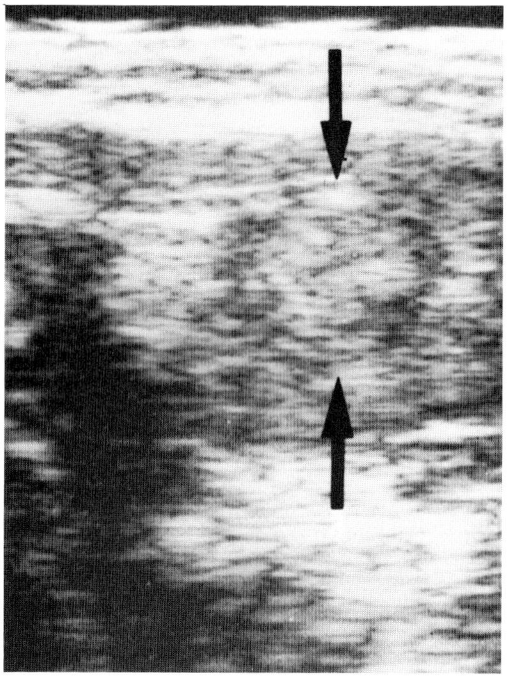

The Parathyroid Gland (18.11 to 18.20)

18.11 Hypercalcemia

Results of routine chemical screening tests identify patients with unsuspected hypercalcemia and hyperparathyroidism more frequently now than in the past. At the Mayo Clinic, the number of cases of hypercalcemia has increased from 1.1 to 7.7:100,000 population since the routine use of chemical screening tests began. While the decision to operate on these patients, especially if they are asymptomatic, is a clinical one, the importance of parathyroid ultrasound is its ability to discover small parathyroid neoplasms.

A 25-year-old patient presented with asymptomatic hypercalcemia. The transverse scan of the left side of the neck (Fig. A) demonstrated the esophagus (E) posteriorly and medially behind the thyroid gland (T). This can occasionally be confused wih a parathyroid neoplasm. (1 marks the trachea, 2 is carotid artery, 3 is the sternocleidomastoid, 4 identifies the sternothyroid and sternohyoid muscles, and 5 identifies the longus colli muscle.)

During a routine thyroid scan, a mass was seen which could represent a normal parathyroid gland (arrowed, Fig. B). The parathyroid gland is usually seen inferior and posterior to the thyroid lobe (T). Most parathyroid glands are too small to be detected.

(Figures from Simeone JF, Mueller PR, Ferrucci JT Jr, et al: High-resolution real-time sonography of the parathyroid. Radiology 141:745–751, 1981.)

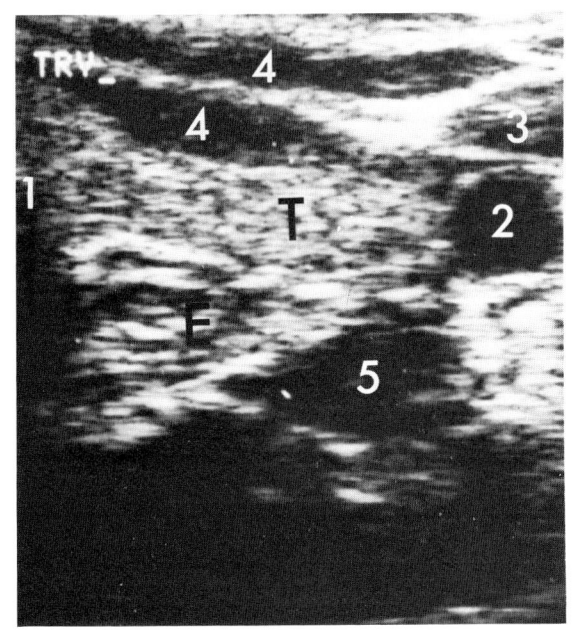

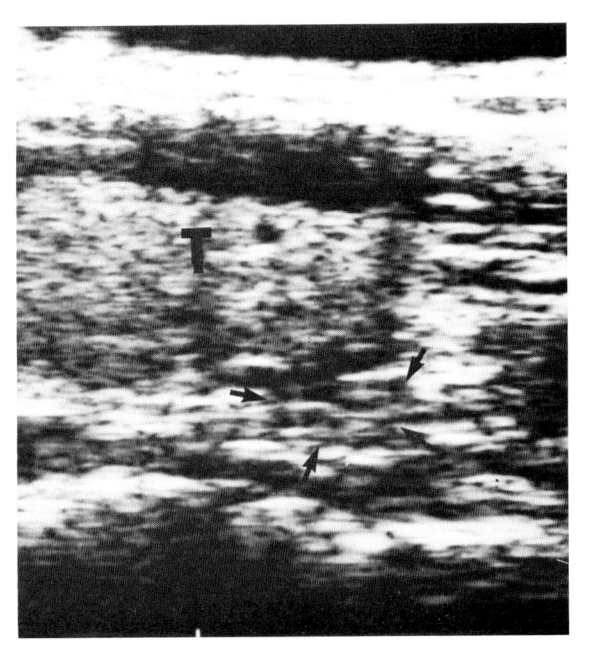

18.12 Adenoma

Following a long history of nephrolithiasis, this patient was discovered to have hypercalcemia. A longitudinal sonogram (Fig. A) demonstrated a parathyroid neoplasm (arrowed) located posterior to the normal thyroid gland. A transverse sonogram (Fig. B) showed a hypoechoic mass (arrowed) medial and posterior to the carotid artery (ca). The strap muscles are identified (M).

Approximately 80 percent of patients with hyperparathyroidism have single adenomas, 18 percent have parathyroid hyperplasia, and 1–2 percent have parathyroid carcinoma. The size of a follicular adenoma can often be correlated with the level of serum calcium. As a general rule, calcium levels of 10.5–11.5 mg/dl are produced by adenomas no larger than 1.5 cm. When the serum calcium exceeds 11.5 mg/dl, the adenomas are larger and therefore easier to find.

(Figures from Simeone JF, Mueller PR, Ferrucci JT Jr, et al: High-resolution real-time sonography of the parathyroid. Radiology 141:745–751, 1981.)

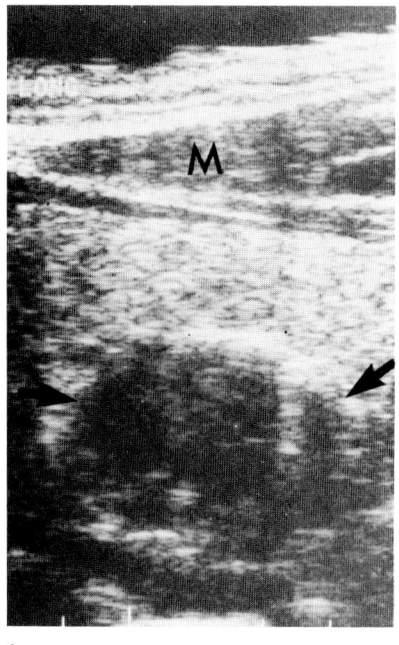

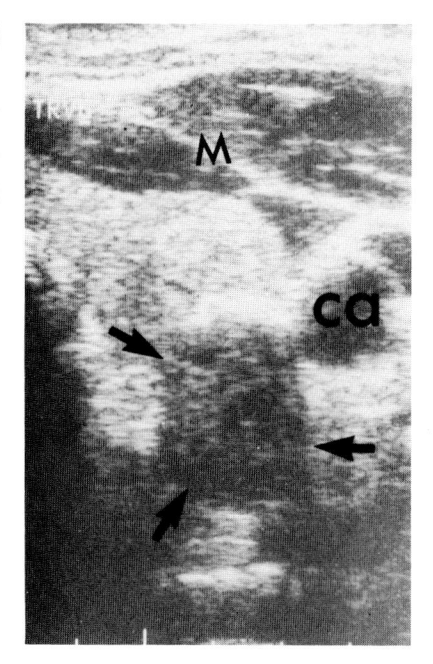

18.13 Prominent Longus Colli Muscle

A patient had documented hyperparathyroidism with elevated serum calcium, elevated serum parathormone levels, and diminishing bone density. A sonogram of the neck was requested in an attempt to identify a parathyroid neoplasm. Transverse sonograms failed to disclose a parathyroid neoplasm (Figs. A and B). However, there was asymmetry of the longus colli muscle; the right side (arrowed, Fig. A) was larger than the left (arrowed, Fig. B). It was therefore suggested that the neoplasm was most likely to be on the right side, where it was, in fact, found at surgery. The right-sided enlargement was probably due to hypertrophy of the thyroid artery supplying the parathyroid neoplasm.

Another patient with documented hyperparathyroidism was scanned. An upper-pole parathyroid neoplasm was diagnosed (arrowed, Fig. C). This false-positive diagnosis of parathyroid neoplasm was due to a colloid nodule of the thyroid mimicking the appearance and location of a parathyroid neoplasm.

The most common causes of false-positive diagnoses include thyroid nodules that mimic parathyroid glands, lymph nodes that mimic parathyroid glands, and on one occasion, thymus tissue in the neck appearing as a parathyroid neoplasm.

(Figures from Simeone JF, Mueller PR, Ferrucci JT Jr, et al: High-resolution real-time sonography of the parathyroid. Radiology 141:745–751, 1981.)

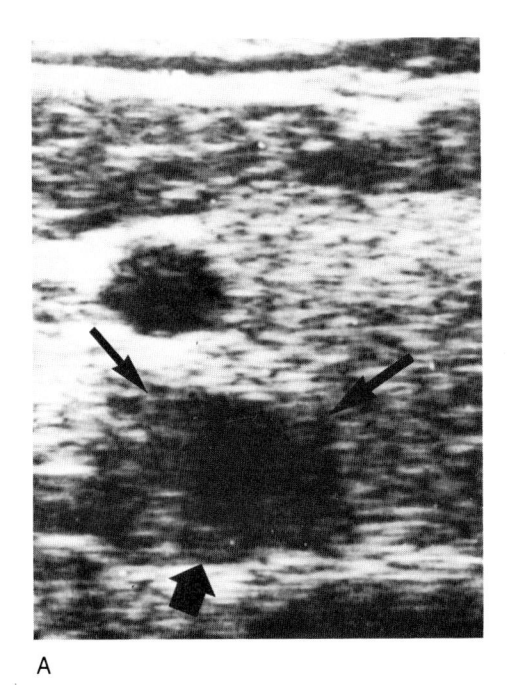

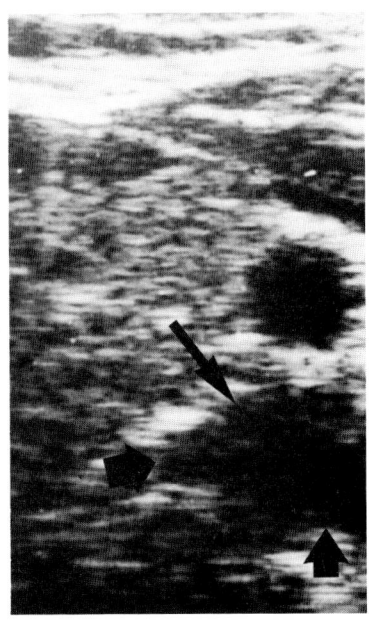

A

B

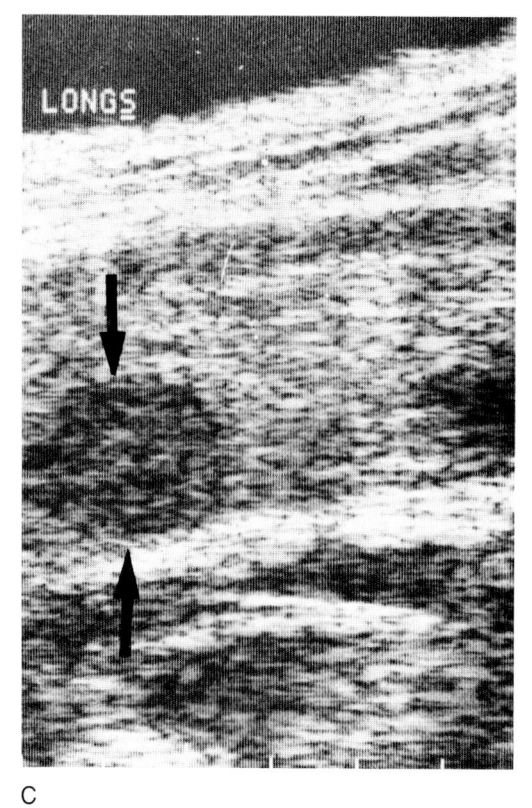

C

18.14 False-Negative Sonogram

Ultrasound examination of the neck of a patient with documented hyperparathyroidism failed to reveal a definite parathyroid neoplasm. A transverse section through the right side of the neck is seen in Figure A and through the left side in Figure B. Surgery revealed a 5-mm parathyroid adenoma on the left side, just medial to the carotid artery. In retrospect, the sonogram showed an asymmetry caused by the nodule (straight arrows in Fig. B) which projected anteriorly from the longus colli muscle (M, curved arrow, Fig. A). In retrospect, this nodule most likely represented a parathyroid neoplasm. Early in our experience, this resulted in a false-negative diagnosis. The highest incidence of false-negative diagnosis occurs in patients with hyperplasia in whom one gland is enlarged and the other three are small and cannot be imaged sonographically.

(Figures from Simeone JF, Mueller PR, Ferrucci JT Jr, et al: High-resolution real-time sonography of the parathyroid. Radiology 141:745–751, 1981.)

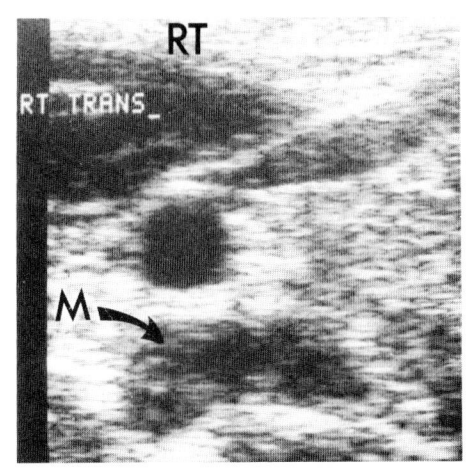

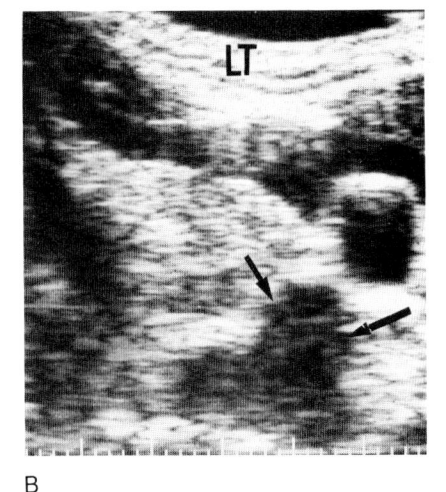

18.15 False-Positive Sonogram

A sonographer experienced in neck and parathyroid ultrasound confidently made the diagnosis of a parathyroid neoplasm in this patient with documented hyperparathyroidism (Figs. A and B). At surgery, no such lesion was found and a neoplasm was discovered on the upper pole of the opposite side. In retrospect, ultrasound showed an echogenic mass (THY) anterior to the longus colli muscles (M) on both the longitudinal (Fig. A) and transverse (Fig. B) scans. The thymus gland occasionally projects into the neck and mimics a parathyroid neoplasm. This echogenic mass was thought to represent a parathyroid neoplasm although the echogenicity was somewhat unusual. At surgery it proved to represent a tongue of thymus tissue.

(Figures from Simeone JF, Mueller PR, Ferrucci JT Jr, et al: High-resolution real-time sonography of the parathyroid. Radiology 141:745–751, 1981.)

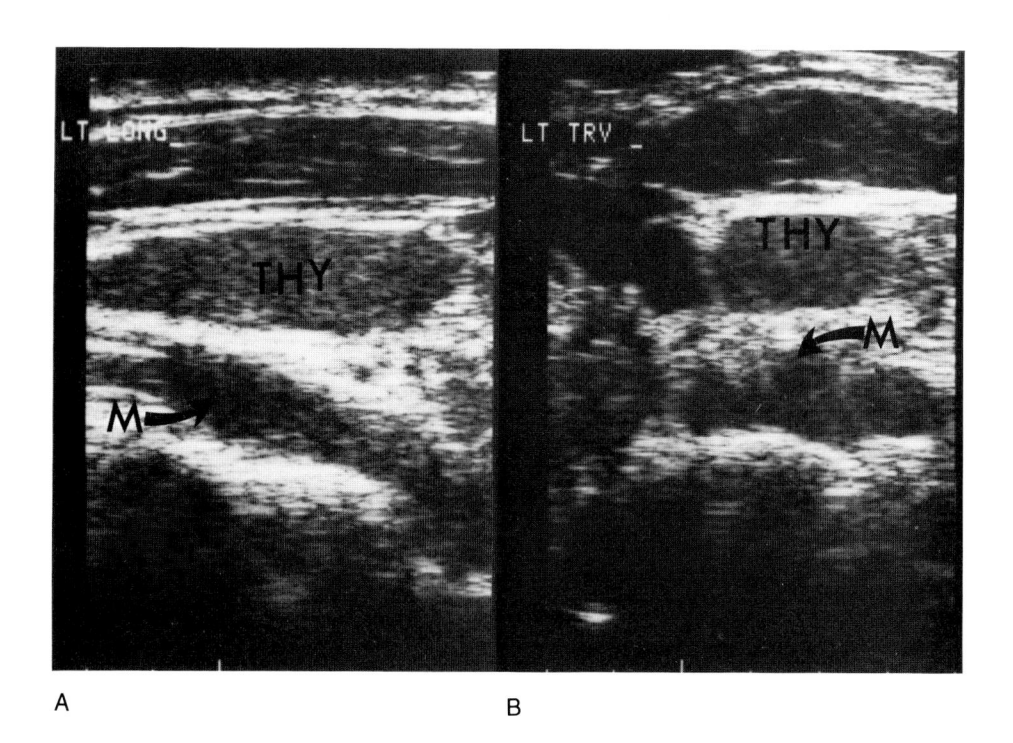

18.16 Hyperplasia

A 50-year-old man presented with a long history of nephrocalcinosis and recent onset of bone pain. Hyperparathyroidism was documented. A longitudinal sonogram (Fig. A) showed a parathyroid mass (N) lying posterior to the thyroid (T). Hyperplasia is a difficult diagnosis to make by ultrasound because of the small size of the hyperplastic glands. In this patient, two parathyroid neoplasms were seen on the ipsilateral side, one at the lower pole (Fig. A) and one nodule (N) at the upper pole of the thyroid (T, Fig. B). When two nodules are seen, a diagnosis of hyperplasia can be suggested.

In the diagnosis of parathyroid hyperplasia, often one of the four glands is enlarged and can generally be appreciated sonographically. The other three glands generally do not exceed 4 or 5 mm and are usually not seen on ultrasound examination. The diagnosis of hyperplasia is based on microscopic examination and can only be made by ultrasound when two or more parathyroid neoplasms are discovered in the neck. However, this is unusual, and generally only one enlarged parathyroid gland is discovered in patients with parathyroid hyperplasia.

(Figures from Simeone JF, Mueller PR, Ferrucci JT Jr, et al: High-resolution real-time sonography of the parathyroid. Radiology 141:745–751, 1981.)

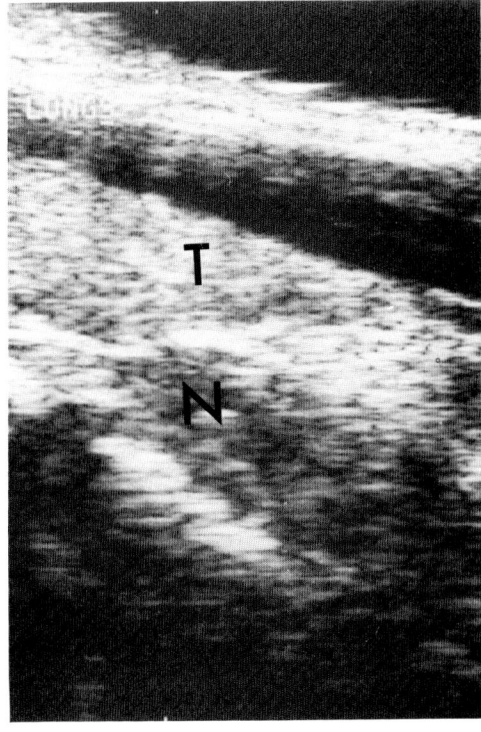

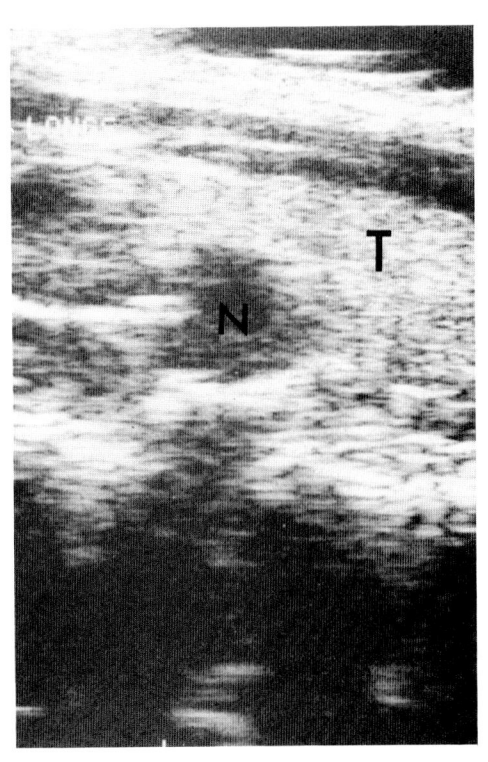

A

B

18.17 Adenoma

An 18-year-old boy had a lifelong history of hypercalcemia. Four previous neck explorations had been performed, resulting in total thyroidectomies and removal of three parathyroid glands, all of which were normal. He presented again with hypercalcemia. A longitudinal ultrasound scan showed a bullet-shaped mass (M in the figure) just anterior to the longus colli muscle (LCM). This was a parathyroid neoplasm which had been missed at all previous surgical operations.

Another important use for ultrasound examination of the parathyroid is in the postoperative patient with signs and symptoms of recurrent hyperparathyroidism. Neck exploration is much more difficult in these patients because of the previous surgery. Preoperative localization of the gland is extraordinarily helpful to the surgeon.
(Figure from Simeone JF, Mueller PR, Ferrucci JT Jr, et al: High-resolution real-time sonography of the parathyroid. Radiology 141:745–751, 1981.)

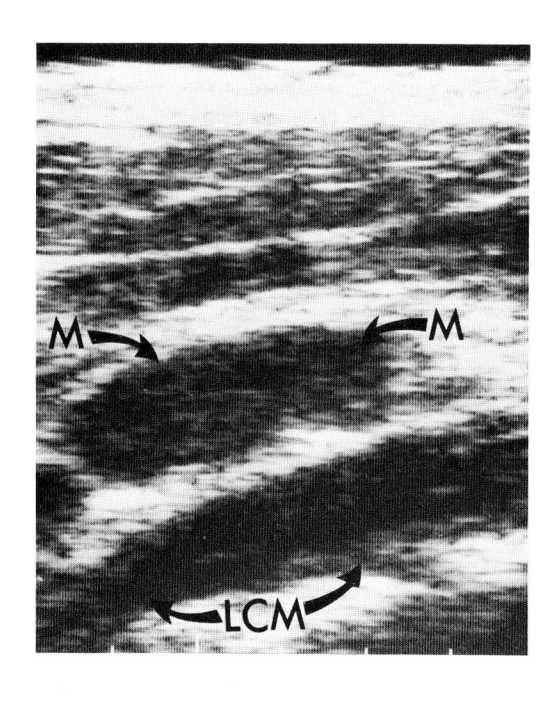

18.18 Migration of Neoplasm

Routine physical examination of a 78-year-old woman showed that her serum calcium was 15.8 mg/dl. A longitudinal ultrasound scan of the neck (shown in the figure) revealed a mass (M) which had migrated from the upper pole to the lower pole. This large, hypoechoic nodule (M) was attached by a vascular pedicle to the upper pole of the thyroid (T).

(Figure from Simeone JF, Mueller PR, Ferrucci JT Jr, et al: High-resolution real-time sonography of the parathyroid. Radiology 141:745–751, 1981.)

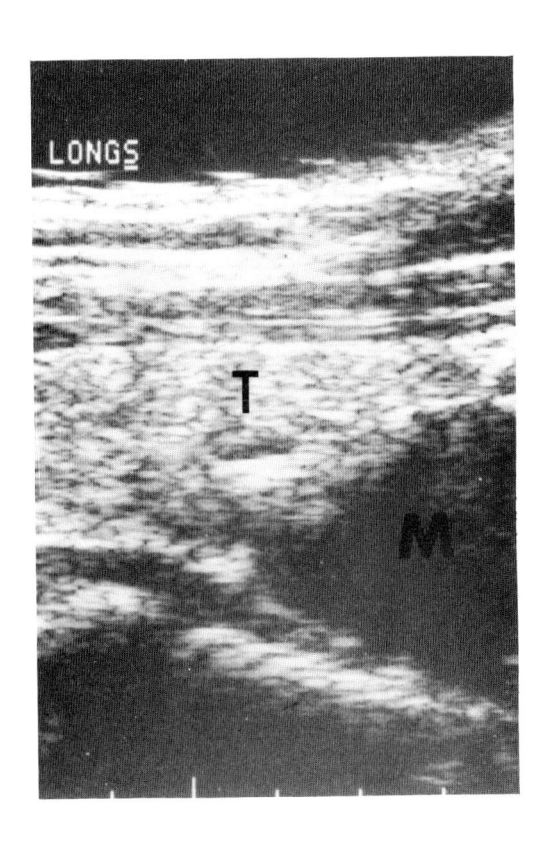

18.19 Ultrasound Appearance of Neoplasms

Almost all parathyroid neoplasms are hypoechoic relative to the adjacent thyroid gland. They may assume many different shapes but for the most part conform to the shape of the neck: they are elongated and shaped like a cigar or bullet. Glands located at the lower poles of the thyroid are generally easier to localize than those of the upper poles. Occasionally, an intrathyroidal parathyroid gland is seen but this is unusual.

Swallowing should be observed in every patient with possible parathyroid abnormality. Swallowing elevates the thyroid gland and neck structures from a subclavicular position into the supraclavicular portion of the neck. Under real-time ultrasound examination, swallowing and elevation can be observed and freeze frames made if the parathyroid gland is seen to emerge from the subclavicular region. Occasionally this may be the only way to discover glands located in the superior mediastinum.

18.20 Summary

While parathyroid sonography can find approximately 75 percent of parathyroid neoplasms,[1] it is a very subjective art. A great deal of practice is needed to discover these masses and often the scanning has to be done by the radiologist rather than the sonographer. Only after examining numerous patients and making the requisite number of false-positive and false-negative diagnoses does one gain experience and confidence in finding parathyroid neoplasms.

However, in experienced hands, one can expect parathyroid ultrasound to localize the parathyroid neoplasm or exclude its presence 75–80 percent of the time. In these patients, this finding is extraordinarily helpful if the surgeon decides that a unilateral neck exploration is all that is indicated in patients with parathyroid adenoma. The savings in operating room time, anesthesia time, and unnecessary surgery are considerable.

In any hospital, the surgeon's attitude toward unilateral neck exploration also determines the importance of parathyroid sonography. If a surgeon is willing to do unilateral neck exploration, ultrasound can be most helpful. In our institution, if a parathyroid neoplasm is found by ultrasound, the neck is explored at the site of the localized neoplasm. That neoplasm is surgically removed as well as the ipsilateral parathyroid gland. If the larger nodule is shown to be a parathyroid adenoma on frozen section and the smaller parathyroid gland is normal, the operation is terminated. If parathyroid hyperplasia is discovered based on examination of frozen section during the unilateral exploration, a bilateral neck exploration must be done. In this latter case, ultrasound scanning did not prevent a bilateral exploration. However, if the surgeon is content to do a unilateral exploration, after a single adenoma is found, at least 1 hour's operating time can be saved. Some surgeons argue that a bilateral exploration is necessary for all patients with hyperparathyroidism because of the presence of bilateral parathyroid adenomas. There is considerable disagreement among various authors regarding the existence of bilateral adenomas.

REFERENCE

1. Wang CA: The anatomic basis of parathyroid surgery. Ann Surg 183:271, 1976

19 The Vascular System

KENNETH J.W. TAYLOR and PAULA JACOBSON

Ultrasound is useful for the display of the larger vessels in the neck, abdomen, and leg. Although in terms of resolution it obviously does not compete with angiography, ultrasound does have the major advantage of being completely noninvasive. When the various modalities are compared, there is a tendency to imply that digital subtraction angiography is not invasive, but the current practice is either to inject a small amount of contrast directly into the artery or to give a large bolus injection of contrast into the central veins or the right atrium. Either practice is highly invasive and contrasts with the innocuous ultrasound evaluation.

The addition of pulsed Doppler provides another dimension to the study of vascular disease and now allows the diagnosis of even minor degrees of stenosis. Doppler ultrasound also promises to be of value in the estimation of blood flow, and the assessment of vascular impedance and its variation in disease. This new modality will require that radiologists readjust their view towards consideration of functional activity instead of structural images.

19.1 Abdominal Vessels

The abdominal aorta may be reliably identified on longitudinal or transverse sonograms in nearly all patients. The upper aorta lying posterior to the liver can always be displayed, but initial attempts to scan the lower aorta may show air-containing gut lying superficial to, and obscuring, the great vessels. Repeated firm scanning movement in the linear plane usually deflects air from the gut and the lower aorta becomes clearly visible. The ability to expel air from gut lying superficial to the great vessels often makes the static manual scanning of the abdominal aorta more successful than dynamic scanning. However, with dynamic scanning firm palpation can still be used to expel air from the viewing field. Caution must obviously be exercised in any firm manipulation of a suspected aortic aneurysm.

A longitudinal section 1 cm to the left of the midline is seen in Figure A. The entire longitudinal extent of the aorta (A) is seen from the level of the diaphragm down to the point of bifurcation at the level of the umbilicus. The celiac trunk is seen (closed arrow) emerging from the anterior surface of the aorta. Slightly lower, the superior mesenteric (open arrow) is seen at its origin from the aorta. A further section in the longitudinal plane (Fig. B) shows both the superior mesenteric artery (SMA) and the inferior mesenteric artery (arrowed) passing inferiorly from their origin into the mesentery. Pulsed Doppler examination of the great vessels shows that each of the major vessels appears to have a specific pattern. Waveform analysis in the aorta (Fig. C) shows that plug flow is present; red cells are moving at the same velocity so that there is a clear window below the velocity time profile.

A lower scan (Fig. D) shows the bifurcation of the common iliac vessels with the external iliac passing superficially, and the internal iliac passing posteriorly into the true pelvis. Beyond the inguinal ligament, the external iliac artery becomes continuous with the femoral artery. Plug flow is also seen in both the common iliac (Fig. E) and the external iliac arteries (Fig. F). Comparing these waveforms, a reverse component is seen which becomes more obvious as the blood passes down towards the leg and becomes maximal in the external iliac artery. This implies that blood actually refluxes up the great vessels during diastole. Thus, blood in the external iliac shows plug flow with a forward component followed by a reverse component as blood rebounds out of the high impedance of the lower limb circulation.

In contrast, the internal iliac artery demonstrates parabolic flow so that there is no window below the waveform (Fig. G). At any instant, cells are moving at many different velocities. Although the internal iliac artery may be seen beyond the bifurcation of the common iliac (Fig. D), it is particularly easily seen on the lateral wall of the pelvis (arrowed) usually lying posterior to the ovary (Fig. H), when the bladder is used as an acoustic window.

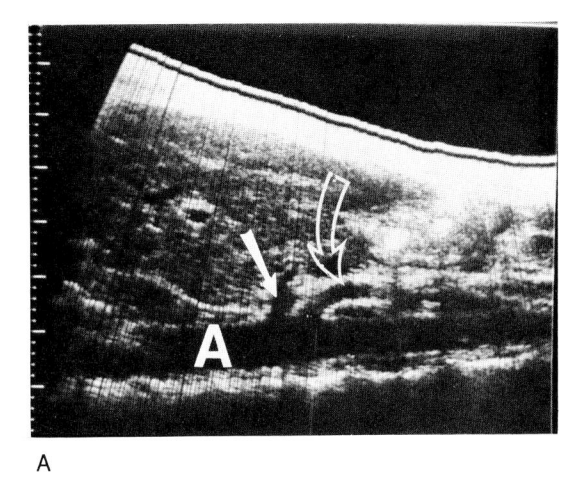

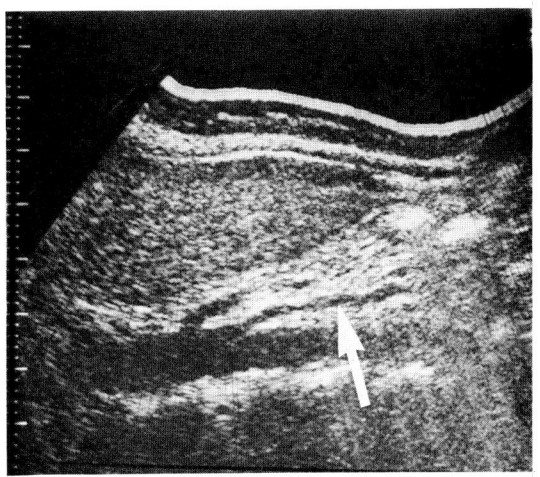

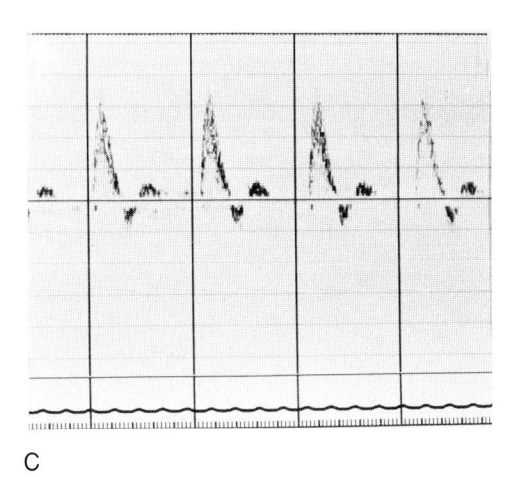

A

B

C

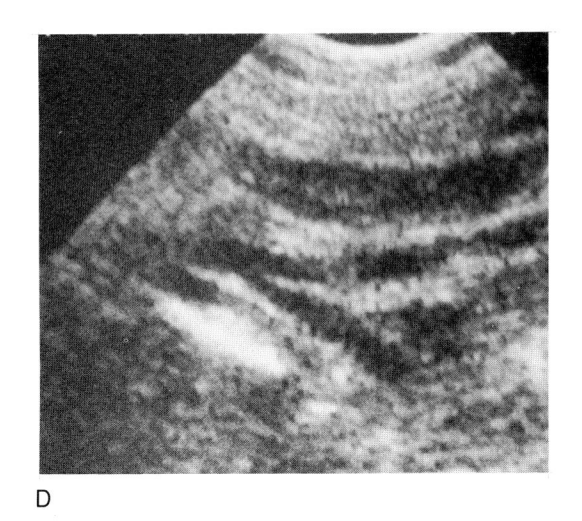

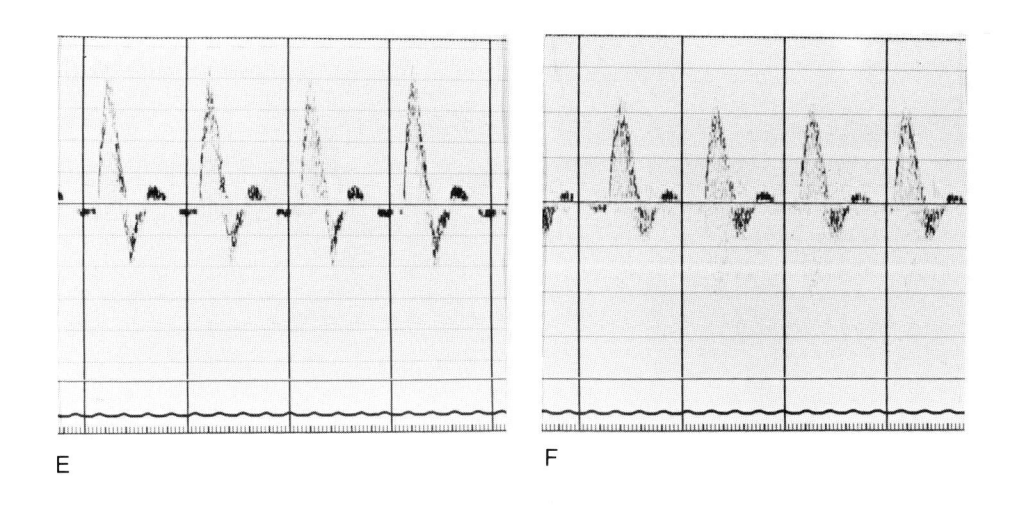

D

E

F

1084

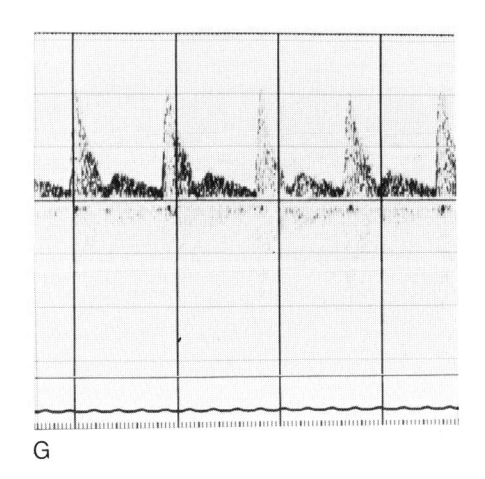

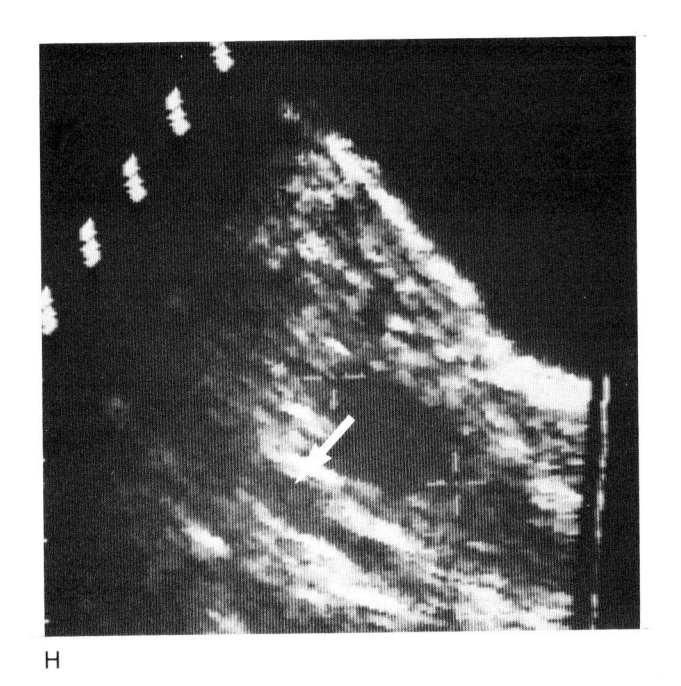

G

H

Anatomy of the Aorta (19.2 and 19.3)

19.2 Transverse

The aorta is imaged by multiple sections at different distances below the xiphisternum. At the origin of the abdominal aorta at the level of the diaphragm, the maximum diameter is 3 cm; this becomes smaller after the origin of the renal arteries and typically is only 2 cm in diameter at the bifurcation, which is at the level of the umbilicus.

Figure A shows the aorta and inferior vena cava immediately below the xiphisternum. The inferior vena cava is more anterior than the aorta, and the wall of the inferior vena cava is thinner than that of the aorta. The lumen of the inferior vena cava varies in size with respiration as well as cardiac pulsations.

A transverse section 8 cm below the xiphisternum (Fig. B) below the origin of the renal arteries shows a vessel only 1.5 cm in diameter. The superior mesenteric artery is seen anterior to the aorta embedded in the fibrofatty tissue in the root of the mesentery, which appears as a highly reflective stroma around the superior mesenteric artery. The splenic vein is seen coursing around the prevertebral region and joins the superior mesenteric vein to form the portal vein.

A transverse section at the level of the umbilicus (Fig. C) reveals the aorta in the midline with the inferior vena cava more posteriorly placed.

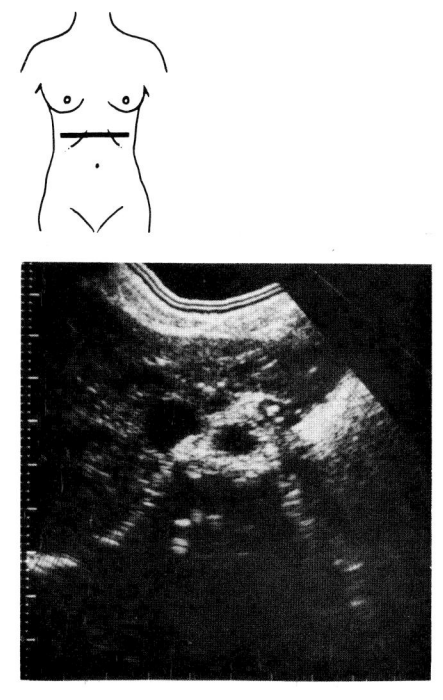

A

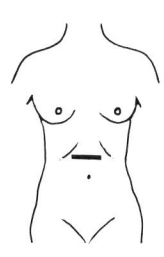

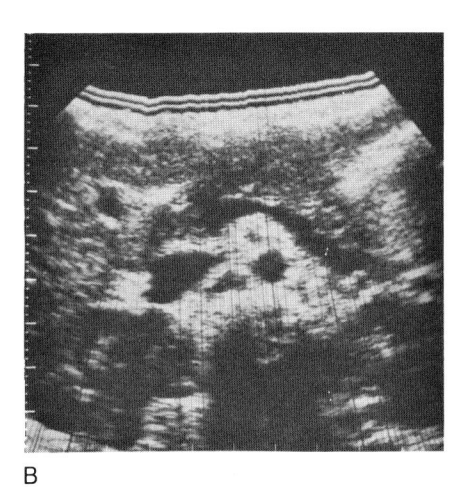

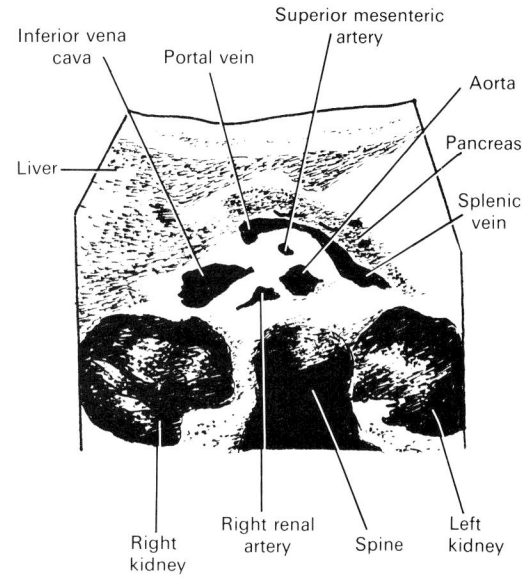

B

| | | Superior mesenteric | |
| Inferior vena cava | Portal vein | artery | Aorta |

Pancreas

Splenic vein

Liver

Right kidney | Right renal artery | Spine | Left kidney

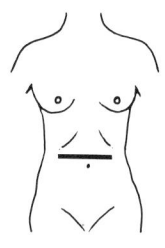

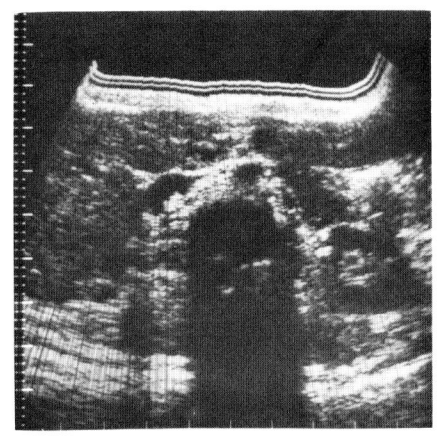

C

1087

19.3 Branches

A longitudinal scan through the aorta reveals the celiac trunk (see Fig. A).

Transverse scans with the transducer directed cephalad show the celiac trunk and its branches (Fig. A). The splenic artery (s) passes to the left and the hepatic artery (h) passes to the right anterior to the portal vein (p). The common duct (d) completes the portal triad. The waveform of the hepatic artery shows a marked diastolic component with cells moving at all velocities (Fig. B). The splenic waveform is extremely turbulent, perhaps associated wih tortuosity commonly found in the splenic artery (Fig. C).

A longitudinal section through the plane of the aorta (A) shows the superior mesenteric vein (arrowed, Fig. D) passing deep to the neck of the pancreas. At the bulbous termination of the superior mesenteric vein, there is confluence with the transverse running splenic vein to form the portal vein. An oblique section (Fig. E) shows the continuity of the splenic vein (arrowed) with the main and right portal vein (P). The plane of the portal vein varies widely in different individuals, but is easily established by altering the angle of the transducer during dynamic scanning.

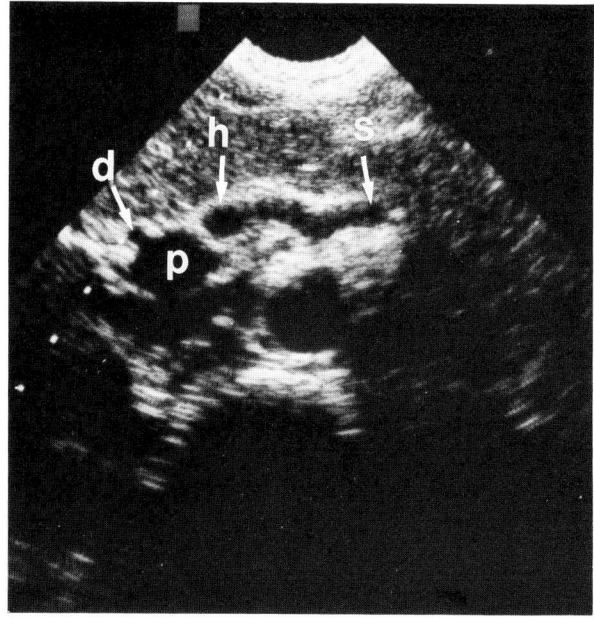

A

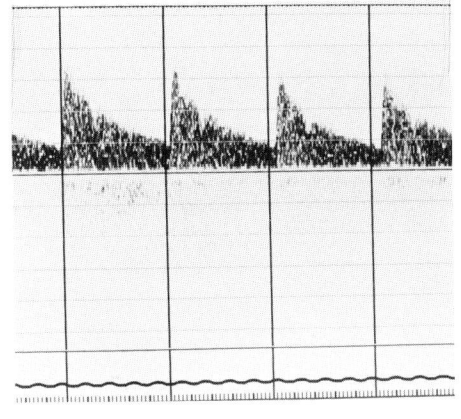

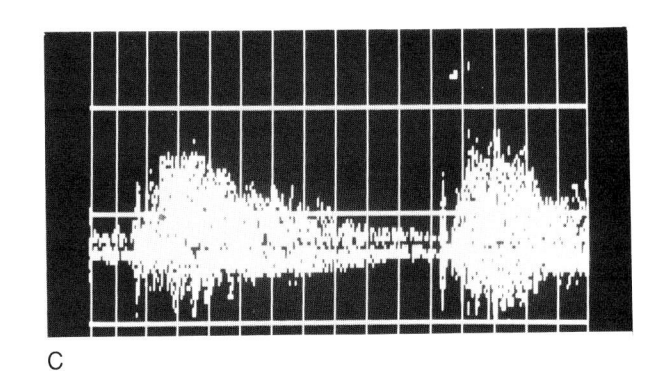

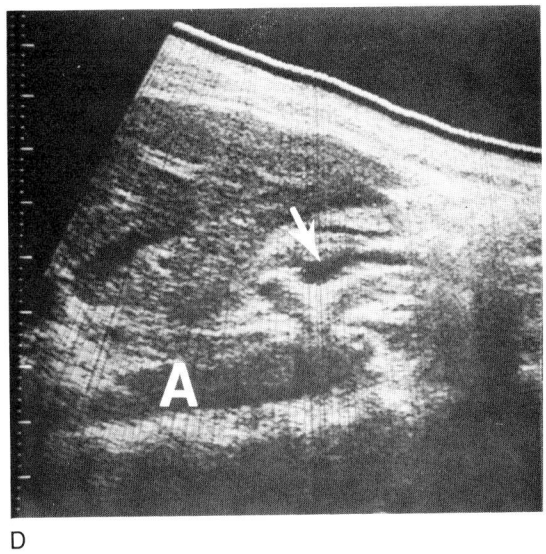

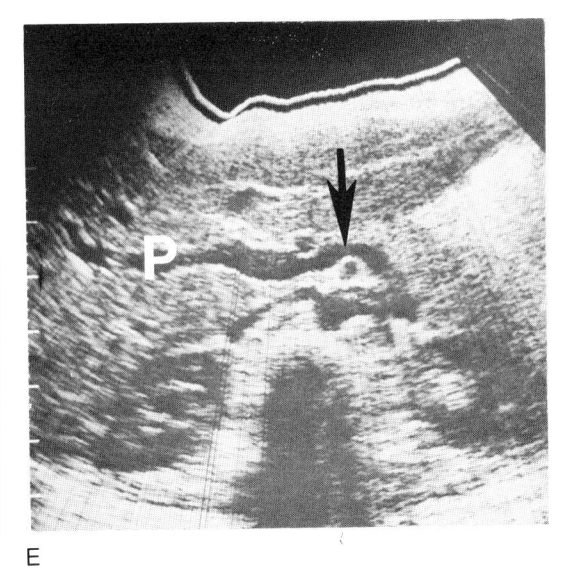

B

C

D

E

19.4 Renal Vessels

Transverse sonograms show the right renal artery (arrowed, Fig. A) and vein (arrowed, Fig. B). These can be seen in virtually every patient since the right lobe of the liver can be used as an acoustic window. Visualization of the left renal vessels requires a gas-free retroperitoneum. A transverse section (Fig. C) demonstrates the left renal artery (L) and the right renal artery (R) arising from the lateral aspects of the aorta. Note that the right renal artery passes posterior to the inferior vena cava and can be seen in this position. Thus, a longitudinal section through the inferior vena cava (V, Fig. D) demonstrates the right renal artery (arrowed) passing posterior to it. The waveform of the renal arteries is characteristic and shows almost a continuous flow with little systolic modulation (Fig. E). This almost continuous flow is seen despite the extreme variations in velocity in the adjacent aorta. The waveform in the renal vessels is the result of a small ostium from a high-pressure large vessel thereby producing almost continuous flow into the low-impedance renal circulation.

The left renal vein (arrowed; Fig. F) is seen on a transverse sonogram passing towards the right in the vascular interval between the aorta and the superior mesenteric artery. There is often a dilatation of the vessel to the left of the vascular space, which must not be mistaken for an aneurysm. The left (L) and right (R) renal veins drain into the inferior vena cava (Fig. G). The pressure fluctuations within the IVC are transmitted to the renal veins. Thus, patent renal veins display cardiac variations in their lumens; such variation indicates patency of the vessels. Therefore, dynamic scanning of the renal vessels is useful in patients with suspected renal thrombosis. The renal vessels, particularly on the right, are amenable to pulsed Doppler examination, which can also be used to document renal vein patency. Estimating absolute blood in the renal vessels is more challenging[1] but waveform analysis may be useful in the diagnosis of renal artery stenosis.[2]

REFERENCES

1. Reid MH, Mackay RS, Lantz BMT: Non-invasive blood flow measurements by Doppler ultrasound with applications to renal artery flow determination. Invest Radiol 15, 323–331, 1980
2. Nichols BT, Rittgers GE, Norris CS, Barnes RW: Non-invasive detection of renal artery stenosis. Bruit 8, 26–29, 1984

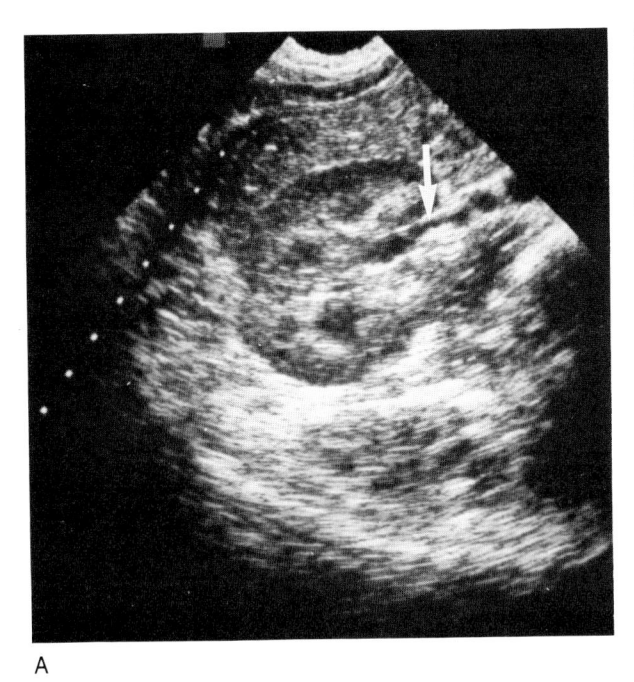

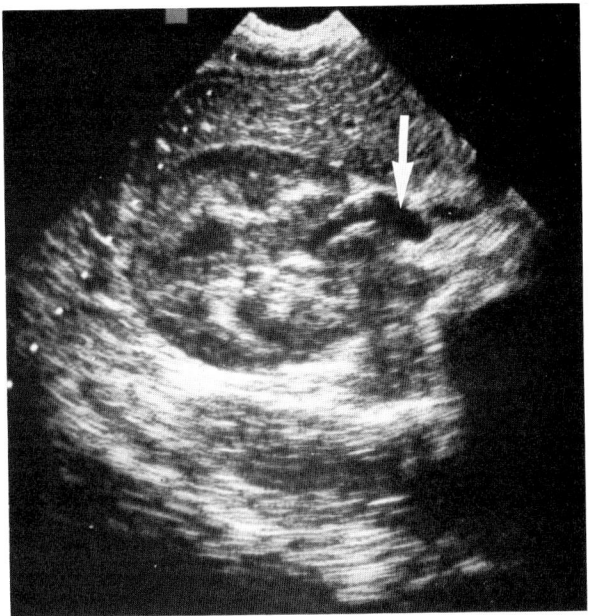

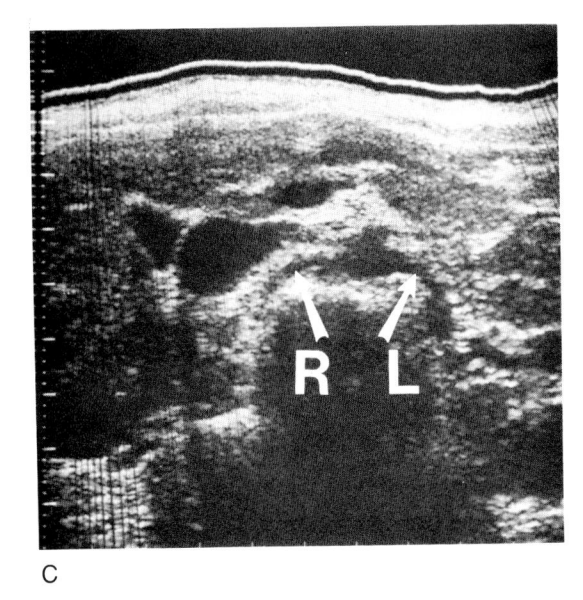

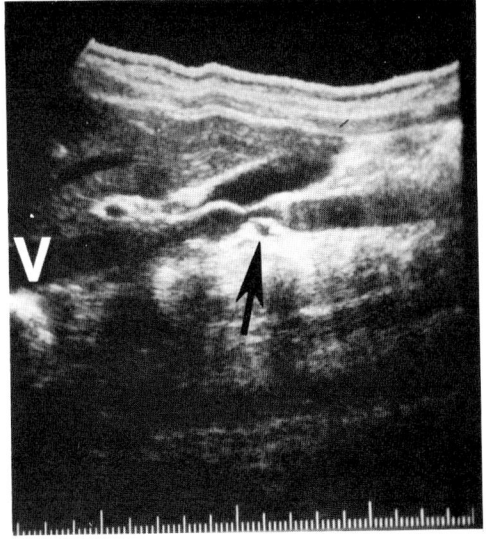

A

B

C

D

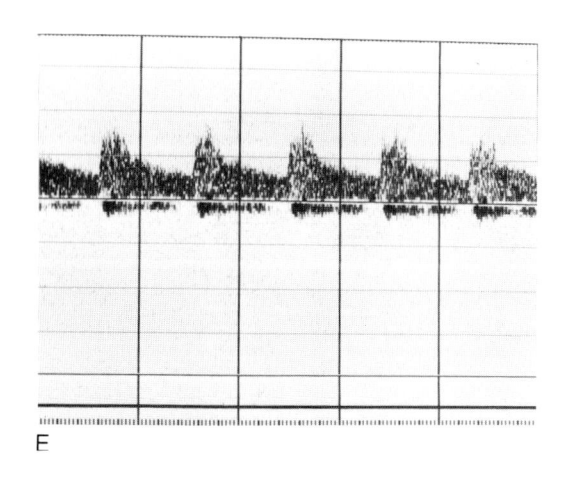

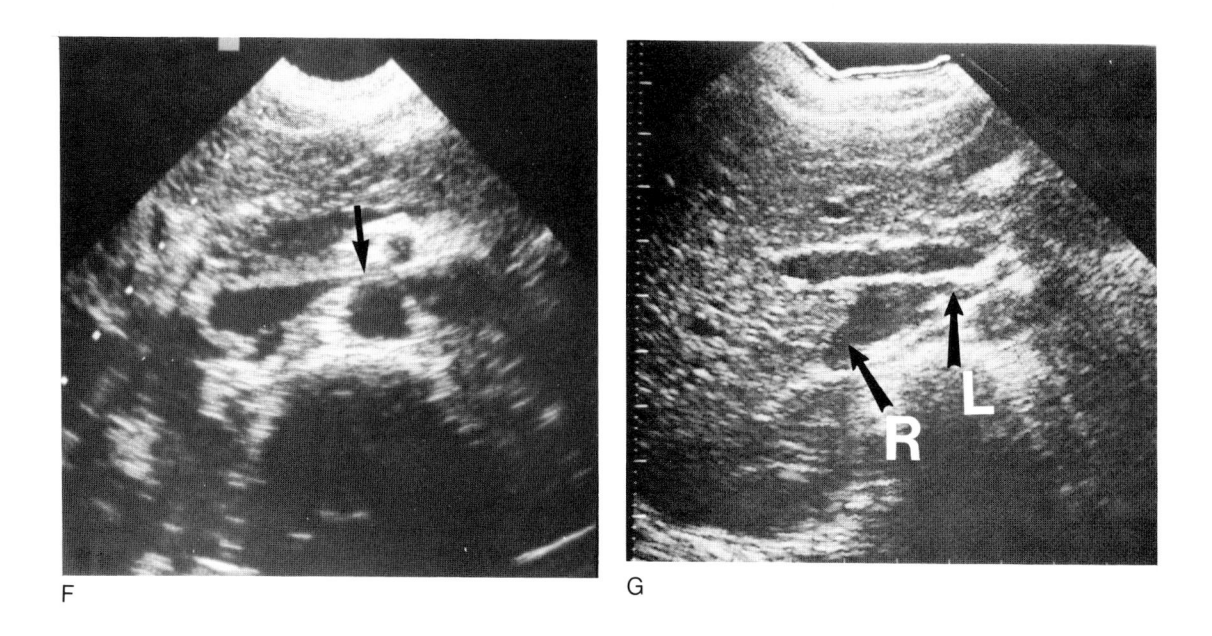

E

F

G

Disorders of the Aorta (19.5 and 19.6)

19.5 Aneurysm

A 56-year-old man was referred for evaluation of a palpable midabdominal mass. Ultrasound examination reveals a localized dilatation of the aorta, on both longitudinal (Fig. A) and transverse sonograms (Fig. B). Note that the intraluminal clot is well-demonstrated, which allows the sonologist to measure both the lumen of the aorta and the size of the aneurysm. Arteriography is not only invasive but also provides only the former measurements.

Eighty percent of abdominal aneurysms involve the lower aorta and spare the origin of the renal arteries. It is, however, important in planning surgery to try to predict when the origin of the renal arteries are involved. This level can usually be identified by either subxiphoid or intercostal sector scanning.

The major advantage of ultrasound in the diagnosis of abdominal aneurysms is its lack of invasion. This permits repeated examinations over the course of months or even years. Aneurysms larger than 5 cm require surgery, since they present an immediate danger to life. Smaller aneurysms may be treated conservatively since death from other manifestations of arterial disease is more common, and in such cases repeated ultrasound examinations form a basis of conservative management.

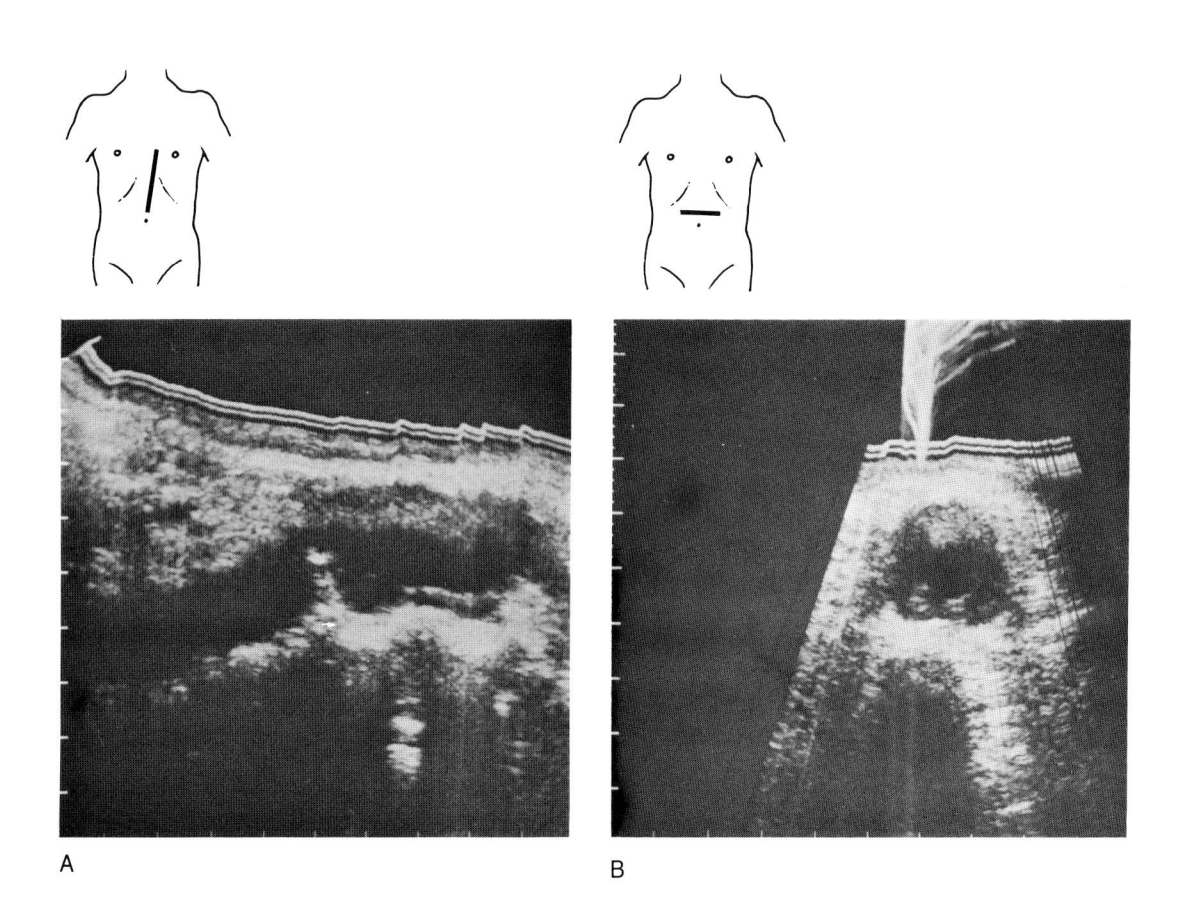

A

B

1094

19.6 Graft

A 60-year-old patient had an aortic aneurysm from the level of the renal arteries to the bifurcation of the abdominal aorta. At surgery, a Dacron graft replacement of the aneurysm was effected and the aneurysm shell sewn around it. A longitudinal songoram 2 cm to the left of the midline shows the entire extent of the abdominal aneurysm, the lower half of which has been replaced by the Dacron graft (Fig. A). There is homogeneous material both anterior and posterior to the graft with some forward angulation of the graft. The transverse sonogram 2 cm above the umbilicus shows the graft and the surrounding homogeneous area (Fig. B). These appearances simulate those of a dissecting aneurysm, but knowledge of the preceding surgery permits differentiation. The homogeneous area around the graft is clearly serous exudate and hematoma within the shell of the aneurysm. There is no evidence of leakage at the suture site, indicating that this is not a false aneurysm.

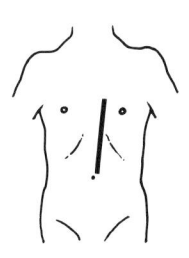

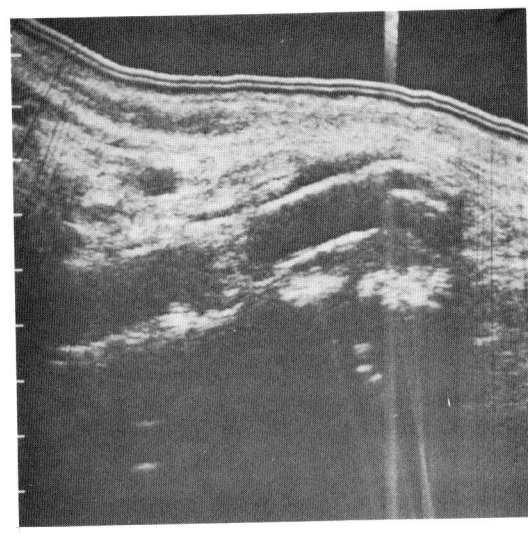

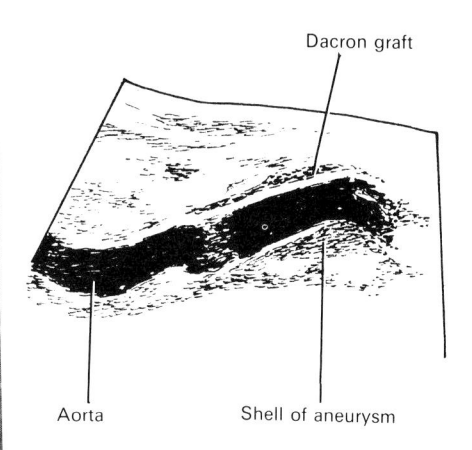

A

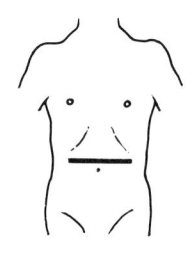

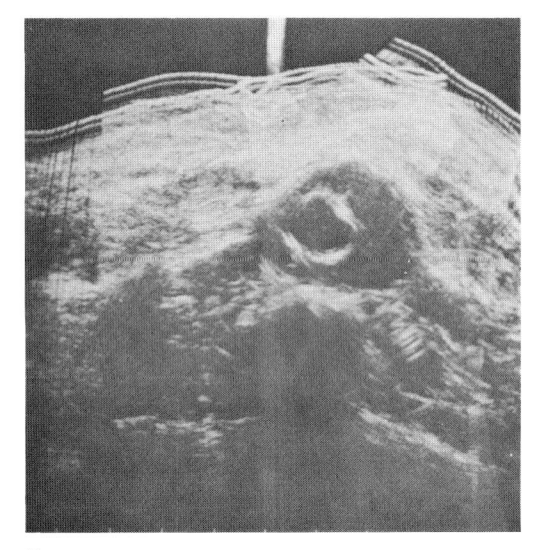

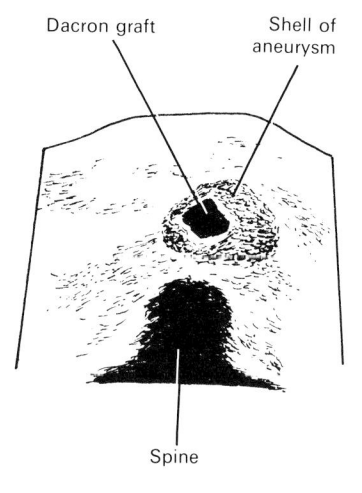

B

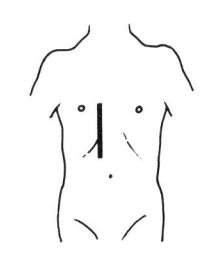

19.7 Inferior Vena Cava

A longitudinal sonogram 2 cm to the right of the midline (Fig. A) shows the inferior vena cava (V) in its longitudinal extent. Unlike the aorta, the walls are thin and the vessel curves anteriorly as it passes through the central tendon of the diaphragm to empty into the right atrium. Since no valves are present in this part of the inferior vena cava or in its termination, the pulsations of the right atrium are transmitted down the inferior vena cava. The vessel therefore displays cardiac pulsations. In addition, there are variations with the respiratory cycle. In inspiration the increased abdominal pressure and decreased thoracic pressure ensure blood flow from the abdomen to the thorax; this constitutes the respiratory pump. Thus a deep breath empties the inferior vena cava while a prolonged Valsalva maneuver distends the normal inferior vena cava.

These variations in the caliber of the inferior vena cava (IVC) can be displayed using the M-mode (Fig. B). The lumen of the inferior vena cava (L) shows large variations which are respiratory, whereas the smaller ones are cardiac in origin. Pulsed Doppler examination also demonstrates the changes in blood velocity and direction associated with respiratory and cardiac excursions (Fig. C). Compare this to the more continuous waveform in the portal vein (Fig. D).

Tumor or thrombus can easily be seen with IVC. They should be excluded by careful real-time examination in any patient with a hypernephroma or evidence of an embolus. Longitudinal scan (Fig. E) and transverse scan (Fig. F) show caval thrombus (arrowed). Recognition of this thrombus and appropriate surgical treatment probably saved this 37-year-old woman from massive pulmonary embolus.

(Scan B from Taylor KJW: Ultrasonic investigation of inferior vena-caval obstruction. Br J Radiol 48:1024–1026, 1975.)

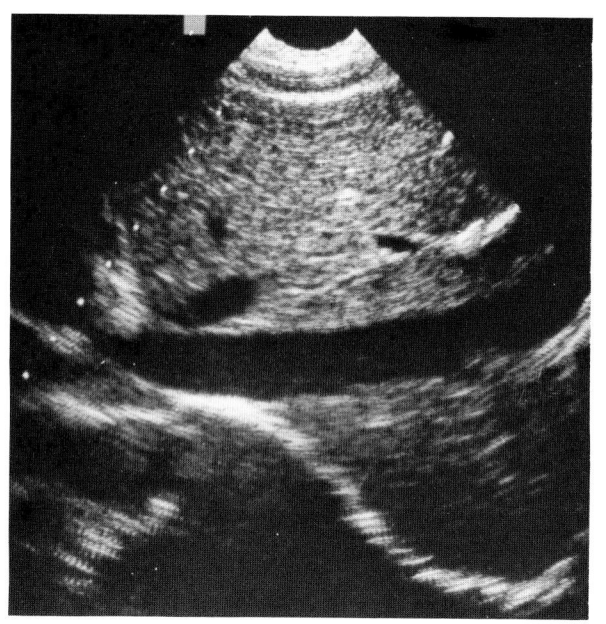

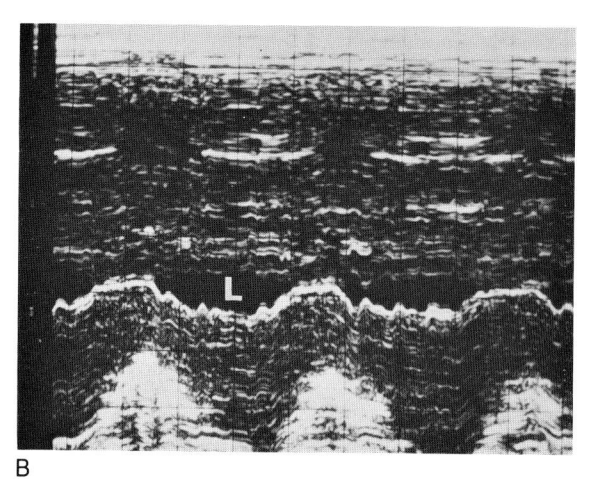

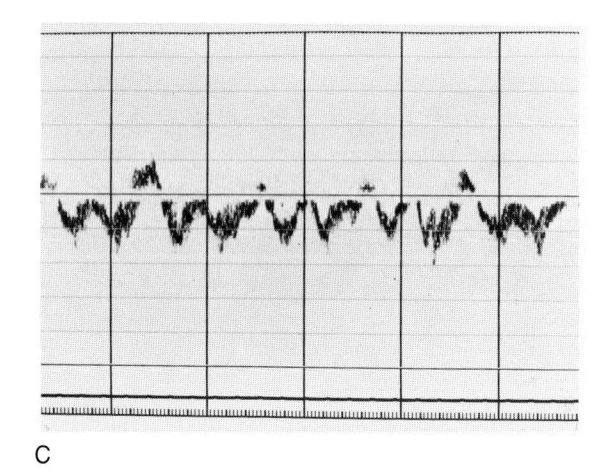

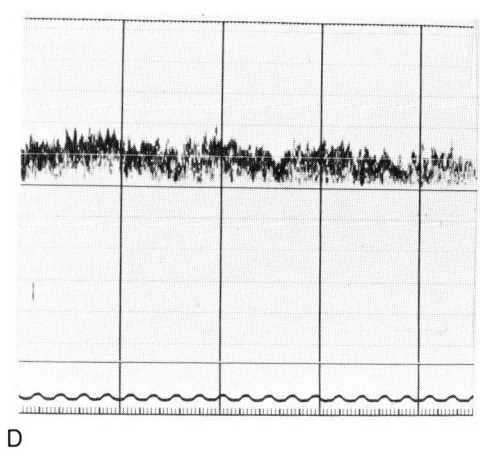

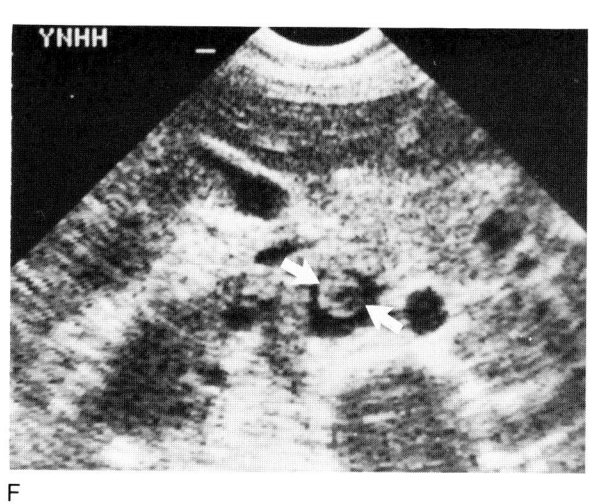

A

B

C

D

E

F

19.8 Intraluminal Echoes

Observation of the portal vein may reveal particulate material moving in the direction of blood flow, and this may be valuable in establishing patency of a vessel.

A longitudinal sonogram is shown in which particulate matter is seen in the portal vein (arrowed). This is not a reverberation echo, and the two are easily differentiated by dynamic scanning.

A similar phenomenon may be seen in the inferior vena cava and renal veins wherever flow is relatively slow. A rational explanation is that the phenomenon is due to red cell aggregation, perhaps due to rouleaux formation.

That this phenomenon is due to reflection of ultrasound by the red cells has been suggested by Wolverson et al.[1] and Shung et al.[2] Alternatively, microbubbles due to absorption of the intestinal air have also been suggested as a physical basis for this phenomenon.[3] Sigel et al.[4,5] conducted experiments in which they found that internal echoes within blood developed within seconds of the onset of stasis. This echogenicity required the presence of red cells and fibrinogen and was increased by the addition of red cells or increased temperature. Prolongation of stasis increased the degree of echogenicity while agitation of the blood caused the echoes to disappear. More obvious echoes were obtained from the blood of patients with myeloma, who readily form rouleaux. All these observations suggest that echogenicity in flowing blood is due to rouleaux formation associated with slow rates of flow and low shear rates.[6]

REFERENCES

1. Wolverson MK, Nouri S, Joist JH, et al: The direct visualization of blood flow by real time ultrasound: clinical observations and underlying mechanism. Radiology 140:443, 1981
2. Shung KPK, Singelman RA, Reid JM: Scattering of ultrasound by blood. IEEE Trans Biomed Eng 23:460, 1976
3. Kort A, Kronzon I: Microbubble formation: in vitro and in vivo observation. J Clin Ultrasound 10:117, 1982
4. Sigel B, Coelho JCU, Spigos DG, et al: Ultrasonography of blood during stasis and coagulation. Invest Radiology 16:71, 1981
5. Sigel B, Coelho JCU, Schade SG, et al: Effect of plasma proteins and temperature on echogenicity of blood. Invest Radiol 17:29, 1982
6. Machi J, Sigel B, Beitler JC, et al: Relation of in vivo blood flow to ultrasound echogenicity. J Clin Ultrasound 11:3–10, 1983

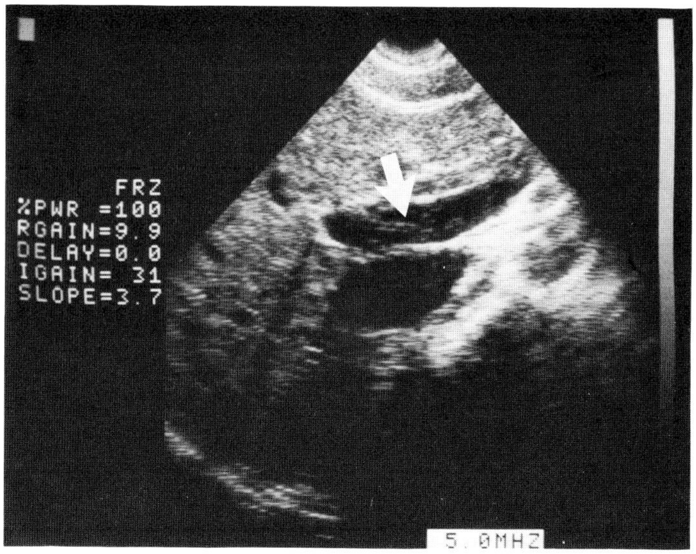
FRZ
%PWR =100
RGAIN=9.9
DELAY=0.0
IGAIN= 31
SLOPE=3.7
5.0MHZ

19.9 Inferior Vena Cava Obstruction by Malignant Liver

A 55-year-old patient who was known to have chronic lymphatic leukemia devleoped hepatomegaly and lymphedema of both legs. It seemed likely that there was pressure on the inferior vena cava. A paramedian sonogram 2 cm to the right of the midline shows a grossly enlarged liver which is abnormally homogeneous, consistent with advanced malignant infiltration (Fig. A). The lumen of the inferior vena cava appears to be abnormally large below, while there is an apparent constriction at a higher level. An M-mode sonogram was taken below the level of the apparent obstruction in the plane shown by the dotted line.

The scan (Fig. B) shows no respiratory variations in the caliber of the inferior vena cava lumen (L), suggesting that the pressure changes in the thorax are not transmitted through the inferior vena cava and indicating obstruction to the cava.

Although M-mode sonography can be used to document the variations in lumen with time, the diagnosis is now more simply made by dynamic scanning.

(Scans from Taylor KJW: Ultrasonic investigation of inferior vena-caval obstruction. Br J Radiol 48:1024–1026, 1975.)

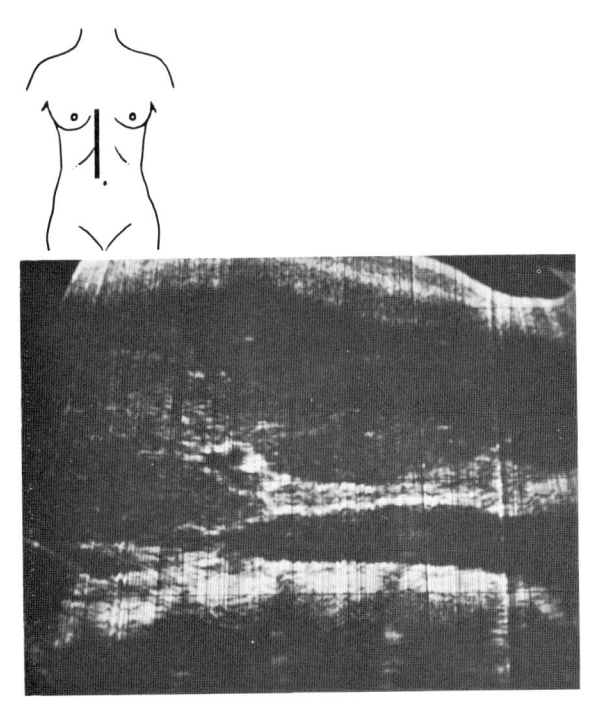

A

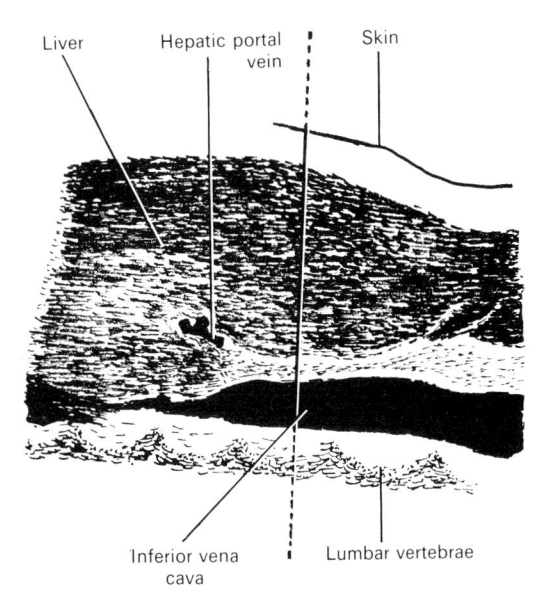

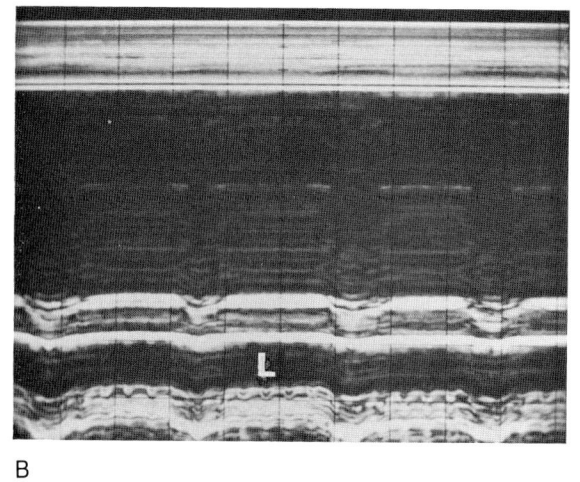

B

19.9 Inferior Vena Cava Obstruction by Malignant Liver

A 55-year-old patient who was known to have chronic lymphatic leukemia devleoped hepatomegaly and lymphedema of both legs. It seemed likely that there was pressure on the inferior vena cava. A paramedian sonogram 2 cm to the right of the midline shows a grossly enlarged liver which is abnormally homogeneous, consistent with advanced malignant infiltration (Fig. A). The lumen of the inferior vena cava appears to be abnormally large below, while there is an apparent constriction at a higher level. An M-mode sonogram was taken below the level of the apparent obstruction in the plane shown by the dotted line.

The scan (Fig. B) shows no respiratory variations in the caliber of the inferior vena cava lumen (L), suggesting that the pressure changes in the thorax are not transmitted through the inferior vena cava and indicating obstruction to the cava.

Although M-mode sonography can be used to document the variations in lumen with time, the diagnosis is now more simply made by dynamic scanning.

(Scans from Taylor KJW: Ultrasonic investigation of inferior vena-caval obstruction. Br J Radiol 48:1024–1026, 1975.)

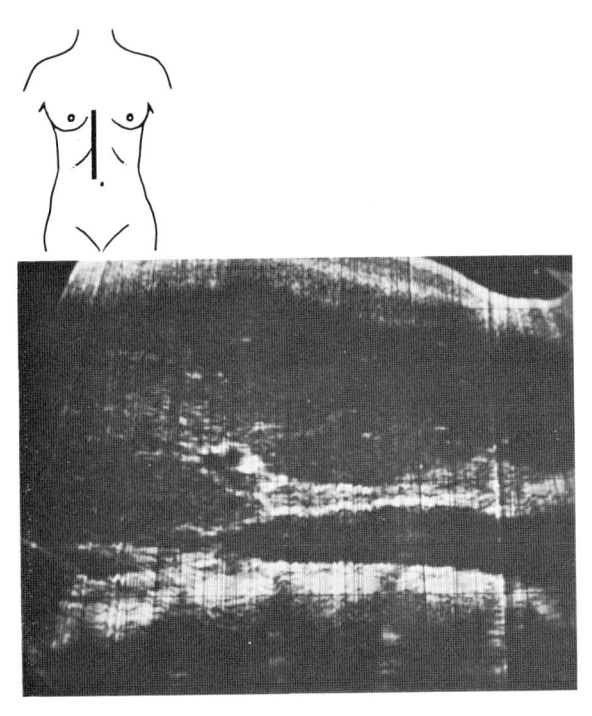

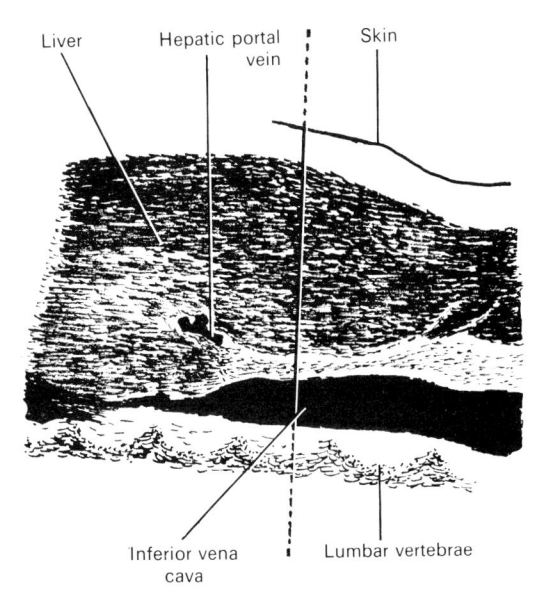

A

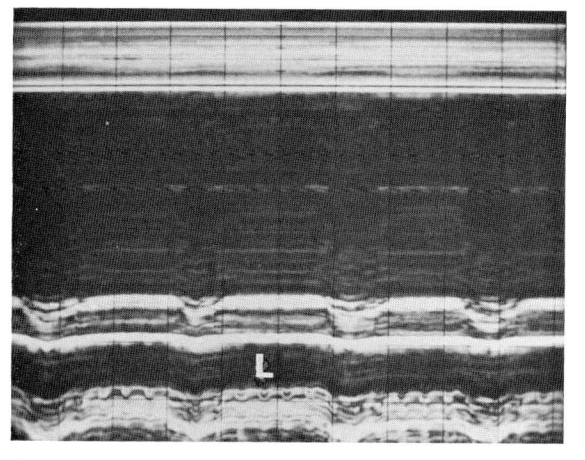

B

19.10 Portocaval Shunt

Portal hypertension is a serious condition resulting from obstruction of the portal flow. The condition results in a 5-year survival of approximately 60 percent, which is often further decreased by excessive alcohol consumption. Although the condition may be due to portal vein obstruction outside the liver, it is most frequently the result of end-stage liver disease, the most prevalent cause of which is alcoholic liver disease. However, it must be recalled that in other countries nonalcoholic liver disease is more prevalent due, for example, to schistosomiasis. These patients, and those with prehepatic causes for portal hypertension, have a much better prognosis than patients with end-stage alcoholic liver disease. The serious effects of portal hypertension are due to the development of portosystemic venous communications. These anastomoses around the lower end of the esophagus form varicose veins which may bleed and become life-threatening.

Hematemasis due to bleeding esophageal varices may be controlled locally by a Sengstaken-Blakemore tube, with circulatory support by transfusions. Since a large number of these patients will subsequently bleed again, the longer-term goal is to relieve the portal hypertension. Liver transplantation is the only permanent method for correcting the condition, but does not have large-scale application without further advances in immunologic research. Thus, efforts are made to decompress the engorged portal venous system by vascular anastomoses. The existence of several different operations for this purpose suggests that none of these techniques is entirely satisfactory; all are associated with considerable morbidity and subsequent mortality.

Currently, the Warren procedure (distal splenorenal anastomosis) is popular. This operation involves the anastomosis of the distal splenic vein to the left renal vein. Particularly in alcoholic patients with calcific pancreatitis, surgical exploration and mobilization of the splenic vein are technically extremely difficult. Some sonologists have reported that such anastomoses may be well-visualized by ultrasound utilizing the spleen as a window. However, the spleen may be removed at surgery and these shunts have not been satisfactorily visualized on a routine basis in our laboratory.

A further operation is the direct portocaval anastomosis. In a minority of patients, these shunts may be visualized directly and pulsed Doppler examination may allow estimation of patency. However, in our experience, these patients are usually very obese with gross postoperative scarring, both in the superficial and deep tissues. It is frequently impossible to visualize the portocaval anastomosis. In these patients, we have utilized a further sign of anastomotic patency.

This alcoholic patient had portocaval anastomosis effected 3 months previously. Scans of the anastomosis were inadequate to establish patency by direct visualization. However, a longitudinal scan in the plane of the IVC demonstrated a dilatation (arrowed) immediately distal to the entrance of the shunt. This appearance, in our experience, has been found to correlate well with patency of the shunt and is presumably due to the turbulence and increased flow associated with the ingress of the portal vein blood flow.

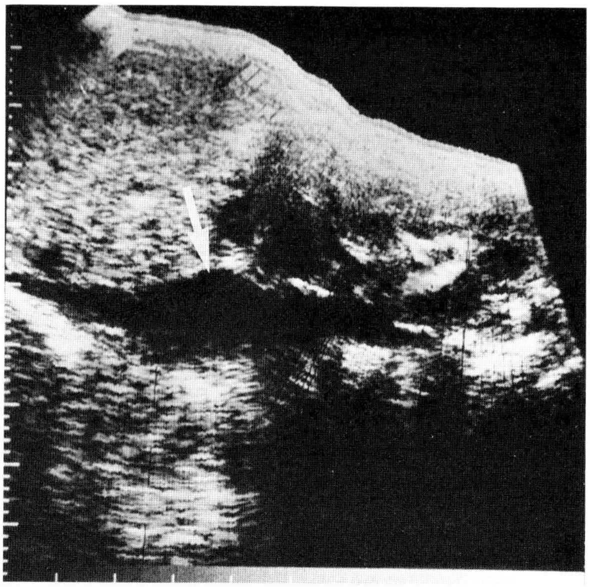

19.11 Portal Vein—Cavernous Transformation

A 62-year-old alcoholic man presented with epigastric pain and an upper GI examination suggested the presence of a pancreatic mass. Ultrasound and CT scans confirmed the presence of this mass and a pseudocyst was noted. A further abnormality was seen.

An oblique ultrasonogram demonstrated multiple tortuous channels surrounding a central structure (Fig. A). Pulsed Doppler examination of the central structure demonstrated no evidence of flow; whereas typical, continuous low velocity flow, characteristic of the portal venous system, was noted in the multiple collateral vessels (Fig. B). The prior CT scan superbly demonstrated these collateral vessels (arrowed in Fig. C) following intravenous contrast material. However, originally, the occluded portal vein had been misinterpreted as an enlarged common duct. Thus, the demonstration of portal venous flow by Doppler examination greatly facilitated the diagnosis of this patient.

Although cavernous transformation of the portal vein was thought to be a primary angiomatous malformation, it is now recognized to be recanalization of the portal vein with periportal collateral channels following portal vein obstruction. Obstruction has been described due to omphalitis, pancreatitis, and alcoholic cirrhosis. Kauzlaric et al.[1] reported two cases describing a diagnostic triad which consisted of failure to visualize the extra-hepatic portal vein, high level echoes in the region of porta hepatis, and visualization of multiple tubular structures in the porta hepatis. The periportal collaterals are beautifully seen on the CT scan in this patient after opacification. However, the diagnosis can be easily made by ultrasound alone when Doppler is utilized. The demonstration of normal almost continuous portal flow in these tortuous collaterals makes a definitive diagnosis of cavernous transformation of the portal vein.

REFERENCE

1. Kauzlaric D, Petrovic M, Barmeir E: Sonograpy of cavernous transformation of the portal vein. AJR 142:382–384, 1984

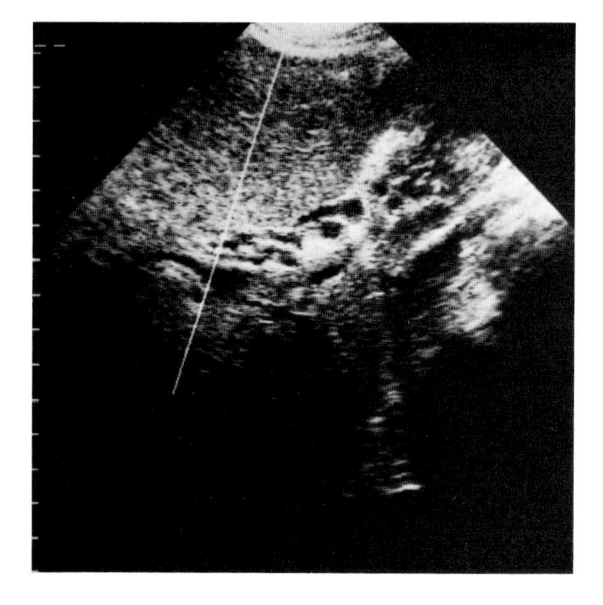

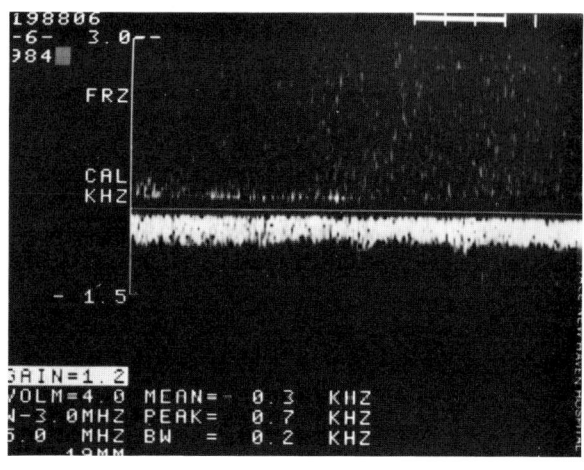

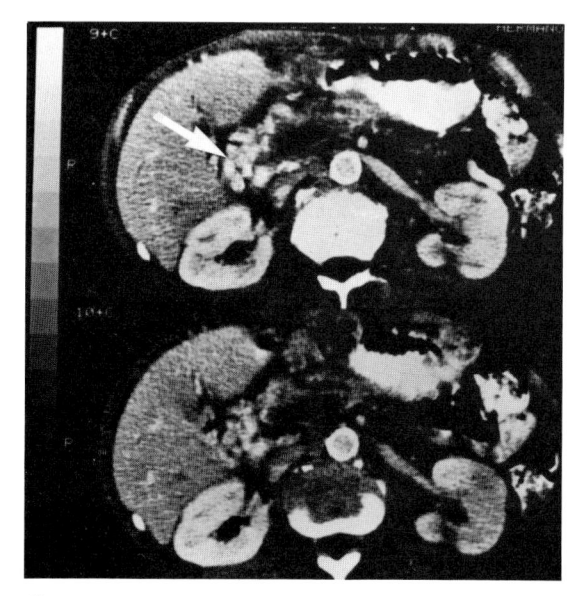

A

B

C

19.12 Popliteal Artery Aneurysm

The popliteal artery is a superficial vessel and any aneurysms derived from it are well-demonstrated by ultrasound. Although these are most aesthetically displayed using a small-parts scanner, they can be adequately imaged using either a static scanner with a 5-MHz transducer, or a linear array with or without a water bag.

An elderly man was referred for investigation of a mass in the popliteal fossa of the right leg. The major differential diagnosis was fluid in a bursa or a popliteal artery aneurysm. A longitudinal sonogram demonstrated a fusiform mass 3.0 cm in maximum diameter (Fig. A), which was continuous with the posterior tibial artery below. The transverse sonogram (Fig. B) was taken through the maximum diameter of the aneurysm. The addition of Doppler ultrasound can also demonstrate arterial flow within to allow definitive diagnosis that such a mass is a popliteal artery aneurysm. Note that there is considerable intraluminal thrombus.

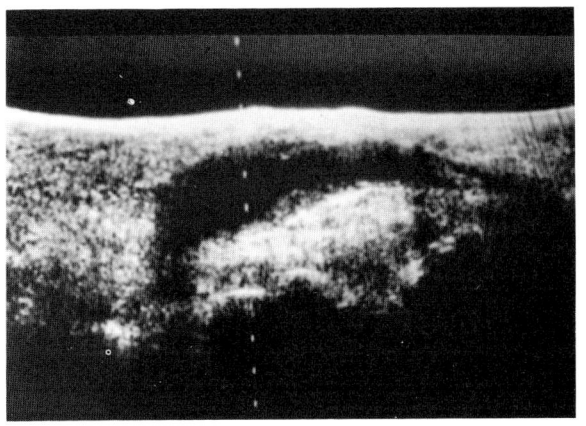

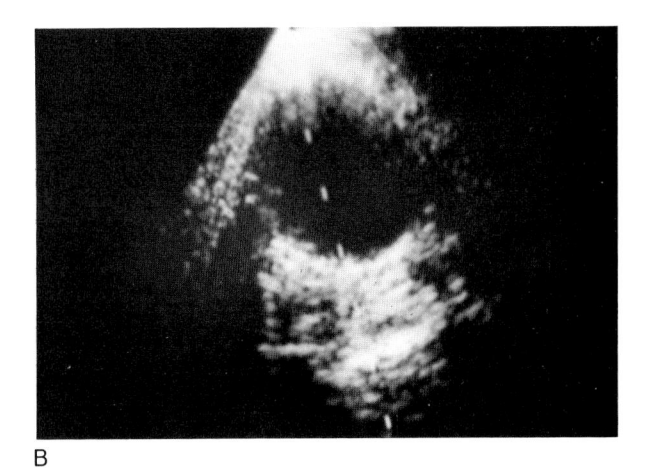

A

B

Carotid Artery (3.13 to 3.17)

19.13 Carotid Artery

NORMAL ANATOMY

The common, internal, or external carotid arteries can be demonstrated using a wide variety of ultrasonic instrumentation. Static scanners can be used with a 5-MHz transducer, either in contact with the skin or with a water bath. Linear arrays may be used, but are difficult to employ when the bifurcation is situated high, because of the proximity of the ramus of the mandible. Rotating sector scanners are most widely used for visualizing carotid vessels. These are usually used in a duplex system with a pulsed Doppler device. The returned Doppler signals are subjected to spectral analysis. A linear mechanical scan is shown in Figure A, with a corresponding normal spectral analysis in Figure B. Note that there is a "window" underneath the curve, indicating that the red cells are moving with simultaneous high velocity ("plug" rather than laminar flow). This can be compared with the spectral analysis seen in patients with even a minor degree of stenosis, in whom this window is lost; this is a sensitive means for detecting minimal stenosis. This "spectral broadening" is due to turbulence associated with stenosis.

STENOSIS

Stroke is a leading cause of death. Forty percent of patients presenting with stroke have occlusion of their carotid arteries. Seventy five percent of these patients have lesions amenable to surgical relief. The availability of successful therapy for carotid artery stenosis by endarterectomy which, in experienced hands, has a mortality of less than 1 percent, raises the possibility of substantially reducing the morbidity, mortality, and the economic burden of stroke. However, when considering the possible benefits of endarterectomy for carotid artery stenosis, it must be recalled that carotid artery disease is but one manifestation of a generalized disease process of atherosclerosis. In many different series, nearly 60 percent of these patients have coexistent coronary artery disease accounting for a high mortality in any follow-up studies. In addition, to establish the significance of carotid artery disease, a careful history must be taken since many cerebral ischemic events in patients with a demonstrated lesion in one artery may be in the areas of distribution of other arteries. Thus, in the follow-up of patients with carotid artery disease, it is important to establish a cause-and-effect relationship between their subsequent clinical course and any demonstrated vascular lesion.

Carotid artery stenosis is a common manifestation of atherosclerotic arterial disease, which has a marked predilection for the bifurcation. Many imaging techniques can be used in the evaluation of carotid bifurcation stenosis. However, the proliferation of noninvasive techniques, in contrast to angiography, has demonstrated the need for careful selection of patients so that maximum diagnostic information can be obtained in a cost-effective way. Symptomatic patients often present with transient ischemic attacks (TIA), which comprise monocular blindness, and temporary sensory or motor disturbance usually affecting only one side of the body. The TIA is distinguished by the transitory nature of the symptoms (less than 24 hours) from a stroke. The occurrence of a TIA has great prognostic significance, since most authors agree that

Table 19-1. Indications for Ultrasound Scanning of Carotid Arteries

Symptomatic	Asymptomatic
Atypical TIA symptoms	Neck bruit
	Preoperative screening
	Postoperative follow-up
	Epidemiologic studies
	Follow-up asymptomatic lesions

the risk of stroke is 40 percent within 5 years; of these, 20 percent will occur in the first year.[1] Twenty percent of that number occur within the first month after the TIA. Thus, TIA increases the risk of stroke by a factor of seventeen times that of the normal population within the next year.[2] Although such patients are often referred for ultrasound evaluation of their carotid arteries, many surgeons believe that prompt arteriography is mandatory in patients with classic TIAs, since the decision to treat using surgery or aspirin requires arteriographic display of the responsible pathology.[3] These authors argue that noninvasive studies evaluate only the degree of carotid stenosis, and that arteriography is required to exclude the possibility of an atheromatous ulcer, which may have provided an embolus. The indications for ultrasound scans of carotid arteries are summarized in Table 19-1.

Ultrasound is useful as a completely noninvasive modality to evaluate the asymptomatic patient or patients with atypical symptoms of TIAs, in whom there is a low clinical suspicion of significant disease. In these patients, our neurologists believe that the risks associated with angiography outweigh the possible benefits.

NECK BRUIT

Neck bruits are usually detected on physical examination of patients over the age of 40. Asymptomatic carotid bruits increase with age from 1 percent at age 45 to 4.4 percent in elderly women.[4] A cervical murmur of some type is much more common, occurring in 12.6 percent of the population aged 45 years and older. The differential diagnosis of such carotid bruits includes physiological murmurs associated with thyrotoxicosis and anemia; venous hum; arteriovenous fistulae; angiomatous malformation; Paget's disease; fever; atherosclerosis in the brachiocephalic, subclavian, vertebral, or carotid arteries; loops; kinks; and fibromuscular dysplasia as well as transmitted cardiac murmurs. In patients with proven carotid stenosis, approximately 53 percent have a bruit.[5] Patients with very tight stenosis or occlusion do not have carotid bruits, thus giving rise to false-negative results. In contrast, a moderate to loud bruit may occur in 10 percent of patients without any carotid stenosis, suggesting that the presence or absence of a bruit is a most fallible indicator of underlying carotid artery disease.[6]

PREOPERATIVE SCREENING

Ultrasound can be used to evaluate the state of the carotid arteries in preparation for major vascular reconstructive surgery, such as coronary arterial revascularization. Patients with significant carotid stenosis have been found to be at risk for perioperative stroke associated with intraoperative hypotension. Such patients can be well-evaluated by ultrasound, since the evaluation is highly sensitive for stenosis greater than 50 percent and morbidity is unlikely with lesser degrees of disease.

POSTOPERATIVE FOLLOW-UP AND EPIDEMIOLOGIC STUDIES

Following endarterectomy, ultrasound can be most valuable for long term follow-up, of both the operated side and the contralateral artery. This is a more rational and cost-effective approach than evaluation by repeated angiography.

Ultrasound could also be invaluable to study both the prevalence of the disease and its natural history. Since the results of numerous surgical series attest that carotid endarterectomy in patients with TIAs dramatically lowers the subsequent incidence of stroke, it may be argued that any person with evidence of carotid artery stenosis should undergo surgery. Ultrasound is the obvious modality to define such patients by widespread screening of the elderly population. However, before ultrasound is used routinely for screening, more work is required on the prevalence of the disease in the normal population.

Martin et al. examined the cervical arteries in 100 consecutive autopsies on patients over the age of 50.[7] Arterial disease was present in all carotid vessels. In 80 percent of these patients, the stenosis exceeded 25 percent, 11 patients had occlusion of at least one artery, and 3 had occlusion of three arteries.

Ultrasound examination using both B-scanning and spectral analysis of the pulsed Doppler signal is the one technique which could be utilized to provide valuable information on the natural history of carotid arterial stenosis. Javid et al. demonstrated by repeated arteriography over 1–9 years that, in 62 percent of patients, atherosclerotic lesions in the carotid bifurcation progressed relentlessly with time.[8] Longitudinal ultrasound studies should allow individuals with progressive disease to be detected and treated, thus minimizing the incidence of stroke.

DOPPLER TECHNIQUES

Numerous Doppler techniques have been utilized to diagnose carotid disease noninvasively. Directional Doppler examination of the supraorbital arteries has been widely used as a simple test. In severe stenosis and occlusion of the internal carotid artery, there is reversal of flow in the supraorbital arteries because of the collateral flow in the external carotid. This technique is grossly insensitive to the presence of moderate degrees of stenosis and is only occasionally useful to detect disease in the carotid siphon, which is not amenable to direct ultrasonic visualization.

Modern techniques for ultrasound diagnosis of carotid artery disease involve direct visualization of the common carotid artery and bifurcation by means of a high-resolution real-time scanner, supplemented by spectral analysis of the pulsed Doppler signal.

A 66-year-old patient presented with transient right-sided weakness. Figure C is a sector scan of the right carotid artery which shows severe stenosis at the bifurcation (arrowed). Spectral analysis of a similar patient shows high frequencies as well as turbulent flow manifested by spectral broadening (Fig. D).

On the left, a calcified plaque is seen (arrowed, Fig. E). A shadow (S) is noted. There is only spectral broadening (Fig. F), indicating moderate stenosis. Despite this, the patient's symptoms emanated from this side. The most severe disease may cause loss of any signal due to complete occlusion of the vessel. In this situation, it is most important that the branches of the external carotid, such as the facial artery, are not mistaken for the internal carotid. This should not be a common problem with the experienced observer, since the internal carotid signal is audibly different from that of the external carotid signal. The internal carotid signal has a diastolic component, as opposed to the purely systolic signal of the external carotid.

The clinical results of modern ultrasonic techniques are encouraging. James et al. demonstrated an 85 percent correlation between angiography and ultrasound, having excluded 10 percent of the ultrasound scans which were technically unsatisfactory.[9] They concluded that ultrasound was satisfactory for detecting atheromatous disease causing stenosis but not for ulceration. They comment that the 10 percent error rate, which was considered to be false-positive for ultrasound, probably reflected false negatives for angiography. This important point of the fallibility of angiography has not been addressed sufficiently. In an arteriographic–pathologic correlation, the accuracy of angiography was only approximately 85 percent so that angiography should not be regarded as the ultimate criterion for determining the accuracy of ultrasound examinations.[10] Fell et al. evaluated 750 patients using combined B-mode imaging with spectral analysis and 135 patients underwent correlative cerebral arteriography. Duplex scanning detected the presence of disease in 97 percent of these patients, but was less accurate for lesions producing less than 10 percent stenosis. Since these patients have a very low incidence of subsequent TIA and stroke, this failure to detect minimal stenoses is clinically irrelevant.

In conclusion, stroke is a devastating disease and preventive surgery is now available for a substantial number of patients. Certainly TIA is an indication for vigorous investigation and treatment. However, the present generation of duplex ultrasound scanners offers the possibility of detecting even minor degrees of stenosis in a completely noninvasive manner. A controlled clinical trial is now required to determine the prevalence of the disease in the asymptomatic population to define those who will benefit from carotid endarterectomy.

(Figs. B, D, and F courtesy of Ms. Jane Shedden, Department of Medical Physics, Cardiff, South Wales.)

REFERENCES

1. Whisnant JP, Matsumoto N, Elveback LR: Transient cerebral ischemic attacks in a community, Rochester, Minnesota, 1955–1969. Mayo Clin Proc 48:194–198, 1973
2. Carlidge NEF, Whisnant JP, Elveback LR: Carotid and vertebral-basilar transient ischemic attacks: a community study, Rochester, Minnesota. Mayo Clin Proc 52:117–120, 1977
3. Janet F, McHugh W: Transient ischemic attacks, asymptomatic bruits, and carotid endarterectomy. JAMA 239:2027–2028, 1978
4. Sandok BA, Whisnant JT, Furlan AJ, et al: Carotid artery bruit: prevalence, surgery and differential diagnosis. Mayo Clin Proc 57:227–230, 1982
5. Riles TR, Lieberman A, Kopelman I, et al: Symptoms, stenosis and bruit: interrelationships in carotid artery disease. Arch Surg 116:218–220, 1981
6. Ziegler BK, Zieli T, Dick A, et al: Correlation of bruit over the carotid artery with angiographically demonstrated lesions. Neurology 21:860–865, 1971
7. Martin MJ, Whisnant JP, Sayre GP, Occlusive vascular disease in the extracranial cerebral circulation Arch Neurol 5:530–538, 1960
8. Javid H, Ostermiller WE, Hengesh JW, et al: Natural history of carotid bifurcation atheroma. Surgery 67:80–86, 1970
9. James EM, Ernest F, Forbes GS, et al: High-resolution dynamic ultrasound imaging of the carotid bifurcation: a prospective evaluation. Radiology 144:853–858, 1982
10. Fell G, Phillips DJ, Chikos PM, et al: Ultrasonic duplex scanning for disease of the carotid artery. Circulation 64:1191–1195, 1981

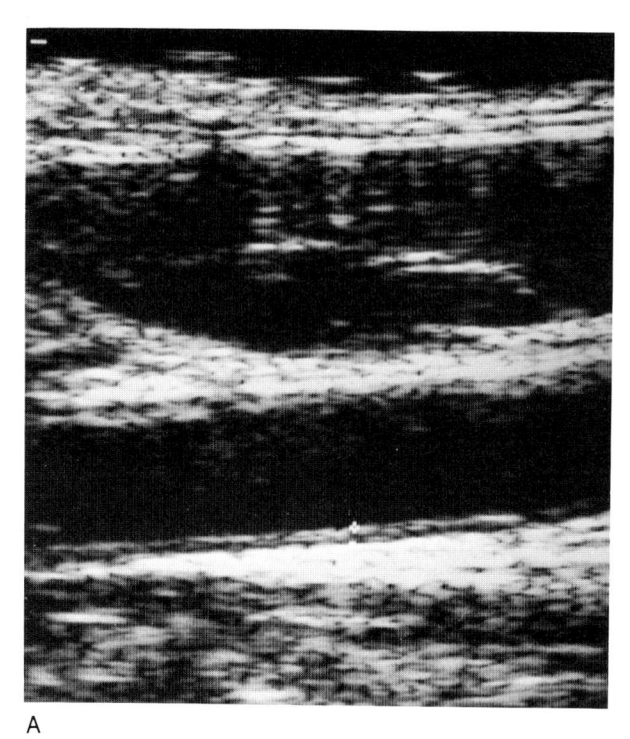

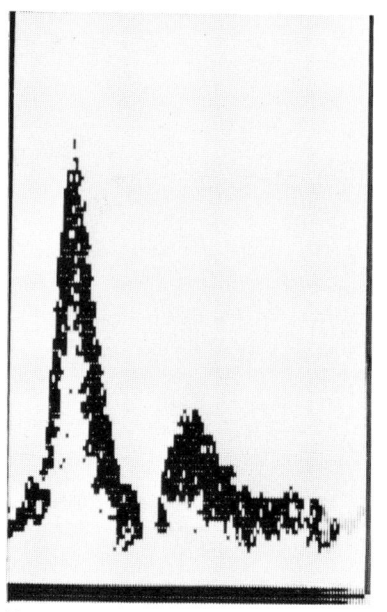

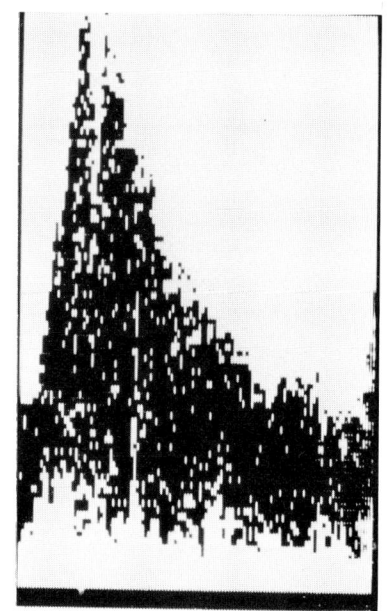

A

B

C

D

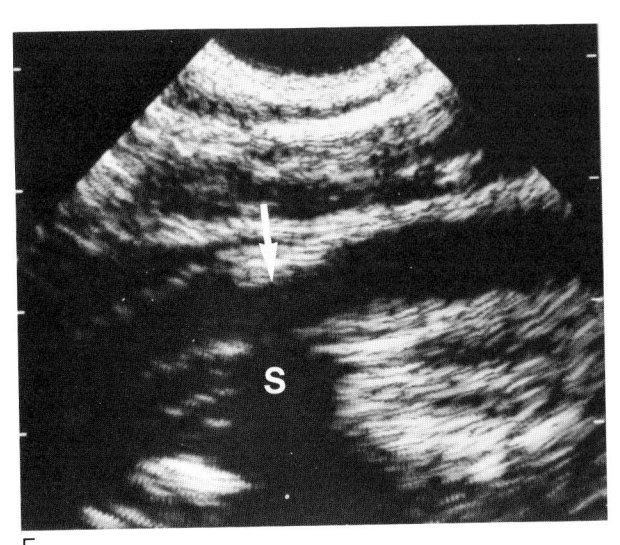

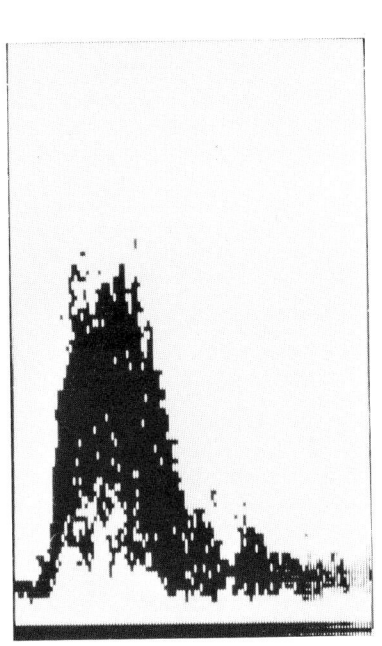

E

S

F

19.14 Normal Carotid Artery

A normal common carotid artery bifurcating into the internal and external carotid arteries is shown in Figure A. There is a slight dilatation, the carotid sinus, at the bifurcation. The presence of the bifurcation causes a predilection for the development of atherosclerosis at this site.

Spectral analysis of the Doppler signal in the common carotid artery (Fig. B) shows the well-defined "window" indicating almost plug flow although with some spectral broadening during the down slope of systole. The peak velocity has been computed to be 107 cm/s after correcting for the angle of attack. The external carotid artery feeds a high impedance vasculature and this is reflected in the waveform (Fig. C). Note that there is little diastolic flow. This should be compared to the waveform in the internal carotid artery (Fig. D). The internal carotid supplies a low impedance circulation so that diastolic flow is present.

The normal range of returned Doppler frequencies is dependent upon many variables including the insonating frequency and the angle between the beam and the vessel. Thus, it is not sufficient to quote 4 kHz as the upper limit of normal as is often done. Some machines now have a cursor which is aligned with the vessel and, with correction for the cosine of the angle, provide estimation of the absolute velocity in the vessel interrogated. However, there is a wide range of velocities in the normal common carotid arteries from 26 to 175 cm per second.[1] Thus, it has been proposed that it is more accurate to use the ratio of the velocities or reflected frequencies between the internal and common carotid artery as a criterion of normal. Normal values include ratios of unity or less, whereas ratios of 1 to 2 indicate up to 50 percent stenosis.[1] Since this is a ratio and is therefore unitless, it may be computed from either the frequency or the velocity providing the angle of incidence is similar. Thus, correction for angle and estimation of absolute velocity is not yet of any proven value.

REFERENCE

1. Blackshear WM, Phillips DJ, Chikos PM, et al: Carotid artery velocity patterns in normal and stenotic vessels. Stroke 11:67–71, 1980

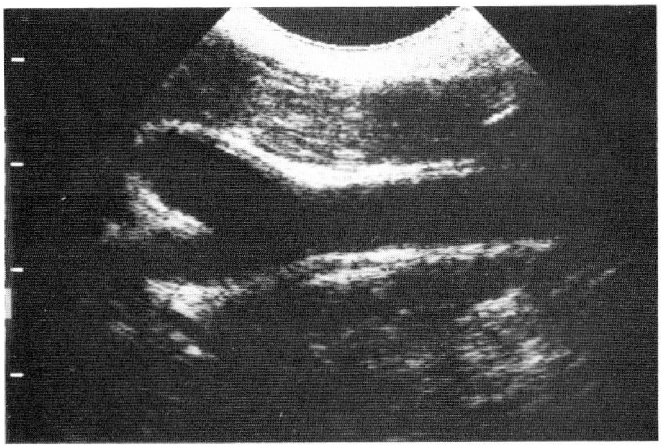

A

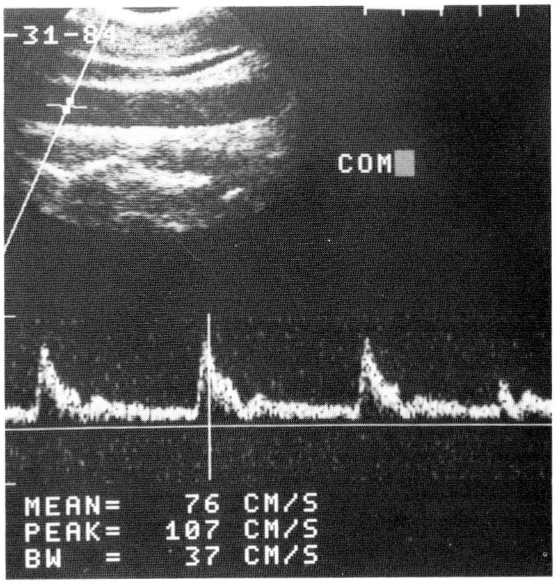
-31-84
COM
MEAN= 76 CM/S
PEAK= 107 CM/S
BW = 37 CM/S

B

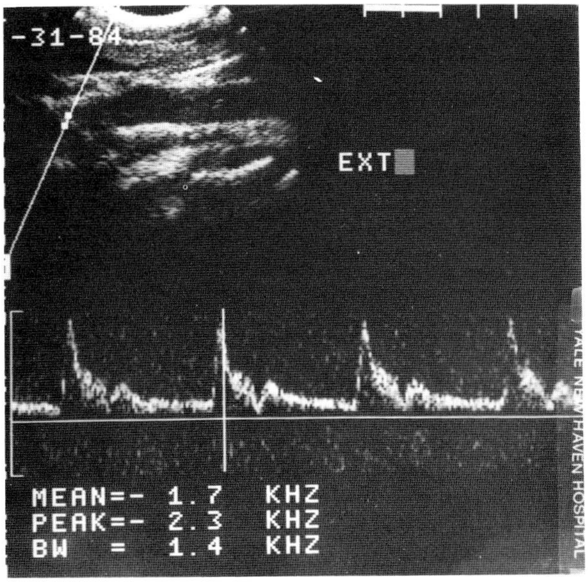
-31-84
EXT
MEAN=- 1.7 KHZ
PEAK=- 2.3 KHZ
BW = 1.4 KHZ

C

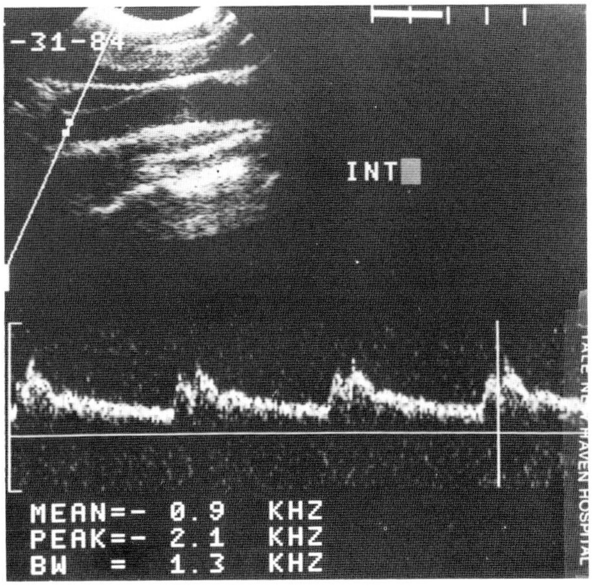
-31-84
INT
MEAN=- 0.9 KHZ
PEAK=- 2.1 KHZ
BW = 1.3 KHZ

D

19.15 Minimal Carotid Disease

A 61-year-old man presented with transient right hemiparesis, which is typical of a left hemispheric transient ischemic attack. Duplex examination showed a calcified plaque in the left common carotid artery with a normal bifurcation and internal carotid (Fig. A). Spectral analysis showed no evidence of abnormally high velocities (Fig. B). This confirmed the absence of significant stenosis. An intra-arterial digital angiogram (Fig. C) was at first reported normal, but on review with the ultrasound scan, the presence of minimal plaque was noted (arrowed).

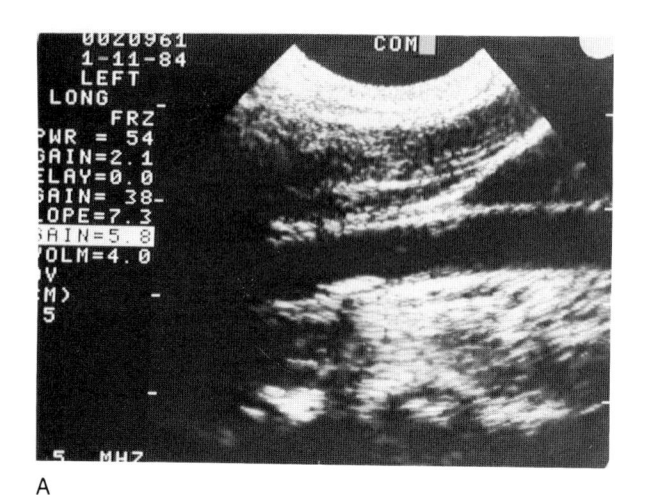

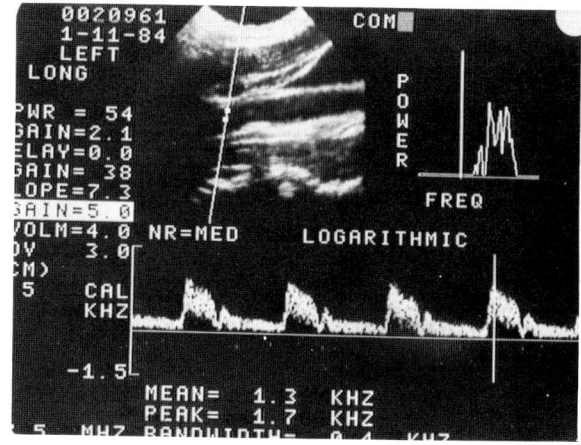

A

B

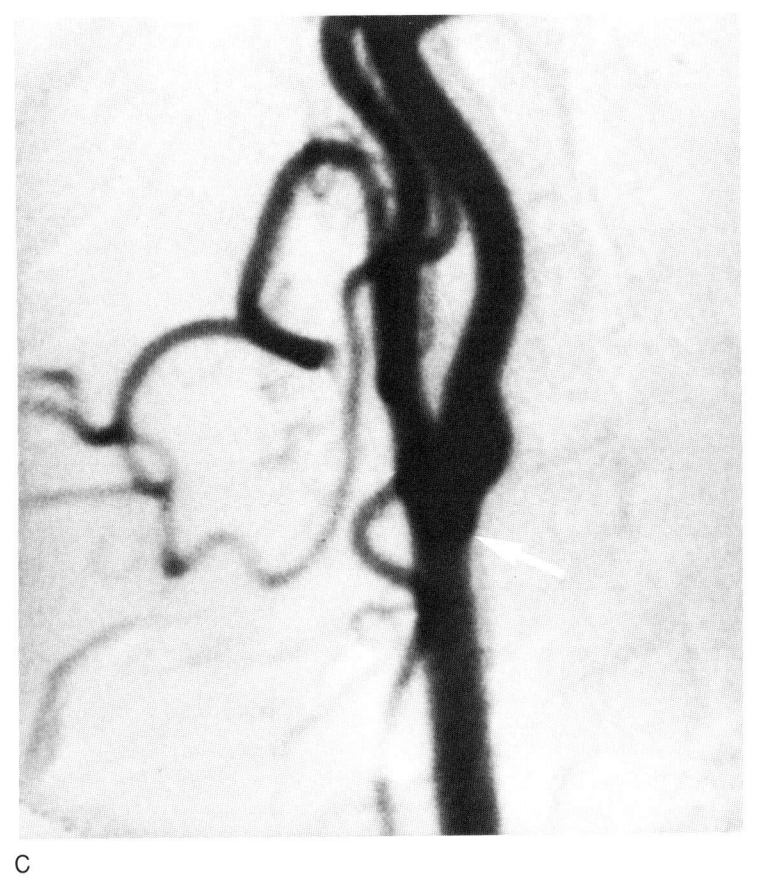

C

19.16 Significant Stenosis

This 55-year-old man was referred for duplex ultrasound examination by his ophthalmologist, who noted a cholesterol embolus on retinoscopy. There was a history of vascular disease, and the patient had undergone a cardiac bypass graft. On the duplex ultrasound scan, the right internal carotid artery (Fig. A) shows significant atheroma with loss of the normal window (spectral broadening) and high frequencies up to 7.5 kHz. On the left, extensive disease is also seen with frequencies up to 5 kHz (Fig. B). An intravenous digital angiogram (Fig. C) shows severe stenosis of the right carotid artery (arrowed), thereby confirming the results of the ultrasound examination. However, overlap on the left prevents adequate diagnosis. This patient proceeded to a intra-arterial digital study, which confirmed the ultrasound findings.

Hoffman et al.[1] reported on the limitations of digital intravenous angiography. They found that the nonsymptomatic side was adequately visualized in only 25 percent of patients in two projections. Without such technical success, significant disease would have been missed in 15 percent of patients. Although some authors remain enthusiastic about the adequacy of digital intravenous techniques to diagnose significant carotid disease,[2] others, including ourselves, have become disillusioned.

James et al.[3] report an 85 percent correlation between angiography and ultrasound, having excluded 10 percent of the ultrasound scans which were technically unsatisfactory. They comment that the 10 percent error rate, which was considered to be a false positive for ultrasound, probably reflects false negative examinations for angiography. The limitation of intravenous angiography remains the large amount of contrast material which must be given to obtain an adequate image. This limits the number of runs which can be performed and this is often inadequate to display both bifurcations in at least two projections. Care is usually taken to ensure that at least the symptomatic side is evaluated in two projections, but this will inevitably lead to missed disease on the nonsymptomatic side.

These reservations do not pertain to the use of intra-arterial digital angiography in which only a small amount of contrast need be used. However, the technique is much more invasive and is not suitable for repeat evaluations which can be performed with ultrasound, for example, in nonsymptomatic patients or in those with nonsignificant disease.

REFERENCES

1. Hoffman MG, Gomes AS, Pais SO: Limitations in the interpretation of intravenous carotid digital subtraction angiography. AJR 142:261–264, 1984
2. Foley WD, Smith DF, Milde MW, et al: Intravenous DSA examination of patients with suspected cerebral ischemia. Radiol 151:651–659, 1984
3. James EM, Ernest F, Forbes GS, et al: High-resolution dynamic ultrasound imaging of the carotid bifurcation: a prospective evaluation. Radiol 144:853–858, 1982

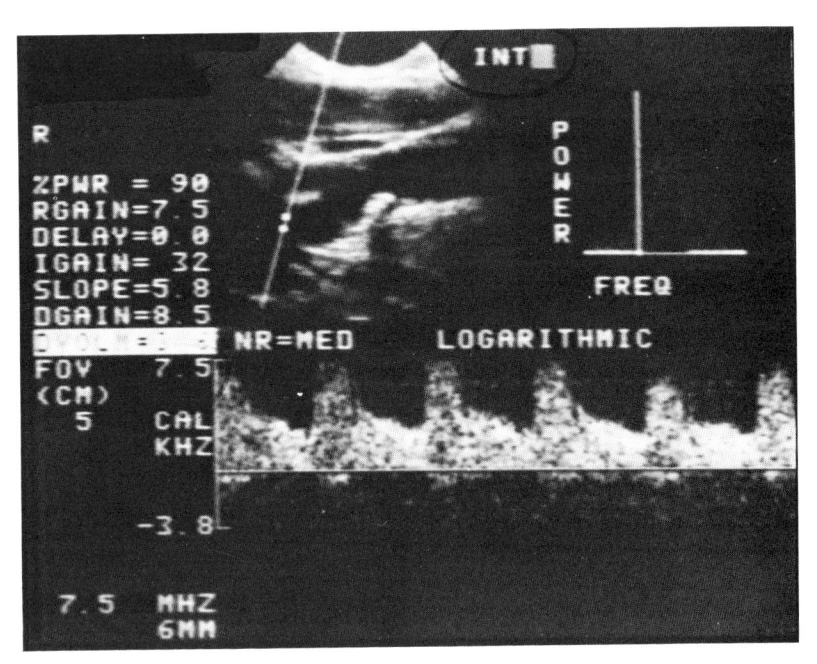

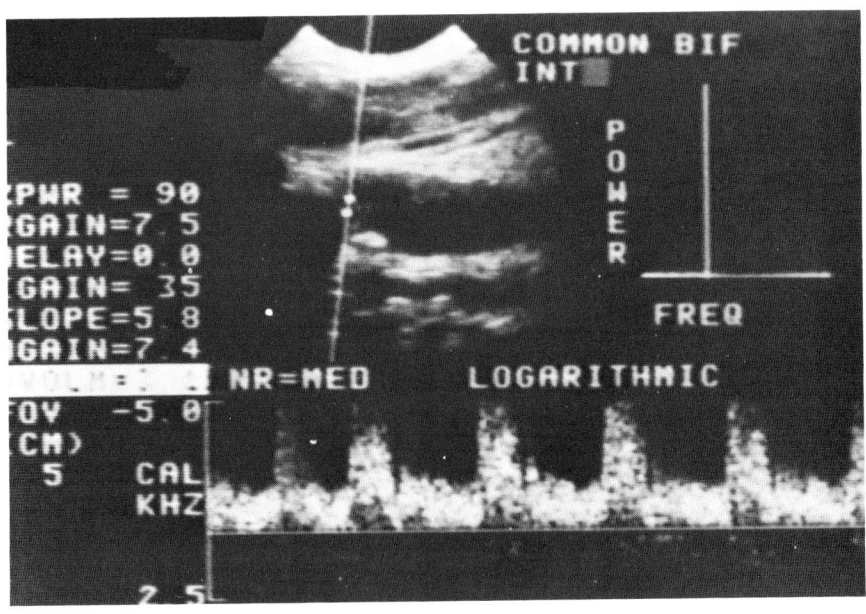

A

B

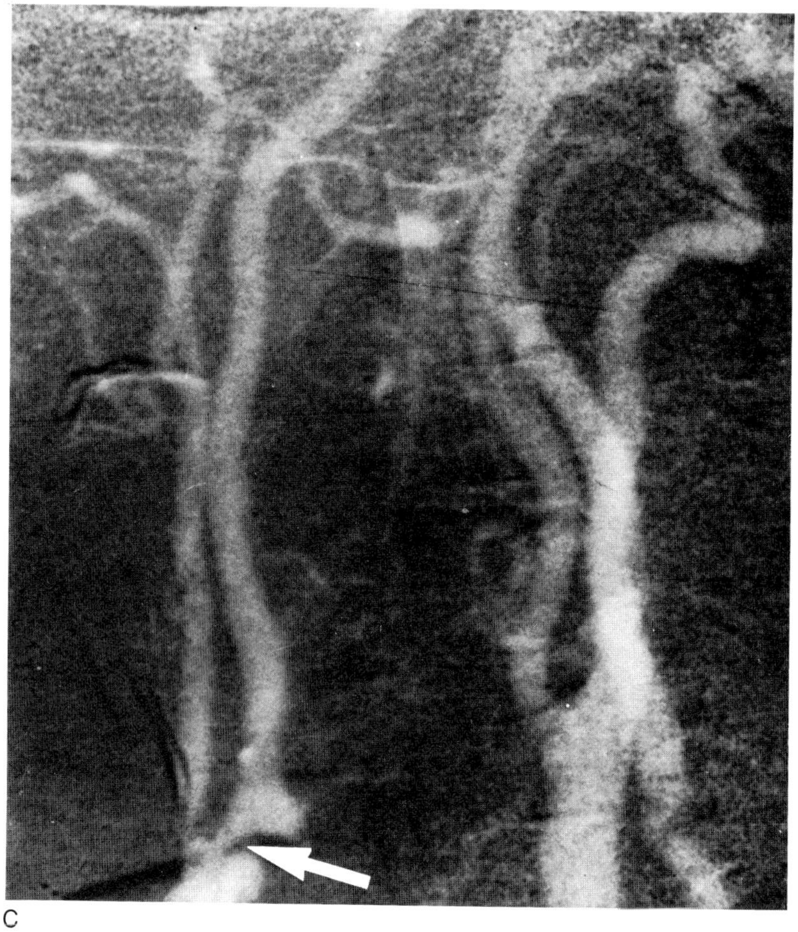

C

19.17 Carotid Artery Occlusion

A 55-year-old man presented with a history of transient right hemiparesis and amaurosis fugax suggesting a left hemispheric ischemic event. A duplex carotid artery examination demonstrated only a very low Doppler shift in the left common carotid artery (Fig. A), probably due to wall movement, and no detectable movement in the internal carotid. The left supra-orbital artery demonstrated reversed flow (Fig. B). Compression of the facial artery caused cessation of flow (Fig. C). These appearances indicated occlusion in the left carotid artery. This was confirmed by an intra-arterial angiogram which showed complete occlusion at the origin of the common carotid artery (Fig. D) with filling of the left anterior and middle cerebral vessels from the right (Fig. E).

This case illustrates a number of useful points. First, many patients with severe disease have minimal symptoms due to good collateral circulation through the circle of Willis from both the contralateral carotid and/or the vertebral arteries. The direction of flow in the ophthalmic artery and its branches is a very insensitive criterion of carotid artery disease. However, when flow is reversed, severe disease is present. Most authors have found that ultrasound is least successful at detecting complete occlusion often due to confusion with other branches of the carotid artery. However, the recognition of reversed flow in the ophthalmic arteries encourages careful re-evaluation to exclude an occlusion.

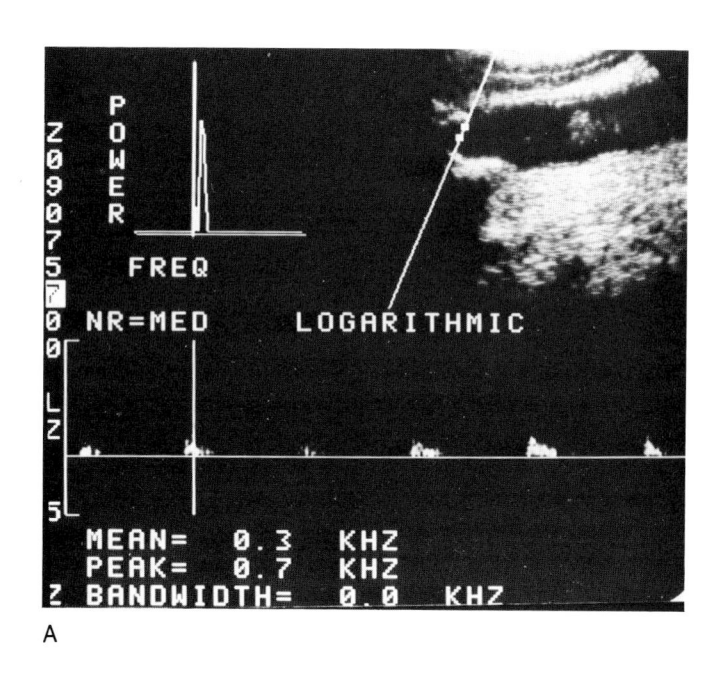

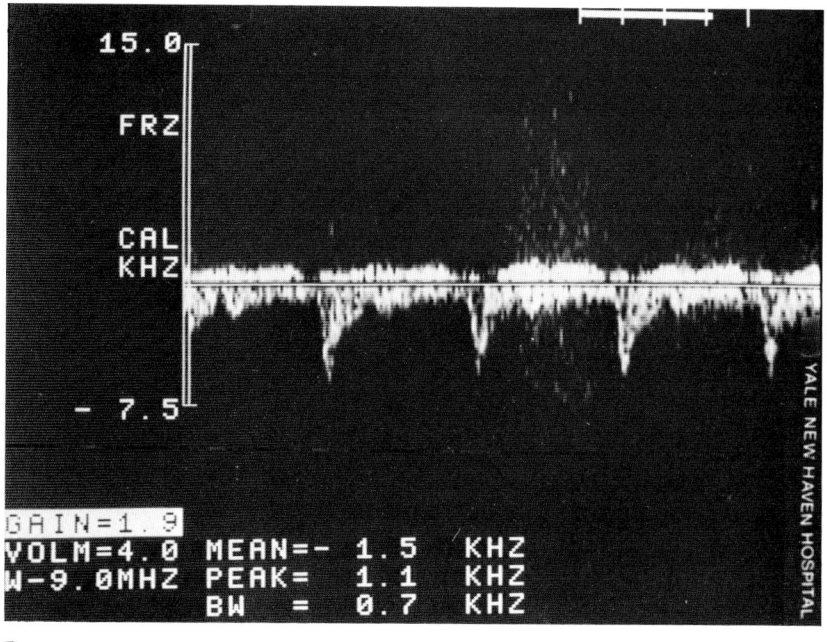

A

B

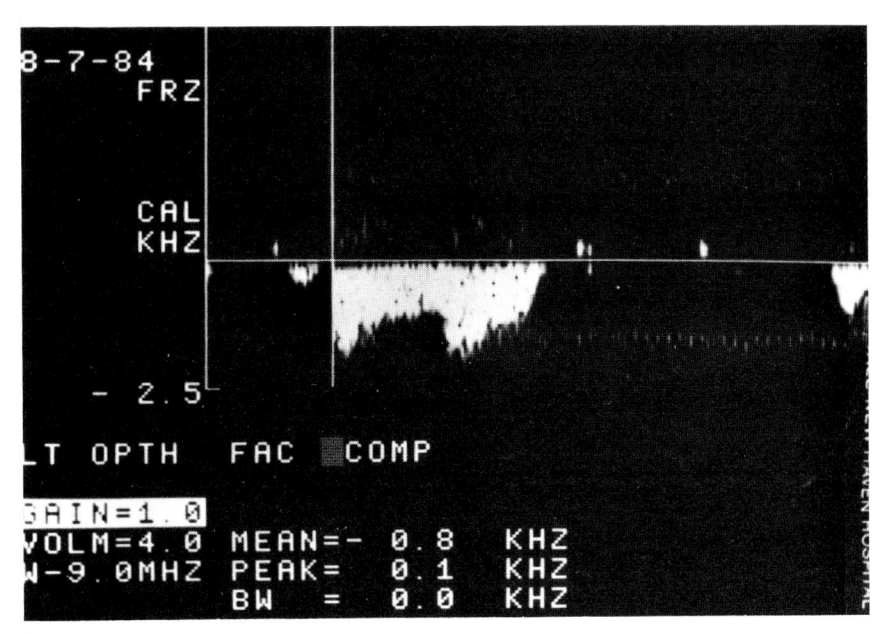

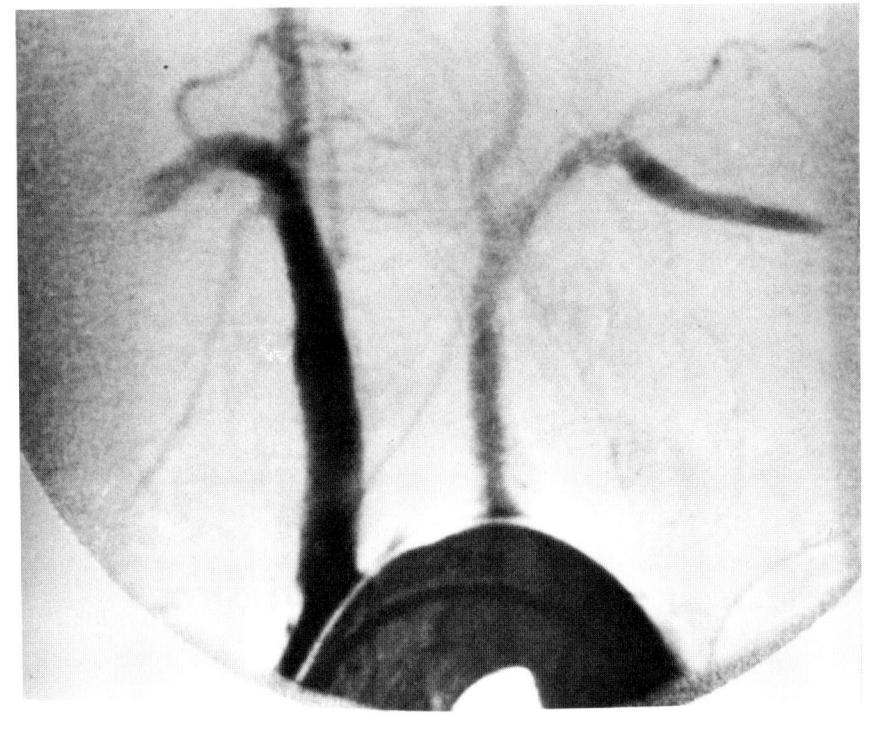

C

D

1123

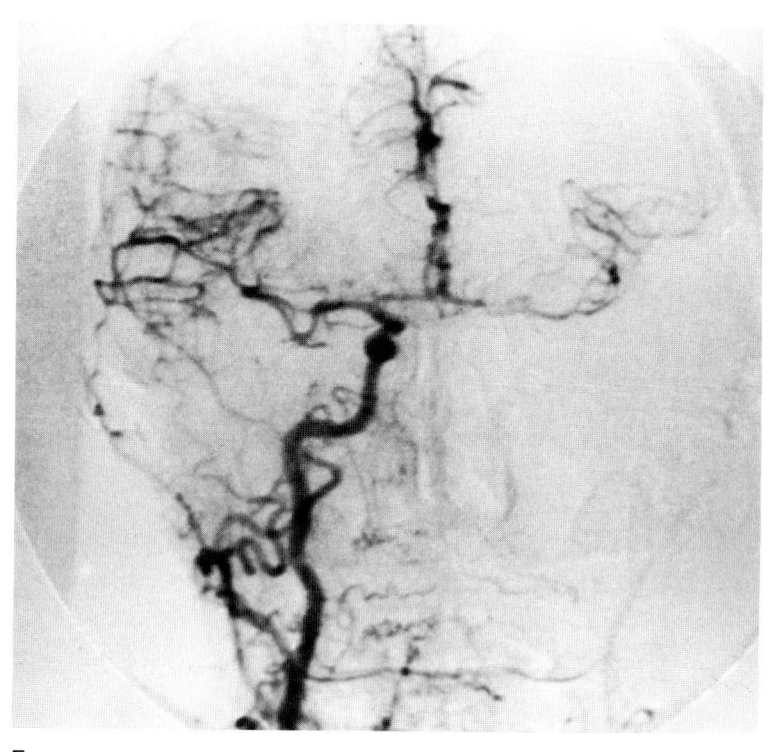

E

20 The Thorax

KENNETH J.W. TAYLOR

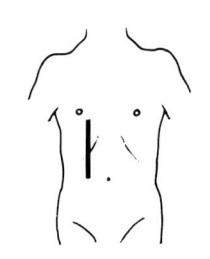

20.1 Pleural Effusion

The chest radiograph shows a patient with both consolidation and a pleural effusion at the right base (Fig. A). The opacity in the left upper lobe was considered to be a bronchogenic carcinoma.

Parasagittal sonograms taken in expiration (Fig. B) and inspiration (Fig. C) show sections through normal liver, diaphragm, pleural effusion, and lung. The base of the lung must be consolidated, since aerated lung does not transmit ultrasound at this frequency. Comparison of the two scans shows that the diaphragm has descended and there has been widening of the costophrenic angle with inspiration. Thus the excursion of the diaphragm can be confirmed and measured. The normal appearance of the liver excludes a subphrenic collection and the absence of echoes from the pleural cavity confirms the presence of an effusion.

A transverse scan (Fig. D) shows a pleural effusion (E) posterior to the liver. The diaphragm is arrowed. This effusion in the posterior costophrenic angle must not be misinterpreted as ascites. Since the liver is in direct contact with the diaphragm at the bare area, no fluid can accumulate between the liver and the diaphragm in this position.

(Scans B and C from Taylor KJW: Use of ultrasound in opaque hemithorax. Br J Radiol 47:199–200, 1974.)

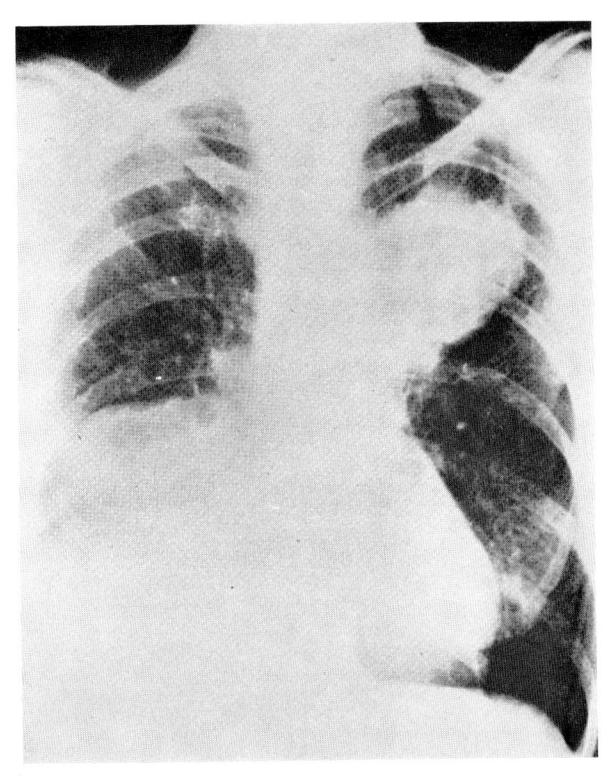

A

1126

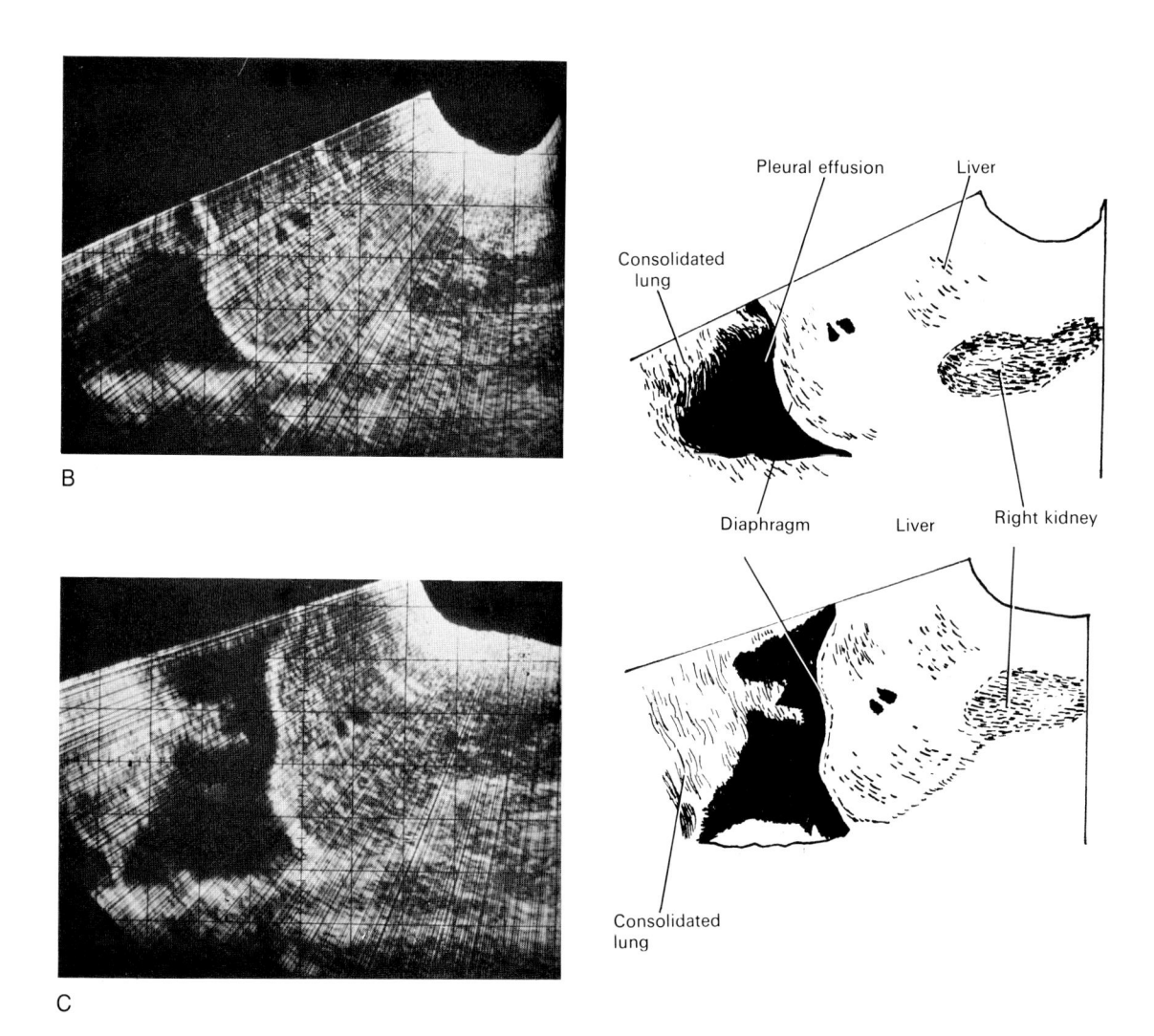

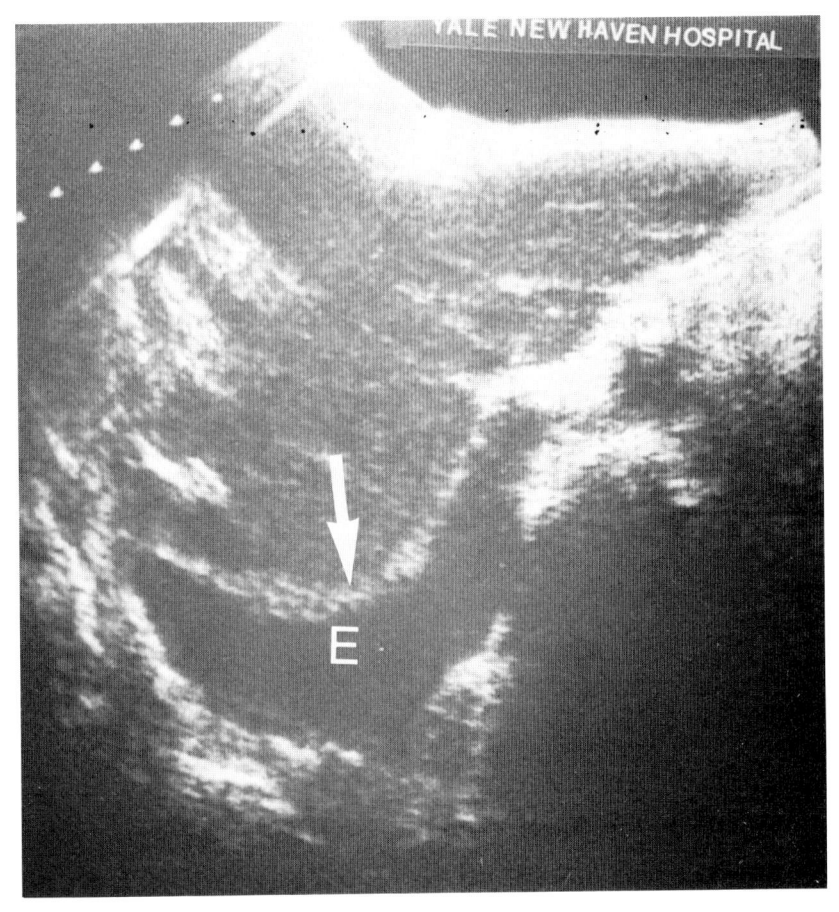

D

20.2 Pleural Empyema

A 4-year-old girl had staphylococcal pneumonia which resulted in a persistent fever, leukocytosis to 23,000/mm^3, and persistent right lung field opacity. No fluid was apparent on decubitus films. She was referred for ultrasound examination to investigate further the cause of her pleural opacity and to exclude an empyema. The child was very active during this procedure. A longitudinal sonogram (Fig. A) through the liver reveals the right hemidiaphragm, which moved with respiration, and definite fluid in the costophrenic angle above the diaphragm below consolidated right lung. Further scanning on the anterior and posterior aspects of the thorax (Fig. B) shows the right kidney with homogeneous material above the kidney in the right hemithorax, but definite echoes are seen in this fluid, indicating cellular debris. Such findings are consistent with an empyema. Aspiration under ultrasound visualization yielded 1 pint of pus.

Laing and Filly[1] reported the absence of any relation between echogenicity of pleural fluid and the success with which it could be aspirated. In 42 patients with echo-free collections, they could obtain fluid in only 74 percent whereas in 17 patients with echogenic collections, aspiration was successful in every one. Clotted blood is probably the most common cause of failure to aspirate an echo-free collection; success in aspirating pleural collections will depend upon the patient population. Failure is more likely in traumatized patients. In our general medical population, it is very rare for us not to obtain fluid for diagnostic purposes.

Real-time examination allows a better assessment of the fluidity of the pleural contents which can be demonstrated by moving the patient. Marks et al.[2] reported a change in the shape of the pleural contents with respiratory motions and observed the motion of septa within the pleural contents.

Hirsch et al.[3] noted that complex septate pleural collections contained an exudative effusion in only 4 percent of their 50 patients while anechoic collections were equally likely to be due to either an exudate or a transudate. They also advocated the use of real-time instrumentation both for speed and ease of use at the bedside of critically ill patients.

REFERENCES

1. Lang FC, Filly RA; Problems in the application of ultrasonography for the evaluation of pleural opacities. Radiology 126:211–214, 1978
2. Marks WN, Filly RA, Callen PW; Real-time evaluation of pleural lesions: new observations regarding the probability of obtaining fluid. Radiology 142:163–164, 1982
3. Hirsch JH, Rogers JV, Mack LA; Real-time sonography of pleural opacities. AJR 136:297–301, 1981

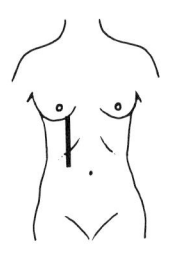

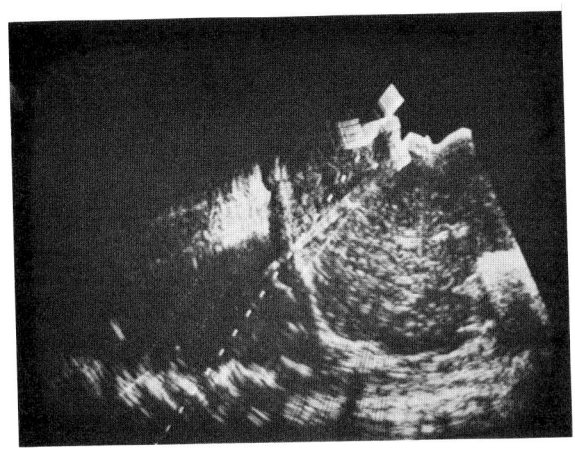

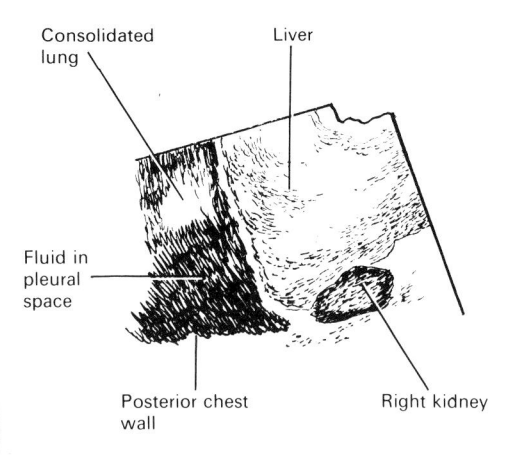

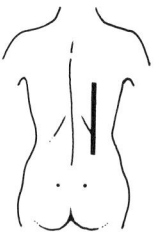

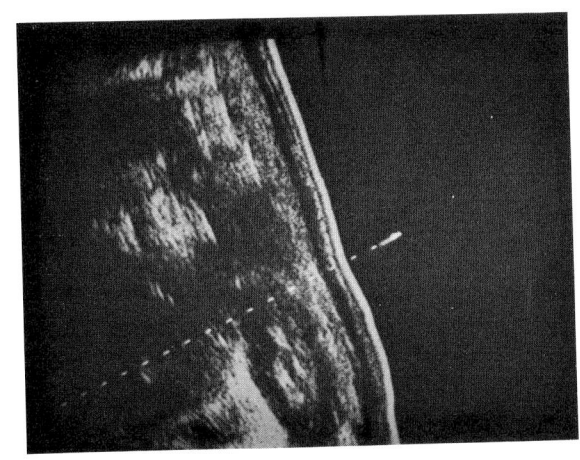

A

Consolidated lung	Liver
Fluid in pleural space	
Posterior chest wall	Right kidney

B

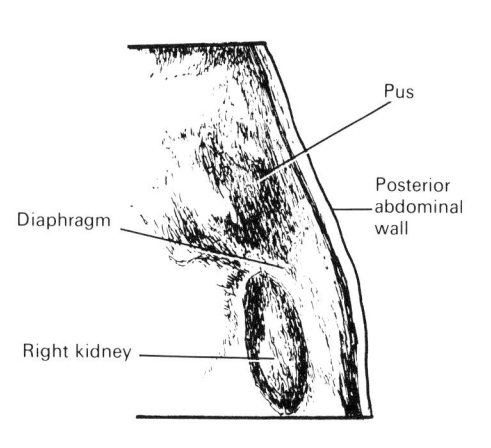

	Pus
Diaphragm	Posterior abdominal wall
Right kidney	

1129

20.3 Pericardial Cyst

A 55-year-old man presented with cough, intermittent low-grade fever, and weight loss. Despite antibiotic therapy, persistent opacities were noted on the posteroanterior (PA) (Fig. A) and lateral (Fig. B) chest radiographs and a tumor was suspected clinically. Radiologically, some features suggested that presence of a pericardial cyst; but, because of the lesion's irregularity on the lateral tomogram, the possibility of tumor was raised. The patient was referred for ultrasound examination.

A transverse sonogram of the thorax (Fig. C) shows an echo-free area (arrowed) immediately to the right of the heart. An A-scan (Fig. D) through this area confirms that this is a cystic lesion. Results of all tests, including bronchoscopy and cytology, were negative for tumor; the patient improved clinically and the infiltrates disappeared. An old chest film was finally traced showing the previous cardiophrenic lesion unchanged, thus confirming its benign nature and the fact that it most likely represented a pericardial cyst. (Case and figures courtesy of Dr. Bruce Simonds.)

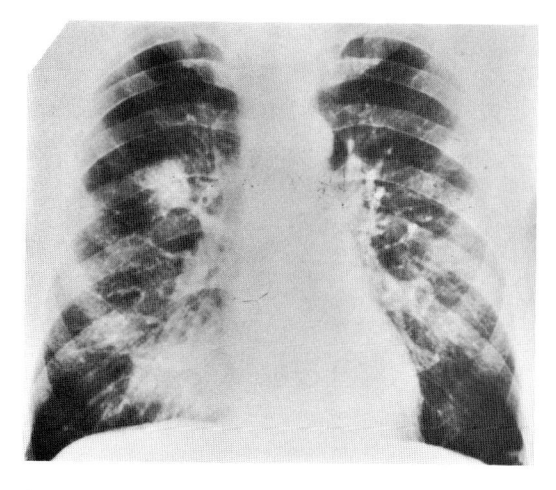

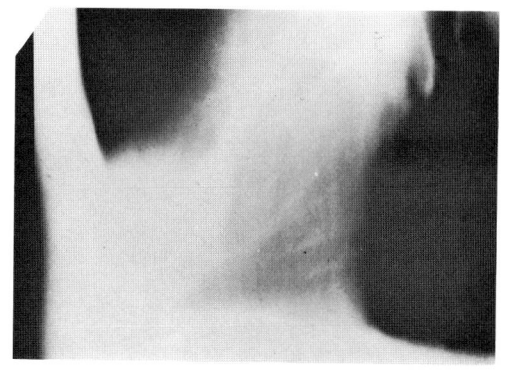

A

B

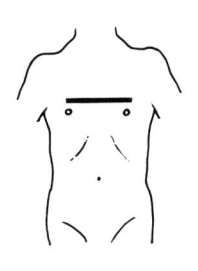

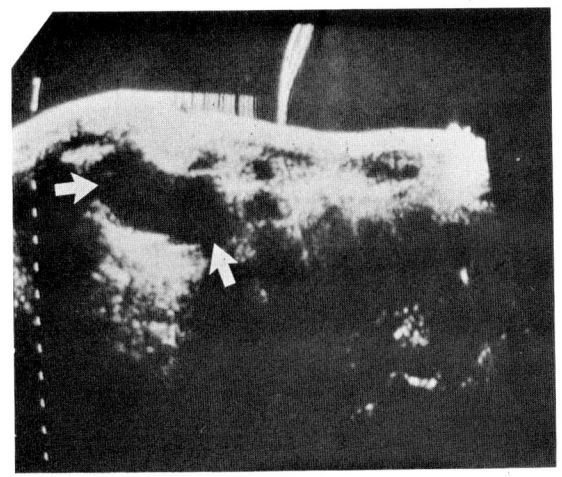

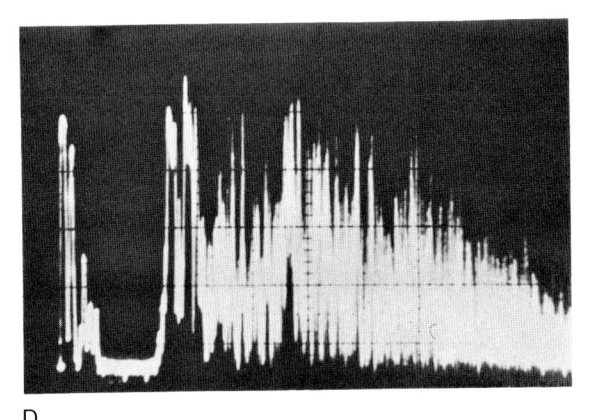

C

D

20.4 Fibrous Mesothelioma

A 45-year-old woman was admitted for diagnostic curettage for postmenopausal bleeding. A preoperative chest radiograph (Fig. A) revealed a huge opacity filling the left side of the chest and displacing the heart toward the right. She was referred for ultrasound evaluation of the heart.

A longitudinal sonogram 7 cm to the right of the midline (Fig. B) showed the right lobe of the liver, the gallbladder, and the right kidney, with the heart immediately above the right hemidiaphragm. This confirmed the massive displacement of the heart.

A transverse sonogram of the left thorax (Fig. C) showed a solid, well-circumscribed mass 14 cm in diameter, returning irregular internal echoes. This was confirmed at thoracotomy and histologic study proved it to be a fibrous mesothelioma.

Mesothelioma is the only primary malignant tumor arising in the pleura and behaves as an invasive sarcoma. This tumor can extend rapidly throughout the pleural space, filling it with gray, fleshy tumor with areas of necrosis. These tumors appear to be associated with asbestosis, raising the possibility of a causal relation. These case histories demonstrate how ultrasound may be used to differentiate between solid and cystic masses within the thorax and, in particular, between pericardial cysts and solid masses arising in the thorax.

(Case and figures courtesy of Mrs. Patricia Donnelly and Dr. Murray Rosenberg, Park City Hospital, Bridgeport, Connecticut.)

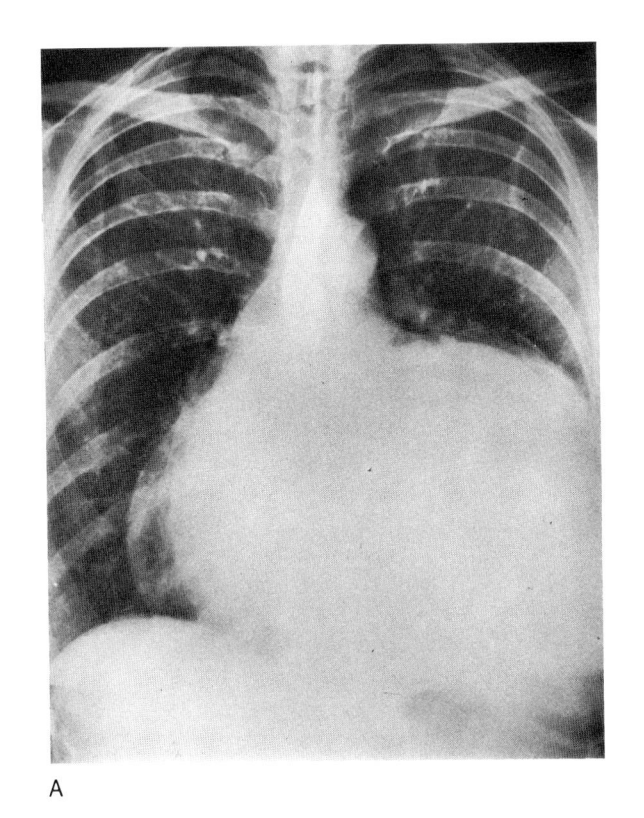

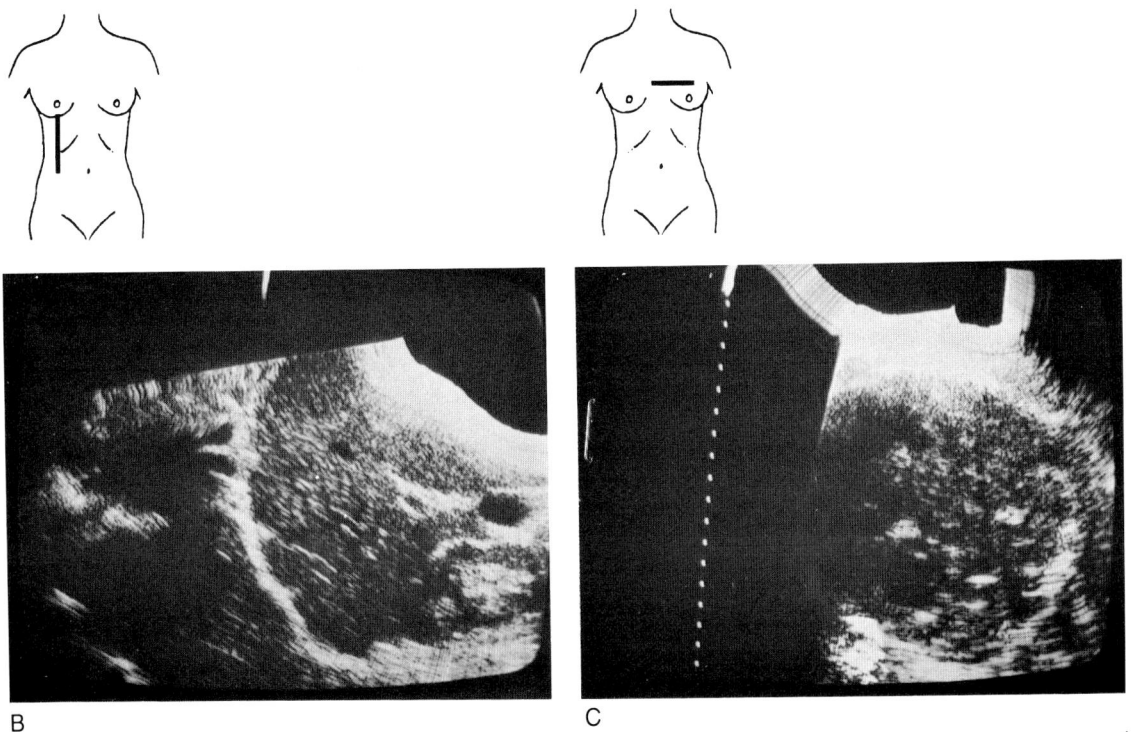

A

20.5 Spindle Cell Sarcoma

A 31-year-old white man presented for evaluation after having undergone multiple previous diagnostic procedures for a known right thoracic mass present since 1976. Previous pathology was reported as fibrous mesothelioma.

PA (Fig. A) and lateral chest radiographs (Fig. B) taken on admission showed a huge right thoracic mass. A CT scan demonstrated a 16 × 10 cm mass above the right diaphragm extending to the left (Fig. C).

A parasagittal sonogram showed a homogeneous mass above the right lobe of the liver, depressing the diaphragm inferiorly (arrowed, Fig. D). A transverse sonogram again showed the mass displacing the diaphragm anteriorly (arrowed, Fig. E). The tumor was resected and proved to be a spindle cell sarcoma.

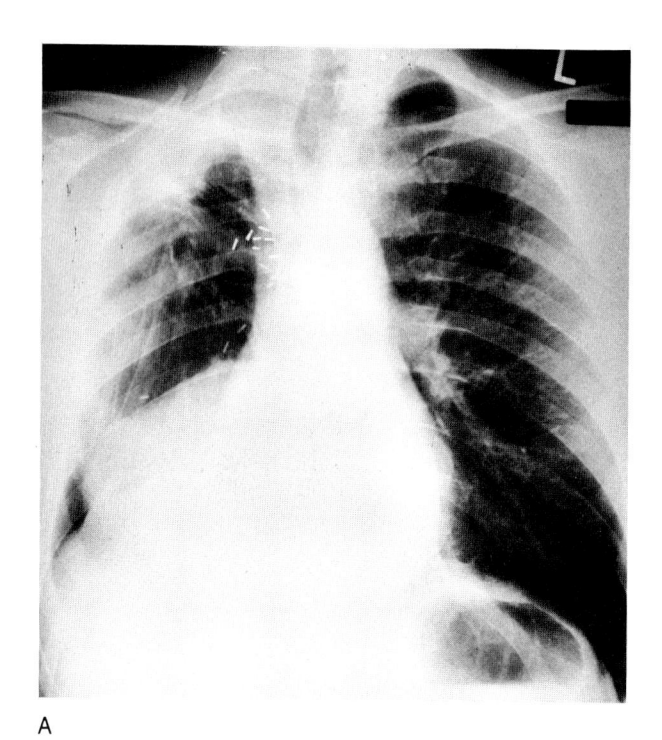

A

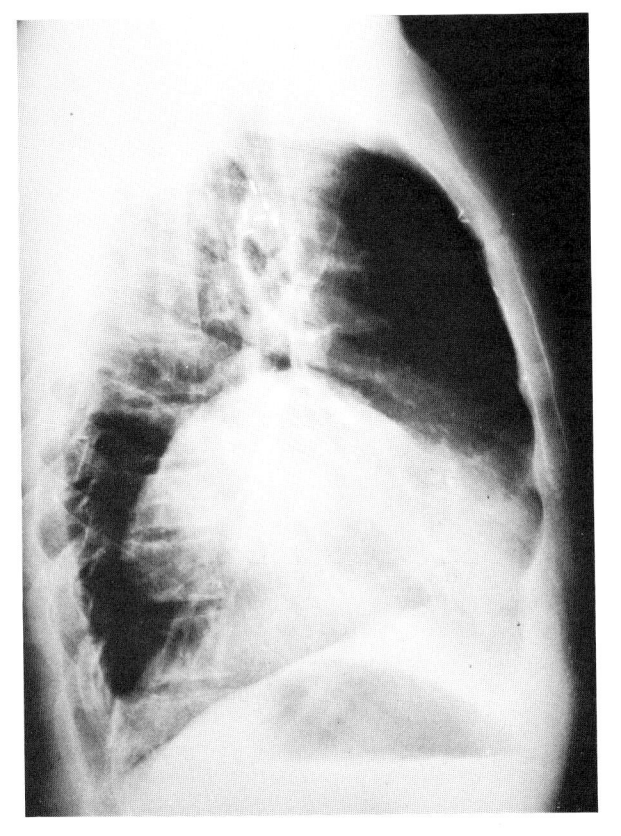

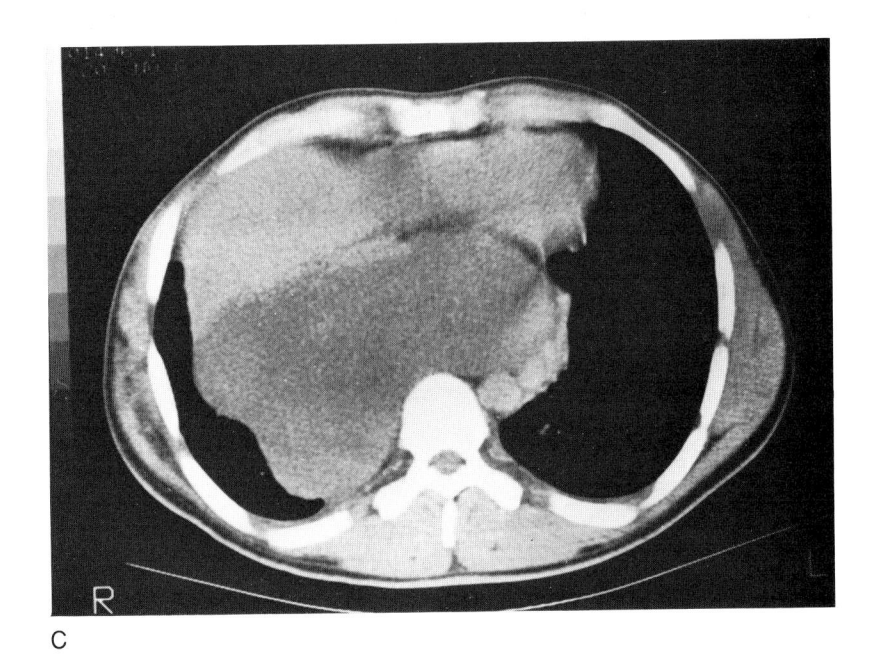

B

C

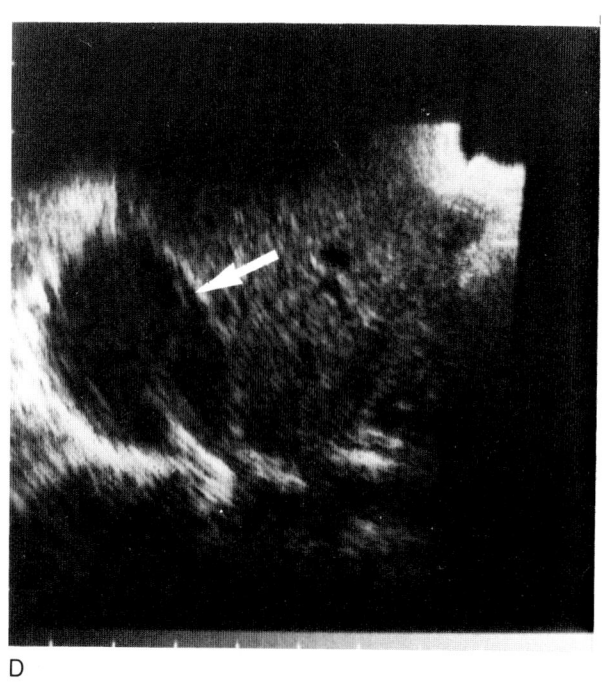

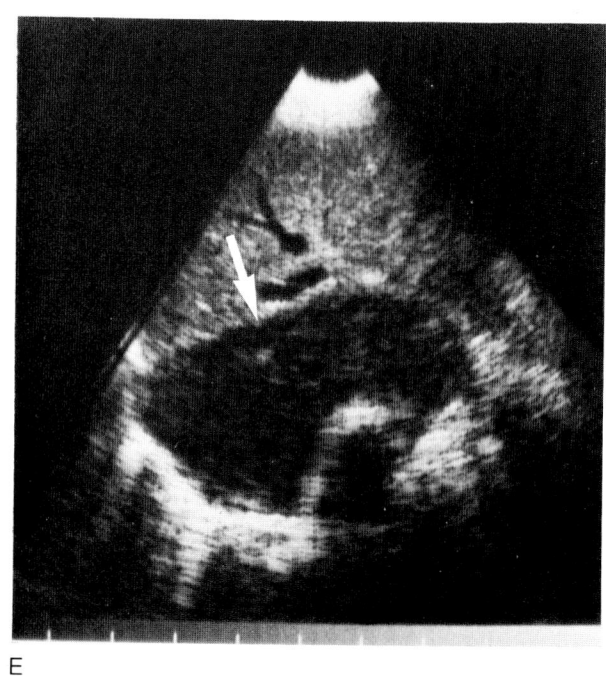

D

E

20.6 Traumatic Rupture of the Diaphragm

A 32-year-old man sustained a stab wound to the left chest 10 months before admission but had been asymptomatic in the interim. He presented with an 8-hour history of increasing epigastric pain associated with vomiting. Examination disclosed a respiratory rate of 48/minute with absent breath sounds over the left chest.

A chest radiograph showed opacification of the left hemithorax with shift of the mediastinum to the right and a healed fracture of the left sixth rib (Fig. A). Air collections in the left chest suggested the presence of bowel. A sonogram in the upright position localized the left hemidiaphragm (arrowed, Fig. B) and showed multiple loops of small bowel (B) above it. Active peristalsis of the herniated bowel could be seen and the valvulae conniventes were clearly seen. The spleen (S) is seen below the diaphragm.

At surgery, 1.5 m of distal jejunum and proximal ileum was reduced into the abdomen. An anterior tear in the left diaphragm (arrowed, Fig. C) was repaired and the patient had an uneventful recovery.

A ruptured diaphragm may remain asymptomatic for a long time after trauma. Sudden herniation of the gut into the chest produces progressive hypotension, cyanosis, and dyspnea, which may be fatal.

Lucido and Wall[1] reviewed 47 patients with rupture of the diaphragm secondary to blunt trauma. The left leaf was ruptured in 43 of these, the right in only 3, and both leaves in 1. Delayed presentation of traumatic diaphragmatic hernias was described in 25 patients by Hegarty et al.[2] Twenty-two of these were due to stab wounds and all but one involved the left leaf of the diaphragm. In this series, four patients had gangrene of their hernias and four patients died. This case demonstrates how the diagnosis can be made easily and expeditiously by real-time ultrasound scanning.

(This case and figures taken from Ammann AM, Brewer WH, Maull KI, Walsh JW: Traumatic rupture of the diaphragm: real-time sonographic diagnosis. AJR 140:915–916, 1983. © 1983 Am Roentgen Ray Soc.)

REFERENCES

1. Lucido JI, Wall CA: Rupture of the diaphragm due to blunt trauma. Arch Surg 86: 131–141, 1963.
2. Hegarty MM, Bryer JV, Angorn IB, Baker LW: Delayed presentation of traumatic diaphragmatic hernia. Ann Surg 188:229–233, 1978

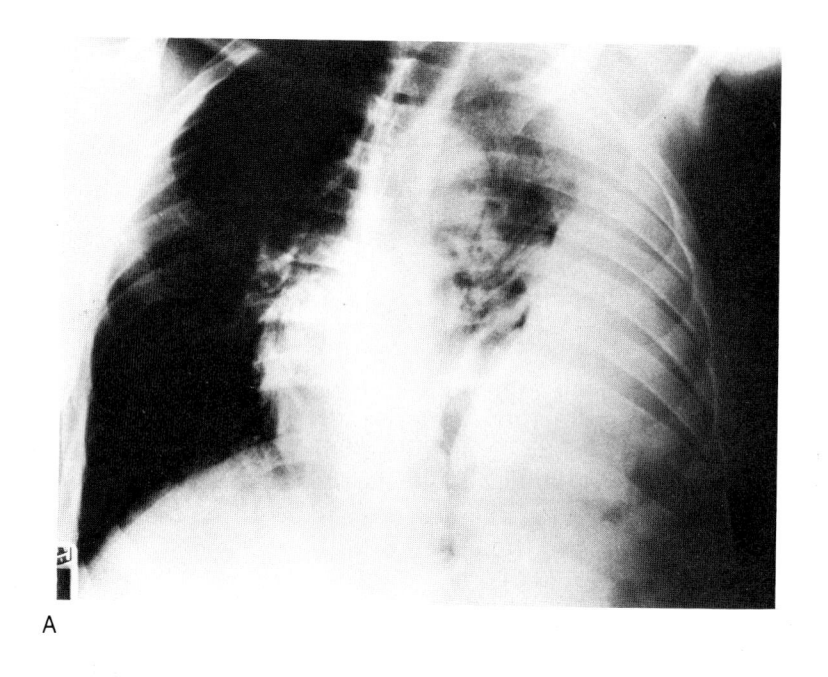

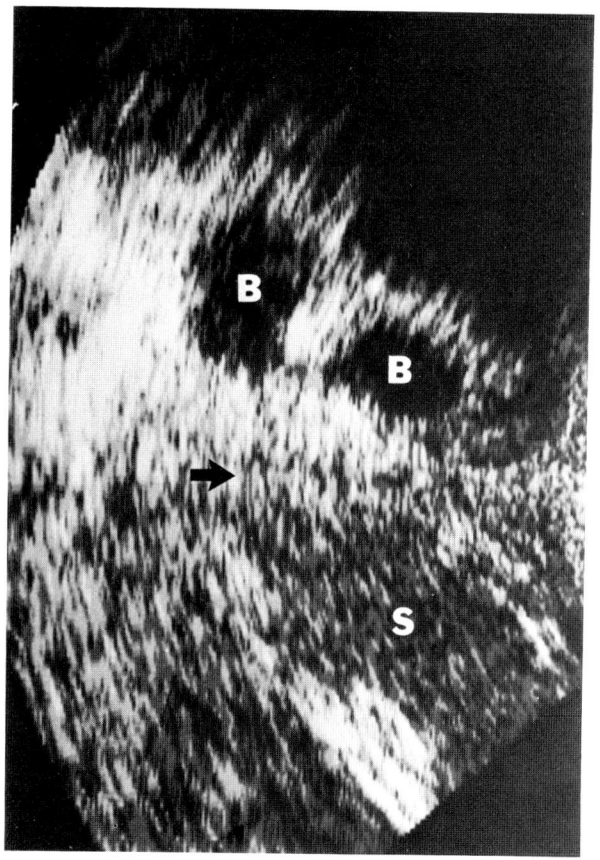

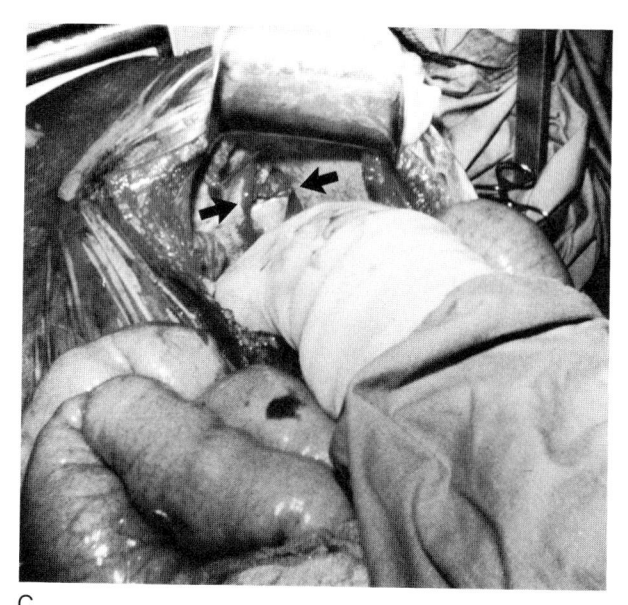

A

B

C

Index

A-scan, amplitude-modulated, 3
Abdomen, fetal, 210–211
Abdominal circumference, for pregnancy dating, 234, 239
Abdominal pregnancy, 319
Abdominal vessels, 1082
Abdominopelvic mass, retroperitoneal, 1006
Abortion
  failed, 157
  inevitable, 156
  missed, 154
Abruptio placenta, 308
Acoustic impedance, 3
Acoustic parameters of biologic media, 7
Acoustic shadow, clean vs dirty, 24–25
Adenoma
  follicular, of thyroid, 1056
  of liver, 482
  parathyroid, 1070, 1076
Adenomatoid tumor, of fetal lung, 268
Adenomyosis, 132
  endometriosis and, 142
Adenopathy, hydronephrosis secondary to, 781
Adrenal gland, 931–943
  hemorrhage of, 934–936
    bilateral, 934
    infected neonatal, 936
  metastases of, 943
  myelolipoma of, 938
  neuroblastoma of, 942
  normal anatomy of, 932
  pheochromocytoma of, 940
Amebic abscess, of liver, 467

Amenorrhea, secondary, in ovarian tumor, 128
Amniocentesis, 186
Anemia, hemolytic, gallstones and, 557
Anencephaly, fetal, 260
Aneurysm
  aortic, 1093
  popliteal artery, 1107
Angiomyolipoma, renal, 869
Aorta
  aneurysm of, 1093
  branches of, 1088
  graft of, 1095
  paraaortic lymphadenopathy of, 993
  transverse, 1086
Appendicitis, subphrenic and pelvic abscess following, 1049
Appendix
  mucocele of, bowel mass, 1038
  ruptured, abscess due to, 1040
Aqueductal stenosis, fetal, 259
Arachnoid cyst, fetal, 266
Arnold-Chiari malformation, neonatal, 425
Artifact, 23–35
  beam width, 28–31
  comet tail, 24, 25
  echogenic focal zone, 29–30
  liver mass, 503–505
  machine-specific, 32–33
  nonshadowing gallstones as, 28–29
  off-axis reflector, 30–31
  partial volume effect as, 29, 30
  phrenic nerve stimulator, 34
  reflection-mirror image, 25–26
  reflection-refraction beam splitting, 27–28

  reflection-reverberation, 23–25
  refraction, 26–27
  resolution, 30
  reverberation, 95
  reverse shadowing, 33, 34
  slice thickness, 31
  sound speed error in, 31–32
  specific location, 33–34
  tissue texture, 32
Ascaris worms, in extrahepatic duct, 607
Axial resolution, 4

B-scan, 3–4
Backscattered echo, 7–9
Beam width artifact, 28–31
Biliary gravel and sludge, 574
Biliary tract. *See also* Extrahepatic ducts.
  anicteric dilatation of, 612
  Caroli's disease of, 616
  choledochal cyst of, 618
  congenital atresia of, 621
  dilatation of, 595
  disparate dilatation of, 602–603
  imaging techniques for, 591–592
  pneumobilia of, 614
Biloma, of liver, 456
Biparietal diameter, 233, 235
Bladder, 888–903. *See also* Urinary bladder.
  ovarian cyst simulating, 92
  rectal, 1047
  replication of, 55
Bowel, 1023–1049. *See also individual parts.*
Bowel contents, ovarian dermoid simulating, 110

Vol. 1: pp. 1–540; Vol. 2: pp. 541–1137

1

Bowel mass, simulating ovarian cyst, 97
Bowel mass mucocele of appendix, 1038
Brain tumor, neonatal, 418
Breast, 329–371
  abscess of, 355
  anatomy of, 333
  cancer of, 329–330
  carcinoma of, 358–362
    impalpable, Doppler ultrasound in, 371
  Doppler ultrasound for, 368–371
  fibroadenoma of, 354
  fibrocystic disease of, 337–352
    aspiration in, 346
    calcified cysts in, 348
    costal cartilage simulating cyst in, 352
    equivocal mammogram in, 349
    equivocal ultrasonogram in, 351
    high-risk patient in, 344
    multiple palpable masses in dense breasts in, 342
    nonpalpable mass in, 340
    spectrum of disease in, 337
  hypertrophy of, 335
  inspissated cyst mimicking carcinoma of, 357
  lactating, 334
  lipoma of, 356
  lymphoma of, 366
  recent growth of mass in, 364
  solid masses of, 353–366. *See also individual masses.*
  vascularity of, 368–369
Bulk modulus of biologic media, 8
Burkitt's lymphoma, of liver, 507

Calculi, urinary, 895
Cancer, of breast, 329–330
Carcinoma
  of breast, 358–362
    Doppler ultrasound in, 371
  of colon, 1045
  endometrial, 152
  of gallbladder, 582–584
  of pancreas, 668–682
  papillary, of thyroid, 1065–1067
  prostatic, 924
  renal cell, 852–860
Caroli's disease, 616
Carotid artery
  Doppler techniques for, 1110–1111
  indications for ultrasound scanning of, 1109
  minimal carotid disease, 1116
  neck bruit at, 1109
  normal, 1114
  normal anatomy of, 1108
  occlusion of, 1121
  postoperative follow-up and epidemiologic studies of, 1109–1110
  preoperative screening of, 1109
  stenosis of, 1108–1109, 1118
Cavernous hemangioma, of liver, 477
Cavum vergae, 381
Cerebral artery infarct, neonatal, 393
Cerebritis, neonatal, 400
Cervical fibroid, 150
Cholecystitis
  acute, 549
  chronic, 559–562
Choledochal cyst, 618
Choledocholithiasis, 605
Chorioangioma, placental, 310
Choriocarcinoma, hydatidiform mole with, 172
Cirrhosis of liver, hepatoma superimposed on, 486
Club foot, 281
Colon
  carcinoma of, 1045
  simulating dermoid cyst, 1043
Comet tail artifact, 24, 25
Common bile duct, anatomy of, 590
Common hepatic duct, anatomy of, 590
Compound scanning, resolution degradation in, 11
Compounding, 9
Compression amplification, 9, 10
Contraction ring, uterine, 321
Contrast resolution, 17, 18
Corpus callosum, neonatal, agenesis of, 412
Costal cartilage, simulating cyst, 352
Cranium, fetal, 192–193
Crown-rump measurement, as determinant of gestational age, 184
Cystadenocarcinoma
  ovarian, 118, 126
  of pancreas, 665
Cystadenoma
  microcystic, of pancreas, 662
  multilocular, endometriosis simulating, 136
Cystic fibrosis, pancreas in, 639
Cystic hygroma, fetal, 263
Cystic teratoma, fetal, 265
Cytoxan (cyclophosphamide) cystitis, 891

Dandy-Walker cyst
  fetal, 267
  neonatal, 423
Dermoid cyst, colon simulating, 1043
Diaphragm
  fetal, hernia of, 271
  traumatic rupture of, 1137
Diethylstilbestrol, 77
Digital instrumentation, 10–11
Doppler shift, angular dependence of, 20, 21
Doppler ultrasound, 17–19
  for breast, 368–371
  frequency spectral analysis in, 19
  imaging in, 18–19
  physical principles of, 17–18
  pulsed, 19–21
    angular dependence of Doppler shift in, 20, 21
    duplex scanners for, 20–21
Double sac sign, of early pregnancy, 166
Duodenal atresia, fetal, 287
Duodenal ulcer, perforated, subphrenic abscess and, 1034
Duodenum, normal, 1023
Duplex scanner, 20–21

Echogenic focal zone artifact, 29–30
Ectopic pregnancy, 159–162
  acute, with ruptured luteal cyst, 168
Electronic scanners, 15, 16
Embryology, of female genital tract, 54
Empyema
  of gallbladder, with pericholecystic abscess, 567
  pleural, 1128
Encephalocele, fetal, 262
Endometrial carcinoma, 152
Endometrioma
  simulating ovarian cancer, 140
  simulating solid ovarian tumor, 134
Endometriosis, 39, 132–144
  adenomyosis and, 142
  simulting fluid in pouch of Douglas, 133
  simulating multilocular cystadenoma, 136
  simulating tubo-ovarian abscess, 138
Epididymitis, 970
Epigastric abscess, perforation of gut and, 1036
Erythroblastosis, fetal, 323
Extrahepatic ducts. *See also* Biliary tract.
  anatomy of, 590
  ascaris worms in, 607
  carcinoma of pancreas and, 599
  cholangiography vs ultrasound for, 592

choledocholithiasis of, 605
disparate dilatation of, 602–603
fatty meal and, 596
imaging techniques for, 591–592
normal caliber of, 590–591
obstruction by tumor in, 610
postcholecystectomy, 591

Fallopian tube, embryology of, 54
Fat, acoustic properties of, 8
Female genital tract, embryology of, 54
Femur measurements for dating pregnancy, 234, 236–237
Fetus
  abnormal anatomy of
    abdominal, 284–291
    chest, 268–274
    cranial, 258–267. See also individual conditions.
    limb, 281–283
    renal, 292–298
    spinal, 275–279
  adenomatoid tumor of lung in, 268
  anencephaly of, 260
  anomaly of, prenatal diagnosis of, 185–186
  aqueductal stenosis in, 259
  arachnoid cyst of, 266
  cystic hygroma of, 263
  cystic teratoma of, 265
  Dandy Walker cyst of, 267
  death of, 317
  diaphragmatic hernia of, 271
  duodenal atresia in, 287
  encephalocele of, 262
  erythroblastosis of, 323
  estimated weight of, for pregnancy dating, 234, 240–241
  gastroschisis in, 284
  hydrocephalus of, 258
  hydrops of, 323
    nonimmune, 326
  jejunal atresia of, 288
  multilocular ovarian cyst of, 290
  normal anatomy of, 187–232
    abdomen, 210–211
    cranium, 192–193
    lower limb, 227
    pelvis, 221
    spine, 188
    thorax, 203
    upper limb, 229
    yolk sac in, 187
  normal and abnormal growth of, 246–249
    head circumference in, 247
    head/abdominal circumference ratio in, 247
    total intrauterine volume in, 246–248
  omental cyst of, 291
  omphalocele in, 285
  osteogenesis imperfecta in, 282
  polycystic kidney disease of, 294
  position of, determination of, 185
  posterior urethral valve in, 296
  renal agenesis in, 298
  rhabdomyosarcoma of, 273
  sacrococcygeal teratoma in, 279
  skeletal dysplasia of, 274
  spina bifida in, 275
    meningomyelocele and, 277
  talipes equina varus in, 281
  thanatophoric dysplasia in, 283
  ureteropelvic junction obstruction in, 292
Fibroadenoma, of breast, 354
Fibrocystic breast, 337–352. See also Breast, fibrocystic disease of.
Fibroid
  cervical, 150
  uterine, 148
    simulating mole, 178
Fibroma, ovarian, simulating tumor, 116
Follicular adenoma, thyroid, 1056
Follicular development, 45
Frequency, 1
Frequency spectral analysis, 19

Gallbladder, 541–621
  carcinoma of, 582–584
    advanced, 584
    occult, 582
  cholecystitis of
    acute, 549
    chronic, cholelithiasis and, 559
    ultrasound and ERCP in, 562
  cystic duct of, distended, 588
  empyema of, with pericholecystic abscess, 567
  gallstones in, 551–557. See also Gallstone.
  gravel and sludge in, 574
  hydrops of, 577–580
    adult, 577
    pediatric, 580
  junctional fold simulating gallstone in, 546
  landmarks and examination technique for, 541–542
  neck of, cystic duct and, 544
  porcelain, 565
  septate, gallstones in, 554
  tumor of wall of, neoplastic or inflammatory, 586
  wall thickening of, 569–572
    nonspecific, 569
    rapid change, 572
Gallstone, 551–557
  classic, 551
  floating, 555
  hemolytic anemia and, 557
  nonshadowing, 28–29
  in septate gallbladder, 554
Gartner's duct cyst, 58
Gastroschisis, fetal, 284
Genital tract, female, embryology of, 54
Germinal matrix hemorrhage, neonatal, 373–374, 383–393
Gestation, multiple, 251, 255
Gestational age. See Pregnancy, dating.
Gestational trophoblastic disease, 170–180. See also Hydatidiform mole.
Glycogen storage disease, liver and, 512
Goiter, multinodular, 1060
Granulomatous disease, splenic, 724
Granulosa-theca cell tumor, 124
Gray-scale ultrasound, 9–10
  scanning techniques in, 11–12
Gut, perforation of, epigastric abscess and, 1036
Gynecology, 37–180. See also individual disorders.
  scanning in, 37
    bladder filling for, 37
    differential diagnosis in, 38–39
    indications for, 37–38
    instrumentation for, 38
    technique for, 38

Hashimoto's thyroiditis, 1062
Head circumference, normal fetal, 247
Head/abdominal circumference ratio, mean fetal, 247
Hemangioendothelioma, of liver, 475
Hemangioma, of liver, 472
  with atypical CT, 480
  cavernous, 477
  with CT correlation, 478
Hematocolpos, 54, 60
Hematoma
  of liver, 452–456
  pelvic, 144
Hemolytic anemia, gallstones and, 557
Hepatic fibrosis, congenital, 882
Hepatic flexure, as right renal imposter, 757
Hepatic vein, anatomy of, 429
Hepatoblastoma, 484
Hepatoma, cirrhosis of liver and, 486

Hernia, diaphragmatic, fetal, 271
Histiocytoma, urachal, 1003
Histoplasmosis, spleen and, 728
Holoprosencephaly, neonatal, 410
Humerus measurements, for dating pregnancy, 234, 236–237
Hunter's syndrome, liver in, 510
Hydatid cyst
  of Morgagni, 102
  renal, 872
Hydatid disease, of liver, 465
Hydatidiform mole
  choriocarcinoma from, pulmonary metastases with, 172
  classic, 170
  degenerating fibroid simulating, 178
  degeneration of, 176
  partial, 174
  pelvic masses simulating, 180
Hydrocele, 973
Hydrocephalus
  fetal, 258
  noenatal, 395–396
Hydronephrosis, 771–788
  incidence and appearance of, 771
  neonatal with ureteropelvic junction obstruction, 775
  partial obstruction and ultrasound Whittaker test in, 777
  of pregnancy, 779
  prune belly syndrome and, 783
  in renal transplantation, antegrade pyelography and Whittaker test for, 829
  secondary to adenopathy, 781
  staghorn calculus with secondary, 786
Hydronephrosis-pyonephrosis, 788
Hydrops, fetal, 323
  nonimmune, 326
Hygroma, cystic, fetal, 263
Hypercalcemia, parathyroid, 1069
Hypertension, portal, 534

In utero therapy, 186
Infantile polycystic kidney disease, 294
Inspissated cyst, breast, mimicking carcinoma, 357
Intestine, 1042. *See also individual parts.*
Intracavity scanners, 16, 17
Intrahepatic duct, anicteric dilatation of, 612
Intraluminal echoes, 1099
Intrauterine device
  localization of, 79
  pregnancy and, 83

Intrauterine volume, total, 246–248
Islet cell tumor, nonfunctioning, 679

Jejunal atresia, fetal, 288
Juxtarenal compartments, normal anatomy of, 747

Keloid formation, retroperitoneal, 1021
Kidney. *See also entries under* Renal.
  horseshoe, 751
  in utero, 746
  malrotation of, 763
  multicystic dysplastic, 886
  neonatal, 744
  nonfunctioning, renal failure and, 766
  normal anatomy of, 735
  pelvic, 765
Klatskin tumor, of liver, 489
Krukenberg's tumor, 123

Lateral resolution, 5–6
Left upper quadrant abscess, 997
Left upper quadrant mass
  CSF collection with, 1015
  as stomach distension or pseudocyst, 1027
Leiomyoblastoma, of retroperitoneum, 1002
Leukemia, chronic myeloid, spleen and, 726
Leukomalacia, periventricular, neonatal, 422
Ligamentum teres, 430
Ligamentum venosum, 430
Linear array, 14
Lipoma, breast, 356
Lipomatosis, pelvic, 927
Liver, 429–539
  abscess of, 458–467
    amebic, 467
    bilateral subphrenic, pelvic abscess and, 459
    gas-containing subhepatic, 463
    subhepatic with ascending cholangitis, 458
  adenoma of, 482
  anatomy of, 429–431
    caudate lobe, 430–431
    hepatic vein, 429
    ligamentum teres, 430
    ligamentum venosum, 430
    portal vein, 429
    Riedel's lobe, 429, 442
    segmental, 429–430
  artifactual mass of, 503–505
    adult, 503
    infantile, 505
  biloma of, 456

  Burkitt's lymphoma of, 507
  cirrhosis of, 525–532
    incidence and diagnosis of, 525
    lobar ratios in, 529
    primary biliary, 532
    regenerating nodules in, 527
  congenital variants of, 442
  fatty infiltration of, 518–520
    diffuse, 518
    focal, 520
  fibrosis of, 514–515
    congenital, 514
    infantile polycystic disease and, 515
  focal lesion of, rapid change in, 522
  focal nodular hyperplasia in, 483
  glycogen storage disease and, 512
  hemangioendothelioma of, 475
  hemangioma of
    with atypical CT, 480
    cavernous, 477
    with CT correlation, 478
    neonatal, 472
  hematoma of, 452–456
    spontaneous, 454
    traumatic, 452
  hepatoblastoma in, 484
  hepatoma superimposed on cirrhosis of, 486
  Hunter's syndrome and, 510
  hydatid disease of, 465
  incidental cyst in, 447
  Klatskin tumor of, 489
  lymphoma of, 509
  malignant, obstructing inferior vena cava, 1101
  metastatic disease of, 490–501
    cystic, from cystadenocarcinoma, 498
    diffuse, 500
    echogenic, from carcinoma of colon, 493
    failure of therapy in, 501
    from islet cell tumor, 497
    necrotic, 496
    simulating Klatskin tumor, 492
  polycystic disease in, 451
  portal hypertension in, 534
  schistosomiasis of, 536
  situs inversus viscerum in, 446
  spontaneous resolution of cyst in, 449
  ultrasound and scintigraphy of, 539
  vascular supply of, 438
  venous congestion in, 444
Lobar nephronia, acute, 875
Long bone lengths, for dating pregnancy, 234, 236–237

Longus colli muscle, prominent, parathyroid gland and, 1071
Lower limb, fetal, 227
Lumbar mass, superficial, 1020
Lung, fetal, adenomatoid tumor of, 268
Luteal cyst, ruptured, with ectopic pregnancy, 168
Lymphadenopathy, paraaortic, 993
Lymphangiectatic cyst, retroperitoneal, 1010
Lymphangiomyomatosis, retroperitoneal, 1008
Lymphocele, in renal transplantation, 832
Lymphoma
  of breast, 366
  Burkitt's, of liver, 507
  focal, of spleen, 719
  of liver, 509
  renal, 866
  of stomach, 1029

M-mode scan, 4, 5
Machine-specific artifact, 32–33
Mammography, ultrasonic, 330–331
  instrumentation for, 330–331
  patient position for, 331
  technique for, 331
Mechanical scanners, 14, 15
Medullary cystic disease, 880
Meningomyelocele, spina bifida and, 277
Mesothelioma, fibrous, 1120
Mirror image artifact, 25–26
Mucocele of appendix, bowel mass, 1038
Multiple gestation, 251, 255
Myelofibrosis, spleen and, 730
Myelolipoma, of adrenal gland, 938

Neck bruit, 1109
Neonatal head, 373–427
  agenesis of corpus callosum in, 412
  Arnold-Chiari malformation in, 425
  brain tumor in, 418
  cavum vergae in, 381
  cerebritis in, 400
  Dandy-Walker cyst in, 423
  germinal matrix hemorrhage in, 373–374, 383–393
    grade I, 383
    grade II, 386
    grade III, 389
    grade IV, 391
    left middle cerebral artery infarct in, 393
  holoprosencephaly in, 410
  periventricular leukomalacia in, 422

posterior fossa subarachnoid cyst in, 406
quadrigeminal plate cyst of, 408
severe porencephaly of, 415
shunt catheter location in, 403
subarachnoid hemorrhage in, 399
subdural collection in, 420
ultrasound technique in, 376
ventriculomegaly and hydrocephalus in, 395–396
Nephritis, acute focal bacterial, 875
Nephroblastoma, 867
Nephrocalcinosis
  cortical, 819
  medullary, 817
Nephrolithiasis, 795
Nephronia, acute lobar, 875
Nephropathy, reflux, 815
Neuroblastoma, of adrenal gland, 942
Neurofibroma, pelvic, 130
Neurofibrosarcoma, of retroperitoneum, 999

Obstetrics, 183–326
  ultrasound in
    applications in, 183
    indications for, 183–186
      amniocentesis as, 186
      bleeding in pregnancy as, 185
      fetal position as, 185
      in utero therapy as, 186
      prenatal diagnosis of fetal anomaly as, 185–186
      uterus too large for dates as, 184
      uterus too small for dates as, 184
Off-axis reflector artifact, 30–31
Omental cyst, fetal, 291
Omphalocele, fetal, 285
Orbital measurement, for pregnancy dating, 234, 238
Osteogenesis imperfecta, fetal, 282
Ovarian cancer, endometrioma simulating, 140
Ovarian cyst, 90–102
  bowel mass simulating, 97
  complicating early pregnancy, 94
  hyperstimulation syndrome with, 98, 100
  multilocular, 96
  fetal, 290
  simulating bladder, 92
  spontaneous resolution of, 90
  in Turner's syndrome, 70
  unilocular, 95
Ovarian dermoid, 103–111
  with calcified elements, 108

with fluid/fluid level, 111
predominantly cystic, 103
simulating bowel contents, 110
Ovarian fibroma, simulating tumor, 116
Ovarian hyperstimultion syndrome, 98, 100
Ovarian mass, differential diagnosis of, 39
Ovarian tumor, 103–130
  cystadenocarcinoma, 118, 126
  cystic pelvic, 120
  dermoid, 103–111. See also Ovarian dermoid.
  endometrioma simulating, 134
  fibroma simulating, 116
  Krukenberg's, 123
  malignant teratoma, 114
  predominantly cystic demoid mass, 103
  secondary amenorrhea due to, 128
  of sex cord origin, 124
Ovary
  normal anatomy of, 40
  pseudotumor of, 72

Pancreas, 623–689
  anatomy and scanning of, 624–625
  carcinoma of, 668–682
    body and tail of pancreas, 677
    head of pancreas, 670
    nonfunctioning islet cell, 679
    tail of pancreas, 675
  cystadenocarcinoma of, 665
  cystadenoma of, microcystic, 662
  cystic fibrosis of, 639
  fatty infiltration of, 638
  hematoma of, 656–659
    infected, 659
    pediatric, 656
  liquefaction necrosis of, 689
  lithiasis of, 646
  normal variants of, 633–636
    bulbous tail simulating tumor, 633
    displacement by hepatomegaly, 635
    superficial location, 636
  pancreatitis or tumor of, 682
  peripancreatic abscess of, 660
  pseudo pseudocyst of, 687
  pseudocyst of, 650–653
    spontaneous drainage of, 650
    traumatic, 653
  pseudopancreatic mass of, 685
  Puestow procedure for, 648
  various imaging modalities for, 626
  water distension of stomach for scanning of, 625–626

Pancreatic sac, 689
Pancreatitis, 641–644
　acute, 641
　acute superimposed on chronic, 643
　chronic, 644
　tumor or, 682
Papillary carcinoma, of thyroid, 1065–1067
Parabolic flow, 19, 20
Parathyroid gland, 1069–1079
　adenoma of, 1070, 1076
　false-negative sonogram of, 1073
　false-positive sonogram of, 1074
　hypercalcemia of, 1069
　hyperplasia of, 1075
　migration of neoplasm of, 1077
　prominent longus colli muscle and, 1071
　ultrasound appearance of neoplasms of, 1078
Partial volume effect, 29, 30
Pelvic abscess
　bilateral subphrenic abscess of liver and, 459
　following appendicitis, 1049
Pelvic hematoma, 144
Pelvic inflammatory disease
　pyohydrosalpinx in, 84
　tubo-ovarian abscess in, 86, 88
Pelvic lipomatosis, 927
Pelvic mass
　palpable, differential diagnosis of, 38–39
　simulating mole, 180
Pelvic neurofibroma, 130
Pelvic tumor, cystic, 120
Pelvis, fetal, 221
Pericardial cyst, 1130
Pericholecystic abscess, empyema of gallbladder with, 567
Perirenal hematoma, 910
Periventricular leukomalacia, neonatal, 422
Pheochromocytoma, of adrenal gland, 940
Phlegmon, splenic, 705
Phrenic nerve stimulator artifact, 34
Pixel, 10
Placenta, 299–304
　chorioangioma of, 310
　development of, 299–300
　grading of, 299
　hydropic degeneration of, 175
　in multiple pregnancy, 309
　position of, 304
　premature separation of, 308
　surface area of, 303
　thickness of, 302

Pleural effusion, 1125
Pleural empyema, 1128
Plug flow, 19
Pneumobilia, 614
Polycystic kidney disease. See Renal cystic disease.
Polyhydramnios, 186
Popliteal artery aneurysm, 1107
Porcelain gallbladder, 565
Porencephaly, neonatal, severe, 415
Portal hypertension, 534
Portal vein, anatomy of, 429
　cavernous transformation, 1105
　Portocaval shunt, 1103
Postprocessing curve, 11
Pouch of Douglas
　endometriosis simulating fluid in, 133
　fluid in, 39
Pregnancy, See also Fetus.
　abdominal, 319
　bleeding in, 185
　　after 20 weeks' gestation, 185
　　before 20 weeks' gestation, 185
　dating, 233–241
　　abdominal circumference for, 234, 239
　　biparietal diameter for, 233, 235
　　crown-rump length for, 184
　　estimated fetal weight for, 234, 240–241
　　femur and humerus measurements for, 234, 236–237
　　orbital measurements for, 234, 238
　double sac sign of, 166
　ectopic, 159–162
　　acute, with ruptured luteal cyst, 168
　　first-trimester complications of, 154–168. See also individual complications.
　hydronephrosis of, 779
　intrauterine device and, 83
　multiple, 251, 255
　　placenta in, 309
　ovarian cyst complicating, 94
Prepubescent normal anatomy, 52
Prostate, 947–964
　anatomy of, 947–948
　cancer of, 958–964
　　clinically confined, 958
　　incidental, 958
　　invasive, 961
　　monitoring, 962
　carcinoma in, 924
　cyst of, 957
　hyperplasia of, 952–953
　　benign, 953
　　nodular, 952

　hypertrophy of, 916–919
　　bladder wall thickening in, 919
　　perabdominal scans in, 916
　incidental bladder cancer and, 964
　normal, 914
　scanning vs digital palpation of, 947
　stones in, 922
Prostatitis, bacterial and nonbacterial, 955
Prune belly syndrome, hydronephrosis and, 783
Pseudocyesis, 316
Pseudogestational sac, 164
Pseudohermaphroditism, 76
Psoas abscess, 1017
Psoas major muscle, normal anatomy of, 749
Puberty, precocious, 72
Puestow procedure, for pancreas, 648
Pulsed Doppler ultrasound, 19–21
Pyelonephritis
　acute, 873
　chronic atrophic, 815
Pyloric stenosis, hypertrophic, 1024
Pylorus, normal, 1023
Pyohydrosalpinx, 84
Pyonephrosis-hydronephrosis, 788

Quadratus lumborum muscle, normal anatomy of, 749
Quadrigeminal plate cyst, neonatal, 408

Rayleigh scattering, 9
Real-time ultrasound, 13
　static vs, 16–17, 18
Recording systems, 12–13
　static image, 12
　video inversion, 13
Rectal bladder, 1047
Rectum, normal, 1046
Rectus sheath hematoma
　bladder deformity secondary to, 906
　old, 908
Reflection-mirror image artifact, 25–26
Reflection-refraction beam splitting, 27–28
Reflection-reverberation artifact, 23–25
Reflector, specular, 7–8
Refraction artifact, 26–27
Renal. See also entries under Kidney.
Renal agenesis, fetal, 298
Renal angiomyolipoma, 869
Renal arteries, normal anatomy of, 743

Renal cell carcinoma, 852–860
  left renal vein and vena cava in, 860
  right renal vein and vena cava in, 857
  solid renal mass in, 852
  tissue necrosis in, 854
Renal cyst, 844–849
  aspiration of, 848–849
  simple, 844
Renal cystic disease, 878–886
  adult (dominant) polycystic disease, 878
  congenital hepatic fibrosis with tubular ectasia in, 882
  in utero, 884
  infantile polycystic disease, 294
  medullary cystic disease, 880
  multicystic dysplastic, 886
Renal disease, medical, 804–808
  acute, 804
  histogram analysis in, 808
Renal failure
  chronic, 810
  nonfunctioning kidney and, 766
Renal hydatid cyst, 872
Renal infection, 873–875
Renal mass, 754–757
  anatomic hepatic flexure as, 757
  anatomic splenic flexure as, 754
  lymphoma as, 866
Renal parenchymal disease, 799–800
Renal sinus, 767–769
  abnormal, 767
  blood clot within, 797
  normal anatomy of, 741
  normal with hydration variation, 769
Renal transitional cell carcinoma, 863
Renal transplantation, 821–835
  acute rejection in, 822
  chronic rejection in, 824
  evaluation in, 821
  hematoma in, 834
  hydronephrosis in, antegrade pyelography and Whittaker test for, 829
  lymphocele in, 832
  obstructive uropathy in, 826
  rejection in, blood clot in renal pelvis secondary to, 835
Renal tubular ectasia, 882
Renal vein
  normal anatomy of, 738
  renal cell carcinoma of, 857–860
Renal vein thrombosis
  acute, 811
  subacute, 813

Renal vessels, 1090
Resolution, 4–6
  axial, 4
  contrast, 17, 18
  lateral, 5–6
  spatial, 17, 18
Resolution artifact, 30
Retroperitoneum, 989–1021
  abdominopelvic mass at, 1006
  cyst of
    in infant, 1013
    lymphangiectatic, 1010
  fat, 989–991
    displacement of, 991
    reflective, 989
  fibrosis of, 792
  keloid formation at, 1021
  left upper quadrant abscess of, 997
  leiomyoblastoma of, 1002
  lymphangiomyomatosis of, 1008
  neurofibrosarcoma of, 999
Reverberation artifact, 23–25, 95
Reverse shadowing, 33, 34
Rhabdomyosarcoma, fetal, 273
Riedel's lobe, 429, 442
Rotating scanners, 14–15

Sacrococcygeal teratoma, fetal, 279
Sarcoma, spindle cell, 1134
Schistosomiasis, of liver, 536
Scrotum. See Testes.
Sector scanning, 14–16
  electronic scanners, 15, 16
  mechanical scanners, 14, 15
  rotating scanners, 14–15
  small-part and intracavitary scanners, 16, 17
Seminal vesicle, normal, 914
Septum of Bertin, 842
Sertoli-Leydig cell tumor, 124
Sex cord, as tumor origin, 124
Side lobes, 30
Situs inversus viscerum, 446
Skeletal dysplasia, fetal, 274
Slice thickness artifact, 31
Small-part scanners, 16, 17
Sonosalpingography, 48
Sound speed error artifact, 31–32
Spatial resolution, 17, 18
Spectral broadening, 19
Specular reflector, 7–8
Spina bifida, 275
  with meningomyelocele, 277
Spindle cell sarcoma, 1134
Spine, fetal, 188
Spleen, 693–730
  abscess of, 707–710
    gas-containing, 710
    related to drug abuse, 707

  autosplenectomy of, 713
  congenital cysts of, 699
  echogenic metastases of, 721
  focal lymphoma of, 719
  granulomatous disease of, chronic, 724
  histoplasmosis and, 728
  infarct of, 712
  leukemia and, chronic myeloid, 726
  myelofibrosis of, 730
  phlegmon of, 705
  psuedocyst of, 703
  pseudospleen, 717
  rupture of, 714
  scanning techniques for, 693–697
    A-scan, 693
    coronal scan, 697
    oblique intercostal scans, 695
  splenomegaly of, 722–723
  traumatic hematoma of, 701
Splenic flexure, as left renal imposter, 754
Splenomegaly, 722–723
  congestive, 722
  inflammatory, 723
Staghorn calculus, with secondary hydronephrosis, 786
Static image recording, 12
Static scanning, real-time vs, 16–17, 18
Stein-Leventhal syndrome, 74
Stomach, lymphoma of, 1029
Subarachnoid cyst, posterior fossa, neonatal, 406
Subarachnoid hemorrhage, neonatal, 399
Subdural fluid collection, neonatal, 420
Suphrenic abscess
  following appendicitis, 1049
  perforated duodenal ulcer and, 1034

Talipes equina varus, 281
Tampon, 50
Teratoma
  cystic, fetal, 265
  malignant ovarian, 114
  sacrococcygeal, fetal, 279
Testes, 965–986
  benign hyperechoic lesion of, 986
  examination technique for, 965–966
  extratesticular pathology of, 970–976
    cyst of, 972
    epididymitis as, 970
    hydrocele as, 973

Testes (Continued)
    tumor as, 976
    varicocele as, 975
  indications for scanning of, 965
  instrumentation for scanning of, 965
  mass of, differential diagnosis of, 966
  normal anatomy of, 967
  torsion of, 982
  trauma to, 984
  tumor of, 978–980
Thanatophoric dysplasia, fetal, 283
Thorax, 1125–1137. *See also individual parts.*
  fetal, 203
Thyroid, 1053–1067
  adenomatous nodules of, 1058
  anatomy of, 1054
  application of ultrasound to, 1053
  equipment for ultrasound of, 1053
  follicular adenoma of, 1056
  hemorrhagic cyst of, 1063
  multinodular goiter of, 1060
  papillary carcinoma of, 1065–1067
  simple cyst of, 1064
Thyroiditis, Hashimoto's, 1062
Time gain control, 6–7
Tissue attenuation, 6–7
Tissue texture artifact, 32
Total intrauterine volume, 246–248
Transducer, function of, 1–2
Transient ischemic attack, 1108–1109
Transitional cell carcinoma
  renal, 863
  of urinary bladder, 903
Trichobezoar, 1033
Triplets, 251
Tubo-ovarian abscess, 86, 88
  endometriosis simulating, 138
Turner's syndrome
  mosaic, ovarian cyst in, 70
  uterine response to exogenous hormones in, 67
Twins, 251
  conjoined, 255

Ultrasound
  backscattered echoes in, 7, 8–9
  digital instrumentation in, 10–11
  Doppler, 17–19
  frequencies in, 1
  gray-scale, 9–10
    scanning techniques in, 11–12
  intensity of, 2–3
  production of, 1–2
  Rayleigh scattering in, 9
  real-time, 13
    static vs, 16–17, 18
  reflection process in, 3–4
  resolution in, 4–6
  specular reflectors for, 7–8
  tissue attenuation and time gain control in, 6–7
  transducers in, 1–2
Umbilical cord
  abnormal, 314
  normal, 312
Upper limb, fetal, 229
Urachal histiocytoma, 1003
Ureteropelvic junction obstruction
  fetal, 292
  neonatal, hydronephrosis with, 775
Urethral valves, posterior, fetal, 296
  secondary bladder outlet obstruction and, 925
Urinary bladder, 888–903
  anatomy of, 888
  anterior deformity of, secondary to rectus sheath hematoma, 906
  blood clot in, 897
  calculi in, 895
  cancer of, prostate scan and, 964
  Cytoxan (cyclophosphamide) cystitis of, 891
  diverticulum containing stone in, 899
  duplication of, 891
  old rectus sheath hematoma and, 908
  outlet obstruction of, posterior urethral valves and, 925
  perirenal hematoma and, 910

  transitional cell carcinoma of, 903
  wall thickening in, prostatic hypertrophy with, 919
Urinary tract, 733–835. *See also entries under* Kidney; Renal.
  duplication of, 760
Urinoma, infected, 912
Uropathy, obstructive, in renal transplantation, 826
Uterine fibroid, 148
  degenerating, 151
  simulating mole, 178
Uterine masses, 146–152
  degenerating fibroid, 151
  fibroid, 148
  Nabothian cyst, 146
Uterus
  agenesis of, 63
  bicornuate, 64
  contraction ring of, 321
  double, 55
  embryology of, 54
  exogenous hormones for Turner's syndrome and, 67
  large for dates, 184
  normal anatomy of, 40
  prepubescent, 52
  retroverted, 43
  small for dates, 184

Vagina
  agenesis of, 63
  embryology of, 54
Vaginal mass, due to tampon, 50
Varicocele, testicular, 975
Vascular system, 1081–1124. *See also individual vessels.*
Vena cava, inferior, 1097
  malignant liver obstructing, 1101
Ventriculomegaly, neonatal, 395–396
Video inversion, 13

Whittaker test, 829
  in hydronephrosis, 777
Wilms' tumor, 867

Yolk sac, fetal, 187

NO LONGER THE PROPERTY OF THE UNIVERSITY OF R.I. LIBRARY